Anxiety Disorders

Theory, Research, and Clinical Perspectives

To my husband David and my children Tal and Rufus, for your love and support (HBS)

To Mariana, my wife, my children Maya, Oren, and Michal, and my parents Yaacov and Zipora, for everything (YN)

To Goretti, my wife, and my children Maria Raquel and Robert Manuel, for your love and generosity (RLF)

To Carol, my wife, my children Gabe and Ben, and my parents, for all you've taught me (FS)

Anxiety Disorders

Theory, Research, and Clinical Perspectives

Edited by

Helen Blair Simpson

Yuval Neria

Roberto Lewis-Fernández

Franklin Schneier

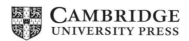

CAMBRIDGE UNIVERSITY PRESS
Cambridge, New York, Melbourne, Madrid, Cape Town, Singapore,
São Paulo, Delhi, Dubai, Tokyo, Mexico City

Cambridge University Press
The Edinburgh Building, Cambridge CB2 8RU, UK

Published in the the United States of America by Cambridge University Press, New York

www.cambridge.org
Information on this title: www.cambridge.org/9780521515573

First published 2010

Printed in the United Kingdom at the University Press, Cambridge

A catalog record for this publication is available from the British Library

Library of Congress Cataloging in Publication data
Anxiety disorders : theory, research, and clinical perspectives / [edited by]
    Helen Blair Simpson ... [et al.].
        p. ; cm.
    Includes bibliographical references and index.
    ISBN 978-0-521-51557-3 (hardback)
    1. Anxiety disorders.   I. Simpson, Helen Blair, 1960–   II. Title.
    [DNLM: 1. Anxiety Disorders. WM 172]
    RC531.A614 2010
    616.85'22–dc22
    2010027379

ISBN 978-0-521-51557-3 Hardback

Contents

Contributors

Avishek Adhikari, MA, MPhil
Graduate Student,
Department of Biological Sciences,
Columbia University,
New York, NY, USA

Susanne E. Ahmari, MD, PhD
Postdoctoral Clinical Fellow,
Columbia University College of
Physicians and Surgeons and New York
State Psychiatric Institute,
New York, NY, USA

Anne Marie Albano, PhD, ABPP
Associate Professor of Clinical Psychology
(in Psychiatry); Director,
Columbia University Clinic for Anxiety
and Related Disorders,
Columbia University College of
Physicians and Surgeons
New York State Psychiatric Institute,
New York, NY, USA

Carlos Blanco, MD, PhD
Professor of Clinical Psychiatry, Columbia
University College of
Physicians and Surgeons,
Anxiety Disorders Clinic, Division of Clinical
Therapeutics, New York State
Psychiatric Institute, New York, NY, USA

Desiree K. Caban, MA
Senior Research Worker,
Division of Clinical Phenomenology,
New York State Psychiatric Institute,
New York, NY, USA

Jonathan S. Comer, PhD
Chief Research Fellow in Child
and Adolescent Psychiatry,
Columbia University College
of Physicians and Surgeons
Clinician, Columbia University

Clinic for Anxiety and Related Disorders,
New York, NY, USA

Jeremy D. Coplan, MD
Professor of Psychiatry;
Director, Primate Behavioral Facility;
Director, Division of Neuropsychopharmacology,
State University of New York,
SUNY-Downstate Medical Center,
Brooklyn, NY, USA

Ana Alicia De La Cruz, MA
Assistant Research Scientist,
Division of Clinical Therapeutics,
New York State Psychiatric Institute,
New York, NY, USA

Emily R. Doherty
Research Assistant, Division of Clinical
Therapeutics, New York State
Psychiatric Institute,
Doctoral Candidate,
St. John's University,
New York, NY, USA

Bruce Dohrenwend, PhD
Professor of Social Science,
Department of Psychiatry,
College of Physicians and Surgeons,
Columbia University,
Professor of Epidemiology,
Mailman School of Public Health,
Columbia University,
Chief of Research,
Division of Social Psychiatry,
New York State Psychiatric Institute,
New York, NY, USA

Amit Etkin, MD, PhD
Assistant Professor,
Department of Psychiatry and Behavioral
Sciences, Stanford University,
Stanford, CA, USA

Brian A. Fallon, MD, MPH, M.Ed
Professor of Clinical Psychiatry,
Columbia University College
of Physicians and Surgeons,
Director of the Center for the
Study of Neuroinflammatory Disorders and
Biobehavioral Medicine,
Division of Clinical Therapeutics,
New York State Psychiatric Institute,
New York, NY, USA

Michael B. First, MD
Professor of Clinical Psychiatry,
Columbia University College of Physicians
and Surgeons Research Psychiatrist,
Division of Clinical Phenomenology,
New York State Psychiatric Institute,
New York, NY, USA

Abby J. Fyer, MD
Professor of Clinical Psychiatry,
Columbia University College of
Physicians and Surgeons, Division of
Clinical Therapeutics,
New York State Psychiatric Institute,
New York, NY, USA

Angela Ghesquiere, MSW
PhD student, Columbia University
School of Social Work,
New York, NY, USA

Jay A. Gingrich, MD, PhD
Associate Professor of Clinical Psychiatry;
Director, Basic Science Division of the Sackler
Institute, Columbia University College of
Physicians and Surgeons,
New York State Psychiatric Institute,
New York, NY, USA

Robert A. Glick, MD
Professor of Clinical Psychiatry,
Columbia University College
of Physicians and Surgeons,
New York, NY, USA

Joshua A. Gordon, MD, PhD
Assistant Professor of Psychiatry,
Columbia University College of
Physicians and Surgeons,
New York State Psychiatric Institute,
New York, NY, USA

Ethan E. Gorenstein, PhD
Associate Clinical Professor of Psychology,
Columbia University College of
Physicians and Surgeons,
Clinical Director,
Behavioral Medicine Program,
Department of Psychiatry,
Columbia University,
New York, NY, USA

Marco A. Grados, MD, MPH
Associate Professor,
Department of Psychiatry
and Behavioral Sciences,
Johns Hopkins University School of Medicine,
Baltimore, MD, USA

James P. Hambrick, PhD
Instructor in Clinical Psychology in Psychiatry,
Columbia University College of Physicians and
Surgeons,
Clinician, Columbia University Clinic for Anxiety
and Related Disorders,
New York, NY, USA

James Hanks
Research Foundation for
Mental Hygiene, Columbia University,
New York, NY, USA

Kelli Jane K. Harding, MD
Assistant Professor of Clinical Psychiatry,
Columbia University College of
Physicians and Surgeons,
Division of Medical Education,
New York State Psychiatric Institute,
New York, NY, USA

Richard G. Heimberg, PhD
Director, Adult Anxiety Clinic,
David Kipnis Distinguished Faculty
Fellow and Professor,
Department of Psychology,
Temple University,
Philadelphia, PA, USA

Rene Hen, PhD
Professor of Neuroscience,
Psychiatry, and Pharmacology,
Columbia University College of
Physicians and Surgeons,

Director, Division of Integrative Neuroscience,
New York State Psychiatric Institute,
New York, NY, USA

Devon E. Hinton, MD, PhD
Associate Professor of Psychiatry,
Harvard Medical School,
Research Scientist, Center for Anxiety and
Traumatic Stress Disorders, Massachusetts
General Hospital,
Boston, MA, USA

Myron A. Hofer, MD
Sackler Professor of Developmental
Psychobiology, Department of Psychiatry,
Columbia University,
New York, NY, USA

Matthew J. Kaplowitz, PhD
Clinical Researcher,
Anxiety Disorders Clinic,
Division of Clinical Therapeutics,
New York State Psychiatric Institute,
New York, NY, USA

Sharaf S. Khan, BS
Project Director,
Research Study, Anxiety Disorders Clinic,
Division of Clinical Therapeutics,
New York State Psychiatric Institute,
New York, NY, USA

Donald F. Klein, MD, DSc
Professor of Psychiatry, Emeritus,
Columbia University College of Physicians and
Surgeons,
Research Professor,
Department of Child and Adolescent Psychiatry,
New York University School of Medicine,
Nathan Kline Institute,
New York, NY, USA

Karestan C. Koenen, PhD
Associate Professor of Society,
Human Development,
and Health and Epidemiology,
Harvard School of Public Health,
Boston, MA, USA

E. David Leonardo, MD, PhD
Assistant Professor of Clinical Psychiatry,
Columbia University College
of Physicians and Surgeons,

New York State Psychiatric Institute,
New York, NY, USA

Roberto Lewis-Fernández, MD
Associate Professor of Clinical Psychiatry,
Columbia University College
of Physicians and Surgeons,
Director of the NYS Center
of Excellence for Cultural Competence
and the Hispanic Treatment Program of the
Anxiety Disorders Clinic,
Division of Clinical Therapeutics,
New York State Psychiatric Institute,
New York, NY, USA

Jeffrey A. Lieberman, MD
Lawrence C. Kolb Professor and Chairman,
Department of Psychiatry,
Columbia University College
of Physicians and Surgeons,
Director, New York State
Psychiatric Institute,
Psychiatrist-in-Chief, New York Presbyterian
Hospital & Columbia University
Medical Center,
New York, NY, USA

Michael R. Liebowitz, MD
Professor of Clinical Psychiatry,
Columbia University,
Former Director, Anxiety
Disorder Clinic,
New York State Psychiatric Institute,
New York, NY, USA

Sarah H. Lisanby, MD
Professor of Clinical Psychiatry,
Director of the Division of Brain Stimulation
and Therapeutic Modulation,
Columbia University College
of Physicians and Surgeons,
New York State Psychiatric Institute,
New York, NY, USA

Antonio Mantovani, MD, PhD
Associate Research Scientist,
Division of Brain Stimulation and
Therapeutic Modulation,
Columbia University College of
Physicians and Surgeons,
New York State Psychiatric Institute,
New York, NY, USA

Research Scientist, Unit of Psychiatry,
Department of Neuroscience, Siena University
Hospital, Siena, Italy

John C. Markowitz, MD
Professor of Clinical Psychiatry,
Columbia University College of
Physicians and Surgeons,
Research Scientist,
Anxiety Disorders Clinic,
Division of Clinical Therapeutics,
New York State Psychiatric Institute,
New York, NY, USA

Patrick J. McGrath, MD
Professor of Clinical Psychiatry,
Columbia University College of
Physicians and Surgeons,
Co-Director,
Depression Evaluation Service, Division of
Clinical Therapeutics,
New York State Psychiatric Institute,
New York, NY, USA

Caitlin McOmish, PhD
Postdoctoral Fellow,
Research Foundation for
Mental Hygiene, Columbia University,
New York, NY, USA

Jeffrey M. Miller, MD
Assistant Professor of Clinical Psychiatry,
Columbia University Research Scientist,
Research Foundation for Mental Hygiene,
New York State Psychiatric Institute,
New York, NY, USA

Jan Mohlman, PhD
Assistant Professor of Psychology,
Department of Psychology,
Rutgers University,
Piscataway, NJ, USA

Elizabeth Sagurton Mulhare, MBA, LMSW
Social Worker and Treatment Care Coordinator,
Personality Disorders Unit,
New York Presbyterian Hospital,
Payne Whitney Westchester,
White Plains, NY, USA

Philip R. Muskin, MD, MA
Professor of Clinical Psychiatry,
Chief, Consultation-Liaison Psychiatry,

Columbia University College of
Physicians and Surgeons,
Research Psychiatrist,
Division of Clinical Therapeutics,
New York State Psychiatric Institute,
New York, NY, USA

Navin Arun Natarajan, MD
Geriatric Psychiatry Fellow,
North Shore–Long Island Jewish
Medical Center,
The Zucker Hillside Hospital,
Glen Oaks, NY, USA

Yuval Neria, PhD
Associate Professor of Clinical Psychology
Columbia University College of Physicians
and Surgeons,
Director of the Trauma and PTSD Program,
Anxiety Disorders Clinic, Division of Clinical
Therapeutics, New York State Psychiatric
Institute, Anxiety Disorders Clinic,
New York, NY, USA

Nicole R. Nugent, PhD
Assistant Professor, Department of Psychiatry
and Human Behavior,
Alpert Medical School,
Brown University,
Staff Psychologist,
Bradley/Hasbro Children's Research Center,
Rhode Island Hospital,
Providence, RI, USA

Mayumi Okuda, MD
Assistant Research Scientist,
Anxiety Disorders Clinic,
Division of Clinical Therapeutics,
New York State Psychiatric Institute,
New York, NY, USA

Mark Olfson, MD, MPH
Professor of Clinical Psychiatry, Columbia
University College of Physicians and Surgeons,
Research Psychiatrist, Division of Epidemiology,
New York State Psychiatric Institute,
New York, NY, USA

Laszlo A. Papp, MD
Associate Professor of Clinical Psychiatry,
Columbia University College of
Physicians and Surgeons,
Director, Biological Studies Unit,

Division of Clinical Therapeutics,
New York State Psychiatric Institute,
New York, NY, USA

Sapana R. Patel, PhD
Assistant Professor of Psychology
(in Psychiatry), Columbia
University College of Physicians
and Surgeons,
Research Scientist, Anxiety Disorders Clinic,
Division of Clinical Therapeutics,
New York State Psychiatric Institute,
New York, NY, USA

Anthony Pinto, PhD
Assistant Professor of Clinical Psychology
(in Psychiatry), Columbia University
College of Physicians and Surgeons,
Research Scientist, Anxiety Disorders Clinic,
Division of Clinical Therapeutics,
New York State Psychiatric Institute,
New York, NY, USA

Kristin Pontoski MA
Graduate Student, Adult Anxiety Clinic,
Department of Psychology,
Temple University,
Philadelphia, PA, USA

Jesse W. Richardson-Jones, PhD
Postdoctoral Fellow,
Department of Psychiatry,
Columbia University College
of Physicians and Surgeons,
New York, NY, USA

Carolyn I. Rodriguez, MD, PhD
Postdoctoral Research Fellow and
Assistant in Clinical Psychiatry,
Columbia University College of
Physicians and Surgeons,
Anxiety Disorders Clinic,
Division of Clinical Therapeutics,
New York State Psychiatric Institute,
New York, NY, USA

Steven P. Roose, MD
Professor of Clinical Psychiatry,
Columbia University of
Physicians and Surgeons,
New York, NY, USA

Moira A. Rynn, MD
Associate Professor of Clinical Psychiatry,
Columbia University College of
Physicians and Surgeons,
Deputy Director of Research,
Division of Child and Adolescent Psychiatry,
New York State Psychiatric Institute,
New York, NY, USA

Franklin Schneier, MD
Professor of Clinical Psychiatry, Columbia
University College of
Physicians and Surgeons,
Research Scientist, Anxiety Disorders Clinic,
Division of Clinical Therapeutics,
New York State Psychiatric Institute,
New York, NY, USA

M. Katherine Shear, MD
Marion E. Kenworthy Professor of Psychiatry,
Columbia University School of Social Work and
Columbia University College of Physicians
and Surgeons,
New York, NY, USA

Ranjeeb Shrestha, MD
Fellow, Child and Adolescent Psychiatry,
The Children's Hospital of Philadelphia,
Philadelphia, PA, USA

Helen Blair Simpson, MD, PhD
Professor of Clinical Psychiatry, Columbia
University College of Physicians and Surgeons,
Director of the Anxiety Disorders
Clinic and the OCD Research Program,
Division of Clinical Therapeutics,
New York State Psychiatric Institute,
New York, NY, USA

Smit S. Sinha, MD
Assistant Professor of Clinical Psychiatry,
Columbia University College of Physicians
and Surgeons,
Research Scientist, Anxiety Disorders Clinic,
Division of Clinical Therapeutics,
New York State Psychiatric Institute,
New York, NY, USA

Natalia Skritskaya, PhD
Research Scientist, Division of Clinical
Therapeutics,

New York State Psychiatric Institute,
New York, NY, USA

Jami Socha, MA
Department of Psychology, Rosalind Franklin
University of Medicine and Science,
North Chicago, IL, USA

Eun Jung Suh, PhD
Assistant Professor of Clinical Psychology,
Department of Psychiatry,
Columbia University College of Physicians and
Surgeons, Anxiety Disorders Clinic,
Division of Clinical Therapeutics,
New York State Psychiatric Institute, New York,
NY, USA

Gregory M. Sullivan, MD
Assistant Professor of Clinical Psychiatry,
Columbia University College of Physicians and
Surgeons,
Research Scientist,
New York State Psychiatric Institute,
New York, NY, USA

Anthony J. Tranguch, MD, PhD
Assistant Clinical Professor of Psychiatry,
Columbia University College of Physicians and
Surgeons,
New York, NY, USA

Hilary B. Vidair, PhD
Research Fellow, Divisions of Child and
Adolescent Psychiatry and Epidemiology,
Clinical Psychologist, Columbia University,
New York State Psychiatric Institute,
New York, NY, USA

Tor D. Wager, PhD
Associate Professor and Director, Cognitive
and Affective Control Laboratory, Department
of Psychology and Neuroscience, University of
Colorado, Boulder, CO, USA
Associate Professor, Department of Psychology,
Columbia University,
New York, NY, USA

Myrna M Weissman, PhD
Professor of Epidemiology in Psychiatry,
Columbia University College of Physicians and
Surgeons
Chief, Division of Epidemiology, New York State
Psychiatric Institute
New York, NY, USA

Noelia V. Weisstaub, PhD
Research Scientist
New York State Psychiatric Institute,
New York, NY, USA

Foreword

Writing a book about anxiety disorders seems deceptively simple. However, nothing could be further from the truth. There are many challenges in this task, and they begin with the terminology. Anxiety is a term used to describe a mental state that has characterized the human condition since the beginning of the human race, and it derives from the fundamental emotion of fear. It is also a word that has been used to describe people and society in certain circumstances from different perspectives by diverse disciplines. Many historians, including Haynes Johnson and Arthur Schlesinger, described the twentieth century as the "Age of Anxiety"; philosophers beginning with Søren Kierkegaard described "Existential Angst," and Paul Tillich wrote of the "Anxiety of Meaninglessness"; and W. H. Auden's poem and Leonard Bernstein's symphony artistically expressed an "Age of Anxiety." Apart from the apotheosis of anxiety in these great works of scholarship and art, at a more mundane level, anxiety is a mental state that affects everyman and is part of the normative range of mental experiences. In addition to being a ubiquitous state of the human mind, anxiety is also a symptom that occurs in many mental disorders ranging from depression to schizophrenia to dementia. When it rises to the level of being the dominant symptom, or where fear is the primary emotional disturbance in a person's distressed mental state, anxiety defines a group of disorders that are believed to be nosologically valid, etiologically distinct, and pathologically disabling. Hence, we use the term anxiety to describe a normative mental state (like happiness, sadness, anger), a symptom, and a group of disorders. No wonder the voluminous literature on this topic (or group of topics). While this book is titled *Anxiety Disorders: Theory, Research, and Clinical Perspectives*, it could just as well be called "The Columbia Guide to Understanding and Treating Anxiety Disorders" or "Understanding Anxiety Disorders: the Columbia Way." It represents the current and cumulative state of the science and art of clinical conceptualization, assessment, and treatment of anxiety in contemporary psychiatry from the perspectives of faculty from the Columbia University Department of Psychiatry and the New York State Psychiatric Institute. Columbia Psychiatry's faculty is well positioned to provide uniquely informative guidance on anxiety disorders for healthcare providers. The Columbia University's Department of Psychiatry is one of the oldest departments in the USA and is the largest, in sheer number of faculty and range of programs, in the country. It also has a long tradition of seminal work, which has involved many figures who have made important contributions to our understanding of and current treatments for anxiety disorders. Early work was conducted by individuals such as Don Klein, Michael Liebowitz, Abby Fyer, Jack Gorman, and Rachel Klein; their mentorship led to new generations of anxiety researchers, including the editors and many of the contributors to this volume. Because of the complexity of their phenomenology, and the suspected etiologic heterogeneity of anxiety disorders, as well as the multimodal range of therapeutic approaches, a multidisciplinary approach to elucidating its mysteries is the best bet for rapid progress. The sheer size of the Columbia faculty focusing on anxiety disorders has enabled the researchers who are the contributors to this book to utilize a multidisciplinary approach, ranging from cross-cultural studies and epidemiology to transgenic mouse models, from descriptive phenomenology to diagnostic imaging, from clinical trials that examine treatment efficacy to community studies that examine treatment effectiveness, and from psychotherapies to pharmacology. I believe that this volume – and its authors, of whom I am extremely proud – adds real value as a unique source of knowledge to clinicians and researchers alike. The book clarifies rather than complicates, and provides a unique and coherent perspective on this complex but prevalent group of disorders, which are integral to the practice of psychiatry.

Jeffrey A. Lieberman

Preface

Anxiety disorders, including phobias, social anxiety disorder, obsessive–compulsive disorder, panic disorder, generalized anxiety disorder, and acute and posttraumatic stress disorders, are the most common class of mental disorders. Research into the causes and treatments of these disorders has exploded over the past few decades, yielding a wealth of new information ranging from brain chemistry to cultural influences to evidence-based treatments. In this book, leading researchers from the Columbia University Department of Psychiatry offer clinicians, researchers, and students a variety of perspectives on new developments and important controversies relevant to the theory, research, and treatment of anxiety disorders.

Clinicians will find reviews of state-of-the-art treatments for anxiety disorders, as well as controversies over diagnostic and treatment issues. Researchers will find in-depth consideration of important selected topics, including genetics of anxiety, neuroimaging, animal models of anxiety disorders, contemporary psychoanalytic theory, and the impact of stressors. By bringing experts representing a variety of approaches together in one volume, this book offers a broad selection of critical overviews of research and clinical topics that capture the ferment of this field of science as it exists today. It communicates the enormous advances that have occurred in anxiety research and provides readers with some of the latest thinking that is shaping the future of this field.

This book represents a unique compilation of research on anxiety and anxiety disorders from the faculty working in the Department of Psychiatry at Columbia University and the New York State Psychiatric Institute. It brings together in one volume recent research on diagnosis and assessment, pathophysiology and etiology, and epidemiology and treatment. Unlike standard textbooks on anxiety disorders, this book provides in-depth selected reviews on controversial topics and outlines important future directions by leading researchers writing about their own field of expertise. Unlike clinical manuals, this book's chapters about assessment and treatment of anxiety disorder delve into the underlying research studies and theories that support current practice and raise important questions about the development of future effective therapies.

The principal audience for the book is psychiatrists, psychologists, social workers, and other providers of mental health who are interested in advancing their knowledge of some of the latest thinking about anxiety and anxiety disorders. In addition, basic scientists and health science students (e.g., medical, nursing, public health, neuroscience graduate students) who want to learn about the latest thinking about anxiety disorders will benefit. A basic knowledge of the field is assumed in most chapters.

We would like to thank our Anxiety Disorders Clinic colleagues, past and present, for their dedication, hard work, and friendship. Our understanding of anxiety and related disorders has evolved over many stimulating scientific conversations and shared projects.

We are also grateful to Sara Putnam, MPH, our Editorial Coordinator, who provided superb help in all stages of the development of this book. Without her dedication and full attention to all details this book would have never materialized.

Chapter

1

Introduction: the need for interdisciplinary approaches

Helen Blair Simpson, Yuval Neria, Roberto Lewis-Fernández, Franklin Schneier

1.1 Introduction

Anxiety research has exploded over the past few decades, yielding a wealth of new information in multiple domains. These domains include underlying neurobiology, risk and protective factors, patterns of expression of normal and pathological anxiety, cultural determinants of this expression, and the delineation of specific anxiety disorders and their evidence-based treatments. As areas of research become increasingly specialized, the need to integrate our understanding across these different domains has become increasingly more important, calling for an interdisciplinary approach. This book brings together research relevant to anxiety disorders from a variety of disciplines into one volume, with the hope that it will encourage readers to bridge these disciplines to further advance our understanding of anxiety and the treatment of anxiety disorders.

Anxiety is a universal human emotion. It alerts us to potential threats and motivates us to prepare for challenges. However, a surprisingly large proportion of the population experiences an excess of anxiety that is counterproductive or even debilitating. This excess often takes the form of prototypical syndromes, which have been termed "anxiety disorders." In the fourth edition of the *Diagnostic and Statistical Manual* (DSM-IV), the anxiety disorders include panic disorder, agoraphobia, social anxiety disorder (SAD, also known as social phobia), specific phobia, posttraumatic stress disorder (PTSD), acute stress disorder, obsessive–compulsive disorder (OCD), and separation anxiety disorder. These disorders are distinguished by their characteristic triggers (e.g., social situations in SAD), distinctive symptoms (e.g., re-experiencing traumas in PTSD), course of illness, and response to treatment.

Typically appearing by young adulthood, the anxiety disorders are the most common class of mental disorders in the United States, with a 29% lifetime prevalence that exceeds that of mood (20%) and substance use disorders (15%) (Kessler *et al.* 2005). As a group, anxiety disorders cost society tens of billions of dollars per year (Greenberg *et al.* 1999). Thus, understanding the causes of these disorders and determining how better to treat them can significantly impact public health.

In 1982, the Anxiety Disorders Clinic, one of the first research clinics in the world to focus on anxiety disorders, was established by Michael Liebowitz and Abby Fyer at Columbia University/New York State Psychiatric Institute (NYSPI). Initial research objectives included improving diagnostic criteria, probing the physiology of panic attacks, examining novel medications, and investigating the presumed genetic basis of these disorders through family studies. At the time, brain functioning was commonly inferred from techniques such as electroencephalographic recordings from the scalp, pharmacologic challenges, or neurotransmitter metabolites accessible in peripheral locations (e.g., platelets, urine and in cerebral spinal fluid). Cognitive–behavioral approaches were available but uncommon in routine clinical practice. Additionally, the US Food and Drug Administration (FDA) had approved no medications for anxiety disorders other than alprazolam for panic disorder in 1981.

Since that time, the scope of anxiety research in general, and in the Anxiety Disorders Clinic in particular, has greatly expanded. Our group, like other research teams around the world, has developed research portfolios that require collaborations with investigators from a wide array of disciplines. We conduct studies in a wide range of fields, including animal models, brain imaging, randomized

Anxiety Disorders: Theory, Research, and Clinical Perspectives, ed. Helen Blair Simpson, Yuval Neria, Roberto Lewis-Fernández, Franklin Schneier. Published by Cambridge University Press. © Cambridge University Press 2010.

clinical trials, epidemiology, and treatment dissemination and implementation in the community. Research has transformed how we treat anxiety disorders: evidence-based practices have been developed and are being disseminated not only to mental health settings but also to primary care practices. Cognitive–behavioral approaches reign among psychotherapies, and the FDA has approved several classes of medication for the treatment of anxiety disorders. The focus has shifted away from identifying a treatment that can beat a placebo or usual care to developing better and novel treatments for those who do not fully respond to our first-line treatments. Increasingly, these novel treatments are based on sophisticated theories of the mechanisms underlying the symptoms.

When Cambridge University Press approached us with the idea of writing a treatment manual on the Columbia University/NYSPI approach to the diagnosis and treatment of anxiety disorders, we welcomed the challenge. However, rather than preparing a treatment manual or textbook, of which there are already several excellent examples for anxiety disorders (e.g., Barlow 2004, Antony & Stein 2008, Stein *et al.* 2009), we aimed to do something different. We chose to design a book that would not only provide a critical overview for clinicians but that would also capture the ferment of science as it exists today. For this approach, we turned to our colleagues at Columbia University/NYSPI and asked them to share their perspectives on the most promising new developments and important controversies in their areas of expertise. Our goal was to illustrate what is most novel in the field of anxiety disorders, focusing on areas in which our institution has made a significant contribution, including nosology, assessment, mechanisms, and treatment.

In sum, this book represents a selective review of the work undertaken over the last three decades to advance our understanding of anxiety and of anxiety disorders. Due to the longevity of the Anxiety Disorders Clinic, we have had the opportunity to work with most of the authors over many years. They are our mentors, our colleagues, our collaborators, and our friends. By honoring where we have come from while focusing on where we are going, we hope that this book will communicate the enormous advances that have occurred in the field of anxiety research, and will provide the reader the opportunity to review, in one volume, some of the latest thinking that is shaping the future of this field.

1.2 Content and structure

We have organized the chapters into four sections.

1.2.1 Section 1: Evolving concepts of anxiety

The first section considers a variety of perspectives on evolving concepts of the nature of anxiety. Comer and Olfson (Chapter 2) set the stage by reviewing the prevalence and distribution of DSM-IV anxiety disorders across the life span, drawing predominantly on large-scale epidemiologic surveys conducted in developed regions of the world. They systematically describe evidence for rates, distributions, correlates, and course of DSM-IV anxiety disorders in the general population. They also describe patterns of comorbidity and service use.

Next, First, Caban, and Lewis-Fernández (Chapter 3) trace the evolution of diagnostic criteria for the anxiety disorders over six decades, from DSM-I in 1952 to the dilemmas facing DSM-5, scheduled for 2013. They discuss the theoretical and empirical findings that led to the refining of these categories, and they detail nosological changes introduced by each successive revision.

Liebowitz (Chapter 4) provides a personal perspective on the evolution of diagnostic approaches to anxiety by describing the development of his research on social anxiety disorder. He discusses initial efforts to classify its phenomenology and relationship to other disorders, such as avoidant personality disorder and atypical depression, and the development of assessment measures. He also documents early steps in developing collaborations between the fields of psychiatry and psychology that have led to state-of-the-art comparative clinical trials of medication and psychotherapy.

Glick and Roose (Chapter 5) provide a concise history of psychoanalytic perspectives on anxiety. They describe the concept of "signal anxiety" and trace changes in this concept from Freudian psychology to ego psychology, object relations, and self psychology. They then describe the emerging integration of psychodynamic concepts with research on temperament, gene–environment interactions, and brain imaging, as well as the relevance of a psychodynamic perspective to general treatment of anxiety disorders.

Finally, Hofer (Chapter 6) applies advances in our understanding of evolution, from Darwin to epigenetics, to consider the origins of adult anxiety and its disorders. He illustrates these concepts with examples from more than three decades of his own research on early separation-induced anxiety in young rats, and highlights the evolutionary clues that processes of early development provide for understanding the roots of human panic disorder.

1.2.2 Section 2: Challenges in diagnosing pathological anxiety

The second section reviews selected topics in the clinical assessment and classification of anxiety pathologies, focusing on current controversies over the commonalities and differences between different diagnostic constructs. Pinto, Grados, and Simpson (Chapter 7) review efforts to identify clinically meaningful subtypes of OCD and to understand obsessive–compulsive symptoms in terms of a dimensional model. In addition, they discuss methods that may enable a shift from phenotypic classification to characterization of biomarkers or endophenotypes as the "next frontier" in OCD research, and the corresponding implications for improving understanding and treatment.

Schneier and Socha (Chapter 8) assess the relationship of SAD to trait phenomena of shyness, behavioral inhibition, and avoidant personality. They explore the concept that these constructs lie on a spectrum of socially anxious temperaments, are essential and adaptive for group-living species, and influence, to a variable extent, a much broader spectrum of psychopathology.

McGrath and Miller (Chapter 9) review the phenomenology, epidemiology, and neurobiology of co-occurring anxious and depressive symptoms and disorders. They also address the clinical relevance of this comorbidity, including its implications for prognosis, ranging from medication response to risk of suicidality.

Harding, Skritskaya, Doherty, and Fallon (Chapter 10) review the latest research on the classification, epidemiology, etiology, assessment, and treatment of health anxiety (also known as illness worry). Health anxiety is a subtype of anxiety that is not currently identified as a specific anxiety disorder and is seen instead as a component of various DSM-IV categories, including hypochondriasis, OCD, and delusional disorder, among others. The authors suggest that nosological recognition of this anxiety subtype could advance its neurobiological characterization and lead to improved and more focused treatment.

Next, Kaplowitz and Markowitz (Chapter 11) critically examine three decades of research on the interrelationships between anxiety disorders and personality disorders. This work documents high levels of comorbidity, challenges assumptions of the independence of Axis I and II disorders, and raises new questions about assessment of anxious states, related traits, and approaches to understanding their interactions.

Finally, Hinton and Lewis-Fernández (Chapter 12) focus on cultural factors in the diagnosis of anxiety disorders. They describe the critical importance of cultural syndromes in cross-cultural assessment, as these syndromes pattern and even modulate the emergence of various anxiety disorders, such as panic disorder and PTSD. The clinical relevance of cultural syndromes is discussed, illustrating the role of environmental factors in the etiology and course of specific subtypes of anxiety.

1.2.3 Section 3: Understanding the causes of anxiety

The third section presents diverse approaches to understanding what causes anxiety and anxiety disorders. These chapters draw on both human and animal studies, and they encompass biological and psychosocial domains. Nugent, Weissman, Fyer, and Koenen (Chapter 13) begin this section by reviewing current evidence for genetic factors in the etiology of human anxiety disorders. They address whether anxiety disorders share heritability, consider intermediate phenotypes and candidate genes that might account for the shared risk, and discuss how emerging technological advances in the field of genetics will affect future research.

Richardson-Jones, Leonardo, Hen, and Ahmari (Chapter 14) review recent strategies for developing animal models of anxiety, focusing on genetic manipulation in mice. They illustrate how state-of-the-art genetic methods have been used to probe the role of a specific serotonin receptor (the 5-HT_{1A} receptor) in anxiety-related behaviors.

In the next chapter, Weisstaub, McOmish, Hanks, and Gingrich (Chapter 15) also discuss how mouse models can help elucidate the causes of anxiety. They review the cortical systems that modulate the expression of anxiety and illustrate how genetic strategies have been used to elucidate the role that different aspects of the serotonin system, including the serotonin transporter, 5-HT_{1A} receptors, and 5-HT_{2A} receptors, play in the generation and modulation of anxiety.

Gordon and Adhikari (Chapter 16) summarize research that has mapped the brain circuits underlying learned fear, bringing the amygdala to the forefront of our understanding of fear responses and suggesting neurobiological underpinnings of cognitive–behavioral therapy (CBT) techniques. They also discuss new animal models of innate anxiety, and consider the relevance of both conditioned and innate fear models to understanding the pathophysiology of human anxiety disorders.

Etkin and Wager (Chapter 17) review the burgeoning literature using functional human neuroimaging to clarify what is known about the neural basis of anxiety in healthy and clinical populations. They present evidence for a neurocircuitry model of anxiety that includes a core limbic–prefrontal circuit for affective reactivity (identified in animal and human studies of fear conditioning) and that is modulated by executive working memory and affect appraisal systems.

Hambrick, Comer, and Albano (Chapter 18) present the cognitive–behavioral model of anxiety, focusing on the core feature of anxious apprehension and how it can lead – through a combination of biological vulnerability, developmental experiences, and life events – to the generation of anxiety disorders. They illustrate how this model informs cognitive–behavioral treatments and continues to evolve over time.

Dohrenwend (Chapter 19) focuses on the controversy over the relative importance of the traumatic stressor versus vulnerability factors in the etiology of PTSD. He reviews the historical broadening of the definition of traumatic stressor (Criterion A) as well as the accumulating evidence for the appearance of PTSD after subthreshold stressors.

Mulhare, Ghesquiere, and Shear (Chapter 20) consider the fundamental role of attachment and separation in the generation of anxiety. They also review recent data on the role of attachment security and anxiety sensitivity in the development of a number of anxiety disorders.

Last, Natarajan, Shrestha, and Coplan (Chapter 21) present findings from studies of non-human primates that inform our understanding of the development of human anxiety disorders. They review primate data on neurobiological mechanisms by which genetic predisposition can interact with early deprivation to generate anxious behavior. They also discuss how some types of stress may promote resilience.

1.2.4 Section 4: Treatment of anxiety: current status and controversial issues

The final section describes evidence-based and novel treatment approaches for anxiety disorders. Rodriguez and Simpson (Chapter 22) review evidence-based treatment strategies for OCD, including both medications and cognitive–behavioral therapy, as well as first-line and augmentation strategies. They also discuss novel treatment approaches that are based on increasingly sophisticated theories about the brain mechanisms underlying obsessions and compulsions.

Schneier, Pontoski, and Heimberg (Chapter 23) review the evidence for first-line and alternative medication and psychotherapeutic treatments for social anxiety disorder. They also probe what is understood and what remains unknown about widely used but little-studied approaches to combining medication and cognitive–behavioral treatments, such as the relative efficacy of concurrent versus sequential treatments.

Sullivan, Suh, and Neria (Chapter 24) review data from randomized controlled trials to address the optimal treatment of PTSD. In particular, they consider the evidence for the efficacy of established medication and psychosocial treatments (e.g., serotonin reuptake inhibitors and prolonged exposure), experimental approaches (e.g., pharmacological strategies to prevent the disorder), and widely used but controversial treatments (e.g., benzodiazepines, eye movement desensitization reprocessing).

Sinha and Klein (Chapter 25) evaluate findings on medication and cognitive–behavioral treatment of panic disorder. They raise methodological concerns about this literature and challenge some prevailing views on the efficacy of treatments for panic disorder, while also addressing practical issues such as appropriate dosing and duration of treatments.

Papp, Gorenstein, and Mohlman (Chapter 26) review evidence-based treatments for generalized anxiety disorder (GAD) and focus on the specific challenges of treating the growing population of older patients. They discuss the importance of modifying approaches to both pharmacotherapy and psychosocial therapy in the elderly, and propose treatment guidelines that emphasize flexibility and multimodal approaches.

Next, Vidair and Rynn (Chapter 27) address how to assess and treat anxiety disorders in children. They provide a comprehensive review of the literature supporting the use of both CBT and medications in children with anxiety disorders, discuss the controversial issue of whether medication treatment is associated with increased risk of suicidal behavior in children, and highlight future research questions.

Mantovani and Lisanby (Chapter 28) review current data on electromagnetic modalities in the treatment of anxiety disorders. The approaches range from one of the oldest (electroconvulsive therapy) to some of the newest modalities (vagal nerve stimulation and transcranial magnetic stimulation).

Patel, Tranguch, and Muskin (Chapter 29) review a spectrum of complementary and alternative treatments of anxiety disorders, including mind–body medicine (e.g., meditation), biologically based practices (e.g., dietary supplements), manipulative and body-based practices (e.g., massage), and energy medicine (e.g., acupuncture). Focusing on the most rigorous studies, their critical review lays out the current state of knowledge in these areas, as well as directions for future research.

Finally, Okuda, Khan, De La Cruz, and Blanco (Chapter 30) review current evidence on the treatment of anxiety disorders in primary care settings, including effectiveness of medication and psychosocial therapies. They describe studies of organizational and educational interventions aimed at improving quality of care for anxiety disorders in primary care, such as the collaborative care model, and critically discuss gaps and future directions.

1.3 Conclusion

In the final chapter (Chapter 31), we summarize some of the key observations from the variety of approaches to anxiety and anxiety disorders presented in this book, highlight the potential and limitations of current research, and offer recommendations for future research directions. We believe that an interdisciplinary approach to anxiety will lead to the greatest progress in this field, and the multiple perspectives brought together, integrated, and assembled in this book are intended as a step in that direction. The ultimate goal is to generate an ongoing and productive dialogue between researchers and clinicians with these different perspectives in order to transform how we understand anxiety and treat anxiety disorders.

References

Antony, M. M., & Stein, M. B., eds. (2008). *Oxford Handbook of Anxiety and Related Disorders*. Oxford: Oxford University Press.

Barlow, D. H., ed. (2004). *Anxiety and Its Disorders: the Nature and Treatment of Anxiety and Panic*, 2nd edn. New York, NY: Guilford Press.

Greenberg, P. E., Sisitsky, T., Kessler, R. C., *et al.* (1999). The economic burden of anxiety disorders in the 1990s. *Journal of Clinical Psychiatry*, **60**, 427–435.

Kessler, R. C., Chiu, W. T., Demler, O., Merikangas, K. R., & Walters, E. E. (2005). Prevalence, severity, and comorbidity of 12-month DSM-IV disorders in the National Comorbidity Survey Replication. *Archives of General Psychiatry*, **62**, 617–627.

Stein, D. J., Hollander, E., & Rothbaum, B. O., eds. (2009). *Textbook of Anxiety Disorders*, 2nd edn. Arlington, VA: American Psychiatric Publishing.

The epidemiology of anxiety disorders

Jonathan S. Comer, Mark Olfson

2.1 Introduction

Psychiatric epidemiology uses population-based survey methods to inform understanding of the prevalence, course, and correlates of mental disorders. Whereas the focus of clinical practice is on the individual patient, psychiatric epidemiology studies the manifestation and distribution of mental disorders in the general population in order to evaluate the public health burden and economic impact of psychiatric conditions, and to provide clues to etiology.

Over the past three decades, advances in psychiatric epidemiology and population-based sampling methodology have enhanced our understanding of the public health burden of psychiatric disorders. Measurement in epidemiology has progressed from reliance on unsystematic reports from hospitals and other service facilities to employment of highly structured interviews that reliably assess well-defined diagnostic entities in representative household samples (Dohrenwend & Dohrenwend 1982). In the United States, almost three decades ago the Epidemiological Catchment Area (ECA) study documented rates of DSM-III conditions in five US communities in household and institutional settings (Robins & Regier 1991). Since this landmark study, a number of large-scale US surveys have expanded on the ECA findings to provide nationally representative data using broad structured diagnostic interviews that reflect evolving iterations of the DSM (e.g., Kessler *et al.* 1994, 2005a, Grant *et al.* 2004a). During this period, there have also been rigorous epidemiologic surveys documenting distributions of disorders throughout Europe, Australia, South America, parts of Asia, Africa, and the Middle East (e.g., ESEMeD/MHEDEA 2000 Investigators 2004a, Kessler & Ustun 2008, Stein *et al.* 2008). Advances have also occurred in evaluating the prevalence and associated public health burden of

psychiatric disorders in youth, although these surveys have been limited to narrower geographical regions (Costello *et al.* 2005). Progress in household survey methods – including improvements in diagnostic nomenclature, the advent and availability of reliable structured diagnostic instruments, and developments in probability sampling – has enhanced our understanding of the prevalence, distribution, correlates, and course of anxiety disorders across the life span.

Anxiety disorders are the most prevalent class of mental disorders (Kessler *et al.* 2005b), and collectively they impose a substantial public health burden on society. This burden is reflected among persons with anxiety disorders in elevated rates of general medical disorders (Kessler & Greenberg 2002), high healthcare utilization and costs (Rice & Miller 1998, Greenberg *et al.* 1999, Wittchen 2002), loss of worker productivity (Kessler & Frank 1997), increased risk of suicide attempts and suicidal ideation (Kessler *et al.* 1999, Pilowsky *et al.* 2006), and poor health-related quality of life (Mendlowicz & Stein 2000, Comer, Blanco, Hasin, *et al.* in press).

In this chapter, we review the prevalence and distribution of DSM-IV anxiety disorders across the life span, drawing predominantly on large-scale epidemiologic surveys conducted in developed regions of the world, where the most rigorous work has been conducted. We refer to relevant DSM-III and DSM-III-R literatures only where DSM-IV research is lacking, or to assess temporal trends. Our review is organized around (a) rates, distributions, correlates, and course of the DSM-IV anxiety disorders in the general population; (b) comorbidity patterns; (c) anxiety disorders in primary care; and (d) service use patterns associated with the anxiety disorders. We conclude by highlighting areas in need of empirical attention and laying out an agenda for future epidemiologic research in this area.

Anxiety Disorders: Theory, Research, and Clinical Perspectives, ed. Helen Blair Simpson, Yuval Neria, Roberto Lewis-Fernández, Franklin Schneier. Published by Cambridge University Press. © Cambridge University Press 2010.

2.2 Anxiety disorders in the general population

Epidemiologic surveys consistently document that anxiety disorders are the most prevalent class of mental disorders. In the USA, almost 30% of Americans meet diagnostic criteria for at least one anxiety disorder in their lifetime (Kessler *et al.* 2005a), with 11–18% of adults meeting criteria for an anxiety disorder within the past year (Grant *et al.* 2004a, Kessler *et al.* 2005b). Prevalence rates of anxiety disorders are roughly equivalent across major US racial/ethnic groups (Breslau *et al.* 2004).

Lifetime prevalence rates of anxiety disorders appear to be somewhat lower outside of the USA, ranging roughly from 9% to 16% across Europe and throughout parts of Africa and Asia (ESEMeD/MHEDEA 2000 Investigators 2004a, Cho *et al.* 2007, Stein *et al.* 2008). Similarly, 12-month prevalence rates of anxiety disorders are notably lower in Mexico, Nigeria, Korea, and across Europe, than in the USA, ranging roughly from 4% to 7% (ESEMeD/MHEDEA 2000 Investigators 2004a, Medina-Mora *et al.* 2005, Gureje *et al.* 2006, Cho *et al.* 2007). At present, it is not clear whether such geographic differences reflect true differences in the prevalence of anxiety disorders, differences across cultures in willingness to endorse emotion-related symptoms, or methodological differences across surveys.

Interestingly, research in the USA shows lower lifetime rates of anxiety disorders among immigrants than among US-born natives of the same national origins (Vega *et al.* 1998, Grant *et al.* 2004b). Early age at immigration and longer duration residing in the USA are both associated with increased risk for mental disorders among immigrants relative to natives (Breslau *et al.* 2007), perhaps highlighting the important roles of early socialization and acculturation in conferring increased risk.

Sex differences in the prevalence of anxiety disorders are consistent across cultures and survey methods. Lifetime and 12-month prevalence rates of anxiety disorders among women are roughly twice the rates found among men (ESEMeD/MHEDEA 2000 Investigators 2004a, Jacobi *et al.* 2004, Kessler *et al.* 2005a, Pirkola *et al.* 2005). In children, girls generally report higher rates of anxiety disorders than boys (Costello *et al.* 2003).

Onset of anxiety disorders typically occurs in early adolescence and young adulthood, and they usually manifest before mood or substance use disorders (Kessler *et al.* 2005a). Approximately 2–4% of youth between the ages of 5 and 15 currently meet criteria for an anxiety disorder (Costello *et al.* 2003). Substantial rates of anxiety disorders have also been reported in preschool children (Egger & Angold 2006), although such findings should be met with caution given the lack of consensus in distinguishing normal and abnormal preschool behavior, sole reliance on parent report, and absence of data on the predictive validity of early childhood diagnoses.

Although anxiety disorders on average have an earlier onset than most other classes of mental disorders, the age-of-onset distribution varies across individual anxiety disorders. Based on recall of community-dwelling adults, specific phobias and separation anxiety disorder have the earliest median age of onset (at about 7 years of age), followed by social anxiety disorder (about 13 years), panic disorder and agoraphobia (about 21 years), and generalized anxiety disorder (early thirties) (Kessler *et al.* 2005a).

Cross-sectional work supports a decline in lifetime prevalence of anxiety disorders in older adulthood. Whereas roughly one-third of US adults between the ages of 18 and 59 report meeting lifetime criteria for an anxiety disorder, only one-sixth of US adults over the age of 60 similarly report the presence of a lifetime anxiety disorder (Kessler *et al.* 2005a). It is not clear whether this pattern reflects a true cohort effect, a methodological artifact, or a combination of the two. Lower lifetime prevalence of anxiety disorders among older adults may also reflect earlier mortality associated with psychiatric disorders. That is, those who live into the upper reaches of human life expectancy are less likely to suffer from mental disorders.

When left untreated, anxiety disorders are typically unremitting and persist as chronic conditions associated with reduced quality of life, including decrements in social functioning, role functioning, educational attainment, financial independence, and mental health (see Mendlowicz & Stein 2000). Many of the DSM-IV anxiety disorders are associated with poorer overall mental well-being than cancer, heart disease, arthritis, hypertension, and a host of other chronic general medical conditions (Comer, Blanco, Hasin, *et al.* in press). Anxiety disorders are also associated with decrements in educational achievement. Anxiety disorders are significant predictors of failure to complete high school, failure to enter college among high-school completers, and failure to complete college among college entrants (Kessler *et al.* 1995a).

Beyond these general trends in the epidemiology of *any* anxiety disorder, in this chapter we next consider patterns associated with several specific anxiety disorders: social anxiety disorder (SAD), generalized anxiety disorder (GAD), panic disorder/agoraphobia (PD/AG), obsessive–compulsive disorder (OCD), posttraumatic stress disorder (PTSD), separation anxiety disorder (SepAD), and specific phobia (SP).

2.2.1 Social anxiety disorder (SAD)

Social fears are relatively common. Roughly one-quarter of US residents report at least one lifetime social fear. The most common of these fears are public speaking (21.2% lifetime prevalence) and speaking up in meetings (19.5%) (Ruscio *et al.* 2008). A diagnosis of social anxiety disorder (SAD), also referred to as social phobia, is appropriate when such social fear is excessive and persistent and accompanied by situational avoidance or substantial distress, as well as functional impairment. Lifetime prevalence estimates of SAD range from 5% to 12%, with 1–7% of adults reporting SAD in the past year (Lampe *et al.* 2003, Grant *et al.* 2004a, 2005a, Kessler *et al.* 2005b, Medina-Mora *et al.* 2005, Ruscio *et al.* 2008). Within the USA, 12-month prevalence of SAD is somewhat lower among Hispanic, Asian, and African Americans than among non-Hispanic White Americans (Smith *et al.* 2006).

Prevalence estimates of DSM-IV SAD are slightly lower than those for earlier DSM criteria, in which the disorder was conceptualized as more akin to a simple phobia. In addition, 12-month SAD prevalence estimates appear to be somewhat higher in the USA (about 7%) (Kessler *et al.* 2005b, Ruscio *et al.* 2008) than in Mexico (1.7%) (Medina-Mora *et al.* 2005), Australia (2.3%) (Lampe *et al.* 2003), South Africa (2.8%) (Stein *et al.* 2008), and across Europe (1.2%) (ESEMeD/MHEDEA 2000 Investigators 2004a).

Across cultures, epidemiologic work typically finds women to be at greater risk for SAD than men (Wittchen *et al.* 1998, ESEMeD/MHEDEA 2000 Investigators 2004a, Grant *et al.* 2005a), although in an exception, Stein and colleagues (2000) did not identify a gender effect. In a nuanced set of gender analyses accounting for the number of reported social fears, Ruscio and colleagues (2008) found that women are at higher risk for more generalized forms of SAD (five or more social fears), whereas men are at higher risk for less generalized forms (four or fewer social fears).

Developmental patterns suggest that the average onset of SAD is in adolescence or young adulthood.

Retrospective data find that the onset of social fears (median onset 10–13 years of age) typically precedes the systematic avoidance of social situations (median onset 12–14 years of age) by about 1–2 years (Ruscio *et al.* 2008), with the mean age of full SAD onset at roughly 15 years of age (Grant *et al.* 2005a). Earlier onset is associated with more pervasive social anxiety in adulthood. For example, those with more generalized forms of SAD (i.e., five or more social fears) typically report onset between early childhood and mid-adolescence, whereas those with less generalized SAD (i.e., four or fewer social fears) are more likely to report cases of onset well into the mid-twenties (Ruscio *et al.* 2008). Although social fears are fairly common in youth, the presence of four or more social fears in childhood or adolescence seems to distinguish SAD youth from their non-anxious counterparts (Puliafico *et al.* 2007).

SAD typically displays a persistent course, with only 20–40% of cases remitting within 20 years of onset, and only 40–60% remitting within 40 years. Compared with matched unaffected controls, individuals with SAD report impaired social functioning, diminished social support (Hambrick *et al.* 2003, Eng *et al.* 2005), lower levels of educational attainment, poorer occupational function (Schneier *et al.* 1994, Wittchen *et al.* 1999, Stein & Kean 2000), and decreased rates of marriage (Schneier *et al.* 1992). Merikangas and colleagues (2007) found that after controlling for comorbid conditions, SAD is associated with an average of 14.9 yearly disability days in the USA.

2.2.2 Generalized anxiety disorder (GAD)

Across several DSM iterations, generalized anxiety disorder (GAD) has evolved from a non-specific residual anxiety category to its current status as a primary anxiety disorder. It is characterized by excessive and uncontrollable worry together with associated somatic symptoms. The shifts in GAD criteria have likely resulted in considerable heterogeneity in studies examining the epidemiology of GAD, and have hampered long-term investigations of the course of the disorder (Kessler *et al.* 2004, Holaway *et al.* 2006).

Despite the changing focus of GAD across DSM refinements, a coherent portrait of DSM-IV GAD is now beginning to emerge. It is a highly prevalent anxiety disorder associated with an unremitting course and considerable life impairment. Lifetime prevalence estimates of DSM-IV GAD range from 3% to 6%, with 1–4% of adults reporting DSM-IV GAD in the past year (Carter *et al.* 2001, ESEMeD/MHEDEA 2000 Investigators 2004a, Jacobi *et al.* 2004, Grant *et al.* 2005b, 2005c, Kessler *et al.* 2005a, 2005b, Lieb *et al.* 2005, Cho *et al.* 2007). Lifetime prevalence rates in the USA (about 4–6%) (Grant *et al.* 2005c, Kessler *et al.* 2005a) are somewhat higher than those reported outside the USA (about 2–3%) (ESEMeD/MHEDEA 2000 Investigators 2004a, Cho *et al.* 2007, Stein *et al.* 2008). Within the USA, 12-month prevalence of GAD is somewhat lower among Hispanic and Asian Americans than among non-Hispanic White Americans (Smith *et al.* 2006). Across cultures, GAD is roughly twice as common among women as among men (Wittchen *et al.* 1994, ESEMeD/MHEDEA 2000 Investigators 2004a, Jacobi *et al.* 2004). However, there is some evidence that gender differences attenuate in middle and older adult cohorts (Hunt *et al.* 2002).

Among the anxiety disorders, GAD has the latest mean and median age at onset (early thirties) (Grant *et al.* 2005c, Kessler *et al.* 2005a, Lieb *et al.* 2005), although substantial numbers of children and adolescents do meet full criteria (Albano & Hack 2004, Comer *et al.* 2004, Robin *et al.* 2005, Alyahri & Goodman 2008). Early GAD onset is associated with greater excessiveness and uncontrollability of worry, as well as a more chronic course with more severe life impairment (Ruscio *et al.* 2005). Although the 12-month prevalence of GAD is significantly lower among older adults than among middle-aged adults (1.6% versus 4–5%) (Hunt *et al.* 2002), GAD may nonetheless be the most common anxiety disorder in the elderly (Beekman *et al.* 2000).

Across the anxiety disorders, GAD may be the most profound and have the most deleterious effect on functioning and health-related quality of life (Grant *et al.* 2005c, Comer, Blanco, Hasin, *et al.* in press). Individuals with GAD are at significantly increased risk of impaired social and role functioning, mental health, and overall physical and mental well-being (Mendlowicz & Stein 2000, Stein & Heimberg 2004, Henning *et al.* 2007). In the National Survey of Functional Health Status, overall mental well-being for individuals with 12-month GAD was almost two standard deviations below that identified for "healthy" individuals (i.e., those with no chronic conditions) (Comer, Blanco, Hasin, *et al.* in press). GAD is also associated with poor marriage stability, as afflicted individuals are almost twice as likely to have their first marriage end in divorce (Kessler *et al.* 1998). Occupational impairment is also common (Merikangas *et al.* 2007).

2.2.3 Panic disorder (PD) with and without agoraphobia

Panic attacks are discrete periods of intense fear or discomfort accompanied by at least four DSM-IV specified symptoms (e.g., palpitations, sweating, shortness of breath, nausea, derealization, paresthesias), reaching peak intensity within 10 minutes. Roughly one-fifth of the general US population has experienced an isolated panic attack (Kessler *et al.* 2006). When panic attacks recur and are accompanied by persistent concern over future attacks, worry about attack implications, or significant behavioral changes to prevent future attacks, a diagnosis of panic disorder (PD) is warranted. When PD is accompanied by intense anxiety about being in places or situations from which escape may be difficult or in which help may not be available in the event of an unexpected panic attack, and such situations are avoided or else endured with marked distress, a diagnosis of PD with agoraphobia is applied.

Across cultures, lifetime PD rates range roughly from 2% to 4%, and 1–3% report the presence of PD within the past year (ESEMeD/MHEDEA 2000 Investigators 2004a, Grant *et al.* 2004a, Jacobi *et al.* 2004, Goodwin *et al.* 2005, Medina-Mora *et al.* 2005, Kessler *et al.* 2006). PD with agoraphobia appears to be somewhat less frequent, with 12-month and lifetime prevalence rates both at roughly 1% (Grant *et al.* 2004a, Kessler *et al.* 2006). Rates for PD and PD with agoraphobia are twice as high in females as in males (Goodwin *et al.* 2005, Jacobi *et al.* 2004, Kessler *et al.* 2006). Within the USA, 12-month prevalence of PD is somewhat lower among Hispanic and Asian Americans than among non-Hispanic White and African Americans (Smith *et al.* 2006).

PD and agoraphobia typically begin in young adulthood (at about 21 years) (Kessler *et al.* 2005a) and only rarely before adolescence. Cross-sectional work suggests that the mean onset of PD is roughly one year following the mean onset of an initial panic attack (Kessler *et al.* 2006), although this has yet to be confirmed by prospective, longitudinal work. A vast majority of initial panic attacks are reported as occurring outside of the home – while on a bus, plane, or subway, or while walking, driving, or at school or work (Craske *et al.* 1990, Shulman *et al.* 1994).

PD with and without agoraphobia tends to persist and interfere with family and occupational functioning (Kessler *et al.* 1998). In the workplace, PD and agoraphobia are associated with approximately 18–21 yearly disability days (Merikangas *et al.* 2007). Quality of life is poor among individuals with PD (Mendlowicz & Stein 2000), and recent analyses of the National Survey of Functional Health Status find that individuals with PD exhibit considerably poorer overall mental well-being compared to individuals with a number of chronic general medical conditions (Comer, Blanco, Hasin, *et al.* in press).

2.2.4 Obsessive–compulsive disorder (OCD)

Few large-scale epidemiologic surveys have assessed obsessive–compulsive disorder (OCD). Consequently, our understanding of the distribution, course, and correlates of OCD in the general population lags behind our understanding of community patterns associated with SAD, GAD, and PD. Lifetime prevalence estimates across household surveys that have assessed OCD range from 1.6% to 2.5% (Canino *et al.* 1987, Weissman *et al.* 1994, Kessler *et al.* 2005a). Twelve-month prevalence rates have been documented at 0.7–2.0% (Jacobi, *et al.* 2004, Kessler *et al.* 2005b, Torres *et al.* 2006, Cho *et al.* 2007). In contrast with several other anxiety disorders, there do not appear to be significant cohort effects in the prevalence of OCD (Kessler *et al.* 2005a).

As with other anxiety disorders, OCD prevalence rates are generally higher among women than among men (Horwath & Weissman 2000), although the pattern may be reversed among youth (Comer *et al.* 2004). At the symptom level, there is evidence that females with OCD are more likely to present with obsessions regarding contamination and aggression, whereas males with OCD are more likely to present with sexual obsessions, checking/repeating compulsions, and needs for symmetry (Lensi *et al.* 1996, Bogetto *et al.* 1999, de Mathis *et al.* 2008). In youth, boys appear to be at greater risk for earlier onset of OCD (Hanna 1995, Gellar *et al.* 1998, de Mathis *et al.* 2008).

OCD typically develops in mid to late adolescence (Riddle 1998, Comer *et al.* 2004) with a median age at onset of 19 years (Kessler *et al.* 2005a). Earlier onset is associated with a more complex and intractable course in adulthood (de Mathis *et al.* 2008). Individuals with OCD report markedly reduced quality of life and general well-being (Mendlowicz & Stein 2000), diminished occupational attainment, impaired family functioning (Koran 2000), and higher rates of suicidal thoughts and attempts (Torres *et al.* 2006). Severity of OCD is inversely correlated with social functioning (Koran *et al.* 1996).

2.2.5 Posttraumatic stress disorder (PTSD)

Since its formal introduction as an anxiety disorder in 1980 (DSM-III), PTSD remains one of only a handful of diagnostic entities in the DSM taxonomy that directly and causally links symptoms to a preceding event/experience. Field trials document three reliable symptom clusters among individuals exposed to diverse traumatic events: (a) re-experiencing symptoms, which are the most common, (b) avoidance/numbing symptoms, and (c) physiological hyperarousal.

Lifetime and 12-month prevalence estimates for PTSD are substantial in the general population, though much lower than the prevalence of exposure to potentially traumatic events. Whereas surveys find that lifetime prevalence of traumatic exposure in the USA falls between 50% and 60%, lifetime and 12-month prevalence estimates for PTSD are roughly 7% and 4%, respectively (Kessler *et al.* 2005a, 2005b). Intriguingly, prevalence rates of traumatic exposure are somewhat higher outside of the USA, whereas rates of PTSD tend to be somewhat lower (Creamer *et al.* 2001, Zlotnick *et al.* 2006, Cho *et al.* 2007, Stein *et al.* 2008). Reported rates of PTSD following traumatic exposure are considerably lower in youth than in adults (Copeland *et al.* 2007; see also Egger & Angold 2006, Alyahri & Goodman 2008). This latter finding may reflect true age-related differences in PTSD rates following traumatic exposure or delayed onset of PTSD following traumatic exposure in youth. Alternatively, this finding may call into question the developmental appropriateness of DSM-IV PTSD criteria for capturing maladaptive child reactions to trauma.

Rates of PTSD are higher among women than men, despite the higher prevalence of exposure to traumatic events reported among men (Kessler *et al.* 1995b, Creamer *et al.* 2001). Women are at greater risk for developing PTSD following exposure to all forms of potentially traumatic events except sexual assault, for which conditional risks are equivalent across gender (Kessler *et al.* 1995b, Stein *et al.* 1997). Across men and women reporting traumatic exposure, approximately 75% report exposure to more than one traumatic event. Among potentially traumatic events, sexual assault, which is more commonly reported by women, is the most highly linked to subsequent development of PTSD (Creamer *et al.* 2001, Zlotnick *et al.* 2006). Similar gender patterns are found in children (Copeland *et al.* 2007).

A substantial number of individuals exposed to traumatic events initially endure remarkably well, though they subsequently develop delayed-onset PTSD in the second post-event year (Solomon 1989, McFarlane 2004, Andrews *et al.* 2007). Such findings highlight the critical importance of prospective, longitudinal work and long-term follow-up evaluations in revealing the course of PTSD.

PTSD follows a persistent course for a substantial proportion of cases. Perkonigg and colleagues (2005) followed a community sample of young adults diagnosed with PTSD across several years. Although 52% of cases remitted, 48% showed no substantial remission. Compared with remitted individuals, unremitted adults were five times more likely to experience new traumatic events. PTSD is also associated with increased risk of divorce (Kessler *et al.* 1998) and occupational impairment (Merikangas *et al.* 2007).

Community PTSD rates can increase greatly in the aftermath of a natural or man-made disaster, which collectively affect on average as many as 33 million individuals each year (International Federation of Red Cross and Red Crescent Societies 1998). Historically, studies of disaster-exposed individuals have focused on clinic and various other convenience samples. Epidemiologic research on disaster-affected samples using population-based sampling methods is rare but has steadily increased over the past eight years.

In the aftermath of the September 11, 2001, terrorist attacks, Schlenger and colleagues (2002) showed in a US national probability sample that post-attack PTSD rates were considerably higher in New York City (11%) than in the rest of the country (4%). Among Americans who lost a loved one in the attacks, an estimated 43% of those who suffered complicated grief met criteria for PTSD 2–3 years later (Neria *et al.* 2007). In a New York City primary-care sample, Neria and colleagues (2006) found that one-year post-attack, roughly 20% of patients met DSM-IV criteria for PTSD. Knowing someone killed in the attacks was associated with twice the odds of developing PTSD (Neria *et al.* 2008). Regarding youth, Hoven and colleagues (2005), employing population-based sampling methods, estimated that 11% of New York City public-school children showed PTSD six months post-attack (compared to about 3% typically found in child samples). Direct exposure was associated with substantially increased odds of PTSD, and Comer, Fan, Duarte, and colleagues (in press) found that in addition to traumatic exposure, attack-related life disruption (i.e., parental job loss; parental restriction of child's post-attack freedom to travel throughout the city) was associated with

increased odds of PTSD (see also Comer & Kendall 2007).

Following Hurricane Katrina, Galea, and colleagues (2007) estimated the prevalence of PTSD to be roughly 30% among residents of the New Orleans metropolitan area, and roughly 16% among residents of other directly affected regions. As in general population studies, females are more likely than males to suffer PTSD in the aftermath of a disaster. Despite the advances in researching post-disaster mental health in industrialized regions of the world, future epidemiologic efforts are needed to document rates of PTSD in developing countries affected by disasters – particularly as research shows it is developing countries that are most affected by disasters and suffer the greatest numbers of disaster-related lives lost (International Federation of Red Cross and Red Crescent Societies 2004).

Epidemiologic research on war-related trauma and posttraumatic stress reactions has increased considerably, and research documents the very heavy mental health toll that wartime deployment can exact on military personnel. Long-term follow-up of veterans of the Vietnam War found that as many as 30% of veterans could be diagnosed with PTSD at some point following their combat experience (Kulka *et al.* 1990), with rates even higher in medical-treatment-seeking samples. Among current US service men and women seen in VA facilities, roughly one quarter of veterans returning from Iraq or Afghanistan are receiving a diagnosis of a mental disorder (Seal *et al.* 2007). Analyses of data from the Department of Defense OEF/OIF post-deployment health screening efforts show that psychiatric symptom reports increase with the passage of time from initial homecoming (Milliken *et al.* 2008). Clinicians in the Post Deployment Health Assessment and Reassessment (Milliken *et al.* 2008) identified roughly 20% of active and 40% of reserve soldiers returning from Iraq and Afghanistan as requiring mental health treatment. In a survey of Israeli veterans of the Yom Kippur War, Neria and Koenen (2003) found combat-related stress and PTSD predicted physical health almost two decades post-combat.

2.2.6 Separation anxiety disorder (SepAD)

Separation anxiety disorder (SepAD) refers to persistent, developmentally inappropriate anxiety concerning separation from major attachment figure(s) or home. It is the only DSM-IV anxiety disorder classified under "disorders usually first diagnosed in infancy, childhood, or adolescence." Lifetime rates of

SepAD in the USA are roughly 5–6% in adults and 4% in youth (Kessler *et al.* 2005a). Across cultures, roughly 2–3% of children meet current diagnostic criteria for SepAD, with prevalence rates declining with age (Egger & Angold 2006, Adewuya *et al.* 2007, Alyahri & Goodman 2008). Although SepAD has historically been believed to occur predominantly in childhood, recent epidemiologic work suggests that the 12-month prevalence of adult SepAD is as much as 2% (Kessler *et al.* 2005b, Shear *et al.* 2006). Approximately one-third of childhood SepAD cases persist into adulthood, and roughly 25% of adult SepAD cases first occur in childhood (Shear *et al.* 2006). Females are consistently at higher risk for SepAD than males across child and adult samples.

2.2.7 Specific phobia (SP)

Specific phobia (SP) refers to a marked and persistent fear of a specific object or situation that causes substantial life interference or distress. Lifetime SP prevalence estimates range from 4% to 13%, with 6–9% of adults reporting SP in the past year (Grant *et al.* 2004a, Kessler *et al.* 2005a, 2005b, Cho *et al.* 2007, Stinson *et al.* 2007). As with most anxiety disorders, 12-month prevalence estimates appear to be somewhat higher in the USA (7–9%) (Grant *et al.* 2004a, Kessler *et al.* 2005b) than outside of the USA (about 4%) (Medina-Mora *et al.* 2005, Cho *et al.* 2007). SP typically starts in childhood (median age about 7–10 years) (Kessler *et al.* 2005a, Stinson *et al.* 2007), during which prevalence rates are roughly 2–3% (Egger & Angold 2006, Alyahri & Goodman 2008). Within the USA, 12-month prevalence of SP is somewhat lower among Hispanic and Asian Americans than among non-Hispanic White and African Americans (Smith *et al.* 2006). As with most other anxiety disorders, SP is more common among females than males, and it tends to run a persistent and disabling course with low rates of spontaneous remission (Wittchen 1988).

2.3 Psychiatric comorbidity

Psychiatric comorbidity, the co-occurrence of multiple mental disorders, is particularly high among individuals diagnosed with an anxiety disorder. Isolated cases of "pure" anxiety disorders (i.e., unaccompanied by additional DSM-IV diagnoses) are relatively rare. Roughly 70–80% of individuals with a lifetime anxiety disorder and 60–90% of individuals with an anxiety disorder in the past year meet criteria for at least one additional disorder (Wittchen *et al.* 1994, Kessler *et al.*

1995b, 2006, Lampe *et al.* 2003, ESEMeD/MHEDEA 2000 Investigators 2004b, Jacobi *et al.* 2004, Torres *et al.* 2006). The most common pattern of comorbidity among individuals with anxiety disorders is meeting criteria for multiple anxiety disorders. For example, individuals with SP, GAD, and SAD are at roughly 15, 9, and 6 times increased odds, respectively, for having a co-occurring anxiety disorder (Grant *et al.* 2005c, Stinson *et al.* 2007, Ruscio *et al.* 2008). Among individuals with lifetime PD with agoraphobia, for example, 94% have another anxiety disorder, most commonly SP (75%) or SAD (67%) (Kessler *et al.* 2006).

Anxiety disorders are also highly comorbid with mood disorders (Brady & Kendall 1992, Costello *et al.* 2003). Individuals diagnosed with 12-month GAD, SAD, and SP are at roughly 19, 5, and 3 times increased odds, respectively, for having a co-occurring mood disorder (Merikangas *et al.* 2002, Grant *et al.* 2005c, Stinson *et al.* 2007, Ruscio *et al.* 2008). Among the mood disorders, individuals with SAD, PTSD, PD, and OCD are at greatest risk for co-occurring major depressive disorder, while individuals with GAD or SP are at greatest risk for co-occurring bipolar disorder. In cases of co-occurring anxiety and mood disorders, onset of anxiety disorders typically occurs prior to mood disorders (Brady & Kendall 1992).

Higher rates of substance use disorders are reported among individuals with anxiety disorders (Creamer *et al.* 2001, Merikangas *et al.* 2002, Chartier *et al.* 2003). Approximately 15% of individuals reporting an anxiety disorder in the past year meet criteria for a co-occurring substance use disorder (Grant *et al.*, 2004a). Individuals with PD with agoraphobia and GAD are at greatest risk.

Rates of personality disorders are also significantly elevated among individuals with anxiety disorders. Roughly 40% of those with anxiety disorders meet a DSM-IV Axis II diagnosis, most commonly dependent personality disorder, avoidant personality disorder, or obsessive–compulsive personality disorder (Grant *et al.* 2005c). Among the anxiety disorders, SAD and GAD have the highest rates of comorbidity with personality disorders (Grant *et al.* 2005b, Stinson *et al.* 2007).

2.4 Anxiety disorders in primary care

Anxiety disorders are highly prevalent among patients in primary care settings (Olfson *et al.* 1997, Kuehn 2008). Roughly one-fifth of primary care patients meet criteria for an anxiety-disorder diagnosis (Kroenke *et al.* 2007), a rate slightly higher than that found in the general population (Grant *et al.* 2004a). In particular, rates of PTSD (at about 9%), GAD (about 8%), and PD (about 7%) are considerably elevated (Kroenke *et al.* 2007), perhaps reflecting the high rates of unhealthy behaviors and risk factors associated with the anxiety disorders (e.g., smoking, physical inactivity, obesity, and binge drinking) (Strine *et al.* 2008), which themselves increase medical treatment seeking. Physical and somatic symptoms that accompany PTSD, GAD, and PD may also lead more individuals with anxiety disorders to seek medical treatment. In contrast, SAD patients are somewhat underrepresented in primary care settings (Gross *et al.* 2005), perhaps reflecting socially avoidant patterns characteristic of SAD and/or negative beliefs about the social implications of seeking treatment.

As in the general population, comorbidity among the anxiety disorders is high in primary care settings. Among primary care patients with anxiety disorders, over 80% suffer from at least one other mental disorder, with more than 40% suffering from a concurrent mood disorder (Rodriguez *et al.* 2004). Over two-thirds of primary care patients with an anxiety disorder report a mood disorder at some time in their life. As in the general population, comorbidity is associated with increased disability in social and occupational functioning (Olfson *et al.* 1997).

In primary care settings, individual anxiety disorders are associated with substantially increased alcohol and substance use and disability. For example, PTSD in primary care settings is associated with three times the odds of heavy drinking (i.e., three drinks at least two times per week), and PD is associated with twice the odds of frequent alcohol use (i.e., four or more times drinking per week). Primary care patients with PD are at twice the odds of reporting suicidal ideation (Pilowsky *et al.* 2006), and primary care patients with GAD report increased pain intensity and healthcare costs (Olfson & Gameroff 2007).

2.5 Service use

A majority of adults with anxiety disorders do not receive treatment for their symptoms during the course of one year (Kessler *et al.* 2005c). Across Europe, only one-quarter of individuals reporting an anxiety disorder in the last year consulted a formal health service regarding emotional problems – a rate significantly lower than rates of treatment seeking reported among individuals suffering from mood or substance use disorders (ESEMeD/MHEDEA 2000 Investigators

2004c). Earlier age at disorder onset is associated with reduced odds of making treatment contact (Wang *et al.* 2007). Mental health service use is particularly low in less-developed regions of the world, with the proportion of individuals in a country receiving services tending to correspond with the country's percentage of gross domestic product spent on health care (Wang *et al.* 2007).

In the USA, epidemiologic surveys document long delays in treatment seeking and low rates of treatment among individuals with anxiety disorders. Only 1–7% of individuals with SAD, PTSD, SP, or SepAD, and only one-third of individuals with GAD or PD, make contact with a service provider within the first year of disorder (Wang *et al.* 2005). The median delay of treatment initiation after initial onset of anxiety disorder ranges from 9 years (GAD) to 20 years (SP), with PD (10 years), PTSD (12 years), and SAD (16 years) having intermediate delays (Wang *et al.* 2005).

Given the availability of highly effective treatments for the anxiety disorders (Heimberg *et al.* 1998, Albano & Kendall 2002, Barlow *et al.* 2007, Roy-Byrne & Cowley 2007, Kendall *et al.* 2008), low rates and long delays in service use underscore the need for greater efforts to increase disorder awareness, enhance treatment access, and improve clinical recognition.

2.6 Conclusion and future directions

Roughly one in three Americans and one in seven individuals in developed regions outside of the USA suffer from an anxiety disorder in their lifetime. In comparison with the general population, these individuals tend to have lower personal income, increased rates of physical problems, and greater numbers of other psychiatric disorders. Individuals with anxiety disorders also tend to report poorer overall well-being, as well as impaired social, occupational, and role functioning. Such findings underscore the magnitude of the disease burden associated with anxiety disorders and bring a renewed sense of urgency to efforts to improve treatment access for these disorders.

High rates of comorbidity among the anxiety disorders call into question key boundary tensions in the current diagnostic system. In recent years, there has been increasing consensus for nosological systems to move beyond current categorical definitions to incorporate a more dimensional approach to classification (Helzer *et al.* 2008). Moreover, although research has done much to document the descriptive epidemiology of psychiatric comorbidity, prospective longitudinal work is needed to examine key issues of temporal precedence and the meaning of and mechanisms underlying such comorbidity. Cross-sectional work cannot reliably determine whether apparent comorbidity represents two manifestations of the same disorder, two stages of the same underlying condition, origins in the same or correlated risk factors, or one condition predisposing an individual to the other (Rutter 1994, 1997).

Most epidemiologic research in this area has relied on retrospective accounts and cross-sectional analyses to answer key questions concerning the course and stability of disorders. Such work is limited due to recall biases and cohort effects. Prospective, longitudinal research is needed to reveal the natural sequencing and trajectory of anxiety disorders, and to determine the direction of associations among anxiety disorders, comorbid conditions, and life quality. Long-term follow-up evaluations in population-based samples are needed to provide information regarding the natural course of disorders over the life span.

Increased efforts are needed to document population-based prevalence estimates of childhood anxiety disorders. In the assessment of childhood psychopathology, the strategy of gathering data from multiple informants, including parents and teachers, has become standard practice (Comer & Kendall 2004, De Los Reyes & Kazdin 2005). These requirements make child diagnostic procedures more time- and labor-intensive.

Psychiatric epidemiologic investigations of anxiety disorders have until recently been largely confined to industrialized regions of the world. Understanding patterns and predictors of anxiety disorders in regions beset by economic, educational, wartime, and health-related hardships is critical to understanding the global burden of anxiety disorders and to planning mental-health service delivery in these areas. Future efforts are needed to advance epidemiologic survey methods in developing countries and refugee populations, and to advance effective care and mental-health literacy in resource-poor regions of the world.

In conclusion, anxiety disorders are the most prevalent class of mental disorders. They collectively impose a substantial public health burden on society. Given the availability of effective interventions for anxiety disorders, and their contrast with documented long delays and low treatment rates, epidemiologic findings underscore the critical importance of accelerating the flow of affected individuals into treatment, improving clinical recognition of anxiety disorders, and reducing financial barriers to effective mental health care.

References

Adewuya, A. O., Ola, B. A., & Adewumi, T. A. (2007). The 12-month prevalence of DSM-IV anxiety disorders among Nigerian secondary school adolescents aged 13–18 years. *Journal of Adolescence*, **30**, 1071–1076.

Albano, A. M., & Hack, S. (2004). Children and adolescents. In R. G. Heimberg, C. L. Turk, & D.S. Mennin, eds., *Generalized Anxiety Disorder: Advances in Research and Practice*. New York, NY: Guilford.

Albano, A. M., & Kendall, P. C. (2002). Cognitive behavioural therapy for children and adolescents with anxiety disorders: Clinical research advances. *International Review of Psychiatry*, **14**, 129–134.

Alyahri, A., & Goodman, R. (2008). The prevalence of DSM-IV psychiatric disorders among 7–10 year old Yemini schoolchildren. *Social Psychiatry and Psychiatric Epidemiology*, **43**, 224–230.

Andrews, B., Brewin, C. R., Phipott, R., & Stewart, L. (2007). Delayed-onset posttraumatic stress disorder: a systematic review of the evidence. *American Journal of Psychiatry*, **164**, 1319–1326.

Barlow, D. H., Allen, L. B., & Badsen, S. L. (2007). Psychological treatments for panic disorders, phobias, and generalized anxiety disorder. In P. E. Nathan & J. M. Gorman, eds., *A Guide to Treatments that Work*, 3rd edn. New York, NY: Oxford University Press.

Beekman, A. T. F., Debeurs, E., van Balkom, A. J. L. M., *et al.* (2000). Anxiety and depression in later life: Co-occurrence and communality of risk factors. *American Journal of Psychiatry*, **157**, 89–95.

Bogetto, F., Venturello, S., Albert, U., Maina, G., & Ravizza, L. (1999). Gender-related clinical differences in obsessive–compulsive disorder. *European Psychiatry*, **14**, 434–441.

Brady, E. U., & Kendall P. C. (1992). Comorbidity of anxiety and depression in children and adolescents. *Psychological Bulletin*, **111**, 244–255.

Breslau, J., Kendler, K. S., Su, M., Gaxiola-Aguilar, S., & Kessler, R. C. (2004). Lifetime risk and persistence of psychiatric disorders across ethnic groups in the United States. *Psychological Medicine*, **35**, 317–327.

Breslau, J., Aguilar-Gaxiola, S., Borges, G., *et al.* (2007). Risk for psychiatric disorder among immigrants and their US-born descendants: Evidence from the National Comorbidity Survey Replication. *Journal of Nervous and Mental Disease*, **195**, 189–195.

Canino, G. J., Bird, H. R., Shrout, P. E., *et al.* (1987). The prevalence of specific psychiatric disorders in Puerto Rico. *Archives of General Psychiatry*, **44**, 727–735.

Carter, R. M., Wittchen, H. U., Pfister, H., & Kessler, R. C. (2001). One-year prevalence of subthreshold and threshold DSM-IV generalized anxiety disorder in a nationally representative sample. *Depression and Anxiety*, **13**, 78–88.

Chartier, M. J., Walker, J. R., & Stein, M. B. (2003). Considering comorbidity in social phobia. *Social Psychiatry and Psychiatric Epidemiology*, **38**, 728–734.

Cho, M.J., Kim, J.-K., Jeon, H.J., *et al.* (2007). Lifetime and 12-month prevalence of DSM-IV psychiatric disorders among Korean adults. *Journal of Nervous and Mental Disease*, **195**, 203–210.

Comer, J. S., & Kendall, P. C. (2004). A symptom-level examination of parent–child agreement in the diagnosis of anxious youths. *Journal of the American Academy of Child and Adolescent Psychiatry*, **43**, 878–886.

Comer, J. C., & Kendall, P. C. (2007). Terrorism: the psychological impact on youth. *Clinical Psychology*, **14**, 178–212.

Comer, J. S., Kendall, P. C., Franklin, M. E., Hudson, J. L., & Pimentel, S. S. (2004). Obsessing/worrying about the overlap between obsessive–compulsive disorder and generalized anxiety disorder in youth. *Clinical Psychology Review*, **24**, 663–683.

Comer, J. S., Blanco, C., Hasin, D. S., *et al.* (in press). Health-related quality of life and clinical correlates across the anxiety disorders. *Journal of Clinical Psychiatry*.

Comer, J. S., Fan, B., Duarte, C., *et al.* (in press). Attack-related life disruption and child psychopathology in New York City public schoolchildren 6-months post-9/11. *Journal of Clinical Child and Adolescent Psychology*.

Copeland, W. E., Keeler, G., Angold, A., & Costello, E. J. (2007). Traumatic events and posttraumatic stress in childhood. *Archives of General Psychiatry*, **64**, 577–584.

Costello, E. J., Mustillo, S., Erkanli, A., Keeler, G., & Angold, A. (2003). Prevalence and development of psychiatric disorders in childhood and adolescence. *Archives of General Psychiatry*, **60**, 837–844.

Costello, E. J., Egger, H., & Angold, A. (2005). 10-year research update review: the epidemiology of child and adolescent psychiatric disorders: I. Methods and public health burden. *Journal of the American Academy of Child and Adolescent Psychiatry*, **44**, 972–986.

Craske, M. G., Miller, P. P., Rotunda, R., & Barlow, D. H. (1990). A descriptive report of features of initial unexpected panic attacks in minimal and extensive avoiders. *Behaviour Research and Therapy*, **28**, 395–400.

Creamer, M., Burgess, P., & McFarlane, A. C. (2001). Posttraumatic stress disorder: findings from the Australian National Survey of Mental Health and Well-Being. *Psychological Medicine*, **31**, 1237–1247.

De Los Reyes, A., & Kazdin, A. E. (2005). Informant discrepancies in the assessment of childhood psychopathology: a critical review, theoretical framework, and recommendations for further study. *Psychological Bulletin*, **131**, 483–509.

de Mathis, M. A., do Rosario, M. C., Diniz, J. B., *et al.* (2008). Obsessive–compulsive disorder: influence of age at onset on comorbidity patterns. *European Psychiatry*, **23**, 187–194.

Dohrenwend, B. P., & Dohrenwend, B. S. (1982). Perspectives on the past and future of psychiatric epidemiology: the 1981 Rema Lapouse lecture. *American Journal of Public Health*, **72**, 1271–1279.

Egger, H. L., & Angold, A. (2006). Common emotional and behavioral disorders in preschool children: presentation, nosology, and epidemiology. *Journal of Child Psychology and Psychiatry*, **47**, 313–337.

Eng, W., Coles, M. E., Heimberg, R. G., & Safren, S. A. (2005). Domains of life satisfaction in social anxiety disorder: Relation to symptoms and response to cognitive–behavioral therapy. *Journal of Anxiety Disorders*, **19**, 143–156.

ESEMeD/MHEDEA 2000 Investigators (2004a). Prevalence of mental disorders in Europe: Results from the European Study of the Epidemiology of Mental Disorders (ESEMeD) project. *Acta Psychiatr Scand*, **109** (Suppl. 420), 21–27.

ESEMeD/MHEDEA 2000 Investigators (2004b). 12-month comorbidity patterns and associated factors in Europe: Results from the European Study of the Epidemiology of Mental Disorders (ESEMeD) project. *Acta Psychiatr Scand*, **109** (Suppl. 420), 28–37.

ESEMeD/MHEDEA 2000 Investigators (2004c). Use of mental health services in Europe: Results from the European Study of the Epidemiology of Mental Disorders (ESEMeD) project. *Acta Psychiatr Scand*, **109** (Suppl. 420), 47–54.

Galea, S., Brewin, C. R., Gruber, M., *et al.* (2007). Exposure to hurricane-related stressors and mental illness after Hurricane Katrina. *Archives of General Psychiatry*, **64**, 1427–1434.

Gellar, D., Biederman, J., Jones, J., *et al.* (1998). Is juvenile obsessive–compulsive disorder a developmental subtype of the disorder? A review of pediatric literature. *Journal of the American Academy of Child and Adolescent Psychiatry*, **37**, 420–427.

Goodwin, R. D., Faravelli, C., Rosi, S., *et al.* (2005). The epidemiology of panic disorder and agoraphobia in Europe. *European Neuropsychopharmacology*, **15**, 435–443.

Grant, B. F., Stinson, F. S., Dawson, D. A., *et al.* (2004a). Prevalence and co-occurrence of substance use disorders and independent mood and anxiety disorders: results from the National Epidemiologic Survey on Alcohol and Related Conditions. *Archives of General Psychiatry*, **61**, 807–816.

Grant, B. F., Stinson, F. S., Hasin, D. S., *et al.* (2004b). Immigration and lifetime prevalence of DSM-IV psychiatric disorders among Mexican Americans and non-Hispanic whites in the United States: results from the National Epidemiologic Survey of Alcohol and Related Conditions. *Archives of General Psychiatry*, **61**, 1226–1233.

Grant, B. F., Hasin, D. S., Blanco, C., *et al.* (2005a). The epidemiology of social anxiety disorder in the United States: results from the National Epidemiologic Survey on Alcohol and Related Conditions. *Journal of Clinical Psychiatry*, **66**, 1351–1361.

Grant, B. F., Hasin, D. S., Stinson, F. S., *et al.* (2005b). Co-occurrence of 12-month mood and anxiety disorders and personality disorders in the U.S.: results from the National Epidemiologic Survey on Alcohol and Related Conditions. *Journal of Psychiatric Research*, **39**, 1–9.

Grant, B. F., Hasin, D. S., Stinson, F. S., *et al.* (2005c). Prevalence, correlates, co-morbidity, and comparative disability of DSM-IV generalized anxiety disorder in the USA: results from the National Epidemiologic Survey on Alcohol and Related Conditions. *Psychological Medicine*, **35**, 1747–1759.

Greenberg, P. E., Sisitsky, T., Kessler, R. C., *et al.* (1999). The economic burden of anxiety disorders in the 1990s. *Journal of Clinical Psychiatry*, **60**, 427–435.

Gross, R., Olfson, M., Gameroff, M. J., *et al.* (2005). Social anxiety disorder in primary care. *General Hospital Psychiatry*, **27**, 161–168.

Gureje, O., Lasebikan, V. O., Kola, L., & Makanjuola, V. A. (2006). Lifetime and 12-month prevalence of mental disorders in the Nigerian Survey of Mental Health and Well-Being. *British Journal of Psychiatry*, **188**, 465–471.

Hambrick, J. P., Turk, C. L., Heimberg, R. G., Schneier, F. R., & Liebowitz, M. R. (2003). The experience of disability and quality of life in social anxiety disorder. *Depression and Anxiety*, **18**, 46–50.

Hanna, G. L. (1995). Demographic and clinic features of obsessive compulsive disorder in children and adolescents. *Journal of the American Academy of Child and Adolescent Psychiatry*, **34**, 19–27.

Heimberg, R. G., Liebowitz, M. R., Hope, D. A., *et al.* (1998). Cognitive behavioral group therapy vs phenelzine therapy for social phobia: 12-week outcome. *Archives of General Psychiatry*, **55**, 1133–1141.

Helzer, J. E., Kraemer, H. C., Krueger, R. F., *et al.* (2008). *Dimensional Approaches in Diagnostic Classification: Refining the Research Agenda for DSM-IV*. Washington, DC: American Psychiatric Association.

Henning, E. R., Turk, C. L., Mennin, D. S., Fresco, D. M., & Heimberg, R. G. (2007). Impairment and quality of life in individuals with generalized anxiety disorder. *Depression and Anxiety*, **24**, 342–349.

Holaway, R. M., Rodebaugh, T. L., & Heimberg, R. G. (2006). The epidemiology of worry and generalized anxiety disorder. In G. C. L. Davey and A. Wells, eds., *Worry and Its Psychological Disorders: Theory, Assessment, and Treatment*. Hoboken, NJ: Wiley.

Horwath, E., & Weissman, M. M. (2000). The epidemiology and cross-national presentation of obsessive–compulsive disorder. *Psychiatric Clinics of North America*, **23**, 493–507.

Hoven, C. W., Duarte, C. S., Lucas, C. P. *et al.* (2005). Psychopathology among New York City public school children 6 months after September 11. *Archives of General Psychiatry*, **62**, 545–552.

Hunt, C., Issakidis, C., & Andrews, G. (2002). DSM-IV generalized anxiety disorder in the Australian National Survey of Mental Health and Well-Being. *Psychological Medicine*, **32**, 649–659.

International Federation of Red Cross and Red Crescent Societies (1998). *World Disasters Report*. New York, NY: Oxford University Press.

International Federation of Red Cross and Red Crescent Societies (2004). *World Disasters Report*. New York, NY: Oxford University Press.

Jacobi, F., Wittchen, H. U., Holting, C., *et al.* (2004). Prevalence, comorbidity and correlates of mental disorders in the general population: results from the German Health Interview and Examination Survey (GHS). *Psychological Medicine*, **34**, 597–611.

Kendall, P. C., Hudson, J. L., Gosch, E., Flannery-Schroeder, E., & Suveg, C. (2008). Cognitive–behavioral therapy for anxiety disordered youth: a randomized clinical trial evaluating child and family modalities. *Journal of Consulting and Clinical Psychology*, **76**, 282–297.

Kessler, R. C., & Frank, R. G. (1997). The impact of psychiatric disorders on work loss days. *Psychological Medicine*, **27**, 861–873.

Kessler, R. C., & Greenberg, P. E. (2002). The economic burden of anxiety and stress disorders. In K. Davis, ed., *Neuropsychopharmacology: the Fifth Generation of Progress*. Baltimore, MD: American College of Neuropsychopharmacology and Lippincott Williams & Wilkins.

Kessler, R. C., & Ustun, T. B. (2008). *The WHO World Mental Health Surveys: Global Perspectives on the Epidemiology of Mental Disorders*. New York, NY: Cambridge University Press.

Kessler, R. C., McGonagle, K. A., Zhao, S., *et al.* (1994). Lifetime and 12-month prevalence of DSM-III-R psychiatric disorders in the United States: results from the National Comorbidity Survey. *Archives of General Psychiatry*, **51**, 8–19.

Kessler, R. C., Foster, C. L., Saunders, W. B., & Stang, P. E. (1995a). Social consequences of psychiatric disorders, I: Educational attainment. *American Journal of Psychiatry*, **152**, 1026–1032.

Kessler, R., Sonnega, A., Bromet, E., Hughes, M., & Nelson, C. (1995b). Posttraumatic stress disorder in the National Comorbidity Survey. *Archives of General Psychiatry*, **52**, 1048–1060.

Kessler, R. C., Walters, E. E., & Forthofer, M. S. (1998). The social consequences of psychiatric disorders, III: Probability of marital stability. *American Journal of Psychiatry*, **155**, 1092–1096.

Kessler, R. C., Borges, G., & Walters, E. E. (1999). Prevalence and risk factors of lifetime suicide attempts in the National Comorbidity Survey. *Archives of General Psychiatry*, **56**, 617–626.

Kessler, R., Walters, E., & Wittchen, H. U. (2004). Epidemiology. In R. Heimberg, C. Turk, & D. Mennin (Eds.), *Generalized anxiety disorder: Advances in Research and Practice*. New York, NY: Guilford Press, pp. 29–50.

Kessler, R. C., Berglund, P., Demler, O., *et al.* (2005a). Lifetime prevalence and age-of-onset distributions of DSM-IV disorders in the National Comorbidity Survey Replication. *Archives of General Psychiatry*, **62**, 593–602.

Kessler, R. C., Chiu, W. T., Demler, O., Merikangas, K. R., & Walters, E. E. (2005b). Prevalence, severity, and comorbidity of 12-month DSM-IV disorders in the National Comorbidity Survey Replication. *Archives of General Psychiatry*, **62**, 617–627.

Kessler, R. C., Demler, O., Frank, R. G., *et al.* (2005c). Prevalence and treatment of mental disorders, 1990 to 2003. *New England Journal of Medicine*, **352**, 2515–2523.

Kessler, R. C., Chiu, W. T., Jin, R., *et al.* (2006). The epidemiology of panic attacks, panic disorder, and agoraphobia in the National Comorbidity Survey Replication. *Archives of General Psychiatry*, **63**, 415–424.

Koran, L. M. (2000). Quality of life in obsessive–compulsive disorder. *Psychiatric Clinics of North America*, **23**, 509–517.

Koran, L. M., Thienemann, M. L., & Davenport, R. (1996). Quality of life for patients with obsessive–compulsive disorder. *American Journal of Psychiatry*, **153**, 783–788.

Kroenke, K., Spitzer, R. L., Williams, J. B. W., Monahan, P. O., & Lowe, B. (2007). Anxiety disorders in primary care: prevalence, impairment, comorbidity, and detection. *Annals of Internal Medicine*, **146**, 317–325.

Kuehn, B. M. (2008). Scientists examine primary care based screening and treatments for anxiety. *JAMA*, **16**, 1886–1887.

Kulka, R. A., Fairbank, W. E., Hough, R. I., *et al.* (1990). *Trauma and the Vietnam War Generation: Report of findings from the National Vietnam Veterans Readjustment Study*. New York, NY: Brunner/Mazel.

Lampe, L., Slade, T., Issakidis, C., & Andrews, G. (2003). Social phobia in the Australian National Survey of Mental Health and Well-Being. *Psychological Medicine*, **33**, 637–646.

Lensi, P., Cassano, G. B., Correddu, G., Ravagli, J. L., & Akiskal, H. S. (1996). Obsessive–compulsive disorder: familial-developmental history, symptomatology, comorbidty and course with special reference to gender-related differences. *British Journal of Psychiatry*, **169**, 101–107.

Lieb, R., Becker, E., & Altamura, C. (2005). The epidemiology of generalized anxiety disorder in Europe. *European Neuropsychopharmacology*, **15**, 445–452.

McFarlane, A. (2004). The contribution of epidemiology to the study of traumatic stress. *Social Psychiatry and Psychiatric Epidemiology*, **39**, 874–882.

Medina-Mora, M. E., Borges, G., Lara, C., *et al.* (2005). Prevalence, service use, and demographic correlates of 12-month DSM-IV psychiatric disorders in Mexico: results from the Mexican National Comorbidity Survey. *Psychological Medicine*, **35**, 1773–1783.

Mendlowicz, M. V., & Stein, M. B. (2000). Quality of life in individuals with anxiety disorders. *American Journal of Psychiatry*, **157**, 669–682.

Merikangas, K. R., Avenevoli, S., Acharyya, S., Zhang, H., & Angst, J. (2002). The spectrum of social phobia in the Zurich Cohort Study of Young Adults. *Biological Psychiatry*, **51**, 81–91.

Merikangas, K. R., Ames, M., Cui, L., *et al.* (2007). The impact of comorbidity of mental and physical conditions on role disability in the U.S. adult population. *Archives of General Psychiatry*, **64**, 1180–1188.

Milliken, C. S., Auchterlonie, J. L., & Hoge, C. W. (2008). Longitudinal assessment of mental health problems among active and reserve component soldiers returning from the Iraq War. *JAMA*, **298**, 2141–2148.

Neria, Y., & Koenen, K. C. (2003). Do combat stress reaction and posttraumatic stress disorder relate to physical health and adverse health practices? An 18-year follow-up of Israeli war veterans. *Anxiety, Stress, & Coping*, **16**, 227–239.

Neria, Y., Gross, R., Olfson, M., *et al.* (2006). Posttraumatic stress disorder in primary care one year after the 9/11 attacks. *General Hospital Psychiatry*, **28**, 213–222.

Neria, Y., Gross, R., Litz, B., *et al.* (2007). Prevalence and psychological correlates of complicated grief among bereaved adults 2.5–3.5 years after September 11th attacks. *Journal of Traumatic Stress*, **20**, 251–262.

Neria, Y., Olfson, M., Gameroff, M. J., *et al.* (2008). The mental health consequences of disaster-related loss: Findings from primary care one year after the 9/11 terrorist attacks. *Psychiatry: Interpersonal and Biological Processes*, **71**, 339–348.

Olfson, M., & Gameroff, M. J. (2007). Generalized anxiety disorder, somatic pain and health care costs. *General Hospital Psychiatry*, **29**, 310–316.

Olfson, M., Fireman, B., Weissman, M. M., *et al.* (1997). Mental disorders and disability among patients in a primary care group practice. *American Journal of Psychiatry*, **154**, 1734–1740.

Perkonigg, A., Pfister, H., Stein, M. B., *et al.* (2005). Longitudinal course of posttraumatic stress disorder and posttraumatic stress disorder symptoms in a community sample of adolescents and young adults. *American Journal of Psychiatry*, **162**, 1320–1327.

Pilowsky, D. J., Olfson, M., Gameroff, M. J., *et al.* (2006). Panic disorder and suicidal ideation in primary care. *Depression and Anxiety*, **23**, 11–16.

Pirkola, S. P., Isometsa, E., Suvisaari, J., *et al.* (2005). DSM-IV mood-, anxiety- and alcohol use disorders and their comorbidity in the Finnish general population: results from the Health 2000 Study. *Social Psychiatry and Psychiatric Epidemiology*, **40**, 1–10.

Puliafico, A. C., Comer, J. S., & Kendall, P. C. (2007). Social phobia in youth: The diagnostic utility of feared social situations. *Psychological Assessment*, **19**, 152–158.

Rice, D. P., & Miller, L. S. (1998). Health economics and cost implications of anxiety and other mental disorders in the United States. *British Journal of Psychiatry Supplement*, (34), 4–9.

Riddle, M. (1998). Obsessive–compulsive disorder in children and adolescents. *British Journal of Psychiatry*, **173**, 91–96.

Robin, J. A., Puliafico, A. C., Creed, T. A., *et al.* (2005). Generalized anxiety disorder. In R.T. Ammerman, ed., *Comprehensive Handbook of Personality and Psychopathology, Volume 3: Child Psychopathology.* Hoboken, NJ : Wiley.

Robins, L. N., & Regier, D. A. (1991). *Psychiatric Disorders in America: the Epidemiologic Catchment Area Study.* New York, NY: Free Press.

Rodriguez, B. F., Weisberg, R. B., Pagano, M. E., *et al.* (2004). Frequency and patterns of psychiatric comorbidity in a sample of primary care patients with anxiety disorders. *Comprehensive Psychiatry*, **45**, 129–137.

Roy-Byrne, P. P., & Cowley, D. S. (2007). Pharmacological treatments for panic disorder, generalized anxiety disorder, specific phobia, and social anxiety disorder. In P. E. Nathan & J. M. Gorman, eds., *A Guide to Treatments that Work*, 3rd edn. New York, NY: Oxford University Press.

Ruscio, A. M., Lane, M., Roy-Byrne, P., *et al.* (2005). Should excessive worry be required for a diagnosis of generalized anxiety disorder? Results from the U.S. National Comorbidity Survey Replication. *Psychological Medicine*, **35**, 1761–1772.

Ruscio, A. M., Brown, T. A., Chiu, W. T., *et al.* (2008). Social fears and social phobia in the USA: results from the National Comorbidity Survey Replication. *Psychological Medicine*, **38**, 15–28.

Rutter, M. (1994). Comorbidity: meaning and mechanisms. *Clinical Psychology: Science and Practice*, **1**, 100–103.

Rutter, M. (1997). Comorbidity: concepts, claims and choices. *Criminal Behaviour and Mental Health*, **7**, 265–285.

Schlenger, W. E., Caddell, J. M., Ebert, L., *et al.* (2002). Psychological reactions to terrorist attacks: findings from the National Study of Americans' Reactions to September 11. *JAMA*, **288**, 581–588.

Schneier, F. R., Johnson, J., Hornig, C. D., Liebowitz, M. R., & Weissman, M. W. (1992). Social phobia: Comorbidity and morbidity in an epidemiologic sample. *Archives of General Psychiatry*, **49**, 282–288.

Schneier, F. R., Heckelman, L., Garfinkel, R., *et al.* (1994). Functional impairment in social phobia. *Journal of Clinical Psychiatry*, **55**, 322–331.

Seal, K. H., Bertenthal, D., Miner, C. R., Sen, S., & Marmar, C. (2007). Bringing the war back home: mental health disorders among 103,788 U.S. veterans returning from Iraq and Afghanistan seen at Department of Veterans Affairs facilities. *Archives of Internal Medicine*, **167**, 476–482.

Shear, K., Jin, R., Ruscio, A. M., Walters, E. E., & Kessler, R. C. (2006). Prevalence and correlates of estimated DSM-IV child and adult separation anxiety disorder in the National Comorbidity Survey Replication. *American Journal of Psychiatry*, **163**, 1074–1083.

Shulman, I. D., Cox, B. J., Aqinaon, R. P., Kuch, K., & Reichman, J. T. (1994). Precipitating events, locations and reactions associated with initial unexpected panic attacks. *Behaviour Research and Therapy*, **32**, 17–20.

Smith, S. M., Stinson, F. S., Dawson, D. A., *et al.* (2006). Race/ethnic differences in the prevalence and co-occurrence of substance use disorders and independent mood and anxiety disorders: results from the National Epidemiologic Survey on Alcohol and Related Conditions. *Psychological Medicine*, **36**, 987–998.

Solomon, Z. (1989). Characteristic psychiatric symptomatology in PTSD veterans: a three year follow-up. *Psychological Medicine*, **19**, 927–936.

Stein, D. J., Seedat, S., Herman, A., *et al.* (2008). Lifetime prevalence of psychiatric disorders in South Africa. *British Journal of Psychiatry*, **192**, 112–117.

Stein, M., & Heimberg, R G. (2004). Well-being and life satisfaction in generalized anxiety disorder: Comparison to major depressive disorder in a community sample. *Journal of Affective Disorders*, **79**, 161–166.

Stein, M., & Kean, Y. (2000). Disability and quality of life in social phobia: epidemiologic findings. *American Journal of Psychiatry*, **157**, 1606–1613.

Stein, M., Walker, J., Hazen, A., & Forde, D. (1997). Full and partial posttraumatic stress disorder: findings from a community survey. *American Journal of Psychiatry*, **154**, 1114–1119.

Stein, M. B., Torgrud, L. J., & Walker, J. R. (2000). Social phobia symptoms, subtypes, and severity: findings from a community survey. *Archives of General Psychiatry*, **57**, 1046–1052.

Stinson, F. S., Dawson, D. A., Chou, S. P., *et al.* (2007). The epidemiology of DSM-IV specific phobia in the USA: results from the National Epidemiologic Survey on Alcohol and Related Disorders. *Psychological Medicine*, **37**, 1047–1059.

Strine, T. W., Mokdad, A. H., Dube, S. R., *et al.* (2008). The association of depression and anxiety with obesity and unhealthy behaviors among community-dwelling U.S. adults. *General Hospital Psychiatry*, **30**, 127–137.

Torres, A. R., Prince, M. J., Bebbington, P. E., *et al.* (2006). Obsessive–compulsive disorder: prevalence, comorbidity, impact, and help-seeking in the British National Psychiatric Morbidity Survey of 2000. *American Journal of Psychiatry*, **163**, 1978–1985.

Vega, W. A., Kolody, B., Aguilar-Gaxiola, S., *et al.* (1998). Lifetime prevalence of DSM-III-R psychiatric disorders among urban and rural Mexican Americans in California. *Archives of General Psychiatry*, **55**, 771–778.

Wang, P. S., Berglund, P., Olfson, M., *et al.* (2005). Failure and delay in initial treatment contact after first onset of mental disorders in the National Comorbidity Survey Replication. *Archives of General Psychiatry*, **62**, 603–613.

Wang, P. S., Aguilar-Gaxiola, S., Alonso, J., *et al.* (2007). Use of mental health services for anxiety, mood, and substance disorders in 17 countries in the WHO world mental health surveys. *Lancet*, **370**, 841–850.

Weissman, M. M., Bland, R. C., Canino, G. J., *et al.* (1994). The cross national epidemiology of obsessive compulsive disorder: The Cross National Collaborative Group. *Journal of Clinical Psychiatry*, **55** (Suppl. 3), 5–10.

Wittchen, H. U. (1988). Natural course and spontaneous remissions of untreated anxiety disorder: results of the Munich Follow-up Study (MFS). In I. Hand & H. U. Wittchen, eds., *Panic and Phobias*. Berlin: Springer.

Wittchen, H. U. (2002). Generalized anxiety disorder: prevalence, burden, and cost to society. *Depression and Anxiety*, **16**, 162–171.

Wittchen, H. U., Zhao, Z., Kessler, R. C, & Eaton, W. W. (1994). DSM-III-R generalized anxiety disorder in the National Comorbidity Survey. *Archives of General Psychiatry*, **51**, 355–364.

Wittchen, H. U., Neslon, C. B., & Lachner, G. (1998). Prevalence of mental disorders and psychosocial impairments in adolescents and young adults. *Psychological Medicine*, **28**, 109–126.

Wittchen, H., Fuetsch, M., Sonntag, Muller, N., & Liebowitz, M. R. (1999). Disability and quality of life in pure and comorbid social phobia: findings from a controlled study. *European Psychiatry*, **14**, 118–131.

Zlotnick, C., Johnson, J., Kohn, R., *et al.* (2006). Epidemiology of trauma, post-traumatic stress disorder (PTSD) and co-morbid disorders in Chile. *Psychological Medicine*, **36**, 1523–1533.

Development of the nosology of anxiety disorders

Michael B. First, Desiree K. Caban, Roberto Lewis-Fernández

3.1 Introduction

Changes in the nosology of anxiety disorders over the past 50 years reflect the evolution of the various editions of the *Diagnostic and Statistical Manual of Mental Disorders* (DSM). The initial two editions of the DSM were thin volumes used by clinicians primarily for coding purposes and were largely ignored by the research community. Given that focus, the nosology mirrored the way clinicians conceptualized anxiety disorders, i.e., as symptomatic manifestations of neurotic conflicts. Thus the provision of descriptive, operationalized definitions of the anxiety disorders in the third DSM edition (DSM-III) in 1980 allowed for reliable diagnostic assessments, which paved the way for a rapid expansion in scientific studies into the pathophysiology and treatment of anxiety disorders. Successive editions of the DSM were modified based on empirical data derived from these research studies, resulting in adjustments to the definitions of anxiety disorders aimed at increasing both diagnostic validity and clinical utility in terms of improving patient care.

Despite these successes, the nosology is still hampered by significant problems, such as excessive diagnostic comorbidity, the arbitrariness of the diagnostic thresholds leading to excessive rates of not otherwise specified (NOS) diagnoses, and the lack of treatment specificity (Kupfer *et al.* 2002). With the preparation of the fifth DSM edition (DSM-5) under way, one of the main challenges facing its developers is whether there are sufficient empirical data available to justify grounding the diagnostic definitions in pathophysiological terms, or whether it continues to make more sense to have the definitions remain descriptive. This chapter follows the evolution of the nosology of the anxiety disorders through the various editions of the APA's *Diagnostic and Statistical Manuals*, and culminates with a summary of some of the possible changes that

might occur in the classification of anxiety disorders in DSM-5. Before summarizing the key features and evolution of the anxiety disorders classification in the DSMs, we begin with a historical précis of theoretical conceptualizations of anxiety that have informed the development of the DSM.

3.2 Historical conceptualiztions

While symptomatic anxiety has been noted in the medical literature as far back as the eighteenth century, anxiety symptoms were then understood as non-psychiatric clinical conditions or included as part of other medical illnesses (Berrios 1996). The nineteenth century ushered in Sigmund Freud's psychoanalytic theories of the mind, which had an enormous influence on psychiatric concepts of illness and diagnosis in the mid twentieth century. Freud viewed anxiety as resulting from sexual libido unable to find discharge either because of inadequate sexual activity or by inhibitions due to repression (Haggard *et al.* 2008). He proposed distinguishing what he later conceptualized as anxiety neurosis from neurasthenia, a condition first described by George Beard in 1868. Neurasthenia at the time was a common diagnosis that broadly included anxiety symptoms among other symptoms (e.g., easy fatigability), many of which are now characteristics of chronic fatigue syndrome. The *International Classification of Diseases* (ICD) contrarily includes a category of neurasthenia (F48) among the neurotic, stress-related, and somatoform disorders, which also includes the anxiety disorders.

Freud subsequently modified his theory, suggesting that "anxiety was more closely related to fear, occurring in response to perceived dangers, either external or internal. This led [Freud] to focus on the ego, one of whose functions is to anticipate and negotiate danger situations" (Haggard *et al.* 2008, p. 471). The introduction to the first edition of the DSM's psychoneurotic

Anxiety Disorders: Theory, Research, and Clinical Perspectives, ed. Helen Blair Simpson, Yuval Neria, Roberto Lewis-Fernández, Franklin Schneier. Published by Cambridge University Press. © Cambridge University Press 2010.

disorders section reveals the underlying influences of Freud's ego psychology model, which "focused more on bringing to the patient's awareness both repressed and disavowed mental content and the role of the unconscious defense mechanisms of the ego as it mediated conflict" (Kay & Kay 2008, p. 1858).

3.3 DSM-I

Aiming to overcome a polyglot of diagnostic labels and systems, the American Psychiatric Association's Committee on Nomenclature and Statistics published the first edition of the *Diagnostic and Statistical Manual of Mental Disorders* (DSM-I) (American Psychiatric Association 1952). DSM-I was originally developed as the mental disorders section of the American Medical Association's fourth edition of the *Standard Nomenclature of Diseases and Operations* (American Medical Association 1952). The manual is broadly organized into three main overarching categories of psychopathology: disorders caused by or associated with impairment of brain functioning (organic brain syndromes), mental deficiency, and disorders of psychogenic origin or without clearly defined physical cause or structural changes in the brain (functional disorders). The latter section was divided into five subsections: psychotic disorders, psychophysiologic autonomic and visceral disorders, psychoneurotic disorders, personality disorders, and transient situational personality disorders. Definitions of disorders in DSM-I were considerably influenced by etiological theories of the time, most significantly psychoanalytic theories of causality. This is in direct contrast to the descriptive, largely atheoretical approach adopted since DSM-III, to be elaborated further below. Consequently, in DSM-I the entire psychoneurotic disorders grouping was defined with "anxiety" presumed as the underlying etiology. The introductory text of the psychoneurotic disorders section noted:

> The chief characteristic of these disorders is "anxiety" which may be directly felt and expressed or which may be unconsciously and automatically controlled by the utilization of various psychological defense mechanisms (depression, conversion, displacement, etc.) (American Psychiatric Association 1952).

The text goes on to explain that

> "anxiety" in psychoneurotic disorders is a danger signal felt and perceived by the conscious portion of the personality. It is produced by a threat from within the personality (e.g., by supercharged repressed emotions, including such aggressive impulses as hostility and resentment), with or without stimulation from such external situations as loss of love, loss of prestige or threat of injury (American Psychiatric Association 1952).

The seven psychoneurotic disorders in DSM-I were then subclassified into what were called "reactions," representing the "various ways in which the patient attempts to handle this anxiety" (American Psychiatric Association 1952) (Table 3.1). From the descriptive perspective established in DSM-III, it is important to note that only "anxiety reaction," "phobic reaction," and "obsessive–compulsive reaction" correspond to what are now classified as anxiety disorders. The use of the term "reaction" reflected the influence of Adolf Meyer's psychobiological view that mental disorders represented reactions of the personality to psychological, social, and biological factors.

Present-day anxiety disorders were also covered in some of the other DSM-I groupings. Transient situational personality disorders is a classification group for transient anxiety symptoms that develop in response to a stressor. Within this section is a category called "gross stress reaction," which represented a precursor to the current categories posttraumatic stress disorder (PTSD) and acute stress disorder (ASD) for reactions to extreme stressors. Gross stress reaction is defined as follows:

> Under conditions of great or unusual stress, a normal personality may utilize established patterns of reaction to deal with overwhelming fear … This diagnosis is justified only in situations in which the individual has been exposed to severe physical demands or extreme emotional stress, civilian catastrophe (fire, earthquake, explosion, etc.) (American Psychiatric Association 1952).

Notably, the definition did not include descriptions of the types of symptoms that may occur in reaction to the stressor.

Other categories incorporated in this section that include anxiety among their examples (e.g., adult situational reaction and adjustment reaction of childhood, adjustment reaction of adolescence, and adjustment reaction of late life) now correspond to the current category of adjustment disorder with anxiety. For instance, the definition of adult situational reaction explained:

> This diagnosis is to be used when the clinical picture is primarily one of superficial maladjustment to a difficult situation or to newly experienced environmental factors with no evidence of any serious underlying personality defects or chronic patterns. It may be manifested by anxiety, alcoholism, asthenia, poor efficiency, low morale, unconventional behavior, etc. (American Psychiatric Association 1952).

Table 3.1. Summary of psychoneurotic disorders included in DSM-I

000-x01	Anxiety reaction	In this kind of reaction, anxiety is diffuse and not restricted to definite situations or objects. It is characterized by anxious expectation and is frequently associated with somatic symptomatology.
000-x02	Dissociative reaction	This reaction represents a type of gross personality disorganization, the basis of which is neurotic disturbance, although diffuse dissociation may at times appear psychotic …The repressed impulse giving rise to the anxiety may be discharged by, or deflected into, various symptomatic expressions, such as depersonalization, dissociated personality, stupor, fugue, amnesia, dream state, somnambulism, etc.
000-x03	Conversion reaction	Instead of being experienced consciously (either diffusely or displaced, as in phobias), the impulse causing the anxiety is "converted" into functional symptoms in organs or parts of the body, usually those that are mainly under voluntary control.
000-x04	Phobic reaction	The anxiety of these patients becomes detached from a specific idea, object, or situation in the daily life and displaced to some symbolic idea or situation in the form of a specific neurotic fear. Commonly observed forms include fear of syphilis, dirt, closed places, high places, open places, animals, etc. The patient attempts to control anxiety by avoiding the phobic object or situation.
000-x05	Obsessive–compulsive reaction	In this reaction, the anxiety is associated with persistence of unwanted ideas and repetitive impulses to perform acts that may be considered morbid by the patient. The patient himself may regard these ideas and behaviors as unreasonable, but is nevertheless compelled to carry out the rituals.
000-x06	Depressive reaction	The anxiety in this reaction is allayed, and hence partially relieved, by depression and self-deprecation. The reaction is precipitated by a current situation, frequently by some loss sustained by the patient, and is often associated with feelings of guilt for past failures or deeds.
000-x0y	Psychoneurotic reaction, other	All reactions considered psychoneurotic and not elsewhere classified.

Psychophysiologic autonomic and visceral disorders, the so-called "organ neuroses," was yet another relevant DSM-I grouping. These categories were for "reactions that represent the visceral expression of affect, which may be thereby largely prevented from being conscious," and the DSM-I text later explained that "the symptoms are due to a chronic and exaggerated state of the normal physiological expression of emotion with the feeling, or subjective part, repressed. Such long continued visceral states may eventually lead to structured changes" (American Psychiatric Association 1952). Similar to the psychoneurotic reactions described earlier, unconscious anxiety experienced by the individual somatically was the presumed etiology. In DSM-I, these conditions were distinguished from anxiety reactions "primarily by predominant, persistent involvement of a single organ system." Disorders included in this section were as follows: psychophysiologic skin reaction (e.g., pruritis "in which emotional factors play a causative role"); psychophysiologic musculoskeletal reaction (e.g., backache); psychophysiologic respiratory reaction (e.g., bronchial spasm); psychophysiologic cardiovascular reaction (e.g., paroxysmal tachycardia); psychophysiologic hemic and lymphatic reaction; psychophysiologic gastrointenstinal reaction (e.g., irritable bowel); psychophysiologic genitourinary reaction (e.g.,

dysuria); psychophysiologic endocrine reaction; psychophysiologic nervous system reaction (e.g., neurasthenia); psychophysiologic reaction of organs of special sense (American Psychiatric Association 1952).

Given our understanding that anxiety is often manifested in somatic terms (e.g., palpitations, sweating, tremor), some cases of what are now classified as anxiety disorders (e.g., panic disorder and generalized anxiety disorder, which include such symptoms in their definition) might have been considered a psychophysiologic autonomic and visceral disorder in DSM-I.

3.4 DSM-II

The second edition of the DSM (DSM-II) was published in 1968 (American Psychiatric Association 1968). DSM-II included ten overarching groupings: mental retardation; organic brain syndromes; psychoses; neuroses; personality disorders and other non-psychotic mental disorders; psychophysiologic disorders; special symptoms (e.g., speech, learning, tic, sleep disorders); transient situational disturbances; behavior disorders of childhood and adolescence; conditions without manifest psychiatric disorder (e.g., marital maladjustment).

The neuroses grouping, a modification of the DSM-I psychoneuroses, was expanded from seven to ten categories (Table 3.2). With few exceptions, the DSM-II definitions of equivalent categories were very similar to those in DSM-I, both versions being informed by Freud's understanding of the causative role of anxiety in the development of a neurosis. In its definition of the neuroses grouping, the DSM-II text noted that

> anxiety is the chief characteristic of the neuroses. It may be felt and experienced directly, or it may be controlled unconsciously and automatically by conversion, displacement, and various other psychological mechanisms. Generally, these mechanisms produce symptoms experienced as subjective distress from which the patient desires relief (American Psychiatric Association 1968).

Regarding specific changes in DSM-II, the DSM-I categories of dissociative reaction and conversion reaction were combined to form hysterical neurosis, a new category, with two subtypes. Three additional types of neuroses were also added: neurasthenic neurosis (in which unconscious anxiety manifests as complaints of chronic weakness, easy fatigability, and sometimes exhaustion), depersonalization neurosis (in which anxiety manifests as feeling of unreality and estrangement from the self, body, or surroundings), and hypochondriacal neurosis (in which anxiety manifests as preoccupation with the body and fear of presumed diseases).

With respect to changes in those neuroses that also appeared in DSM-I, the definition of anxiety neurosis in DSM-II more closely resembles the present-day classification of panic disorder, i.e., "the neurosis is characterized by anxious over-concern extending to panic and frequently [is] associated with somatic symptoms" (American Psychiatric Association 1968), as opposed to the more generalized anxiety-disorder-like description in DSM-I. Similarly, the description of phobic neurosis was more phenomenologically based ("characterized by intense fear of an object or situation which the patient consciously recognizes as no real danger to him") (American Psychiatric Association 1968).

Within the transient situational disturbances grouping, the category gross stress reaction was altogether eliminated. Instead, such severe reactions to extreme stress were featured in the category for adjustment reaction of adult life that included as an example "fear associated with military combat and manifested by trembling, running, and hiding" (American Psychiatric Association 1968).

Given increased attention to disorders specifically related to children and adolescents, a new grouping, behavior disorders of childhood and adolescence, was added in DSM-II, and this included some childhood anxiety disorders. In particular, two categories were added: withdrawing reaction of childhood or adolescence, and overanxious reaction of childhood or adolescence. Withdrawing reaction is for children who are detached, sensitive, shy, timid, and generally unable to form close interpersonal relationships. (This category corresponds to the current category social anxiety disorder, as well as some cases of autism.) Overanxious reaction is for children with chronic anxiety, excessive and unrealistic fears, sleeplessness, nightmares, and exaggerated autonomic responses, and would likely correspond to the DSM-III category and the current category of separation anxiety disorder.

Changes to the major grouping, psychophysiologic disorders, were mostly limited to the removal of psychophysiologic nervous system reaction, which is equivalent to the neurasthenic neurosis category included under the major grouping of neuroses in Table 3.2.

3.5 DSM-III

With final publication in 1980, DSM-III proved to be groundbreaking (American Psychiatric Association 1980). Arising from an emerging recognition of the importance of common diagnostic terms for both clinical practice and research, two new innovations relevant to the classification of anxiety disorders were introduced in DSM-III: the reliance on a descriptive approach to classification and the provision of explicit diagnostic criteria for each of the disorders.

The descriptive approach adopted in DSM-III defines disorders in terms of their shared descriptive features rather than relying on unproven hypotheses about underlying etiology, except for those disorders in which etiology or pathophysiological processes are included as part of the defining criteria (e.g., posttraumatic stress disorder, organic mental disorders, or adjustment disorder). An important goal of the descriptive approach was to allow clinicians with very different theoretical orientations to communicate with one another about psychiatric diagnosis. For example, a cognitive–behavioral therapist might believe that panic attacks arise from cognitive distortions about the significance of normal physical sensations. These distortions ("these sensations mean I'm having a heart attack") set off a vicious cycle, leading to increasingly intense physical sensations that subsequently lead to more anxiety, culminating in a

Table 3.2. Summary of neuroses included in DSM-II

300.0	Anxiety neurosis	This neurosis is characterized by anxious over-concern extending to panic and frequently associated with somatic symptoms. Unlike phobic neurosis, anxiety may occur under any circumstances and is not restricted to specific situations or objects. This disorder must be distinguished from normal apprehension or fear, which occurs in realistically dangerous situations.
300.1	Hysterical neurosis	This neurosis is characterized by an involuntary psychogenic loss or disorder of function.
300.13	Conversion type	In the conversion type, the special senses or voluntary nervous system are affected, causing such symptoms as blindness, deafness, anosmia, anesthesias, paresthesias, paralyses, ataxias, akinesias, and dyskinesias.
300.14	Dissociative type	In the dissociative type, alterations may occur in the patient's state of consciousness or in his identity to produce such symptoms as amnesia, somnambulism, fugue, and multiple personality.
300.2	Phobic neurosis	This condition is characterized by intense fear of an object or situation that the patient consciously recognizes as no real danger to him. His apprehension may be experienced as faintness, fatigue, palpitations, perspiration, nausea, tremor, and even panic. Phobias are generally attributed to fears displaced to the phobic object or situation from some other object of which the patient is unaware. A wide range of phobias has been described.
300.3	Obsessive–compulsive neurosis	This disorder is characterized by the persistent intrusion of unwanted thoughts, urges, or actions that the patient is unable to stop. The thoughts may consist of single words or ideas, ruminations, or trains of thought often perceived by the patient as nonsensical. The actions vary from simple movements to complex rituals such as repeated handwashing. Anxiety and distress are often present either if the patient is prevented from completing his compulsive ritual or if he is concerned about being unable to control it himself.
300.4	Depressive neurosis	This disorder is manifested by an excessive reaction of depression due to an internal conflict or to an identifiable event such as the loss of a love object or cherished possession.
300.5	Neurasthenic neurosis (neurasthenia)	This condition is characterized by complaints of chronic weakness, easy fatigability, and sometimes exhaustion. Unlike hysterical neurosis, the patient's complaints are genuinely distressing to him, and there is no evidence of secondary gain.
300.6	Depersonalization neurosis (depersonalization syndrome)	This syndrome is dominated by a feeling of unreality and of estrangement from the self, body, or surroundings.
300.7	Hypochondriacal neurosis	This condition is dominated by preoccupation with the body and with fear of presumed diseases of various organs.

panic attack. Alternatively, a biologically oriented clinician might believe that a panic attack primarily represents overactivity of the locus ceruleus. Despite these divergent understandings of etiology, the two clinicians can agree on what a panic attack looks like and thus both utilize the DSM-III definition of panic disorder. Consequently, diagnostic groupings in DSM-III were based on presenting symptomatology (i.e., psychotic disorders, mood disorders, etc.) rather than etiology.

Due to the importance of anxiety as a presenting symptom, a new grouping specifically for anxiety disorders was formed, and this included several disorders that had been listed in the DSM-II neuroses grouping. A number of disorders that had been considered to be "anxiety disorders" in prior DSM editions because of their presumed underlying etiology were now placed in other diagnostic groupings based on their presenting

symptomatology. Hysterical neurosis, conversion type, and hypochrondrical neurosis were both placed within the newly formed somatoform disorders grouping, created for presentations characterized by physical symptoms suggesting physical disorders for which there are no demonstrable organic findings. Hysterical neurosis, dissociative type, and depersonalization neurosis were placed within the newly created dissociative disorders grouping. Depressive neurosis was included in the affective disorders grouping, while neurasthenic neurosis was eliminated due to limited use by clinicians practicing in the United States.

The remaining DSM-II neuroses – anxiety neurosis, phobic neurosis, and obsessive–compulsive neurosis – were placed within the newly formed anxiety disorders grouping. In each of these, anxiety is either the predominant presenting symptom or, in the case of

Table 3.3. Diagnostic criteria for panic disorder in DSM-III

A	At least three panic attacks within a three-week period in circumstances other than during marked physical exertion or in a life-threatening situation. The attacks are not precipitated only by exposure to a circumscribed phobic stimulus.
B	Panic attacks are manifested by discrete periods of apprehension or fear, and at least four of the following symptoms appear during each attack:
	(1) dyspnea
	(2) palpitations
	(3) chest pain or discomfort
	(4) choking or smothering sensations
	(5) dizziness, vertigo, or unsteady feelings
	(6) feelings of unreality
	(7) paresthesias (tingling in hands or feet)
	(8) hot or cold flashes
	(9) sweating
	(10) faintness
	(11) trembling or shaking
	(12) fear of dying, going crazy, or doing something uncontrolled during an attack
C	Not due to a physical disorder or another mental disorder, such as major depression, somatization disorder, or schizophrenia.
D	The disorder is not associated with agoraphobia.

Table 3.4. Diagnostic criteria for generalized anxiety disorder in DSM-III

A	Generalized persistent anxiety is manifested by symptoms from three of the following four categories:
	(1) *Motor tension*: shakiness, jitteriness, jumpiness, trembling, tension, muscle aches, fatigability, inability to relax, eyelid twitch, furrowed brow, strained face, fidgeting, restlessness, easy startle
	(2) *Autonomic hyperactivity*: sweating, heart pounding or racing, cold, clammy hands, dry mouth, dizziness, light-headedness, paresthesias (tingling in hands or feet), upset stomach, hot or cold spells, frequent urination, diarrhea, discomfort in the pit of the stomach, lump in the throat, flushing, pallor, high resting pulse and respiration rate
	(3) *Apprehensive expectation*: anxiety, worry, fear, rumination, and anticipation of misfortune to self or others
	(4) *Vigilance and scanning*: hyperattentiveness resulting in distractibility, difficulty in concentrating, insomnia, feeling "on edge," irritability, impatience
B	The anxious mood has been continuous for at least one month.
C	Not due to another mental disorder, such as a depressive disorder or schizophrenia.
D	At least 18 years of age.

obsessive–compulsive neurosis, it is experienced if the individual attempts to resist the need to act out the compulsions. Anxiety neurosis was split into two categories, panic disorder and generalized anxiety disorder.

Based on research showing that imipramine, a tricyclic antidepressant, blocked recurrent panic attacks (Klein 1964) but had no effect on phobic anxiety not associated with panic attacks (Zitrin *et al*. 1978), a separate panic disorder category was created for conditions characterized by recurrent panic attacks (Table 3.3). The DSM-III diagnostic criteria for panic disorder were based on the Feighner criteria for anxiety neurosis. The Feighner criteria were developed by a team of researchers at Washington University in St. Louis in 1972 with the stated purpose of "provid[ing] common ground for different research groups so that diagnostic definitions can be emended constructively

as further studies are completed" (Feighner *et al*. 1972, p. 57). Anxiety neurosis was the only anxiety disorder included among the 16 disorders for which inclusion and exclusion criteria were presented. Therefore, diagnostic criteria for the other DSM-III anxiety disorders had to be developed by expert consensus de novo as part of the DSM-III development process. The second category, generalized anxiety disorder, was newly created for cases that would have received a DSM-II diagnosis of anxiety neurosis, in which the anxiety was free-floating yet did not present with recurrent panic attacks. This category was defined as generalized, persistent anxiety of at least one-month duration that does not meet the symptoms of the other anxiety disorders (Table 3.4).

In DSM-III, phobic neurosis was subdivided into separate categories based on "differing clinical pictures,

25

Table 3.5. Diagnostic criteria for phobic disorders in DSM-III

Agoraphobia

A	The individual has marked fear of and thus avoids being alone or in public places from which escape might be difficult or help not available in case of sudden incapacitation, e.g., crowds, tunnels, bridges, public transportation.
B	There is increasing constriction of normal activities until the fears or avoidance behavior dominate the individual's life.
C	Not due to a major depressive episode, obsessive–compulsive disorder, paranoid personality disorder, or schizophrenia.

Social phobia

A	A persistent, irrational fear of, and compelling desire to avoid, a situation in which the individual is exposed to possible scrutiny by others and fears that he or she may act in a way that will be humiliating or embarrassing.
B	Significant distress because of the disturbance and recognition by the individual that his or her fear is excessive or unreasonable.
C	Not due to another mental disorder, such as major depression or avoidant personality disorder.

Simple phobia

A	A persistent, irrational fear of, and compelling desire to avoid, an object or situation other than being alone, or in public places away from home (agoraphobia), or of humiliation or embarrassment in certain social situations (social phobia). Phobic objects are often animals, and phobic situations frequently involve heights or closed spaces.
B	Significant distress from the disturbance and recognition by the individual that his or her fear is excessive or unreasonable.
C	Not due to another mental disorder, such as schizophrenia or obsessive–compulsive disorder.

ages at onset, and differential treatment responses" (American Psychiatric Association 1980, p. 371). Accordingly, "the essential feature of the phobias is persistent and irrational fear of a specific object, activity, or situation that results in a compelling desire to avoid the dreaded object, activity, or situation (the phobic stimulus)." Subdivided into three types, phobic disorders include agoraphobia, social phobia, and simple phobia (Table 3.5). Agoraphobia is the most severe and pervasive form of phobic disorder and is characterized by a marked fear of being in public places from which escape might be difficult or help not available in case of sudden incapacitation. Two subtypes of agoraphobia were provided, indicating whether or not there is an associated history of panic attacks. Social phobia is characterized by a persistent, irrational fear of social situations in which the individual fears that he or she may act in a way that will be humiliating or embarrassing. Simple phobia is characterized by a persistent, irrational fear of objects or situations other than those described by agoraphobia or social phobia, such as fear of snakes, fear of seeing blood, fear of flying, and so forth.

While separation anxiety disorder can be considered to be a form of phobia (i.e., the phobic stimulus is separation from major attachment figures) because it characteristically begins in infancy or childhood and rarely persists into adulthood, it was included in the section "disorders usually first evident in infancy, childhood or adolescence" (American Psychiatric Association 1980, p. 377). Separation anxiety disorder is characterized by excessive anxiety upon separation from major attachment figures or from home or other familiar surroundings. Other anxiety disorders in the childhood section included avoidant disorder of childhood or adolescence and overanxious disorder.

In DSM-III, obsessive–compulsive disorder (OCD) was characterized by the same features found in the description of DSM-II's obsessive neurosis, i.e., recurrent obsessions or compulsions. The DSM-III definition operationalized this concept into diagnostic criteria that can be reliably applied in research settings. Initially, the developers of DSM-III were unsure in which major diagnostic grouping to include OCD; it was eventually decided that

> even though the predominant symptoms are obsessions or compulsions rather than anxiety itself, anxiety is almost invariably experienced if the individual attempts to resist the obsessions or compulsions. In addition, most patients with the disorder also experience anxiety apart from the obsessions and compulsions (Spitzer & Williams 1985, p. 762).

A new category of posttraumatic stress disorder was added to the anxiety disorders grouping to cover responses to severe traumatic stressors. Having first been identified in veterans who had returned to the USA following the Vietnam War, PTSD was originally termed "post-Vietnam syndrome" or "delayed-stress syndrome" (Spitzer & Williams 1985, pp. 762–763). The characteristic symptoms involved re-experiencing a traumatic event generally outside the scope of usual human experience with numbing of responsiveness to,

Table 3.6. Diagnostic criteria for posttraumatic stress disorder in DSM-III

A	Existence of a recognizable stressor that would evoke significant symptoms of distress in almost everyone.
B	Re-experiencing of the trauma as evidenced by at least one of the following:
	(1) recurrent and intrusive recollections of the event
	(2) recurrent dreams of the event
	(3) sudden acting or feeling as if the traumatic event were reoccurring because of an association with an environmental or ideational stimulus
C	Numbing of responsiveness to or reduced involvement with the external world, beginning some time after the trauma, as shown by at least one of the following:
	(1) markedly diminished interest in one or more significant activities
	(2) feeling of detachment or estrangement from others
	(3) constricted affect
D	At least two of the following symptoms that were not present before the trauma:
	(1) hyperalertness or exaggerated startle response
	(2) sleep disturbance
	(3) guilt about surviving when others have not, or about behavior required for survival
	(4) memory impairment or trouble concentrating
	(5) avoidance of activities that arouse recollection of the traumatic event
	(6) intensification of symptoms by exposure to events that symbolize or resemble the traumatic event

or reduced involvement with, the external world. See Table 3.6 for PTSD diagnostic criteria.

Unlike DSM-II's unspecified neurosis, which was not a diagnosis but rather a category for medical record librarians and statisticians to code incomplete diagnoses, DSM-III's atypical anxiety disorder was a diagnostic category used for situations where an individual presents with anxiety disorder symptoms that do not meet the criteria for any of the other specified anxiety disorders.

3.6 DSM-III-R

Work began on a revision to the third edition in 1983 (DSM-III-R), which was subsequently published in 1987 (American Psychiatric Association 1987). Perhaps the most important change in the DSM-III-R classification of anxiety disorders was the elimination of the DSM-III hierarchy that had prevented the diagnosis of panic or any other anxiety disorder if these occurred concurrently with an affective disorder (Frances *et al.* 1990). This change was made in response to several studies that questioned the validity of the DSM-III hierarchical relationship giving affective disorders precedence over anxiety disorders. For example, a case–control study by Leckman and colleagues (1983) examined lifetime psychiatric diagnoses of relatives of individuals with major depression. They found that the relatives of probands with comorbid major depression and anxiety were at greater risk for both depression and anxiety

disorders than the probands of relatives with depression alone. The rates were equally high whether the anxiety symptoms were separate from the depressive episodes or always associated with the depressive episodes, a finding that was at odds with what would be predicted from the DSM-III hierarchical relationship.

DSM-III-R field trials were conducted for agoraphobia without history of panic disorder (AWOPD) and generalized anxiety disorder (GAD). The field trial indicated that agoraphobia is most typically seen as a complication of panic disorder. Consequently, DSM-III-R changed the relationship between agoraphobia and panic disorder, making panic disorder the primary disorder, which was then subtyped as to whether or not it is associated with agoraphobic avoidance. Given the rarity of agoraphobia occurring in the absence of panic in clinical samples, there was controversy concerning whether agoraphobia in the absence of panic disorder should even be included in DSM-III-R. Evidence from the Epidemiological Catchment Area Study, however, showed that agoraphobia without panic attacks may be encountered fairly often in non-psychiatric samples (Regier *et al.* 1988). AWOPD was still conceptualized as phobic avoidance occurring in response to the development of unexpected physical symptoms that may take the form of a subthreshold panic attack. Therefore, this category was provided with a specifier for *limited-symptom attacks*. See Table 3.7 for AWOPD diagnostic criteria.

Table 3.7. Diagnostic criteria for agoraphobia without history of panic disorder (AWOPD) in DSM-III-R

A	Agoraphobia: fear of being in places or situations from which escape might be difficult (or embarrassing) or in which help might not be available in the event of suddenly developing a symptom(s) that could be incapacitating or extremely embarrassing. Examples include: dizziness or falling, depersonalization or derealization, loss of bladder or bowel control, vomiting, or cardiac distress. As a result of this fear, the person either restricts travel or needs a companion when away from home, or else endures agoraphobic situations despite intense anxiety. Common agoraphobic situations include being outside the home alone, being in a crowd or standing in a line, being on a bridge, and traveling in a bus, train, or car.
B	Has never met the criteria for panic disorder.

Specify with or without limited symptom attacks

Changes were made to the GAD criteria set in order to make it more diagnostically specific. GAD was defined as excessive and/or unrealistic worry in two or more domains (e.g., finances, health of family members) unrelated to another Axis I disorder. Furthermore, the minimum duration was lengthened from one to six months in order to help clarify the boundary between GAD and non-pathological worry and adjustment disorders. See Table 3.8 for GAD criteria.

The criteria set for PTSD also underwent revision. The nature of the traumatic stressor was further clarified to include "natural disasters (e.g., floods, earthquakes), accidental disasters (e.g., car accidents with serious physical injury, airplane crashes, large fires, collapse of physical structures), or deliberately caused disasters (e.g., bombing, torture, death camps)" (American Psychiatric Association 1987). The grouping for numbing symptoms (i.e., Criterion C) was expanded to include symptoms of avoidance and amnesia, and the miscellaneous-symptoms grouping (i.e., Criterion D) was replaced with a category of physiologic arousal symptoms. A duration criterion of at least one month was added to exclude transient and non-pathological reactions to extreme stress. Finally, examples of symptoms specific to children were also incorporated, as was a *delayed onset* specifier for cases where the onset of symptoms was at least six months after exposure to the trauma. See Table 3.9 for PTSD diagnostic criteria.

Other DSM-III-R changes included the addition of a new specifier, *generalized type*, to social phobia if the phobic avoidance is generalized to include most social situations. With the exception of minor editorial clarifications or elimination of exclusion criteria in some cases, simple phobia and OCD remained essentially the same. Revisions were made to the criteria for separation anxiety disorder to raise the threshold for diagnosis by adding the terms "persistent" and "recurrent" to the diagnostic criteria. Finally, as part of a system-wide change to replace the residual "atypical" category with an NOS category, DSM-III's atypical anxiety disorder was changed to anxiety disorder not otherwise specified.

3.7 DSM-IV

Having the benefit of a decade of research on DSM-III diagnostic entities to inform the revision process, the fourth DSM edition (DSM-IV: American Psychiatric Association 1994) was developed using a three-stage process of empirical review that included comprehensive and systematic reviews of the published literature, re-analyses of secondary datasets, and issue-focused field trials (Frances *et al.* 1989). Four of the DSM-IV field trials focused on anxiety disorders.

One field trial was conducted in consideration of the possibility of adding a new category to DSM-IV, mixed anxiety–depressive disorder, which the World Health Organization (WHO) had already decided to add to the tenth edition of the *International Classification of Diseases* (ICD-10). The field trial found that patients who presented with a mixture of anxious and depressed symptoms but who did not meet DSM-III-R definitional thresholds for an Axis I anxiety or mood disorder often report associated significant impairment. Due to the limited available empirical data for this category, most particularly information about potential rates of false positives, developers decided that this category should be included in DSM-IV's Appendix B (Criteria Sets and Axes Provided for Further Study) in order to stimulate further research.

Based on findings from the OCD field trial (Foa *et al.* 1998), changes were made to the diagnostic criteria so that obsessions were defined in terms of their functionality (i.e., obsessions cause marked anxiety or distress, and compulsions prevent or reduce that anxiety or distress) rather than on whether they were thoughts or behaviors. Thus, a mental act that is aimed at reducing the anxiety from an obsession (e.g., compulsively counting up to a certain number) would be considered to be a compulsion rather than an obsession in DSM-IV. Furthermore, DSM-IV provided a specifier, *with poor insight*, in order to indicate whether the individual lacks insight into the unreasonableness of his or her obsessive thoughts or compulsive behaviors. See Table 3.10 for DSM-IV criteria for OCD.

Table 3.8. Diagnostic criteria for generalized anxiety disorder (GAD) in DSM-III-R

A	Unrealistic or excessive anxiety and worry (apprehensive expectation) about two or more life circumstances, e.g., worry about possible misfortune to one's child (who is in no danger) and worry about finances (for no good reason), for a period of six months or longer, during which the person has been bothered more days than not by these concerns. In children and adolescents, this may take the form of anxiety and worry about academic, athletic, and social performance.
B	If another Axis I disorder is present, the focus of the anxiety and worry in A is unrelated to it, e.g., the anxiety or worry is not about having a panic attack (as in panic disorder), being embarrassed in public (as in social phobia), being contaminated (as in OCD), or gaining weight (as in anorexia nervosa).
C	The disturbance does not occur only during the course of a mood disorder or a psychotic disorder.
D	At least 6 of the following 18 symptoms are often present when anxious (do not include symptoms present only during panic attacks):

Motor tension
- (1) trembling, twitching, or feeling shaky
- (2) muscle tension, aches, or soreness
- (3) restlessness
- (4) easy fatigability

Autonomic hyperactivity
- (5) shortness of breath or smothering sensations
- (6) palpitations or accelerated heart rate (tachycardia)
- (7) sweating, or cold clammy hands
- (8) dry mouth
- (9) dizziness or lightheadedness
- (10) nausea, diarrhea, or other abdominal distress
- (11) flushes (hot flashes) or chills
- (12) frequent urination
- (13) trouble swallowing or "lump in throat"

Vigilance and scanning
- (14) feeling keyed up or on edge
- (15) exaggerated startle response
- (16) difficulty concentrating or "mind going blank" because of anxiety
- (17) trouble falling or staying asleep
- (18) irritability

E	It cannot be established that an organic factor initiated and maintained the disturbance, e.g., hyperthyroidism, caffeine intoxication.

A number of changes were made to the PTSD criteria (Table 3.11), based on literature review, data re-analyses, and the results of a field trial (Roth *et al.* 1997, Kilpatrick *et al.* 1998). Three changes were made to the stressor criterion. DSM-III-R described the traumatic stressor as being "outside the range of normal human experience" and then went on to provide a list of examples of such experiences. In DSM-IV, this phrase was eliminated, since a number of studies demonstrated that exposure to traumatic stressors in the general population was not uncommon and thus not outside the range of normal human experience. The stressor criterion was replaced by a requirement that the trauma "involve experiencing, witnessing, or being confronted with an event or events that involve actual or threatened death or serious injury or a threat to the physical integrity of self or others" (American Psychiatric Association 2000). DSM-IV also added a requirement that the patient's response to the stressor involve "intense fear, helplessness, or horror" (American Psychiatric Association 2000) in order to screen out stressors not experienced by the person as traumatic. Other changes included moving physiological reactivity upon exposure to cues from Criterion D (increased arousal) to Criterion B (re-experiencing the trauma) and adding a clinical-significance criterion (i.e., the disturbance causes clinically significant distress or

Table 3.9. Diagnostic criteria for posttraumatic stress disorder in DSM-III-R

A	The person has experienced an event that is outside the range of usual human experience and that would be markedly distressing to almost anyone, e.g., serious threat to one's life or physical integrity; serious threat or harm to one's children, spouse, or other close relatives and friends; sudden destruction of one's home or community; or seeing another person who has recently been, or is being, seriously injured or killed as the result of an accident or physical violence.
B	The traumatic event is persistently re-experienced in at least one of the following ways:
	(1) recurrent and intrusive distressing recollections of the event (in young children, repetitive play in which themes or aspects of the trauma are expressed)
	(2) recurrent distressing dreams of the event
	(3) sudden acting or feeling as if the traumatic event were recurring (includes a sense of reliving the experience, illusions, hallucinations, and dissociative (flashback) episodes, even those that occur upon awakening or when intoxicated)
	(4) intense psychological distress at exposure to events that symbolize or resemble an aspect of the traumatic event, including anniversaries of the trauma
C	Persistent avoidance of stimuli associated with the trauma or numbing of general responsiveness (not present before the trauma), as indicated by at least three of the following:
	(1) efforts to avoid thoughts or feelings associated with the trauma
	(2) efforts to avoid activities or situations that arouse recollections of the trauma
	(3) inability to recall an important aspect of the trauma (psychogenic amnesia)
	(4) markedly diminished interest in significant activities (in young children, loss of recently acquired developmental skills such as toilet training or language skills)
	(5) feeling of detachment or estrangement from others
	(6) restricted range of affect, e.g., unable to have loving feelings
	(7) sense of a foreshortened future, e.g., does not expect to have a career, marriage, or children, or a long life
D	Persistent symptoms of increased arousal (not present before the trauma), as indicated by at least two of the following:
	(1) difficulty falling or staying asleep
	(2) irritability or outbursts of anger
	(3) difficulty concentrating
	(4) hypervigilance
	(5) exaggerated startle response
	(6) physiologic reactivity upon exposure to events that symbolize or resemble an aspect of the traumatic event (e.g., a woman who was raped in an elevator breaks out in a sweat when entering any elevator)
E	Duration of the disturbance (symptoms in B, C, and D) of at least one month.
	Specify delayed onset if the onset of symptoms was at least six months after the trauma.

impairment in functioning). Additional modifications describing how PTSD is manifested in children were incorporated throughout the criteria set. For example, repetitive play involving themes of the trauma was provided as an additional example under the item for recurrent and intrusive recollections of the trauma. Finally, two new specifiers were provided to denote the duration of PTSD symptoms: *acute*, for symptom duration of less than three months, and *chronic*, for symptoms lasting three months or more.

Several changes were made to the definition of panic disorder regarding the diagnostic threshold (i.e., number, frequency, and duration) for panic attacks (Fyer *et al.* 1998). The panic attack threshold was changed from four attacks within a four-week period to recurrent unexpected panic attacks accompanied by a month or more of either persistent concern about having additional attacks, worry about the implications of the attack or its consequences, or a significant change in behavior related to the attacks. In addition, freestanding criteria sets were provided for the definitions of panic attack and agoraphobia in order to emphasize that these can occur in the context of a number of different anxiety disorders. See Tables 3.12–3.14 for panic attack, agoraphobia, and panic disorder diagnostic criteria.

A new criterion was added to agoraphobia without history of panic disorder to address an unresolved issue in DSM-III-R as to whether a diagnosis is warranted if avoidance is associated with a general medical condition. DSM-IV recognized that individuals

Table 3.10. Diagnostic criteria for obsessive–compulsive disorder in DSM-IV

A	Either obsessions or compulsions

Obsessions as defined by (1), (2), (3), and (4)

(1) recurrent and persistent thoughts, impulses, or images that are experienced, at some time during the disturbance, as intrusive and inappropriate and that cause marked anxiety or distress

(2) the thoughts, impulses, or images are not simply excessive worries about real-life problems

(3) the person attempts to ignore or suppress such thoughts, impulses, or images, or to neutralize them with some other thought or action

(4) the person recognizes that the obsessional thoughts, impulses, or images are a product of his or her own mind (not imposed from without as in thought insertion)

Compulsions as defined by (1) and (2)

(1) repetitive behaviors (e.g., hand washing, ordering, checking) or mental acts (e.g., praying, counting, repeating words silently) that the person feels driven to perform in response to an obsession, or according to rules that must be applied rigidly

(2) the behaviors or mental acts are aimed at preventing or reducing distress or preventing some dreaded event or situation; however, these behaviors or mental acts either are not connected in a realistic way with what they are designed to neutralize or prevent or are clearly excessive

B	At some point during the course of the disorder, the person has recognized that the obsessions or compulsions are excessive or unreasonable. *Note*: This does not apply to children.
C	The obsessions or compulsions cause marked distress, are time consuming (take more than 1 hour a day), or significantly interfere with the person's normal routine, occupational (or academic) functioning, or usual social activities or relationships.
D	If another Axis I disorder is present, the content of the obsessions or compulsions is not restricted to it (e.g., preoccupation with food in the presence of an eating disorder; hair pulling in the presence of trichotillomania; concern with appearance in the presence of body dysmorphic disorder; preoccupation with drugs in the presence of a substance use disorder; preoccupation with having a serious illness in the presence of hypochondriasis; preoccupation with sexual urges or fantasies in the presence of a paraphilia; or guilty ruminations in the presence of major depressive disorder).
E	The disturbance is not due to the direct physiological effects of a substance (e.g., a drug of abuse, a medication) or a general medical condition.

Specify if:

With poor insight: if, for most of the time during the current episode, the person does not recognize that the obsessions and compulsions are excessive or unreasonable.

with certain general medical conditions might avoid situations due to *realistic concerns* about being incapacitated (e.g., fainting in an individual with transient ischemic attacks). This criterion stipulates that the diagnosis should be given only if the fear or avoidance is clearly in excess of that usually associated with the general medical condition (American Psychiatric Association 2000). See Table 3.15 for diagnostic criteria for AWOPD.

The category simple phobia was re-titled to specific phobia for compatibility with ICD-10. The diagnostic threshold was raised: in addition to persistent fear, the fear must also be marked and excessive or unreasonable. The literature review and data re-analysis indicated certain commonalities and differences between individuals with particular types of phobic stimuli (for example, individuals who fear the sight of blood tend to have a fainting reaction upon exposure to the phobic stimulus). These subgroupings resulted in the inclusion of subtypes indicating the focus of fear or avoidance. These included *animal type*, if the fear is cued by animals or insects; *natural environment type*, if the fear is cued by objects in the natural environment, such as storms, heights, or water; *blood-injection-injury type*, if the fear is cued by seeing blood or an injury or by receiving an injection or other invasive medical procedure; *situational type*, if the fear is cued by a specific situation, i.e., public transportation, tunnels, bridges, etc.; and *other type*, if the fear is cued by other stimuli.

Several changes were also made to the diagnostic criteria for GAD. In addition to having excessive anxiety and worry, DSM-IV required that "the person finds it difficult to control the worry." Based on the results of data re-analyses, the lengthy DSM-III-R 18-item set of somatic anxiety symptoms was simplified to a six-item list. See Table 3.16 for a comparison of DSM-III-R and DSM-IV symptom lists.

As part of the overarching plan to eliminate the word "organic" from DSM-IV (Spitzer *et al.* 1992), Organic anxiety disorder was replaced by two new disorders: anxiety disorder due to a general medical condition, and substance-induced anxiety disorder.

Table 3.11. Diagnostic criteria for posttraumatic stress disorder in DSM-IV

A	The person has been exposed to a traumatic event in which both of the following were present:
	(1) the person experienced, witnessed, or was confronted with an event or events that involved actual or threatened death or serious injury, or a threat to the physical integrity of self or others
	(2) the person's response involved intense fear, helplessness, or horror. *Note*: In children, this may be expressed instead by disorganized or agitated behavior
B	The traumatic event is persistently re-experienced in one (or more) of the following ways:
	(1) recurrent and intrusive distressing recollections of the event, including images, thoughts, or perceptions. *Note*: In young children, repetitive play may occur in which themes or aspects of the trauma are expressed.
	(2) recurrent distressing dreams of the event. *Note*: In children, there may be frightening dreams without recognizable content.
	(3) acting or feeling as if the traumatic event were recurring (includes a sense of reliving the experience, illusions, hallucinations, and dissociative flashback episodes, including those that occur on awakening or when intoxicated). *Note*: In young children, trauma-specific reenactment may occur.
	(4) intense psychological distress at exposure to internal or external cues that symbolize or resemble an aspect of the traumatic event
	(5) physiological reactivity on exposure to internal or external cues that symbolize or resemble an aspect of the traumatic event
C	Persistent avoidance of stimuli associated with the trauma and numbing of general responsiveness (not present before the trauma), as indicated by three (or more) of the following:
	(1) efforts to avoid thoughts, feelings, or conversations associated with the trauma
	(2) efforts to avoid activities, places, or people that arouse recollections of the trauma
	(3) inability to recall an important aspect of the trauma
	(4) markedly diminished interest or participation in significant activities
	(5) feeling of detachment or estrangement from others
	(6) restricted range of affect (e.g., unable to have loving feelings)
	(7) sense of a foreshortened future (e.g., does not expect to have a career, marriage, children, or a normal life span)
D	Persistent symptoms of increased arousal (not present before the trauma), as indicated by two (or more) of the following:
	(1) difficulty falling or staying asleep
	(2) irritability or outbursts of anger
	(3) difficulty concentrating
	(4) hypervigilance
	(5) exaggerated startle response
E	Duration of the disturbance (symptoms in B, C, and D) is more than 1 month.
F	The disturbance causes clinically significant distress or impairment in social, occupational, or other important areas of functioning.

Specify if:
Acute: if duration is less than 3 months
Chronic: if duration of symptoms is 3 months or more
Specify if:
With delayed onset: if onset of symptoms is at least 6 months after the stressor

These were added to the anxiety disorders grouping. Subtypes were provided to indicate the nature of the predominant symptoms: *with generalized anxiety*; *with panic attacks*; *with obsessive–compulsive symptoms*; or *with phobic symptoms* (the latter applying only to substance-induced anxiety disorder).

One new anxiety disorder was added to DSM-IV, acute stress disorder (Table 3.17). Acute stress disorder is characterized by a cluster of anxiety and dissociative symptoms occurring within one month of a traumatic event. The diagnostic criteria were developed to differentiate between time-limited reactions to trauma and PTSD. A diagnosis of acute stress disorder is made only for symptoms that are present for a minimum of two days and a maximum of four weeks, and that occur within four weeks of the

Table 3.12. Diagnostic criteria for panic attack in DSM-IV

A discrete period of intense fear or discomfort, in which four (or more) of the following symptoms developed abruptly and reached a peak within 10 minutes

(1) palpitations, pounding heart, or accelerated heart rate

(2) sweating

(3) trembling or shaking

(4) sensations of shortness of breath or smothering

(5) feeling of choking

(6) chest pain or discomfort

(7) nausea or abdominal distress

(8) feeling dizzy, unsteady, lightheaded, or faint

(9) derealization (feelings of unreality) or depersonalization (being detached from oneself)

(10) fear of losing control or going crazy

(11) fear of dying

(12) paresthesias (numbness or tingling sensations)

(13) chills or hot flushes

Table 3.13. Diagnostic criteria for agoraphobia in DSM-IV

A Anxiety about being in places or situations from which escape might be difficult (or embarrassing) or in which help may not be available in the event of having an unexpected or situationally predisposed panic attack or panic-like symptoms. Agoraphobic fears typically involve characteristic clusters of situations that include being outside the home alone; being in a crowd or standing in a line; being on a bridge; and traveling in a bus, train, or automobile.
Note: Consider the diagnosis of specific phobia if the avoidance is limited to one or only a few specific situations, or social phobia if the avoidance is limited to social situations.

B The situations are avoided (e.g., travel is restricted) or else are endured with marked distress or with anxiety about having a panic attack or panic-like symptoms or require the presence of a companion.

C The anxiety or phobic avoidance is not better accounted for by another mental disorder, such as social phobia (e.g., avoidance limited to social situations because of fear of embarrassment), specific phobia (e.g., avoidance limited to a single situation like elevators), obsessive–compulsive disorder (e.g., avoidance of dirt in someone with an obsession about contamination), posttraumatic stress disorder (e.g., avoidance of stimuli associated with a severe stressor), or separation anxiety disorder (e.g., avoidance of leaving home or relatives).

Table 3.14. Diagnostic criteria for panic disorder with (or without) agoraphobia in DSM-IV

A Both (1) and (2):

(1) recurrent unexpected panic attacks

(2) at least one of the attacks has been followed by 1 month (or more) of one (or more) of the following:

(a) persistent concern about having additional attacks
(b) worry about the implications of the attacks or its consequences (e.g., losing control, having a heart attack, "going crazy")
(c) a significant change in behavior related to the attacks

B The presence (absence) of agoraphobia

C The panic attacks are not due to the direct physiological effects of a substance (e.g., a drug of abuse, a medication) or a general medical condition (e.g., hyperthyroidism).

D The panic attacks are not better accounted for by another mental disorder, such as social phobia (e.g., occurring on exposure to feared social situations), specific phobia (e.g., on exposure to a specific phobic situation), obsessive–compulsive disorder (e.g., on exposure to dirt in someone with an obsession about contamination), posttraumatic stress disorder (e.g., in response to stimuli associated with a severe stressor), or separation anxiety disorder (e.g., in response to being away from home or close relatives).

Table 3.15. Diagnostic criteria for agoraphobia without history of panic disorder (AWOPD) in DSM-IV

A	The presence of agoraphobia related to fear of developing panic-like symptoms (e.g., dizziness or diarrhea).
B	Criteria have never been met for panic disorder.
C	The disturbance is not due to the direct physiological effects of a substance (e.g., a drug of abuse, a medication) or a general medical condition.
D	If an associated general medical condition is present, the fear described in Criterion A is clearly in excess of that usually associated with the condition.

Table 3.16. Comparison of DSM-III-R and DSM-IV symptom lists for generalized anxiety disorder (GAD)

DSM-III-R	DSM-IV
Motor tension	(1) restlessness or feeling keyed up or on edge
(1) trembling, twitching, or feeling shaky	(2) being easily fatigued
(2) muscle tension, aches, or soreness	(3) difficulty concentrating or mind going blank
(3) restlessness	(4) irritability
(4) easy fatigability	(5) muscle tension
	(6) sleep disturbance (difficulty falling or staying asleep, or restless unsatisfying sleep)
Autonomic hyperactivity	
(5) shortness of breath or smothering sensations	
(6) palpitations or accelerated heart rate (tachycardia)	
(7) sweating, or cold clammy hands	
(8) dry mouth	
(9) dizziness or lightheadedness	
(10) nausea, diarrhea, or other abdominal distress	
(11) flushes (hot flashes) or chills	
(12) frequent urination	
(13) trouble swallowing or "lump in throat"	
Vigilance and scanning	
(14) feeling keyed up or on edge	
(15) exaggerated startle response	
(16) difficulty concentrating or "mind going blank" because of anxiety	
(17) trouble falling or staying asleep	
(18) irritability	

traumatic event. By contrast, a PTSD diagnosis is given for disturbances lasting more than one month. The stressors for acute stress disorder are the same as those described for PTSD.

Finally, in keeping with the DSM-IV convention that diagnostic criteria should apply across the developmental age range (e.g., there have never been separate diagnostic criteria for depression occurring in childhood), several of the DSM-III-R childhood anxiety disorders were subsumed under their adult counterparts: DSM-III-R's avoidant disorder of childhood into social anxiety disorder and DSM-III-R's overanxious disorder into generalized anxiety disorder.

3.8 DSM-IV-TR

The fourth edition of the DSM *Text Revision* (DSM-IV-TR), published in 2000, was undertaken to serve as an intermediary between DSM-IV and DSM-5 (American Psychiatric Association 2000). The changes made were limited to the text sections. No new disorders, subtypes, or major changes in the criteria sets were considered. Most of the changes were in sections of the text covering associated features and disorders;

Table 3.17. Diagnostic criteria for acute stress disorder in DSM-IV

A	The person has been exposed to a traumatic event in which both of the following were present:
	(1) the person experienced, witnessed, or was confronted with an event or events that involved actual or threatened death or serious injury, or a threat to the physical integrity of self or others
	(2) the person's response involved intense fear, helplessness, or horror
B	Either while experiencing or after experiencing the distressing event, the individual has three (or more) of the following dissociative symptoms:
	(1) a subjective sense of numbing, detachment, or absence of emotional responsiveness
	(2) a reduction in awareness of his or her surroundings (e.g., "being in a daze")
	(3) derealization
	(4) depersonalization
	(5) dissociative amnesia (i.e., inability to recall an important aspect of the trauma)
C	The traumatic event is persistently re-experienced in at least one of the following ways: recurrent images, thoughts, dreams, illusions, flashback episodes, or a sense of reliving the experience; or distress on exposure to reminders of the traumatic event.
D	Marked avoidance of stimuli that arouse recollections of the trauma (e.g., thoughts, feelings, conversations, activities, places, people).
E	Marked symptoms of anxiety or increased arousal (e.g., difficulty sleeping, irritability, poor concentration, hypervigilance, exaggerated startle response, motor restlessness).
F	The disturbance causes clinically significant distress or impairment in social, occupational, or other important areas of functioning or impairs the individual's ability to pursue some necessary task, such as obtaining necessary assistance or mobilizing personal resources by telling family members about the traumatic experience.
G	The disturbance lasts for a minimum of 2 days and a maximum of 4 weeks and occurs within 4 weeks of the traumatic event.
H	The disturbance is not due to the direct physiological effects of a substance (e.g., a drug of abuse, a medication) or a general medical condition, is not better accounted for by brief psychotic disorder, and is not merely an exacerbation of a pre-existing Axis I or II disorder.

specific culture, age, and gender features; prevalence; course; familial pattern; and differential diagnosis.

3.9 DSM-5

The next edition of the *Diagnostic and Statistical Manual of Mental Disorders*, DSM-5, is due in 2013. As in previous revisions of the manual since 1980, DSM-5 attempts to balance research advances on the anxiety disorders with the need to maintain continuity with preceding DSM editions in the organization and definition of disorders. At this time, substantial changes are being considered for DSM-5, including for the anxiety disorders. Possible areas for change are the grouping of related diagnostic categories into spectra, inclusion of cross-cutting characteristics across disorders in the form of dimensions, further specification of child presentations of disorders, isolation of the impairment criterion from disorder descriptions, clarification of the relationship between Axis I disorders and personality disorders, and greater attention to phenomenological variation between genders and across racial, ethnic, and cultural groups.

The grouping of related disorders into spectra is a novel organizational approach proposed for DSM-5 (Angst 2007). The goal is to cluster in discrete sections of the manual those disorders that share common biological, psychological, and/or epidemiological elements. For the anxiety disorders, two possible spectra are under consideration. The first is whether it makes sense to continue to include obsessive–compulsive disorder in the anxiety disorders section or instead in another diagnostic grouping. Some evidence suggests that OCD shares more neurobiological, genetic, and psychological features in common with other disorders characterized by repetitive behaviors and/or thoughts. One alternative under consideration is the creation of a new diagnostic grouping for obsessive–compulsive spectrum disorders, which might include OCD, body dysmorphic disorder, hypochondriasis, tic disorders, and possibly trichotillomania and obsessive–compulsive personality disorder. The second reorganization of disorders being discussed involves the possibility of grouping trauma-related disorders, such as PTSD and ASD. This "trauma spectrum" may also group other disorders not currently included under the anxiety disorders, such as the dissociative disorders, other reactions to traumatic events not meeting threshold criteria for PTSD or ASD that are currently classified under the adjustment disorders, and possibly acute psychotic states occurring in response to severe stressors.

The inclusion of symptom or trait dimensions as complementary diagnostic elements to the current disorder categories is another potentially new addition in DSM-5 (Brown & Barlow 2005). Current diagnostic categories establish a cutoff point (e.g., six months duration of three out of six generalized anxiety symptoms for GAD). However, the genetic and neurobiological data seem more compatible with dimensional measures of pathology, raising questions about the possible arbitrariness of some of the existing cutoffs and their reduced sensitivity to treatment effect compared to dimensional outcome measures (Pine *et al.* 2002, Andrews *et al.* 2008, Helzer *et al.* 2008a). Moreover, a dimensional approach would permit the inclusion of subthreshold presentations in the definition of disorders, as milder forms on the continuum, facilitating identification and possible treatment of these frequently impairing presentations (Helzer *et al.* 2008b).

In addition, certain symptom dimensions, such as anxiety, are present not only in the anxiety disorders but also characterize other diagnoses, such as major depression, schizophrenia, and some personality disorders. Using one set of global dimensions across DSM-5 as a complementary characterization may help clarify the nosological relationship across disorders and the comorbidity of individual cases, facilitating treatment choices. The relationship between GAD and major depression, for example, may be better understood as the intersection of anxiety and depressive dimensions than as the comorbidity of distinct categories.

Finally, within the anxiety disorders, certain dimensions cut across various specified anxiety disorders, such as fear of anxiety symptoms (anxiety sensitivity), avoidance, fear of negative evaluation, behavioral inhibition, and illness phobia/hypochondriasis, among others. Inclusion in DSM-5 of a subset of these or other intra-anxiety-disorder dimensions may help clarify disorder subtypes and interrelationships (Helzer *et al.* 2008c). It should be noted that a dimensional approach is being considered in DSM-5 as complementary to the usual categorical diagnoses, rather than as a replacement for them.

Another planned innovation in DSM-5 involves expanding its developmental perspective to integrate symptom descriptions encompassing the full life span into all appropriate criteria sets (Pine *et al.* 2002). This will likely entail at least four distinct approaches. First, determining whether it is appropriate to link disorders that are currently listed separately but which may be developmentally connected, such as selective mutism in children and social anxiety disorder in adults. Second, refining criteria for childhood and adolescent presentations of disorders currently listed in the anxiety section – such as PTSD, social anxiety disorder, and generalized anxiety disorder/overanxious disorder – for which greater descriptive evidence has accumulated since DSM-IV-TR, including as possible developmental subtypes of relevant disorders. Third, considering for inclusion of disorders that are currently listed in the childhood section but for which there may be evidence of an adult version, such as adult separation anxiety disorder. Fourth, adding new disorders if evidence indicates that exposure to risk factors during childhood leads to childhood onset and, subsequently, lifelong pathological syndromes. For example, a new category of developmental trauma disorder has been proposed, wherein prolonged and severe physical and/or sexual abuse during childhood or adolescence may result in a stable cluster of posttraumatic pathologies (mood, anxiety, dissociative, and personality symptoms), disruptions in developmental competencies (e.g., emotional labeling, identity formation), maladaptive behaviors (e.g., substance use, suicidality), and marked functional impairment.

Another area under examination throughout DSM-5, which will also affect the anxiety disorders, is whether impairment should continue to be considered as a constitutive element of disorder definition. This was the DSM-IV position, where an impairment criterion ("clinical significance") was included in over 70% of disorders. Instead, an alternative being explored is whether symptom descriptions should be refined further so as to enable diagnosis with or without associated impairment. On one hand, since DSM-IV, the strong linkage of impairment and symptom description has been criticized on the grounds that it does not permit disorder definition prior to the development of impairment, may hinder research on the relationship of impairment and disorder, and may help exclude subjects from research trials who have early forms of the disorder, thereby limiting assessment of etiologies and risk factors in this highly informative population (Lehman *et al.* 2002). On the other hand, the DSM-IV clinical-significance criterion also plays an important role in distinguishing normality from pathology, and there is a question as to whether the field has advanced sufficiently across all diagnostic entities to permit disorder definition without it. If not, eliminating the impairment criterion may have the unintended effect of pathologizing normal coping. An alternative is to retain the distress component of the clinical-significance criterion as part of disorder definition but remove the impairment element. Evaluation of this issue involves all DSM-5 diagnoses and will be considered for the anxiety disorders in relation to the rest of the manual.

Other areas under consideration for the entire manual include the relationship between personality disorders and Axis I disorders. As part of the greater dimensional focus of DSM-5, a proposal under consideration is that personality traits be characterized for all patients, independently of the presence of a personality disorder. In terms of the anxiety disorders, this may help clarify the relationship between long-standing personality patterns of avoidance and the development of social anxiety disorder (Schneier *et al.* 1996). A dimensional approach may also contribute to the decision as to whether long-standing obsessive–compulsive personality traits belong in a new obsessive–compulsive spectrum (Samuels *et al.* 2007).

Greater attention to gender and racial/ethnic and cultural aspects of disorder presentation may include proposed changes to disorder criteria. For instance, higher rates of PTSD in women may be related to the separation of the trauma-exposure criterion in DSM-IV into two subcriteria, which requires a reaction involving intense fear, helplessness, or horror (Criterion A2) in addition to simple exposure (Criterion A1). Since women are more likely to endorse Criterion A2 than men, this may confound gender differences in exposure to traumatic events with gender differences in the conditional probability of PTSD given exposure (Breslau & Kessler 2001). Adjusting or removing Criterion A2 may more accurately describe the relationship between exposure and development of disorder, and thereby lead to a more even gender ratio in PTSD prevalence.

Attending to cultural variation may also lead to suggestions for changes in criteria. For example, lower rates of panic disorder in Asians (Kawakami *et al.* 2005) may be due in part to the mismatch between culturally specific presentations of panic attacks – with symptoms such as neck soreness, tinnitus, headache, or marked dizziness – and the specified list of 13 panic attack symptoms in DSM-IV-TR (Hinton *et al.* 2000). In this case, solutions may include relative despecification of the list of panic symptoms to a more general autonomic-arousal criterion, the addition of alternate symptoms to the list, or a description in the text of

suggested cultural modifications during the diagnostic process. In addition, a revamped cultural formulation guideline, currently included in Appendix I of DSM-IV-TR, may play a more central role in DSM-5. This would provide a standard method for assessing cultural factors in the clinical encounter, facilitating the process of translation between DSM-5 categories and cultural presentations (Lewis-Fernández & Díaz 2002).

Note

Dr. Lewis-Fernández is a member of the DSM-5 Work Group on Anxiety, Obsessive–Compulsive Spectrum, Posttraumatic, and Dissociative Disorders. Information or views expressed in this chapter do not necessarily represent the views of the DSM-5 Work Group.

References

American Medical Association (1952). *Standard Nomenclature of Diseases and Operations*, 4th edn. Philadelphia, PA: Blakistone.

American Psychiatric Association (1952). *Diagnostic and Statistical Manual of Mental Disorders* (DSM-I). Washington, DC: American Psychiatric Association.

American Psychiatric Association (1968). *Diagnostic and Statistical Manual of Mental Disorders*, 2nd edn (DSM-II). Washington, DC: American Psychiatric Association.

American Psychiatric Association (1980). *Diagnostic and Statistical Manual of Mental Disorders*, 3rd edn (DSM-III). Washington, DC: American Psychiatric Association.

American Psychiatric Association (1987). *Diagnostic and Statistical Manual of Mental Disorders*, 3rd edn., revised (DSM-III-R). Washington, DC: American Psychiatric Association.

American Psychiatric Association (1994). *Diagnostic and Statistical Manual of Mental Disorders*, 4th edn (DSM-IV). Washington, DC: American Psychiatric Association.

American Psychiatric Association (2000). *Diagnostic and Statistical Manual of Mental Disorders*, 4th edn, text revision (DSM-IV-TR). Washington, DC: American Psychiatric Association.

Andrews, G., Brugha, T., Thase, M. E., *et al.* (2008). Dimensionality and the category of major depressive episode. In J. E. Helzer, H. C. Kraemer, R. F. Krueger, *et al.*, eds., *Dimensional Approaches in Diagnostic Classification: Refining the Research Agenda for DSM-5*. Arlington, VA: American Psychiatric Press, pp. 35–51.

Angst, J. (2007). The bipolar spectrum. *British Journal of Psychiatry*, **190**, 189–191.

Berrios, G. (1996). *The History of Mental Symptoms: Descriptive Psychopathology Since the Nineteenth Century.* Cambridge: Cambridge University Press.

Breslau, N., & Kessler, R. (2001). The stressor criterion in DSM-IV posttraumatic stress disorder: an empirical investigation. *Biological Psychiatry*, **50**, 699–704.

Brown, T. A., & Barlow, D. H. (2005). Dimensional versus categorical classification of mental disorders in the fifth edition of the Diagnostic and Statistical Manual of Mental Disorders and beyond: comment on the special section. *Journal of Abnormal Psychology*, **114**, 551–556.

Feighner, J. P., Robins, E., Guze, S. B., *et al.* (1972). Diagnostic criteria for use in psychiatric research. *Archives of General Psychiatry*, **26**, 57–63.

Foa, E., Kozak, M., Goodman, W., *et al.* (1998). DSM-IV field trial: obsessive–compulsive disorder. In T. Widiger, A. Frances, H. Pincus, *et al.*, eds., *DSM-IV Sourcebook, Volume 4*. Washington, DC: American Psychiatric Association, pp. 761–778.

Frances, A., Widiger, T., & Pincus, H. A. (1989). The development of DSM-IV. *Archives of General Psychiatry*, **46**, 373–375.

Frances, A., Pincus, H., Manning, D., & Widiger, T. (1990). Classification of anxiety states in DSM-III and perspectives for its classification in DSM-IV. In S. Sartorius, V. Andreoli, G. Cassano, *et al.*, eds., *Anxiety: Psychobiological and Clinical Perspectives*. New York, NY: Hemisphere, pp. 139–146.

Fyer, A., Katon, W., Hollifield, M., *et al.* (1998). DSM-IV panic disorder field trial: panic attack frequency and functional disability. In T. Widiger, A. Frances, H. Pincus, *et al.*, *DSM-IV Sourcebook, Volume 4*. Washington, DC: American Psychiatric Association, pp. 779–802.

Haggard, P., Furman, A., Levy, S. T., *et al.* (2008). Psychoanalytic theories. In A. Tasman, J. Kay, J. Lieberman, M. First & M. Maj, eds., *Psychiatry*, 3rd edn. Chichester: Wiley, pp. 464–485.

Helzer, J. E., Bucholz, K. K., Gossop, M. (2008a). A dimensional option for the diagnosis of substance dependence in DSM-5. In J. E. Helzer, H. C. Kraemer, R. F. Krueger, *et al.*, eds., *Dimensional Approaches in Diagnostic Classification: Refining the Research Agenda for DSM-5*. Arlington, VA: American Psychiatric Press, pp. 19–34.

Helzer, J. E., Kraemer, H. C., Krueger, R. F., *et al.*, eds. (2008b). *Dimensional Approaches in Diagnostic Classification: Refining the Research Agenda for DSM-5*. Arlington, VA: American Psychiatric Press.

Helzer, J. E., Wittchen, H. U., Krueger, R. F., & Kraemer, H. C. (2008c). Dimensional options for DSM-5: the way forward. In J. E. Helzer, H. C. Kraemer, R. F. Krueger, *et al.*, eds., *Dimensional Approaches in Diagnostic Classification: Refining the Research Agenda for DSM-5*. Arlington, VA: American Psychiatric Press, pp.115–127.

Hinton D., Ba, P., Peou, S., & Um, K. (2000). Panic disorder among Cambodian refugees attending a psychiatric clinic: Prevalence and subtypes. *General Hospital Psychiatry*, **22**, 437–444.

Kawakami, N., Takeshima, T., Ono, Y., *et al.* (2005). Twelve-month prevalence, severity, and treatment of common mental disorders in communities in Japan: preliminary findings from the World Mental Health Japan Survey 2002–2003. *Psychiatry and Clinical Neurosciences*, **59**, 441–452.

Kay, J., & Kay, R. (2008). Individual psychoanalytic psychotherapy. In A. Tasman, J. Kay, J. Lieberman, M. First & M. Maj, eds., *Psychiatry*, 3rd edn. Chichester: Wiley, pp. 1851–1874.

Kilpatrick, D. G., Resnick, H. S., Freedy, J.R., *et al.* (1998). The posttraumatic stress disorder field trial: evaluation of the PTSD construct – criteria A through E. In T. Widiger, A. Frances, H. Pincus, *et al.*, *DSM-IV Sourcebook, Volume 4*. Washington, DC: American Psychiatric Association, pp. 803–846.

Klein, D. (1964). Delineation of two drug-responsive anxiety syndromes. *Psychopharmacologia*, **5**, 397–408.

Kupfer, D., First, M., & Regier, D. (2002). Introduction. In D. Kupfer, M. First, & D. Regier, eds., *A Research Agenda for DSM-5*. Washington, DC: American Psychiatric Association, pp. xv–xxiii.

Leckman, J., Merikangas, K., Pauls, D. L., Prusoff, B. A., & Weismann, M. M. (1983). Anxiety disorders and depression: contradictions between family study data and DSM-III conventions. *Archives of General Psychiatry*, **140**, 880–882.

Lehman, A. F., Alexopolous, G. S., Goldman, H., Jeste, D., & Ustun, B. (2002). Mental disorders and disability: time to reevaluate the relationship? In D. J. Kupfer, M. B. First, & D. A. Regier, eds., *A Research Agenda for DSM-5*. Washington, DC: American Psychiatric Association, pp. 201–218.

Lewis-Fernández, R., & Díaz, N. (2002). The cultural formulation: a method for assessing cultural factors affecting the clinical encounter. *Psychiatric Quarterly*, **73**, 271–295.

Pine, D. S., Alegría, M., Cook, E. H., *et al.* (2002). Advances in developmental science and DSM-5. In D. J. Kupfer, M. B. First, & D. A. Regier, eds., *A Research Agenda for DSM-5*. Washington, DC: American Psychiatric Association, pp. 85–122.

Regier, D. A., Boyd, J. H., Burke, J. D., *et al.* (1988). One-month prevalence of mental disorders in the United States: based on five Epidemiologic Catchment Area sites. *Archives of General Psychiatry*, **45**, 977–986.

Roth, S., Newman, E., Pelcovitz, D., van der Kolk, B., & Mandel, F. S. (1997). Complex PTSD in victims exposed to sexual and physical abuse: results from the DSM-IV

Field Trial for Posttraumatic Stress Disorder. *Journal of Trauma and Stress*, **10**, 539–555.

Samuels, J. F., Bienvenu, O. J., Pinto, A., *et al.* (2007). Hoarding in obsessive–compulsive disorder: results from the OCD collaborative genetics study. *Behaviour Research and Therapy*, **45**, 673–686.

Schneier, F. R., Liebowitz, M. R., Beidel, D. C., *et al.* (1996). Social phobia. In T. A. Widiger, A. J. Frances, H. A. Pincus, *et al.*, eds., *DSM–IV Sourcebook, Vol. 2.* Washington DC: American Psychiatric Association, pp. 507–548.

Spitzer, R., & Williams, J. (1985). Proposed revisions in the DSM-III classification of anxiety disorders based on research and clinical experience. In A. Tuma & J. Maser, eds., *Anxiety and the Anxiety Disorders*. Hillsdale: Lawrence Erlbaum Associates, pp. 759–773.

Spitzer, R., First, M., Williams, J. B., *et al.* (1992). Now is the time to retire the term "organic mental disorders". *American Journal of Psychiatry*, **149**, 240–244.

Zitrin, C., Klein, D., & Woerner, M. G. (1978). Behavior therapy, supportive psychotherapy, imipramine, and phobias. *Archives of General Psychiatry*, **35**, 307–316.

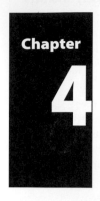

The emergence of social anxiety disorder as a major medical condition

Michael R. Liebowitz

4.1 Development of the modern concept of social anxiety disorder

To properly understand the current concept of *social anxiety disorder*, previously termed *social phobia*, it is necessary to recall the situation surrounding this condition in the early to mid 1980s, after the publication of DSM-III (American Psychiatric Association 1980) but before the revised version, DSM-III-R, was available (American Psychiatric Association 1987).

4.1.1 Background

In DSM-III, the prevailing diagnostic guide when I began my research career, social phobia was considered a subdivision of phobic disorders along with agoraphobia and the specific phobias. This classification reflected the work of investigators like Isaac Marks (Marks & Gelder 1966), whose classic studies of phobias in the 1960s and 1970s made a powerful empirical case – based on symptomatic presentation, course of illness, and family history – for reducing a laundry list of individual phobias into these three major categories. The distinct category of social phobia was found by Marks to include "fears of eating, drinking, shaking, blushing, speaking, writing, or vomiting in the presence of other people," with the core feature being fear of appearing foolish to others, leading to marked avoidance.

Marks's original concept of social phobia was not far from our current thinking about this condition, but the very influential DSM-III classification did not adopt his concept in full. While accepting Marks's major subdivisions of phobic disorders, DSM-III greatly narrowed the definition of social phobia, limiting it to fear and avoidance of performance situations or (at most) one to two interpersonal situations. Individuals with broad interpersonal fears and avoidance were relegated to a

category called *avoidant personality disorder*. This was a new term developed for DSM-III based on the work of Millon (Millon *et al.* 2004) and others who believed that conditions affecting wide areas of adaptive behavior and appearing to be chronic must be personality disorders. Thus, individuals with broad interpersonal fears and avoidance were thought to have avoidant personality disorder rather than an anxiety disorder. However, the DSM-III narrowing of social phobia had no empirical basis and was derived instead purely from this theoretical model.

4.1.2 My first anti-anxiety studies

This was the dogma of the early to mid 1980s when my own work in the anxiety field began. At first I worked with panic-disorder patients, in collaboration with other investigators including Donald Klein and Abby Fyer, and, a bit later, Jack Gorman. We were investigating the biological basis of panic attacks, using techniques like infusions of sodium lactate to precipitate panic attacks in the laboratory in vulnerable individuals (always with their prior informed consent). We studied the physiological characteristics of these panic attacks and looked for ways to block them in the lab as well as in patients' everyday lives. Out of this work came a number of useful findings, such as the recognition that beta-blockers could lower the heart rate during a panic attack but not block one; that extended pretreatment with imipramine would block laboratory-induced as well as clinical panics; and that fluoxetine, the first available selective serotonin reuptake inhibitor (SSRI), was a good anti-panic drug if started in small doses but often made panics worse if started at the usual antidepressant dose of 20 mg per day.

It was in this clinical research setting that my work with what we now refer to as *social anxiety disorder* began. One of my responsibilities as junior researcher was to interview subjects for our clinical trials. One

Anxiety Disorders: Theory, Research, and Clinical Perspectives, ed. Helen Blair Simpson, Yuval Neria, Roberto Lewis-Fernández, Franklin Schneier. Published by Cambridge University Press. © Cambridge University Press 2010.

patient, an unmarried male in his late twenties, presented for treatment with numerous panic attacks that were very frightening to him and that led him to greatly restrict his activity. Because he frequently suffered panic attacks while riding on the subway, he became frightened to do so. In New York City, where most travel is by mass transit, this greatly limited his mobility. We diagnosed him with panic disorder and treated him with imipramine, our best anti-panic drug at the time. I saw him for follow-up every two weeks after that. However, despite taking substantial doses of medication and achieving a good therapeutic blood level, he showed very little improvement. Basically, his panic attacks and avoidant behavior did not improve.

This was a fairly rare event in our experience, and one of the things we routinely did in such situations was to review the patient's clinical features to make sure our diagnosis was correct. We went over this man's history very carefully and discovered that there were some very peculiar aspects to his case. For one, his panic attacks only occurred when he felt people were looking at and evaluating him. On the subway, for example, if he happened to be the only person sitting in a particular subway car, he was relatively comfortable. However, when other people entered the car, and especially when someone sat across from him and began looking at him, he quickly became panicky. This was very unusual in our experience, because typical panic-disorder patients suffered panic attacks somewhat unexpectedly and worried about being incapacitated by them. For this reason, they tended to feel most comfortable with others around who could help in a possible emergency and most uncomfortable when there was no one around to help if they became panicky. However, with this patient the reverse was true. At night, if his street was empty, he could go out comfortably. During the day, when there were others who might look at him or, worse, speak to him, he was terrified. This did not seem like typical panic disorder or agoraphobia.

I clearly remember discussing the case with my colleagues and all of us being quite puzzled by it. We reluctantly concluded that it sounded like some kind of social phobia, but none of us knew very much about this condition. We decided that someone needed to review the literature on social phobia, and I volunteered. I believe this was sometime in 1983.

4.1.3 First review paper on social phobia

I spent the next six months or so using my spare time to review the literature on social phobia. I looked at the history of its classification; what was know about prevalence; anything I could find about pathophysiology, assessment, and treatment; and whatever had been written about its severity and impairment. From this review my colleagues and I came up with a number of interesting impressions, conclusions, and questions.

One conclusion was that social phobia was a relatively neglected anxiety disorder that had received little systematic research attention, except from behavior therapists who were beginning to use desensitization and exposure treatment strategies with these patients. Secondly, while DSM-III limited social phobia essentially to performance anxiety, and relegated more widespread interpersonal fear and avoidance to the newly created category of avoidant personality disorder, there did not seem to be any empirical basis for this. The DSM-III formulation represented a distinct narrowing of Marks's conception. Moreover, it struck me that there was a risk associated with this approach. Patients with more widespread interpersonal fears and avoidance would be regarded as having personality rather than anxiety disorders. If so, given the state of the field at that time, then clinicians would be more likely to treat them with some form of dynamic psychotherapy rather then behavior therapy or medication.

A third conclusion was that while DSM-III held that social phobia was a rather uncommon disorder, there was little empirical basis to support this. As it turned out in subsequent epidemiological surveys like the Epidemiological Catchment Area Study (ECA) (Regier *et al.* 1984) and the National Comorbidity Survey (NCS) (Kessler *et al.* 1994), social phobia was found to be a very common anxiety disorder, and one of the most common psychiatric conditions.

We also found that there was a striking paucity of medication treatment studies for social phobia. This was due to several factors. Some researchers considered it part of normal shyness or a manifestation of a personality problem, both cases suggesting medication treatment would not be helpful. Others regarded it as a variant of agoraphobia and thus not in need of independent study.

The limited pharmacological research that had been done, however, actually offered several promising leads. Researchers had studied the use of beta-adrenergic blockers in analogues of social phobia (e.g., musicians who were anxious on stage but had not undergone formal diagnostic assessment) and found them to be helpful in improving performance. The one placebo-controlled trial of a beta-blocker in a clinical population of social phobics had a very small sample size and gave concomitant behavior therapy to all study participants; it did not find a drug–placebo difference (Falloon *et al.*1981). There were also placebo-controlled trials of the monoamine oxidase inhibitor (MAOI) phenelzine in mixed populations of patients with agoraphobia and social phobia, where a positive medication effect was found. However, outcomes for the two subpopulations were not analyzed separately, so it was unclear if the social phobic patients benefited from the MAOI. This was an important distinction because prior trials had already demonstrated phenelzine's efficacy for agoraphobia.

The accepted view on the severity of social phobia was especially troubling. DSM-III held that social phobia was not a highly disabling condition. In this it was wrong on two counts. First, even within the limits of the DSM-III definition, public speaking or performance anxiety can be highly distressing and at times disabling. In the two decades since I started my research on social phobia, many of my patients have come for treatment because of a fear of public speaking or performance. In the days and weeks leading up to their performance they become terrified, cannot sleep, and consider canceling engagements or quitting their jobs. Most of these individuals are otherwise highly socially competent and functional, but their performance anxiety can make their lives a nightmare.

Social phobia turned out to be an even more severe clinical problem, however, for patients whose fear of evaluation and scrutiny by others interfered with social functioning as well as performance. For example, we evaluated people who could not go to a party, talk to a colleague, ask a stranger for directions, or interact with a cashier in a store. Some did this with difficulty and maintained the façade of a normal life, although they struggled with enormous personal anguish on a daily basis. Others gave up the struggle, dropped out of school, stopped working, or took jobs where little interaction with the public was required. Moreover, their anxiety problems made them vulnerable to other conditions such as alcohol abuse (an attempt at self-medication) and depression.

At this juncture we did several very useful things. One was to publish a paper entitled "Social phobia: review of a neglected anxiety disorder," which laid out all the issues we have just discussed (Liebowitz *et al.* 1985). This paper, published in the *Archives of General Psychiatry* in 1985, greatly helped to raise professional awareness about social phobia and was influential in bringing much-needed research and clinical attention to the disorder. As described in more detail below, we also developed and validated measures for assessing social phobia, and organized clinical trials to examine how best to treat social phobia.

4.1.4 Early clinical trials in social phobia

Because so little was known about the pharmacological treatment of social phobia, we spearheaded clinical trials using the MAOI phenelzine and the beta-adrenergic blocker atenolol. Our goals were threefold. One was to find medications that would be useful for treating social phobia. A second was to see if we could find support for a broader conceptualization of the condition than was contained in DSM-III. If for a sample of patients who fit a broader definition of social phobia we showed that symptoms could respond to a short-term medication intervention, we would also be validating the view that these symptoms were manifestations of an anxiety rather than a personality disorder, opening the way for testing of many other medication and psychotherapy modalities.

A third goal of the clinical trial program was to gain some insights into the pathophysiology of social phobia. Atenolol is a cardioselective beta-blocker that does not readily penetrate the blood–brain barrier. To the degree that it was helpful in social phobia, it would be implicating peripheral autonomic activation in the disorder. In addition, by this time our views had evolved to the point that we thought that there were two distinct subtypes of social phobia, a non-generalized form and a generalized form. The non-generalized form encompassed patients whose primary problem was performance anxiety but who were comfortable in most social situations. The generalized subtype, on the other hand, described a disorder in which affected individuals feared most social as well as performance situations. We believed that the non-generalized but not the generalized subtype of social phobia would respond to beta-blockers, and such a finding would support our proposed distinction between the two hypothesized subtypes. A positive finding for beta-blockers in social phobia would also support its distinctiveness from panic disorder, where beta-blockers were not helpful.

The choice of phenelzine as one of our first study drugs deserves a bit more discussion. Phenelzine was selected for several reasons. As mentioned previously, prior studies had identified phenelzine as useful in heterogeneous samples of phobic patients, suggesting but not proving that it might be useful in social phobia.

There was also another line of evidence that suggested MAOIs might be useful in social phobia. Before joining the anxiety research program at the New York State Psychiatric Institute, I had worked in its Depression Evaluation Service (DES), where we studied atypical depression. The DES director, Fred Quitkin, and his mentor, Don Klein, both had a long-standing interest in MAOIs, believing that they were superior to tricyclic antidepressants like imipramine in atypical depression, a subtype of major depression. The term *atypical depression* had been applied by British investigators in the 1950s and 1960s to depressed patients who lacked the typical melancholic traits of insomnia, loss of appetite, and diurnal variation with early-morning worsening, and who also seemed to respond poorly to electroconvulsive therapy. When depressed, these patients often overslept and overate, had prominent anxiety symptoms and neurotic traits, and were not anhedonic. However, no criteria for atypical depression had ever been operationalized or validated. In the DES, we came up with an operational definition of atypical depression and then demonstrated in controlled trials that such patients did better on phenelzine than imipramine or placebo (Liebowitz *et al.* 1988). Our set of criteria for atypical depression was incorporated into DSM-IV (American Psychiatric Association 1994) as a cross-sectional modifier for major depression.

The relevance of atypical depression to social phobia is as follows. The key requirement for atypical depression was mood reactivity, the ability to be fully cheered up temporarily by pleasant events in the midst of a depressive episode. We also required at least two of the following four features: overeating, oversleeping, extreme leaden fatigue, and rejection hypersensitivity. This last feature was a trait rather then a state feature, that is, characteristic of the patient even when not depressed. Individuals who are hypersensitive to rejection overreact to criticism, rejection, or even lack of positive attention by becoming excessively hurt, enraged, and depressed. Over time they also often become avoidant of situations where such rejection is likely to occur, and the condition thus bears some similarity to social phobia. In our treatment studies of atypical depression, phenelzine had proven helpful in reducing rejection hypersensitivity so that successfully treated patients became more resilient to the vicissitudes of interpersonal relationships. They also became less avoidant of situations where criticism or rejection might occur, further suggesting this medication might be useful in social phobia. Due to the resemblance between these features of atypical depression and social phobia, we wanted to examine whether phenelzine might be similarly effective in social phobia.

Our first trials were open rather than placebo-controlled, so that we could get a feel for the dose and time course for drug response in our social phobia patients. If the studies were positive, we would then move on to the placebo-controlled trials that were necessary for a definitive finding. If they were negative, there would be no need to proceed further. This is an approach to drug development that I still believe in but that, unfortunately, has been largely abandoned by the pharmaceutical industry. Most new drug development programs now proceed directly from phase I safety trials in normal volunteers to large placebo-controlled phase II trials in patient populations without ever establishing optimum doses or time course to response, let alone identifying which patient subtypes might be most responsive to a particular drug.

The open trials with phenelzine (Liebowitz *et al.* 1986) and atenolol (Gorman *et al.* 1985) were both positive, leading us to design a controlled trial comparing phenelzine and atenolol to placebo in social phobia (Liebowitz *et al.* 1992). We intentionally included patients with a broad range of interpersonal fears and avoidance, as well as those with more discrete performance fears, and made prospective determinations of the subtype to which each patient belonged.

The findings were quite informative. Among the 74 patients who completed the eight-week trial, the response rate to phenelzine was 64.5%, versus 30% for atenolol and 23% for placebo. Phenelzine was significantly better than atenolol or placebo, with no difference between the latter two. Patients with the generalized form of social phobia constituted 76% of the sample, and as a subgroup they were more responsive to phenelzine then to atenolol or placebo, confirming one of our major hypotheses.

The finding that phenelzine was useful for generalized social phobia helped to validate a broader definition of social phobia. The designation of a generalized subtype of social phobia was first included in DSM-III-R, and further elaborated in DSM-IV, which recognized two subtypes of the condition: a non-generalized form, consisting mainly of discrete performance anxiety, and a generalized form with more wide-ranging interpersonal anxiety and avoidance. Increasing recognition of the importance of the generalized subtype led to adoption in the DSM-IV of the term *social anxiety disorder* as an alternative name for social phobia.

The new term was thought to better reflect the clinical situation, common in child patients but also seen in adults, in which social or performance situations were dreaded but not necessarily avoided. The two terms are considered interchangeable, but since the mid 1990s *social anxiety disorder* has increasingly become the preferred terminology, and I will use it in the remainder of this chapter.

The non-generalized sample in our clinical trial comparing phenelzine and atenolol was unfortunately too small for separate outcome analyses, so it remained unclear as to whether atenolol or phenelzine were helpful for such patients. At the same time, clinical experience suggests that less cardiospecific beta-blockers such as propranolol are helpful for social phobic patients with predominantly public-speaking and other performance fears. The drugs help most if taken shortly before the performance and appear to reduce tremor, tachycardia, palpitations, and cracking of the voice. This helps lower overall anxiety, further reducing physical symptoms. Beta-blockers do not seem helpful for the anticipatory anxiety that often occurs the night before an important lecture; here benzodiazepines seem more helpful. To my knowledge, however, there have not been any placebo-controlled trials testing these clinical observations.

4.1.5 Development of the Liebowitz Social Anxiety Scale

To conduct clinical trials of social anxiety disorder, we also had to develop valid and reliable rating scales for this condition. The most important of these turned out to be the Liebowitz Social Anxiety Scale (LSAS), a 24-item measure that assesses anxiety and avoidance related to the performance and social situations that are commonly troubling to social anxiety disorder patients (Liebowitz 1987). As it assesses both anxiety and avoidance, the LSAS avoids the problem that has plagued the panic disorder field, where investigators have not known whether to make panic attacks or agoraphobia their primary outcome measure. Also, looking at both the experience of anxiety and the behavior of avoidance allows a rater to assess patients from several vantage points at the same time and to query any seeming inconsistencies in their responses. The LSAS has demonstrated good inter-rater reliability and high external validity (Heimberg *et al.*1999). It also allows for finer-graded assessments, where subscores for performance fear and avoidance versus social fear and avoidance can be determined. Masia, Klein, and Liebowitz have also

adapted the LSAS for children and adolescents; this instrument is called the Liebowitz Social Anxiety Scale for Children and Adolescents (LSAS-CA) (Masia-Warner *et al.* 2003). The LSAS and LSAS-CA have come to be used as the primary outcome measure for most pharmacological studies of social anxiety disorder over the past two decades.

4.2 Evolution of evidence-based treatment for social anxiety disorder

4.2.1 Subsequent medication trials in social anxiety disorder

Our study comparing phenelzine, atenolol, and placebo in social anxiety disorder became a model to be followed by subsequent trials. The acute phase was eight weeks long, which is probably sufficient to see improvement in social anxiety disorder, although current trials have extended this to 12 weeks. We also specified social anxiety disorder subtype, but most of our patients turned out to have the generalized form of the disorder. Virtually all subsequent medication trials in social anxiety disorder have primarily or exclusively studied patients with the generalized subtype.

Along with our trial there were several other placebo-controlled trials of phenelzine in social anxiety disorder, one comparing it to the benzodiazepine alprazolam (Gelernter *et al.* 1991), and another to the reversible MAO-A selective MAOI moclobemide (Versiani *et al.* 1992). Both found phenelzine to be highly effective. These were followed by several other moclobemide trials, which unfortunately did not confirm the strongly positive findings of the initial trial. There were also open trials with the tricyclic imipramine (Simpson *et al.* 1998a), with the anti-anxiety agent buspirone (Schneier *et al.* 1993), and with low doses of the MAO-B inhibitor selegiline (Simpson *et al.* 1998b). In each case investigators were looking for a medication as effective as phenelzine without the potential toxicity of a non-selective, irreversible MAOI. Unfortunately, none of these alternatives to phenelzine proved to be as useful for social anxiety disorder. While I was not the principal investigator on any of these trials, I was involved as a co-investigator in the first and one of the subsequent moclobemide trials, as well as in the trials of buspirone, selegiline, and imipramine.

What did turn out to be useful were the selective serotonin reuptake inhibitors (SSRIs) and serotonin–norepinephrine reuptake inhibitors (SNRIs). Following

Mannuzza, S., Schneier, F. R., Chapman, T. F., Liebowitz, M. R., Klein, D. F., & Fyer, A. J. (1995). Generalized social phobia: reliability and validity. *Archives of General Psychiatry* **52**, 230–237.

Marks, I. M., & Gelder, M. G. (1966). Different age of onset in varieties of phobias. *American Journal of Psychiatry*, **123**, 218–221.

Masia-Warner, C., Storch, E. A., Pincus, D. B., *et al.* (2003). Liebowitz Social Anxiety Scale for children and adolescents: an initial psychometric investigation. *Journal of the American Academy of Child and Adolescent Psychiatry*, **42**, 1076–1084.

Millon, T., Meagher, S., & Millon, C. (2004) *Personality Disorders in Modern Life*. Hoboken, NJ: Wiley.

Pande, A. C., Davidson, J. R. T., Jefferson, J. W., *et al.* (1999). Treatment of social phobia with gabapentin: a placebo-controlled study. *Journal of Clinical Psychopharmacology*, **19**, 341–348.

Regier, D. A., Myers, J. K., Kramer, M., *et al.* (1984). The NIMH Epidemiologic Catchment Area program: historical context, major objectives, and study population characteristics. *Archives of General Psychiatry*, **41**, 934–941.

Schneier, F. R., Saoud, J. B., Campeas, R., *et al.* (1993). Buspirone in social phobia. *Journal of Clinical Psychopharmacology*, **13**(4), 251–56.

Schneier, F. R., Heckelman, L. R., Garfinkel, R., *et al.* (1994). Functional impairment in social phobia. *Journal of Clinical Psychiatry*, **55**, 322–331.

Schneier, F. R., Liebowitz, M. R., Abi-Dargham, A., *et al.* (2000). Low dopamine D2 receptor binding potential in social phobia. *American Journal of Psychiatry*, **157**, 457–459.

Simpson, H. B., Schneier, F. R., Campeas, R., *et al.* (1998a). Imipramine in the treatment of social phobia. *Journal of Clinical Psychopharmacology*, **18**, 132–135.

Simpson, H. B., Schneier, F. R., Marshall, R. D., *et al.* (1998b). Low dose selegiline (L-Deprenyl) in social phobia. *Depression and Anxiety*, 7, 126–129.

Stein, M. B., Liebowitz, M. R., Lydiard, R. B., *et al.* (1998a). Paroxetine treatment of generalized social phobia (social anxiety disorder): a randomized, double-blind, placebo-controlled study. *JAMA*, **280**, 708–713.

Stein, M. B., Chartier, M. J., Hazen, A. L., *et al.* (1998b). A direct interview family study of generalized social phobia. *American Journal of Psychiatry*, **155**, 90–97.

Stein, M. B., Fyer, A. J., Davidson, J. R. T., Pollack, M. H., & Wiita, B. (1999). Fluvoxamine treatment of social phobia (social anxiety disorder): a double-blind, placebo-controlled study. *American Journal of Psychiatry*, **156**, 756–760.

Tillfors, M., Furmark, T., Marteinsdottir, I., *et al.* (2001). Cerebral blood flow in subjects with social phobia during stressful speaking tasks: a PET study. *American Journal of Psychiatry*, **158**, 1220–1226.

Versiani, M., Nardi, E., & Liebowitz, M. R. (1992). Phenelzine vs moclobemide in social phobia: a placebo controlled trial. *British Journal of Psychiatry*, **161**, 353–360.

Chapter 5

Anxiety as signal, symptom, and syndrome

Robert A. Glick, Steven P. Roose

5.1 Introduction

Anxiety is both an innate and a constructed response to perceived and anticipated threat. Depending upon the nature of the threat (a danger of what and to whom), on brain structure and function, and on personality organization, anxiety responses can be adaptive or maladaptive, normal or pathological, fleeting or sustained. A psychodynamic theory or any theory of affect, motivation for behavior, and technique in clinical work must offer a comprehensive and cogent framework to understand anxiety. Mental models have deepened in complexity as both clinical work and research have increased our knowledge about mental organization, motivations, memory, affect regulation, and the internalization of interpersonal relationships. Threats or dangers can be unconscious or conscious, internal or external, present or past, real or imagined. A number of variables, including temperament, determine an individual's perception of his or her environment, making it more or less threatening as well as influencing the threshold for and intensity of anxiety. Anxiety is an inescapable human experience and one by which we define our environment and ourselves. As meaning-seeking and meaning-creating creatures, we look to explain our subjective experience, including our sense of danger and vulnerability. Anxiety compels reason for our feelings and demands a response.

This chapter will explore anxiety as signal, symptom, and syndrome. Diagnosis and treatment of anxiety requires an approach that incorporates psychodynamic, genetic, and developmental perspectives. The chapter is divided into three sections. The first section describes the evolution of the major psychodynamic models of signal anxiety. Each model (1) assumes that signal anxiety is a response to an anticipated unconscious, intrapsychic danger, (2) defines the nature of and response to danger, and (3) describes the influence

of signal anxiety on mental development and structure. The next section considers research on temperament, genetics, and early trauma. Collectively, these forces shape the perception of danger and/or the experience of anxiety. Brain structure and function also have a significant impact on character development and adaptation. The final section presents a clinical approach to the diagnosis and treatment of anxiety, as signal, symptom, and syndrome.

5.2 Psychodynamic theories of signal anxiety

The major psychodynamic models of signal anxiety posit anxiety as a signal of unconscious, intrapsychic danger. An explanation of the origins, function, and impact of signal anxiety is nested in a more comprehensive theory of mind. As will be discussed, all models posit an unconscious process that includes (1) a form of threat, (2) signal anxiety, and (3) defense mechanism as response. The clinician infers this process from clinical phenomena such as symptoms, thoughts, affects, and behaviors. However, the psychodynamic clinician may infer this process of threat, signal anxiety, and defense from phenomena that are not considered anxiety symptoms. For example, a person shows up for an important appointment two hours late, having forgotten to check their schedule that morning. When telling this story, they are annoyed at themselves and perplexed but not exhibiting symptoms of anxiety. The psychodynamic clinician infers the unconscious process of defensive avoidance against an unconscious threat and would explore the threat that led to the behavior. This is a clinical application of the model of signal anxiety. The three models most relevant to the concept of signal anxiety in current clinical practice are the Freudian *structural* or *ego psychological*, the *object relations*, and the *self-psychological*.

Anxiety Disorders: Theory, Research, and Clinical Perspectives, ed. Helen Blair Simpson, Yuval Neria, Roberto Lewis-Fernández, Franklin Schneier. Published by Cambridge University Press. © Cambridge University Press 2010.

5.2.1 Freud's first traumatic and topographic models of anxiety

In 1886, when Sigmund Freud opened his clinical practice treating "nervous disorders," many of his patients suffered from "anxiety hysteria," a diagnosis that included patients with conversion symptoms, phobias, obsessive–compulsive disorders, and "anxiety neurosis or actual neurosis," or what we now call panic attacks and generalized anxiety disorders. Freud's trip to Paris in 1884 exposed him to the drama of Charcot's demonstration of hysteria and hypnosis and to the idea of mental dissociation and the unconscious. The concept of the unconscious had been much discussed in France for decades and was fundamental to the ideas of dissociation, trauma, and the use of hypnosis for the treatment of hysteria. The effects associated with traumatic memories could exist as powerful forces that could distort normal psychological function. Charcot assumed that some form of heritable, organic degeneracy predisposed patients to hysteria and made them receptive to the use of hypnosis as treatment. Freud was fascinated but unconvinced.

After 10 years of theorizing about his clinical experience, in which hypnosis had proved to be an ineffective treatment for most patients and the theory of dissociative states as the etiology of mental illness had proved inadequate, Freud made a remarkable conceptual leap. In *The Neuro-Psychoses of Defence* (1894) Freud described the topographic model of the psychical apparatus. This model divides the mind into unconscious, preconscious, and conscious domains. He also proposed the principle of "psychic determinism," which posits that thoughts, feelings, and symptoms are not random but rather arise from antecedent psychological processes and functions, and are therefore not simply meaningless biological events. Freud now believed that for most of his patients it was not a primary failure of brain function that led to phenomena such as the dissociation underlying anxiety hysteria. Instead, it was the failure to defend against the conscious awareness of some painful and morally unacceptable traumatic memory.

Freud initially believed the memories were of traumatic childhood sexual seduction. The conversion symptoms represented a somatic form of the memory and were a final attempt to ward off conscious awareness of the memory and its associated affects. Anxiety signals the dangers associated with the return of the repressed. However, he soon abandoned the universality of traumatic seduction and replaced it with the dangers associated with the expression of the infantile psychosexual drives. Anxiety disorders resulted from failure of repression of these drives, and thus danger was not from outside forces, but from internal pressures. The significance of the shift away from the dangers of memories of actual sexual seduction to the dangers of failure to control the expression of the infantile psychosexual drive was that everyone was vulnerable to the development of anxiety symptoms.

At the same time that Freud was developing new theories of the etiology of anxiety based on psychological defenses and the topographic model, he nonetheless retained a physiological (i.e., non-psychological) model for the etiology of forms of anxiety, called the actual neurosis (Freud 1896). In this model, sexual practices that fail to achieve adequate sexual satisfaction led to toxic build-up and alteration of the sexual drive, like wine turning to vinegar. The toxic derivatives of the drive produced symptoms of anxiety. In this model, the danger was physical, not psychological, and the anxiety was not a signal but a symptom. The anxiety neuroses, the syndromes of anxiety disorders and neurasthenia, were caused by coitus interruptus, anorgasmia, or abstinence, and behavioral modification of these problematic sexual practices was the treatment of choice.

Thus, in Freud's early theories, anxiety is *both* signal and symptom. One of the more subtle, yet far-reaching, implications of the signal anxiety model is that anxiety has an important psychological meaning, and understanding anxiety is a window into the internal structure of the mind. Even more far-reaching than the particulars of the model (which would soon change) is the fact that Freud's attention shifted from explaining forms of psychopathology in his few patients to a model of normal psychological life.

5.2.2 Freud's structural model of signal anxiety and its elaboration in ego psychology

By 1923, Freud had come to appreciate that his topographic model needed revision. Major parts of mental life, such as unconscious defense, transference, narcissism, and aggression, were not adequately addressed in the topographic model. In *The Ego and the Id* (1923) Freud proposed a new defining psychoanalytic theory, the structural theory, where he described the mind as composed of three structures or agencies – the id, ego, and superego. For Freud, each structure had a unique and essential role in mental life, and most of mental life occurred out of conscious awareness. The id was the unrelenting impersonal and irrational source of instinctual, psychosexual drives, the body's energic representative in the mind. The superego was the source of conscience, moral authority (harsh or otherwise), and the ego ideal, or the repository of the parental, societal, and cultural values. The ego was the executive function, the problem solver, dealing with the competing demands of the id, superego, and reality. The threat of intrapsychic conflict, for instance, between the id (drives) and superego (conscience), might generate anxiety that signals the ego to mobilize defenses. Critical to this model is that anxiety is not a symptom experienced by the patient but an unconscious signal to the ego to resolve the conflict. The patient may experience the consequences of the mobilization of defense as inhibitions, obsessions, hysteria, or "normal" asymptomatic life. In this model, when the ego is unable to effectively manage these intrapsychic conflicts, the result is symptom formation, and first among all symptoms is anxiety. The conscious experience of anxiety as a symptom occurs when defenses are insufficient.

Signal anxiety became a central concept in understanding mental life with the publication of *Inhibitions, Symptoms, and Anxiety* (Freud 1926). In this monograph, Freud outlined the developmental dangers that continue as the source of unconscious conflict in adult mental life. They are:

> the danger of psychical helplessness … when his ego is immature [traumatic overstimulation]; the danger of the loss of the object when he is still dependent on others [loss of mother as the source of care and protection]; the danger of castration [loss of genital, masturbatory pleasure]; and the fear of the superego to the latency period. Nevertheless, all these danger-situations and determinants of anxiety can persist side by side and cause the ego to react to them with anxiety at a period later than the appropriate one (Freud 1926, p. 142).

In the topographic model, the mechanism of action of the psychotherapeutic intervention is making conscious traumatic memories. In the structural model, the mechanism of action is making conscious the unconscious conflict between the drive derivative, or wish, and the threat of punishment. In the topographic model there is anxiety as a symptom but not unconscious anxiety. Anxiety as both symptom and signal begins with the structural model.

Anna Freud furthered her father's emphasis on the importance of defense as the ego's response to conflict. On the occasion of her father's 80th birthday in 1936, she published her monograph, *The Ego and the Mechanisms of Defence* (Freud 1936), in which she describes the unconscious defensive strategies and their role in development. This now familiar list of defense mechanisms was the ego's response to signal anxiety; they were the means by which first the child, and then the adult, allow for "safe" drive expression that is compatible with reality.

Following Anna Freud, the structure and function of the ego continued to be the primary focus of clinical work with patients and in theory building. Heinz Hartmann (1939) wrote *Ego Psychology and the Problem of Adaptation*, in which he outlined a comprehensive theory of normal ego structure and development. Hartmann believed the child comes into the world with the capacity to develop adaptive ego functions to fit into an average expectable environment. Signal anxiety remained the central response of the ego. However, Hartmann's emphasis on the adaptive functions of the ego is still clinically relevant to this day. The clinician understands symptomatic anxiety as an indicator of the ego's failure to adapt to the demands of internal and external reality.

5.2.3 Object relations theory and signal anxiety

Object relations theory posits an innate drive for attachment to others, and the expression of this drive creates interactions. Internalization of early interpersonal experience establishes the mental structures defined as internalized object relations. The term *object* refers to the mental representation of the other person in the interpersonal interaction. Internal object relations regulate internal and external adaptation. This model replaces id, ego, and superego with self and object representations as the primary mental structures. In this model, signal and symptomatic anxiety reflect threats to these internal object relations. The threat is to the object relation, not directly to an interpersonal relationship; however, a threat to the object relation may indirectly threaten the interpersonal relationship. For example, unconscious fear of losing the caretaking object can make one either overly dependent on or overly distrustful of others.

The nature of the threat varies with different object relations theorists. Melanie Klein (1964, 1975) believed that innate aggression was the threat to the internal object relations, and that the aggressive drive creates the fantasy of the bad or dangerous mother, which may not reflect the actual mothering. In contrast, D. W. Winnicott (1965), a pediatrician turned psychoanalyst, saw the actual mother–infant dyad as the crucial factor. The "holding environment" created by the mother for this dyad was crucial for stable self and object representations and mental organization, what Winnicott called the "true self," as opposed to the "false self." Insufficient, or "not good enough" mothering created the threat that led to the development of the defensive false self. While Winnicott did not use the term *signal anxiety*, in his model failure of the holding environment created inner distress and uncertainty about safety and self-boundaries. This is equivalent to signal anxiety that leads to the construction of defensive false self.

Finally, Otto Kernberg (1976) offered a model that incorporated drives, object relations, and ego psychology. In this developmental model, the earliest task is the building of stable object relations. The power of early aggressive drives threatens nascent object relations structures. This threat is met with the primitive defenses of denial, splitting, and projection, making the objects dangerous. Once a level of mental organization and structure is securely established, a maturing ego, developing out of early self and object representations, faces the threats of painful or dangerous affects derived from the drives. A maturing and stable ego structure can meet threats with defenses that maintain stable self and object representation structures. Defenses define the level of personality organization, the nature of the full spectrum of psychopathology.

5.2.4 Self psychology and dangers to the self

Self psychology, formulated by Heinz Kohut (1971, 1977) focuses on the concept of the self. Whereas the Freudian ego is a set of adaptive mental functions, and in object relations theory the self is a representation of oneself in relation to others, self psychology has a broader concept of self that subsumes all mental structures, and functions that serve to maintain stable self-esteem and identity. All defensive functions are subservient to the stability of self-organization. In this model, danger to the self comes primarily from the developmental failure of appropriate caregiver empathic response in building stable and robust self-organization. The infant requires caregivers to optimally mirror the infant's developing sense of self. In normal development, empathic failures are inevitable and necessary to promote self-growth and adaptation. When there is either severe or sustained empathic failure, that is, traumatic failures, this constitutes the threat, and signal anxiety prompts a specific pattern of narcissistic defense mechanisms, i.e., idealization and devaluation. The clinician working within the self-psychological model considers clinical phenomena such as empty and disappointing adult relationships, fragile self-esteem, grandiosity, and a pervasive sense of meaninglessness and isolation as consequences of the pathological narcissistic defenses. When these defenses fail, symptoms of intense anxiety, often referred to as disintegration anxiety or loss of the sense of self, occur.

In summary, the psychodynamic models of the mind all include an unconscious process of threat, signal anxiety, and response. The nature of the threat and the pattern of response is defined by the theoretical model of mental structure and function. If the response is not adequate to eliminate the threat, then anxiety as a symptom results. The concept of signal anxiety guides the clinician in uncovering the unconscious conflicts and the threats to mental structures and functions. Helping patients understand that their current problems reflect, in part, maladaptive or ineffective solutions to unconscious conflicts offers potentially effective therapeutic strategies.

5.3 Neurobiological factors in anxiety as signal, symptom, and syndrome

Neurobiological factors also contribute to the development and expression of anxiety symptoms and syndromes. Variables most germane to the psychodynamic theories previously reviewed include "temperament," gene–environment interactions, and the impact of early experiences on brain structure and function. Although early psychodynamic models of the mind do not explicitly cite the role of temperament, i.e., non-dynamic – "biological" – variables, the existence of such variables is implicit in concepts such as ego weakness or strength, and they are explicitly acknowledged by later object relations theorists.

Within neurobiology, there is a differentiation between the fear response and anxiety:

> Like fear, anxiety is a normal and adaptive response that ensures dangers are either avoided or reduced through preparation and vigilance. A well-defined threatening stimulus that is immediately present or imminent in the environment elicits a fear response. When the threat

53

is more poorly defined and temporally remote … the behavioral state it elicits is typically referred to as anxiety (Sullivan *et al.* 2009).

Importantly, anxiety itself is divided into state and trait conditions. State anxiety is provoked by a clear stimulus and is transient. Trait anxiety is continuous and exists irrespective of the presence or absence of a discrete stimulus. Trait anxiety is also often considered to be a dimension of temperament.

With respect to temperament, infant/child research has demonstrated that among young children there is significant variability in reaction to novel social situations (Kagan *et al.* 1987). Some children, approximately 15%, are keenly averse to novelty, whereas at the other extreme 15% are novelty-seeking. This dimension of novelty aversion or novelty seeking is accompanied by differences in autonomic nervous system function, such as heart-rate variability, which represent the moment-to-moment interplay between sympathetic and parasympathetic tone (Kagan *et al.* 1988). That novelty aversion means that the child will have a diathesis to experience greater anxiety is a cogent hypothesis. What is the impact on the development and the experience of the infant/child if he or she interacts with the world through the lens of heightened anxiety? In such circumstances, the infant cannot be adequately reassured or comforted by the interaction between mother and child, and the mother cannot feel confident and effective. The crucial mutual reassurance derived from the interpersonal experience of pleasure is diminished. Thus, trait anxiety, or an increased diathesis to experience anxiety, can shape interactions, and it can create intrapsychic conflict. This can create fears of rejection, abandonment, humiliation, and damage. Anxiety can create events, not simply be a reaction to them. If anxiety-prone temperament predictably influences interactions, it creates the expectation of a negative experience (anticipatory anxiety), and that can lead to patterns of behavior such as avoidance or hostility. However, biology is not destiny. Studies have shown that consistent parental encouragement can significantly modify the child's behavior in children with high aversion to novelty as manifested by extreme shyness.

Thus, temperament contributes to the construction of a structured and replicated pattern of response to perceived internal and external dangers. This response pattern is the very definition of character. There are other dimensions that can manifest as traits, including mood, cognition, perception, etc. All of these dimensions can impact early interpersonal interactions,

internalized object relations, as well as a pattern of ego defense mechanisms in response to signal anxiety.

Studies of gene–environment interaction further support the significant effect of traits on the development of mental structures and psychopathology. Arguably the most germane study with respect to anxiety is that by Caspi and colleagues (2003) where, in a cohort of women, the genotype for the serotonin transporter was determined. Subjects are either homozygous for the short allele, signifying less-than-optimal serotonin function, heterozygous, or homozygous for the long allele, signifying robust serotonin activity (i.e., not an anxious temperament or, in other words, a healthy and flexible ego). Women homozygous for the short allele who suffered no abuse in early life did not develop a higher than expected rate of depression. However, in this same group there was a direct increase in the rate of depression with increasing exposure to abusive experiences. In contrast, women homozygous for the long allele did not express a higher-than-expected rate of depression irrespective of whether or not they had experienced significant abuse. "Good" serotonin function protects against the impact of bad experiences; the long allele serves as a "resilience" gene. In contrast, negative life events interacted with short-allele genotype to express a mood disorder.

The importance of gene–environment interactions cannot be overemphasized, and it is a model that allows for a level of complexity that fits the human condition. It could be argued that abuse is not an independent variable separate from the genotype; for example, an infant homozygous for the short allele may be inconsolable and thus more frustrating to the mother and therefore more likely to elicit an abusive response. The mother herself may be homozygous for the short allele and may have married a man more likely to be homozygous because of assortative mating. The model allows for a bidirectional interaction between infant and mother, between temperament and response, and between life experience and the development of pathology. Perhaps what is most significant about this model is that it can be applied to understanding normal development as well as pathology. Just as Freud sought to develop a theory of mind that explained normal psychological functioning as well as pathology, an understanding of the gene–environment interaction can fulfill the same goal.

The gene–environment interaction model of development is compatible with both Hartmann's concept of adaptation to the average expectable environment and the object relations model of good-enough parenting.

For example, even in the infant homozygous for the long allele, the infant–mother interaction inevitably has moments when the mother misunderstands or cannot adequately meet the demands of the infant, moments of empathic failure. The adaptation of the infant and mother to empathic failures is critical for the development of the self. If empathic failure stimulates the infant to further its own independence in order to achieve an experience of pleasure, then it is a beneficial moment in development. In fact, a dyad in which there is no empathic failure, no frustration, may inhibit normal separation and development. An appreciation of temperament and gene–environment interactions have contributed to a revision of early psychodynamic models of infant–mother interaction in which variation in the infant's temperament and the influence of this variable on the interaction was not sufficiently appreciated.

Another research finding that is now comfortably incorporated into a modern psychodynamic model of anxiety and development is the evidence that early stressful experiences produce enduring effects on brain structure and function (Brown *et al.* 1986, Dawson *et al.* 2000, Heim *et al.* 2000, 2001, Kuhn & Schanberg 1991). This effect is manifest in the response to stressful stimuli throughout adult life. Supporting data come from studies of rodent, non-human primate, and even human subjects. Rodent and non-human primate studies document that infants directly stressed during rearing or raised by a stressed mother have heightened behavioral responses to stress in adulthood (Coplan *et al.* 2001, Gutman & Nemeroff 2002, Hofer 1975, 1996, Mirescu *et al.* 2004). In some experimental paradigms, this heightened reactivity is significantly diminished by the administration of a selective serotonin reuptake inhibitor. Additionally, depressed women who have experienced abuse early in life have a hyperactive response in the amygdala to an experimentally induced stress (Drevets *et al.* 1997, Davis & Whalen 2001). This hyperactive response is not present in normal controls or in depressed women who did not experience early abuse. In clinical language, repeated stressful experiences in early life construct a brain that will respond intensely to stress in adulthood.

Imaging techniques have been used to illustrate the presence of unconscious processes that to date have only been hypothesized, specifically that unconscious affects (signal anxiety) are a crucial determinant of behavior. In a very sophisticated paradigm, Etkin and colleagues (2005) measured baseline anxiety in a group of normal subjects and then exposed them to a series of fearful faces. Fearful faces will reliably stimulate activity in the amygdala, but the unique aspect of this experiment was that the faces were presented in two different ways, one that represented conscious activity and one that represented unconscious processing. The unconscious processing was achieved through a procedure called backward masking, in which the fearful face is presented very rapidly and then is immediately followed by the presentation of a neutral image. The fearful face is presented so briefly that the stimuli cannot be recorded consciously, and, if reacted to, the reaction represents unconscious stimulation. There was an increase in amygdala activity after the presentation of fearful faces, and this increase was directly correlated to the baseline trait anxiety scores. However, this finding was only true when the fearful faces were presented so briefly that they could only be processed unconsciously.

5.4 A clinical approach

Knowledge of the psychobiology of fear, anxiety, and anxiety disorders (as reviewed in section 5.3) deepens the clinician's hypotheses about patients, how they came to be who they are, and why they are coming for help. When patients tell the history of their illnesses, they tell the narratives of their lives. We are the authors of a life narrative, a story that includes a cogent, albeit often significantly incomplete and incorrect, explanation of why and when we feel anxious. These narratives include theories of etiology – the patient's stories of "this is what happened to me, this is what has made me anxious, and this is how I cope." Much of what happens in treatment is a revision of the narrative to include the new story lines that are written when the patient and therapist consider the patient's life using a developmental model that recognizes gene–environment interactions, dimensions of temperament, and structural changes in the brain that result from early experience. This approach enhances the clinician's capacity to assess, hypothesize about, and empathize with the patient.

Many symptomatic patients were forced to make adaptations to internal and external threats in early childhood. The clinician appreciates that the patient retains the best available adaptive response from childhood even though the persistence of this pattern of behavior in adult life may result in disabling symptoms. For many patients, both their anxiety symptoms and their means of coping with anxiety are a familiar, even defining, component of personal identity. For these many reasons, behavior is hard to change.

Ironically, the treatment of symptomatic anxiety may create an anxiety of its own, the anxiety about change. Though there are effective treatments for anxiety disorders, the clinical results are often quite disappointing, and even surprisingly poor. Patients stop taking medications or drop out of treatment; they stop treatment even when, or especially when, they acknowledge it is helpful. Non-compliance with treatment may reflect the patient's experience of the treatment as a threat.

The resistance to treatment is paralleled by the hope of relief. Patient expectancy, which refers to patients' beliefs about how treatment will affect them, is hypothesized to be a major mechanism of the placebo effect. For example, when trying to understand response rates in randomized controlled trials (RCTs) of medication, the clinician needs to consider the patient's "state of mind." A substantial portion of the change observed in patients receiving antidepressants for major depression (MDD) results from the placebo effect rather than the specific effects of medication. A meta-analysis of placebo-controlled RCTs of antidepressants reported that the placebo groups in these trials averaged 1.5 standard deviation units of improvement, which was 75% of the improvement shown in the antidepressant groups (Kim & Holloway 2003).

The magnitude of the placebo effect in antidepressant clinical trials is influenced by what patients know about the study design – what patients are told about the study influences their expectations of effects. Patients who know they have a high probability of receiving an active treatment will have a higher response rate to the active treatment than patients who know they have a 50% chance of receiving a placebo and a 50% chance of receiving an active treatment. In a meta-analysis of 90 antidepressant comparator (i.e., medication vs. medication) or placebo-controlled RCTs, the odds of response and remission were significantly higher if the patient received the same medication in a comparator as opposed to a placebo-controlled trial (Rutherford et al. 2009, Sneed et al. 2008).

Sitting across from the patient, the clinician also has unconscious processes that may effect diagnostic assessment and treatment. Recent studies of patients entering psychoanalysis have used structured interviews and rating scales to assess Axis I mood and anxiety disorders. In a sample of 100 patients applying for treatment to a clinic that offered only psychodynamic

psychotherapy or psychoanalysis, 56% had current major depression or dysthymia, and 25% had either panic attacks, social anxiety disorder (SAD), or generalized anxiety disorder (GAD). The mean Hamilton Rating Scale for Anxiety (HAM-A) score of patients seeking treatment was 14.6 ± 8.1 (Caligor et al. 2009). Thus, this patient population had significant anxiety symptoms as well as a high rate of disorder. However, there was a quite striking difference between the clinician's recognition of Axis I mood versus anxiety disorders. The clinician's diagnosis of mood disorder was concordant with the Structured Clinical Interview for DSM-IV (SCID) diagnosis in 60% of cases. In contrast, the clinician's diagnosis of anxiety disorder was concordant with the SCID diagnosis in only 20% of cases ($\chi^2 = 8.33$, df = 3, $p < 0.005$) (Garfinkle et al. 2009). Thus, the psychodynamic clinicians in this study were significantly more likely to diagnose a mood disorder than an anxiety disorder. The prominent role played by the construct of signal anxiety in psychoanalytic theory may impede the recognition of an anxiety disorder.

Many patients present with the acute onset of anxiety symptoms but do not meet the criteria for an Axis I anxiety disorder. These patients come because the anxiety is a "new thing" in their lives. They have thought of themselves as resilient and not anxious. They often believe they know the source of their anxiety and may feel embarrassed or ashamed at having difficulty and needing help. The source can be something challenging, an anticipated event that represents a developmental milestone, like having a child, or a loss, like failing an exam or suffering a rejection. These patients fear that they will not be able to meet the challenge or deal with the stress. For example, a young married attorney develops anxiety when starting her first job. She fears the stress on her marriage. Evaluation reveals no prior psychopathology and a history of well-functioning relationships. Helping her see that being anxious may be appropriate and "normal" in this life circumstance relieves the anxiety and self-doubt. The most apt diagnosis is often adjustment disorder with anxiety features. For this patient, a consultation that emphasizes clarification, psychoeducation, reassurance, and support may be sufficient.

However, in some patients the anxiety triggered by a life event, e.g., getting a promotion or being fired, can be particularly intense and persistent despite efforts at reassurance and support. The symptoms may result from failure to manage a recurrent unconscious conflict. Consultation may reveal a history of developmental trauma or temperamental vulnerability and a rigid personality structure. For example, a young man presents with recurrent anxiety symptoms and a history of failed relationships. Family history reveals a volatile early home environment, a parental divorce in his adolescence, and a pervasive sense of insecurity. The acute precipitant of the anxiety is a new romantic relationship with an available and appropriate partner. He knows that he is worried about being rejected and feels a need to protect himself. The patient experiences the anxiety as painful and disruptive, but he does not meet criteria for an anxiety disorder. In this patient the defenses in response to the signal anxiety cannot contain the intrapsychic conflict, and symptomatic anxiety erupts.

The first case is an illustration of transient anxiety that is a common experience and should not be considered pathological. The second case illustrates anxiety as symptom, and despite the fact that the patient may not meet criteria for anxiety syndrome, this patient needs treatment.

5.5 Conclusion

Anxiety is a universal experience, a symptom, and a signal. Anxiety warns us of danger, real or imagined, and, paradoxically, treatment can be experienced as threatening. As characterized by Eric Kandel:

> Anxiety is a normal inborn response either to threat – to one's person, attitudes, or self-esteem – or to the absence of people or objects that assure and signify safety. Anxiety has subjective as well as objective manifestations … Anxiety as a signal prepares the individual for fight or flight if the danger is external. For internal danger, Freud suggested that defensive mental mechanisms substitute for actual flight or withdrawal. I would only make a cautionary comment here: simply because aspects of anxiety may be learned and thus acquired does not exclude the possible contribution of a genetic predisposition to anxiety. In fact, what might be inherited is the predisposition to learn certain stimulus relationships (Kandel 1983).

References

Brown, G. W., Harris, T. O., & Bifulco, A. (1986). Long-term effects of early loss of parent. In M. Rutter, C. E. Izard, & P. B. Read, eds., *Depression in Young People: Developmental and Clinical Perspectives*. New York, NY: Guilford Publications.

Caligor, E., Stern, B. L., Hamilton, M., *et al.* (2009). Why we recommend analytic treatment for some patients and not for others. *Journal of the American Psychoanalytic Association*, 57, 677–694.

Caspi, A., Sugden, K., Moffitt, T. E., *et al.* (2003). Influence of stress on depression: moderation by a polymorphism in the 5-HTT gene. *Science*, 301, 386–389.

Coplan, J.D., Smith, E.L.P., Altemus, M., *et al.* (2001). Variable for aging demand rearing: sustained elevations in C1 sternal cerebrospinal fluid corticotropin-releasing factor concentrations in adult primates. *Biological Psychiatry*, 50, 200–204.

Davis, M., & Whalen, P. J. (2001) The amygdala: vigilance and emotion. *Molecular Psychiatry*, 6, 13–34.

Dawson, G., Ashman, S. B., & Carver, L. J. (2000). The role of early experience in shaping behavioral and brain development and its implications for social policy. *Developmental Psychopathology*, 12, 695–712.

Drevets, W. C., Price, J. L., Simpson, J. R., *et al.* (1997). Subgenual prefrontal cortex abnormalities in mood disorders. *Nature*, 386, 824–827.

Etkin, A., Pittenger, C., Polan, H.J., & Kandel, E.R. (2005). Toward a neurobiology of psychotherapy: basic science and clinical applications. *Journal of Neuropsychiatry and Clinical Neuroscience*, 17, 145–158.

Freud, A. (1936). *The Ego and the Mechanisms of Defence*. London: Hogarth Press.

Freud, S. (1894). *The Neuro-Psychoses of Defence*. The Standard Edition of the Complete Psychological Works of Sigmund Freud, Volume III (1893–1899). London: Hogarth Press.

Freud, S. (1896). *Further Remarks on the Neuro-Psychoses of Defence*. The Standard Edition of the Complete Psychological Works of Sigmund Freud, Volume III (1893–1899). London: Hogarth Press.

Freud, S. (1923). *The Ego and the Id*. The Standard Edition of the Complete Psychological Works of Sigmund Freud, Volume IXX, 1–66. London: Hogarth Press.

Freud, S. (1926). *Inhibitions, Symptoms, and Anxiety*. The Standard Edition of the Complete Psychological Works of Sigmund Freud, Volume XX. London: Hogarth Press.

Garfinkle, S., Hamilton, M., Wininger, L., Garfinkle, M., & Roose, S. (2009). Diagnosis and medication of mood disorders vs anxiety disorders by psychoanalytic candidates. New Research, Meeting of the American Psychoanalytic Association of New York.

Gutman, D., & Nemeroff, C. B. (2002). Neurobiology of early life stress: rodent studies. *Seminars in Clinical Neuropsychiatry*, 7, 89–95.

Hartmann, H. (1939). *Ego Psychology and the Problem of Adaptation*. New York, NY: International Universities Press.

Heim, C., Newport, D. J., Heit, S., *et al.* (2000). Pituitary–adrenal and autonomic responses to stress in women after sexual and physical abuse in childhood. *JAMA*, 284, 592–597.

Heim, C., Newport, D. J., Bonsall, R., Miller, A. H., & Nemeroff, C. B. (2001). Altered pituitary-adrenal responses to provocative challenge tests in adult survivors of childhood abuse. *American Journal of Psychiatry*, **158**, 575–581.

Hofer, M. A. (1975). Studies on how early maternal separation produces behavioral change in young rats. *Psychosomatic Medicine*, **37**, 245–64.

Hofer, M. A. (1996). Multiple regulators of ultrasonic vocalization in the infant rat. *Psychoneuroendocrinology*, **21**, 203–217.

Kagan, J., Reznick, J., & Snidman, N. (1987). The physiology and psychology of behavioral inhibition in children. *Child Development*, **58**, 1459–1473.

Kagan, J., Reznick, J., & Snidman, N. (1988). Biological bases of childhood shyness. *Science*, **240**, 167–171.

Kandel, E. (1983). From metapsychology to molecular biology: explorations into the nature of anxiety. *American Journal of Psychiatry*, **40**, 1277–1293. Reprinted in *Psychiatry, Psychoanalysis, and the New Biology of Mind*. Washington, DC: American Psychiatric Publishing, 2005.

Kernberg, O. (1976). *Object Relations Theory and Clinical Psychoanalysis*. New York, NY: Jason Aronson.

Kim, S. Y., & Holloway, R. G. (2003) Burdens and benefits of placebos in antidepressant clinical trials: a decision and cost-effectiveness analysis. *American Journal of Psychiatry*, **160**, 1272–1276.

Klein, M. (1964). *Contributions to Psychoanalysis, 1921–1945*. New York, NY: McGraw-Hill.

Klein, M. (1975) *Envy and Gratitude and Other Works: 1946–1963*. New York, NY: Delacorte.

Kohut, H. (1971). *The Analysis of Self*. New York, NY: International Universities Press

Kohut, H. (1977). *The Restoration of the Self*. New York, NY: International Universities Press

Kuhn, C. M., & Schanberg, S. M. (1991). Stimulation in infancy and brain development. In B. J. Carroll, ed., *Psychopathology and the Brain*. New York, NY: Raven Press.

Mirescu, C., Peters, J. D., & Gould, E. (2004). Early life experience alters response of adult neurogenesis to stress. *Nature Neuroscience*, **7**, 841–846.

Rutherford, B., Sneed, J., & Roose, S. P. (2009). Does study design influence outcome? The effects of placebo control and treatment duration in antidepressant trials. *Psychotherapy and Psychosomatics*, **78**, 172–181.

Sneed, J. R., Rutherford, B. R., Rindskopf, D., *et al.* (2008). Design makes a difference: a meta-analysis of antidepressant response rates in placebo-controlled versus comparator trials in late life depression. *American Journal of Geriatric Psychiatry*, **16**, 65–73.

Sullivan, G., Debiec, J., Bush, D., Lyons, D., & LeDoux, J. (2009). The neurobiology of fear and anxiety. In D. Charney, & E. Nestler, eds., *Neurobiology of Mental Illness*. New York, NY: Oxford University Press.

Winnicott, D. W. (1965). *The Maturational Process and the Facilitating Environment*. London: Hogarth Press.

Chapter

6

New concepts in the evolution and development of anxiety

Myron A. Hofer

6.1 Introduction

Recent advances in our understanding of the relationship between development and evolution provide psychiatry with a unifying theory that can integrate social, psychological, and biological approaches to the understanding of how mental illness develops. These advances have resulted from discoveries in a number of different areas: the regulation of gene expression during development, the fossil record of evolution, the application of DNA mapping to phylogeny, field studies that for the first time have observed and analyzed in detail the process of rapid evolutionary change, the new concept of development as a major source of diversity in evolution, the maturation of the field of sociobiology, and, finally, the discovery of laboratory models of anxiety in a range of organisms representing our phylogenetically distant ancestors.

In addition to the advances in the fields of evolution and development, major changes have taken place in our concept of the emotions, changes that facilitate application of the new evolutionary concepts to anxiety. In traditional theory, emotions were considered as discrete entities, each defined by certain characteristic behavioral and physiological response patterns (Darwin 1872, Izard 1977, Lewis & Brooks-Gunn 1979). In development and in evolution, emotions were believed to emerge as units and to follow the appearance of new cognitive advances or structures. The newer view is a functional or transactional one (Lazarus 1991, Campos *et al.* 1994). Emotions are seen as processes existing at the interface of the organism and its transactions with the environment. They are defined in terms of particular characteristics of the functional relationships between the organism and the environment, serving to regulate (establish, maintain, or disrupt) these relationships. Different families of emotions can be defined in terms of the

nature, dynamics, and adaptive role of those transactions rather than in terms of certain invariant features of the response. In development and in evolution, each family of emotions emerges gradually, together with its cognitive components, following growth in the complexity of the organism.

Thus, in this chapter, I view anxiety as an organized group of adaptive functions by which an organism senses, evaluates, and responds to cues of danger in its external (or internal) environment. Anxiety disorders then can be approached in research and treatment as failures of these adaptive processes at any one of a number of possible points in their development. In the first section, I review recent advances in our understanding of evolution in relation to development as this can be applied to the origins of adult anxiety and its disorders. I then use these conceptual advances to interpret recent research findings on the development of early separation-induced anxiety in young rats, and to search for evolutionary clues in an analysis of human panic disorder and its early developmental roots.

6.2 New advances in understanding evolution and development

The application of evolutionary concepts to our understanding of emotions, begun by Darwin with the publication of *The Expression of the Emotions in Man and Animals* (1872), strongly influenced many later developments in psychology, such as psychoanalysis and ethology. Subsequently, Haldane (1932), Hamilton (1964), Trivers (1974), and finally Wilson (1975) brought about a synthesis of ethology, evolutionary biology, and population genetics, which Wilson called "sociobiology." Comparative psychology and ecology have been transformed as a result (Alcock 2001), but the application of this thinking to psychiatric illness has been delayed, first by a reluctance within the field to accept the idea of genetic influences on aspects of the human mind and personality, and subsequently by a concept of mental illness limited to the medical models of single gene mutations, environmental toxins, and degenerative disease. In the last decade, however, there are signs of an awakening interest within medicine, and particularly psychiatry, in the usefulness of an evolutionary approach (Nesse & Williams 1996, McGuire & Troisi 1998). This approach is becoming more widespread with the discovery of increasingly complex forms of genetic regulation and their roles in psychiatric illness.

The mechanism of evolution, natural selection, is primarily supported by evidence provided in the remarkable variation in domesticated species (Darwin 1868), in the range of available laboratory animals resulting from selective breeding by scientists (De Fries *et al.* 1981), and most recently, in the field studies of rapid evolution under the natural pressures of yearly climatic change (Grant 1986). Because these forms of selection have been convincingly shown to alter behavioral and biological traits of small groups of animals in a rapid and powerful manner over a few generations, this constitutes the most direct evidence we have as to how the emotions, and anxiety itself, may have evolved over geological time (one such study, using repeated selection in our laboratory, will be described below).

The new field of evolutionary developmental biology, or "evo-devo," emphasizes the role of development in creating the variation necessary for selection to act upon, as will be described in the next section. Extreme forms of anxiety may be thought of as a by-product of this property of development. Thus, some individuals with anxiety disorders in civilized society today may represent potentially adaptive variations that would be well suited to extreme conditions of societal disintegration, whereas others are essentially flawed by-products or "failed experiments" of the essential genetic/developmental mechanisms that create variation in evolution. See section 6.2.1 for more on the problem of distinguishing "normal" from "pathological" anxiety.

Discoveries in the genetic mechanisms of early development in the past five years have provided the basis for an integration of the fields of evolutionary and developmental biology (for a review, see Carroll 2005), as predicted many years earlier by Gottlieb (1987). We have learned that genes are not only instruments of inheritance in evolution, but also targets of molecular signals originating both within the organism and in the environment outside it. These epigenetic signals

regulate development. Rapid progress in understanding these molecular genetic mechanisms has revealed an unexpected potential for plasticity that can enable a relatively few evolutionarily conserved cellular processes to be linked together by differential gene expression into a variety of adaptive patterns that respond to environmental changes as well as to genetic mutations. The resulting plasticity allows a variety of developmental pathways, evident in both behavior and physiology, to be generated from the same genome. This discovery of a central role for the regulation of gene expression in development has at last provided a specific mechanism for the familiar, but uninformative, concept of "gene–environment interaction" in the origin of adult behavior patterns and vulnerability to mental illness. An example of this novel developmental process is described in section 6.2.2 below.

We know surprisingly little about the development of anxiety in the individual, and this may well be an area in which new evolutionary concepts can be helpful in gaining an understanding of human anxiety. For it is becoming evident, through molecular/genetic as well as new fossil evidence, that one of the most powerful mechanisms for producing rapid, major changes in evolution is through alterations in the developmental paths of individual traits (West-Eberhard 2003). For example, each system within the organism and each behavioral trait has its own developmental schedule for expression, one strongly shaped by genetic timing mechanisms ("heterochrony"). When one of these regulatory genes is altered by selection or mutation, the developmental schedule for that trait is shifted in relation to others. A single mutation in the timing of gene expression can have major effects on the phenotype that are nevertheless not lethal because of accommodation by the regulatory nature of other developing systems. In this way, the principle of heterochrony serves to unite the processes of evolution with those of development and helps us to understand the heterogeneity of the manifestations of anxiety over the course of development and within individuals of a given age.

Such processes at work during hominid evolution, in response to a varied range of environmental demands at different ages, may help account for the variation in the forms and manifestations of anxiety throughout development in today's population. For example, the appearance of stranger anxiety at about age six months in a broad range of human cultures and child-rearing practices has been related to the appearance of the capacity for rapid crawling and exploratory behavior at that age, which can expose the infant to potentially dangerous strangers (Marks & Nesse 1994). Thus, the appearance of particular forms of anxiety at different ages, along a "developmental path," may be traced back to age-specific evolutionary forces in our distant past. An example of the formation of such a developmental path, using experimental selection over generations in the rat, is described below (section 6.4).

6.2.1 Anxiety as adaptation and illness

One of the major difficulties that psychiatrists have with evolutionary accounts of the origin of major mental illnesses is the apparently incapacitating effects of these conditions, effects that should have led to their disappearance from the gene pool in the more hostile environments of our prehistoric past. It is tempting to suppose that although evolution may have given humans a wide range of adaptive patterns of response, this cannot account for clinical conditions such as panic disorder. How can evolution account for such extreme forms of behavior, without the intervention of a demonstrably pathological process such as infection, or toxin, or a recent single gene mutation?

This question has several possible answers, and one of them goes back to one of the principal lines of evidence used by Darwin in the first chapter of *The Origin of Species by Means of Natural Selection* (1859) and presented in detail in the two volumes he published a decade later (1868) as the most compelling evidence for his theory. Overwhelming evidence indicates that when plant seeds or young animals are brought from their natural environments in the wild into the conditions of domestication, a remarkable increase occurs in the degree of variation between individual members, with the appearance of new traits or the exaggeration of traits seen in the wild. Though he could suggest no mechanism at the time, Darwin reasoned that these new variants appeared because of the relaxation of the harsh and limiting selective pressures on the developing young in the wild and because of the developmental effects of the novel environments of domestication, such as high levels of nutrition, that facilitated the expression of novel traits. Today, we know that such facilitation occurs when developmental plasticity reveals latent developmental pathways and "unmasks" novel genes that had previously remained unexpressed (Kirschner & Gerhart 2005).

With the pervasive relaxation of natural selection pressures brought about by civilization, and in response to the novel environments thrust on humans

by technological change, it appears likely that conditions are present for the expression of great variability in human traits. Thus, patients with incapacitating anxiety may represent extreme examples of the results of the increased variation of humans under the influence of civilization. Since many mechanisms of variation are essentially random, some of these may represent "failed experiments" of evolution that would be maladaptive under any conditions we can imagine. Others could be adaptive to some extreme conditions but are "costly" to survival in current conditions.

The difficulty in distinguishing evolutionarily maladaptive from adaptive anxiety has a parallel in our current diagnostic system, in which the standard for inclusion of a behavior or state of mind as a disorder may simply depend upon whether the individual or caregiver seeks treatment for it from a healthcare professional. Although the distinction between anxiety and its disorders may often reside "in the eye of the beholder," a better understanding of the mechanisms of development in evolution should allow us eventually to separate out disorders as a class of cases that involve highly unusual mechanisms of development – for instance, like those that differentiate the growth processes of (healthy) scar tissue formation from those of cancer.

6.2.2 Developmental plasticity and the evolution of alternative adult phenotypes

Recent research in animals and humans is beginning to reveal some of the mechanisms for the emergence of different patterns of behaviors in adults that are closely associated with anxiety disorders. Clinically, we refer to such patterns as different temperaments or personalities. One of the results of this research has been the discovery of the role of differences in parenting patterns as a crucial "switch" for alternative developmental pathways. The parents' response to their environmental conditions plays a predictive role in the pre-adaptation of the young to the changed conditions. The evidence for this comes from both human and animal studies, and I briefly review the animal research, which is more recent and is beginning to reveal the underlying molecular/genetic mechanisms.

The discovery of specific interactions between mother and infant laboratory rats that regulate individual physiological and behavioral systems of the infant throughout early development, reviewed by Hofer (2003), led to studies on the long-term effects of different patterns and levels of maternal behavior on anxiety-related physiology and behavior in adult offspring. In a series of recent studies, Meaney (2007) and his group (Cameron *et al.* 2005) have found alternative phenotypes in the offspring of two groups of dams within the colony that showed relatively high or low levels of maternal licking, grooming, and arched nursing. The long-term effects of relatively high or low levels of these particular mother–infant interactions were as evident in cross-fostered pups that had been born to mothers of the opposite type, as they were in the mother's own offspring, ruling out a predominantly genetic (or prenatal) mechanism for the phenotypic differences between groups of offspring.

Low levels of these particular maternal interactions resulted in more fearful adult offspring, with heightened startle responses and intense adrenocortical responses to stress. The capacity of these adults to learn to avoid signals of danger was enhanced, whereas their spatial learning and memory were relatively impaired, reflected in slower hippocampal synapse growth. Young adults in this group also showed more rapid sexual maturation (vaginal opening), greater sexual receptivity, more rapidly repeated sexual encounters, and a higher rate of pregnancy following mating, than offspring of high-level-interaction mothers. These differences appear to be suited to a harsh, unpredictable, and threatening environment with few resources, an environment in which intense defensive responses, fearful avoidance of threats, and early, increased sexual activity will be likely to result in maximal survival and more offspring born in the next generation.

In turn, high levels of these mother–infant interactions lead to the development of exploratory behavior, rather than fear of novelty, a predisposition to learn spatial maps rather than avoidance responses, and lower levels of adrenocortical responses and slower sexual development – traits that would be a liability in very harsh environments but allow optimal adaptation to a stable, supportive environment with abundant new opportunities and resources. In non-human primates, Jeremy Coplan has shown that a disturbed mother–juvenile interaction, produced by subjecting the mother to a variable schedule of food delivery, can lead to abnormalities in regulation of the hypothalamic–adrenocortical axis and disturbances of affect and of social relationships later in life (see Chapter 21).

In a remarkable series of cell biological studies, Diorio and Meaney were able to localize the long-term effects of early maternal behaviors to specific molecular mechanisms in the adult's brain (Diorio & Meaney 2007). For example, differences in adrenocortical responses to stress were traced to the hippocampal cell membrane receptors that sense the level of adrenocortical hormone and inhibit the hormonal response to stress in the adult – a form of feedback inhibition, as in a thermostat. They found that the genes responsible for the synthesis of these receptors in the infant offspring of the high or low licking/grooming mothers were differently regulated. The rates of gene expression were in turn modified by "epigenetic" changes within the complex histone protein structure that surrounds DNA and controls which genes will be available for activation at that time. These findings link variation within the range of normally occurring levels of mother–infant interactions to molecular processes regulating gene expression in the developing young. The complex molecular structure, chromatin, that supports and surrounds the long, thin DNA strands includes several mechanisms for silencing some genes and opening others to activation (gene transcription) in response to outside signals. Two genes in the brain regions known to be involved in adrenocortical responses showed evidence of this kind of epigenetic modification (histone methylation and deacetylation) (Weaver *et al.* 2004). Additionally, specifically blocking these epigenetic modifications could reverse the adrenocortical changes.

Champagne and Meaney have gone on to find that mothers with high and low interaction levels pass these different maternal behavior patterns on to their daughters, along with the different levels of adult adrenocortical and fear responses (Champagne *et al.* 2006). This transgenerational effect on maternal behavior appears to be linked to the effects of maternal interaction patterns on her one-week-old infant's developing brain systems (and specifically to the estrogen-induced oxytocin receptors) in the areas that will be central to maternal behavior in adulthood. In evolution, the effects of such transgenerational mechanisms can link environmental stress acting on mothers (predicting a harsh environment for the next generation) to changes in anxiety levels in offspring through stress-induced reductions in a mother's interaction with her pups (Champagne & Meaney 2006).

In summary, the mechanism for the differences in anxiety phenotypes has been shown to be a novel epigenetic process through which lasting and widespread changes in levels of gene expression in specific areas of the offspring's brain are produced through a long-term alteration in the protein structure of the chromatin "packaging" in which the DNA is embedded. Furthermore, these changes can be transmitted to the next generation through maternal behavioral interactions affecting gene expression within the developing brain systems of her infants that will later determine their maternal behavior as adults. In this way, induced developmental change in one generation can be passed on as a pre-adaptation to successive generations through non-Lamarckian mechanisms that do not involve the germ-cell DNA.

New evidence is accumulating that epigenetic mechanisms may well play an important role in human psychiatric disorders (Tsankova *et al.* 2007), and, most directly related to development, Meaney and associates have reported epigenetic modulation of gene expression in the brains of suicide victims with histories of childhood abuse and severe neglect, compared to accident victims without such early histories (McGowan *et al.* 2008).

6.3 The early development of separation anxiety in a small mammal

According to MacLean (1985), the three crucial behavioral attributes that evolved with the mammals are play, parental behavior, and the separation cry – all of which, he points out, are absent in most modern-day reptiles. MacLean provides neuroanatomical and neurophysiological evidence supporting his theory that the presence of these behaviors in modern-day mammals is made possible by the specialized neural networks of the limbic system and their connections to the cerebral cortex and the midbrain. The evolution of social relationships based on mutual attachment in mammals provides a new set of behaviors, motivational systems, and dangers within which a new variant of anxiety can evolve. The infant mammal's separation cry is a communication to the mother with adaptive value; it is also a manifestation of a state of distress that may constitute the first innate anxiety state to have evolved.

6.3.1 The separation call

Of today's small mammals, one of the most successful orders is the rodent. A domesticated strain, the laboratory rat, is the species of animal we know the most about, next to the human. Rat infants respond to their first experienced separation with loud (60–90 dB) ultrasonic calls. Evolution has endowed mammalian infants with a response to a set of cues (isolation from conspecifics) that represent the potential for several actual dangers. The uncertain nature of the dangers,

the sudden loss of the infants' familiar and responsive companions, the prolonged immaturity of offspring and the related period of close parental care seem to resemble the conditions that give rise to the separation anxiety we are familiar with in children and even in adult humans.

I became interested in this calling behavior after I found that preweanling rat pups showed a number of other behavioral and physiological responses to separation from their mother (reviewed in Hofer 1996). In a series of studies, Harry Shair and I first found that pups emitted these calls when isolated, even if they remained untouched in their familiar home cage nest, showing that separation from social companions was a key element in eliciting these vocalizations (Hofer & Shair 1978). Next, we found that if pups were alone in an unfamiliar place, they would greatly reduce or cease calling when a littermate or their mother was placed with them, even if she was completely passive (anesthetized).

We now had a behavioral indicator for a state induced rapidly by separation, one that could be roughly quantified by using an ultrasonic detector commercially available for observing bats. We also had a means of rapidly terminating the state by what appeared to be a form of the well-known human response of "contact comfort." Because the separation-induced state depended on the sudden loss of contact with social companions, we embarked on a search for the sensory cues to which the pup was responding (Hofer & Shair 1980, 1991). We found that after the neonatal period, pups appeared to be responding to texture, odor, and temperature in a cumulative fashion, with contour and size as additional factors.

But do rat pups really experience separation negatively, and does the state induced by separation involve a change in the way the pup responds to new information, as would be expected during an anxiety state? Experiments by researchers interested in early learning have given affirmative answers to both of these questions. Isolated rat pups will learn difficult maze problems to get back to their mothers (Kenny & Blass 1977). Furthermore, cues associated with separation are strongly avoided when encountered subsequently (Smith *et al.* 1985). These findings show that rat pups dislike separation and are strongly predisposed to respond to cues associated with reunion. In addition, Norman Spear's group (1985) found a variety of associations, discriminations, and tasks that rat pups learned less well when they were separated from their home cages than when they were provided with familiar nest cues during the learning experience. This was not a generalized interference with cognitive processing, however. As in human anxiety, rat pups form some associations *more* readily when isolated. They learn to associate novel tastes and odors with illness and then avoid those cues two to three times more strongly when the learning took place when separated than when in the home cage.

6.3.2 Brain mechanisms

For those most interested in the neurobiological mechanisms of anxiety, studies on drugs and neuropeptide modulators have provided the most compelling evidence that the isolation distress state of young rats provides a useful animal model of anxiety (for reviews see Miczek *et al.* 1991, Hofer 1996). Pharmacological studies by a number of different groups have found that most major classes of drugs that are useful in human anxiety have powerful and selective inhibitory effects on isolation-induced ultrasonic calls in rat pups, usually without affecting other behaviors or inducing signs of sedation. Even more convincing is that synthetic compounds known to produce severe anxiety in human volunteers (such as pentylenetetrazol and the inverse agonist benzodiazepines) greatly increase the call rate in isolated pups and can even elicit calling in the home cage when the pup is with its familiar littermates (for reviews see Miczek *et al.* 1991, Hofer 1996).

6.3.3 The evolution of early separation-induced calling

How did vocalization first evolve as a manifestation of the infant's separation state so that the mother's retrieval behavior could then act selectively to enhance survival of vocal young and establish this important mother–infant communication system? In thinking about this question, we recalled the close natural association of cold temperature with displacement from the mother and from the home nest in small mammals, and that cold ambient temperature is a major cue for the elicitation of calling in isolated rat pups. In addition, we found evidence that infant vocalization may not have first evolved as a signal to the mother, but as a respiratory response promoting oxygenation during recovery from severe hypothermia, to which infant mammals are extremely vulnerable (Hofer & Shair 1992). Phrases such as "left out in the cold" and our use of "warm" or "cold" to describe emotional closeness or distance may not simply be modern metaphors, but testimony to an ancient role for the respiratory acts that produce vocalization during a period in mammalian evolution when

thermal stresses were unavoidable. We found evidence that coordinated laryngeal and respiratory function may have been shaped by selection for their physiological roles in survival after severe hypothermia.

The results of more recent evolutionary shaping by natural selection are evident in the sensory and perceptual adaptations of rodent mothers to their infants' vocalizations, such as an auditory frequency response threshold tuned to the exact frequency of infant vocalization, 45 kHz, that underlies the rodent mother's search, retrieval, and care-giving responses (Ehret 1992). However, the infant's vocalization can also alert predators to the location of vulnerable infants. Not surprisingly, predator odors dramatically suppress ultrasonic vocalizations in isolated pups, a specific fear response (Takahashi 1992).

Thus, the evolution of the infant separation cry has apparently involved an "evolutionary trade-off," that is, a ratio of risk to benefit that is thought to have shaped many behaviors throughout evolution. In this case, the theory predicts that in environments with many predators and thus the higher likelihood that vocalization may attract a predator before their mother finds them, infants that show *less* separation-induced vocalization will gradually increase in the population. However, when nest disruption occurs frequently (e.g., through repeated flooding) and fewer predators exist, high rates of isolation calling, ensuring more rapid and certain maternal retrieval, would be more advantageous.

6.4 Evolution and development of an anxious temperament

To explore these hypothetical evolutionary processes, we have been conducting a laboratory experiment that simulates them: selectively breeding adult rats that, as 10-day-old infants, had shown relatively high or relatively low rates of ultrasonic vocalization responses to separation. These will be referred to as "high line" or "low line" pups. We found that in as few as five generations, two distinct lines emerged that differed significantly on this infantile trait from a randomly bred control line when compared at 10 days postnatal. Cross-fostering of high- and low-line pups at birth to mothers of the opposite line showed no evidence of postnatal maternal influences on 10-day-olds' isolation calling rates (Brunelli *et al.* 1997). Clearly, this manifestation of early separation anxiety has a strong hereditary basis.

Since to our knowledge there have been no other systematic studies of selective breeding for an infant behavior trait, we did not know how repeated selection might be expected to affect infant calling rates in descendants during earlier or later developmental periods. Furthermore, we wondered whether other traits related to vocalization or to an underlying anxiety state might also be affected in adults through their genetic, physiological, or behavioral links to the developing systems influencing the infants' vocal response to separation. What we found after 15 generations (Hofer *et al.* 2001) was that infants' calling during isolation was strikingly elevated in high-line pups, starting as early as three days of age, which is the age at which calling develops and a week before the age at which selection had been carried out (10 days of age). Low-line pups, in contrast, moderately decreased their calling rate at this early age. The greatest difference between high and low lines was at the age of repeated selection, 10 days postnatal. Response differences were much less evident in 14-day-olds, and the lines converged as the response ceased to occur in all groups during the weaning period at 18–20 days postnatal. Thus, selection had resulted in high-line pups showing markedly elevated isolation call rates throughout their early development, whereas the lows showed a more rapid decline than normally occurs from neonate to weanling. Thus, selection at 10 days of age appeared to be acting on the whole developmental trajectory of the vocal response to separation, either delaying or hastening the normal developmental decline in response magnitude from 3 to 18 days of age.

In more recent studies, after 25 generations of selection, Brunelli has found a number of other behaviors and physiological responses that have been differentially shaped by selection (Brunelli & Hofer 2007). These differences appear to form coherent groups of traits. In juveniles, at 18 days of age, when separation calling has ceased to occur in any of the lines, both defecation/urination and sympathetically mediated heart-rate acceleration were greater in high-line juveniles than in controls. As 30-day-old adolescents, rough and tumble play behaviors, and the short, high-frequency "play calls" that accompany these interactions, were reduced compared to randomly bred controls. High-line adults were significantly slower to emerge into an open test box, and avoided the center area more completely, than the low-line animals. In addition, high-line adults showed a much more quiet, passive response to the "Porsolt" swim test, a pattern associated with depression-like states in rodents.

The low-line pups, as they developed to 18 days of age, surprisingly showed an even greater heart-rate acceleration than high-line pups in response to isolation testing. They also had a much delayed return to baseline, but through a different autonomic mechanism – vagal withdrawal. Low-line adolescents were deficient on all play behaviors on all days of testing and emitted the fewest play calls. As adults, compared to the highs, the low-lines were quicker to emerge into the open area, explored its center more, and were more active in the swim test. When confronted with another male, 70% of low-line males engaged in aggressive behavior, compared to 30% of randomly bred controls.

In summary, these groups of traits suggest a characterization of the high-line adults as anxious and passive, while the low-line adults were exploratory, active, and aggressive. As weanlings and adolescents, there were significant differences between the lines, but these were more difficult to characterize. Both highs and lows had higher heart-rate responses than controls, but different autonomic mechanisms; both showed reduced play and lower play calls, but the lows showed a near absence of play behaviors. Apparently, repeated selection for high and low rates of infant calling during isolation had selected patterns of genes underlying lifelong developmental paths and involving a number of associated traits. These alternative phenotypes, or temperaments, were created by selective breeding based on a single point early in development, as genetic alleles for the different infantile anxiety traits were gradually recruited by repeated selection over generations.

These results resemble the studies described in the previous section, in which different maternal behavior patterns acting on infants, rather than genetic selection, had long-term effects on the development of a specific group of associated adult traits. Thus, the developmental paths or structures for (at least) two anxiety-related phenotypes, each with adaptive potential, are latent within the genetic/environmental potential for development of this species. One set can be realized through repeated selection of genetic alleles over 15 or 20 generations; the other is realized in a much more rapid transgenerational effect on development, involving changes in the maternal behavior of daughters mediated by epigenetic processes regulating the development of neural regulation of behavior and physiology in that next generation. These findings show us some unexpected ways in which the advancing search for genes related to anxious temperament in humans may be revealing, and may help in our growing understanding of the genetics of anxiety disorders (Smoller & Faraone 2008).

6.5 Evolutionary clues in human panic disorder

Evolutionary approaches to obsessive–compulsive disorder, panic disorder, and other human anxiety disorders have been reviewed by Stein and Bouwer (1997). The findings on the most fully described and best documented of these – panic disorder – suggest that it might have evolved from an adaptive physiological response in our ancestors, similar to the hypothesized evolution of the separation call from an adaptive response to hypothermia in infant rats described earlier. Klein (1993) has proposed that the precipitation of acute symptoms of anxiety in patients with panic disorder (and some persons without panic disorder) by carbon dioxide (CO_2) inhalation may represent an adaptive "suffocation alarm." Klein hypothesized that in some individuals the threshold level of this alarm system is lowered to the point that normal or even low levels of partial pressure of CO_2 (pCO_2) in the circulation can trigger acute anxiety, a "false suffocation alarm." This could be enhanced when other cues to possible suffocation, such as closed exits, crowds, or immobilization, are also present. When further sensitized, through genetic or environmental mechanisms, the alarm and the panic response may occur spontaneously. He proposed that panic may be more primitive than other forms of anxiety, and that it also differs in being a response to an endogenous cue (pCO_2) rather than an external threat. Klein pointed out that the hyperventilation, frequent yawns, and sighs in patients between panic episodes may constitute tests monitoring for signs of rising blood pCO_2. If CO_2 is not rapidly lowered and symptoms eased as a result of these respiratory maneuvers, this triggers a false alarm that suffocation could be imminent. Klein suggested that another distinctive feature of panic attacks, the relative lack of adrenocortical response, may derive from the maladaptive consequences of hypercortisolemia in hypoxic conditions, as would be found in suffocation.

The association of adult panic disorder with separation anxiety in childhood, and with the precipitating conditions of separation and loss in adulthood, is particularly interesting in the light of the previous section on alternate paths in the development of anxious

temperaments. Evolution has given us a variety of genes that are related to expressions of anxiety over the life span, and a variety of environmental/regulatory pathways exist that activate particular groups of genes, leading to adaptive or to maladaptive levels of anxiety at different life stages.

6.6 Clinical implications

Insights into the evolution of anxiety can be clinically useful (Marks & Nesse 1994). The transition from anxious personality to anxiety disorder will result when a combination of genetic vulnerability and life experiences combine to raise anxiety to levels that are nonadaptive and even crippling in the person's present environment. Social and other environmental interactions can either intensify anxiety and/or preserve the life and comfort of the patient with anxiety disorder. Once a patient is led to realize that his or her symptoms are part of the history of human nature, that these responses can even be advantageous in certain situations, and that the real problem lies in their occurrence at the wrong time and place, this understanding can help alleviate the confusion, shame, and hopelessness that burden so many patients with anxiety disorders.

As our understanding of genetic mechanisms involved in the expression of behavior and in predisposition to mental illness grows exponentially in the coming years, so will our insight into the evolution of the behaviors and states of mind that are the subject of this volume. We can begin to see the outlines of what lies ahead, but there is much more to be learned. I hope that we will continue to view this state of affairs with more curiosity and anticipation than anxiety.

Acknowledgments

The work described in this chapter was supported by project grants and a Research Scientist Award from NIMH, and by the Sackler Institute for Developmental Psychobiology at Columbia University.

Permission has been granted by American Psychiatric Publishing Inc. to reproduce and modify portions of the chapter "Evolutionary concepts of anxiety" from the *Textbook of Anxiety Disorders*, 2nd edition (Hofer 2009).

References

Alcock, J. (2001). *The Triumph of Sociobiology*. New York, NY: Oxford University Press.

Brunelli, S. A., & Hofer, M. A. (2007). Selective breeding for infant rat separation-induced ultrasonic

leads to significant distress or impairment, particularly in areas of interpersonal functioning. Individuals with this disorder are often characterized as rigid and overly controlling. They may find it difficult to relax, feel obligated to plan out their activities to the minute, and find unstructured time intolerable (Pinto *et al.* 2008a). The presence of comorbid OCPD has been suggested as a possible OCD subtype (Coles *et al.* 2008).

Studies using DSM-IV criteria have consistently found elevated rates of OCPD in subjects with OCD, with estimates ranging from 23% to 32% (Samuels *et al.* 2000, Albert *et al.* 2004, Pinto *et al.* 2006), compared with rates of 0.9–3.0% in community samples (Torgersen *et al.* 2001, Samuels *et al.* 2002, Albert *et al.* 2004). While OCPD is the most frequently diagnosed personality disorder in OCD (Samuels *et al.* 2000, Pinto *et al.* 2006) and occurs more frequently in individuals with OCD than in individuals with other anxiety disorders (panic disorder, social anxiety disorder) (Skodol *et al.* 1995, Crino & Andrews 1996, Diaferia *et al.* 1997) or major depressive disorder (Diaferia *et al.* 1997), it is important to note that OCPD is not found in most OCD cases and is not a prerequisite for OCD.

There is evidence of a familial association between OCPD and OCD. Several studies have reported increased frequencies of OCPD traits in the parents of children with OCD (Swedo *et al.* 1989, Lenane *et al.* 1990) and a significantly greater frequency of OCPD in first-degree relatives of OCD probands compared to relatives of control probands (11.5% versus 5.8%, respectively) (Samuels *et al.* 2000). In fact, OCPD was the only personality disorder to occur more often in the relatives of OCD probands. More recently, Calvo and colleagues (2008) reported a higher incidence of DSM-IV OCPD in parents of pediatric OCD probands versus the parents of healthy children, even after parents with OCD were excluded. Preoccupation with details, perfectionism, and hoarding were significantly more frequent in parents of OCD children. Counting, ordering, and cleaning compulsions in OCD children predicted elevated odds of perfectionism and rigidity in their parents.

Individuals with both OCD and OCPD present with distinct clinical characteristics, patterns of functioning, and course of OCD. Recent data from 629 individuals with personality disorders indicated that three of the eight DSM-IV OCPD criteria (preoccupation with details, perfectionism, and hoarding) were significantly more frequent in patients with comorbid OCD than in those without OCD (Eisen *et al.* 2006).

The relationship between OCD and these three criteria remained significant after controlling for the presence of other anxiety disorders and major depressive disorder, with odds ratios ranging from 2.71 to 2.99.

Coles and colleagues (2008) were the first to systematically examine a range of clinical characteristics in individuals with and without comorbid OCPD in a primary OCD sample. As compared to subjects without OCPD, the OCD+OCPD subjects had a significantly younger age at onset of first OC symptoms, as well as poorer psychosocial functioning, even though the groups did not differ in overall severity of OCD symptoms. Individuals with OCD+OCPD also had higher rates of comorbid anxiety disorders and avoidant personality disorder. These subjects reported higher rates of hoarding and incompleteness-related symptoms (including symmetry obsessions and cleaning, ordering, repeating compulsions), as compared to OCD–OCPD subjects. Subjects with comorbid OCPD were significantly less likely to partially remit from OCD after two years as compared to those without comorbid OCPD (Pinto 2009). Other studies have reported a poorer OCD response to both serotonin reuptake inhibitor (SRI) medications (Cavedini 1997) and cognitive–behavioral therapy (CBT) (Pinto *et al.* 2009) in patients with comorbid OCPD, further evidence of a distinct clinical presentation for the putative comorbid OCPD subtype.

The relationship between OCD and OCPD may be particularly strong for a subgroup of individuals with OCD with symmetry-related symptoms. In a clinical OCD sample, Baer (1994) found that an OCD symptom factor characterized by symmetry, ordering, repeating, counting, and hoarding was most strongly correlated with the preoccupation with details, perfectionism, and hoarding criteria of OCPD. Similarly, in the Johns Hopkins OCD Family Study, Wellen and colleagues (2007) reported that the ordering and arranging factor of the Leyton Obsessional Inventory (Cooper 1970) was the only one associated with OCPD.

7.2.2 Dimensional approaches

Over the last two decades, there has been great interest in deriving a multidimensional model of OCD based on symptom content. In this time, more than 20 factor analyses (involving > 5000 OCD subjects) have delineated the heterogeneous symptoms of OCD into three to six clinically meaningful dimensions associated with separable patterns of comorbidity, treatment response, and neural correlates (Mataix-Cols *et al.* 2005, Bloch *et al.* 2008). Despite the large number of studies, debate remains regarding the exact factor structure of OCD symptoms, in part because differences in clinical ascertainment, scoring, and statistical methods across studies have sometimes resulted in varying structures.

For example, Baer (1994) applied principal components analysis to categories of current symptoms on the Yale–Brown Obsessive Compulsive Scale – Symptom Checklist (YBOCS-SC). He reported a three-factor solution: (1) *symmetry/hoarding*, which included symmetry and saving obsessions and ordering, hoarding, repeating, and counting compulsions; (2) *contamination/checking*, including contamination and somatic obsessions and cleaning and checking compulsions; and (3) *pure obsessions*, including aggressive, sexual, and religious obsessions. Leckman and colleagues (1997) conducted a principal components analysis on the total number of lifetime symptoms in each of the YBOCS-SC categories in two independent groups of patients. Four factors were identified: (1) *obsessions and checking*, (2) *symmetry and ordering*, (3) *cleanliness and washing*, and (4) *hoarding*. Using current symptoms and applying the same scoring method as Baer, Mataix-Cols and colleagues (1999) reported five factors in their principal components analysis: (1) *symmetry/ordering*, (2) *hoarding*, (3) *contamination/cleaning*, (4) *aggressive/checking*, and (5) *sexual/religious obsessions*.

Pinto and colleagues (2007) applied principal components analysis to the proportion of current symptoms endorsed in each of the YBOCS-SC categories and reported a similar five-factor solution: (1) *symmetry/ordering*, (2) *hoarding*, (3) *doubt/checking*, (4) *contamination/cleaning*, and (5) *taboo thoughts* (aggressive, sexual, and religious obsessions). The resulting five factors corresponded to long-held OCD symptom themes, dating back to Janet's descriptions in 1903 of incompleteness (*les sentiments d'incomplétude*, which corresponds to symmetry/ordering symptoms), forbidden thoughts, and doubt (*folie du doute*) (Pitman 1987).

Bloch and colleagues (2008) presented a meta-analysis of 21 factor analytic studies of OCD and reported four factors: (1) *symmetry/ordering*, (2) *forbidden thoughts and checking*, (3) *contamination/cleaning*, and (4) *hoarding*. The authors noted that the meta-analysis was limited by the use of category-level rather than item-level (symptom) data from the YBOCS-SC. Category-level factor analyses are problematic since they assume the validity of these symptom groupings, restrict the number of items available for analysis, and limit the symptom dimensions that can emerge.

To address the limitations of category-level data, Pinto and colleagues (2008b) independently replicated the five factors derived in Pinto *et al.* (2007), using a separate dataset of lifetime individual symptoms (rather than symptom categories) from 485 adults with lifetime OCD enrolled in a family study. These analyses indicated that the same underlying structure of OCD symptoms holds in both a sample of individuals with OCD and a sample of affected family members. Schooler and colleagues (2008) used a novel item-level confirmatory factor analysis based on structural equation modeling on a modified self-report version of the YBOCS-SC and found support for five factors over four. The five factors noted in this study are consistent with those identified by Pinto and colleagues (2008b).

There have been several attempts to evaluate the familiality of OCD symptom dimensions. Alsobrook and colleagues (1999) reported that the recurrence risk of OCD among first-degree relatives of probands with high scores on either obsessions/checking or symmetry/ordering factors was twice as high as that among relatives of probands with low scores on these factors. The same two factors were correlated between siblings and mother–child pairs in a sample of TS-affected sibling pairs and relatives (Leckman *et al.* 2003). Cullen and colleagues (2007) found significant intrafamilial sib–sib correlations for the symmetry/ordering and hoarding factors. In a study of affected sibling pairs, Hasler and colleagues (2007) reported four factors with significant sib–sib correlations, with hoarding and obsessions/checking demonstrating the strongest familiality. Using the same dataset, Pinto and colleagues (2008b) reported significant sib–sib associations for four of their five factors, with the hoarding and taboo thoughts factors being the most robustly familial.

Two studies support the temporal stability of the symptom dimensions in adult patients over several years (Mataix-Cols *et al.* 2002a, Rufer *et al.* 2005). Both noted the tendency for symptom changes to occur within rather than between dimensions. The strongest predictor of the presence of a particular symptom was having had that symptom at a prior time point.

Data from neuropsychological and neuroimaging studies have suggested that OCD symptom dimensions may differ in their underlying neurobiology. Lawrence and colleagues (2006) reported that OCD patients high on the hoarding dimension showed impaired decision making on a gambling task, and symmetry/ordering symptoms were negatively associated with set shifting. In a PET study, Rauch and colleagues (1998) reported that checking symptoms correlated with increased regional cerebral blood flow (rCBF) in the striatum, symmetry/ordering with reduced rCBF in the striatum, and washing symptoms correlated with increased rCBF in bilateral anterior cingulate and left orbitofrontal cortex. In an fMRI symptom provocation study, patients demonstrated significantly greater activation than controls in bilateral ventromedial prefrontal regions (washing experiment); putamen/globus pallidus, thalamus, and dorsal cortical areas (checking experiment); and left precentral gyrus and right orbitofrontal cortex (hoarding experiment) (Mataix-Cols *et al.* 2004). In a large unmedicated patient sample, van den Heuvel and colleagues (2009) found that scores on the contamination/washing dimension were negatively correlated with gray-matter volume in the bilateral dorsal caudate nucleus and white-matter volume in the right parietal region. Scores on the harm/checking dimension were negatively correlated with gray- and white-matter volume of the bilateral temporal lobes. Scores on the symmetry/ordering dimension were negatively correlated with gray-matter volume of the bilateral parietal cortex and positively correlated with bilateral medial temporal gray- and white-matter volume.

With regard to treatment response, studies show that patients with high scores on the hoarding dimension respond poorly to various SRI medications (Mataix-Cols *et al.* 1999), CBT (Mataix-Cols *et al.* 2002b), and the combination of SRI+CBT (Saxena *et al.* 2002), although a recent study found that hoarding and non-hoarding OCD patients responded equally well to paroxetine (Saxena *et al.* 2007). There is also evidence that patients high on the sexual/religious dimension may have poorer response to CBT (Mataix-Cols *et al.* 2002b) and poorer long-term outcome with combined SRI+CBT (Alonso *et al.* 2001). In contrast, in a placebo-controlled study of citalopram (Stein *et al.* 2007), high scores on the aggressive/religious/sexual dimension predicted better outcome, while high scores on the symmetry/hoarding and contamination/cleaning dimensions predicted worse outcome.

7.3 Exploring endophenotypes of OCD

A strategy that has been successfully applied to other heterogeneous and complex psychiatric disorders is to identify intermediate phenotypes (precursors to symptoms) that are more closely related to neurobiological mechanisms than phenotypes (Gottesman & Gould 2003, Preston & Weinberger 2005). When these unobservable characteristics are found to mediate the relationship between genes and a given behavioral phenotype, they are called "endophenotypes," and they can be neurophysiological, biochemical, endocrinological, neuropsychological, cognitive, and neuroanatomical. Researchers hope that since endophenotypes are less complex and heterogeneous than the associated disorder, they will be linked to fewer genes and thus more amenable to study. Although endophenotypes are seen as a means to overcome barriers to progress in genetic studies, they also have broader use in psychiatry, such as improving diagnosis and classification, the development of animal models, and understanding mechanisms of treatment response.

To maximize the utility of endophenotypes, Gottesman and Gould (2003) outlined criteria for their identification, which were further elaborated by Crosbie and colleagues (2008). A valid endophenotype should have the following characteristics: (a) sensitivity and specificity in relation to the disorder, (b) heritability and genetic specificity, (c) familial aggregation, (d) presence in unaffected relatives, (e) trait-like qualities (i.e., temporally stable), (f) biological plausibility, (g) sound psychometric properties, and (h) feasibility. The distinction between "endophenotypes" and "biological markers" is that a biological marker is not necessarily related to genes and may signify differences that do not have genetic underpinnings, while endophenotypes, on the other hand, are heritable. In OCD, the study of endophenotypes is in its infancy, and to date none of the candidate markers under study satisfy all of the criteria listed here. The most promising candidates – neurocognitive, physiological, and neuroimaging measures – are presented in the sections that follow.

7.3.1 Potential neurocognitive measures

Several neurocognitive measures have been examined in OCD as potential markers of neural dysfunction. These measures have focused on functions associated with the cortical–striatal–thalamic circuits implicated in OCD, including response inhibition, reversal learning, set shifting, and other executive functions.

Because the symptoms of OCD suggest problems inhibiting motor behavior, a deficit in response inhibition, as measured by the stop-signal reaction time (SSRT: the processing time required to inhibit a prepotent motor response), has been proposed as a candidate neurobehavioral marker. The stop-signal task measures a subject's ability to withhold a planned movement in response to an infrequent countermanding signal (Boucher *et al.* 2007). SSRT has been shown to be significantly longer in subjects with OCD and their unaffected first-degree relatives, as compared to healthy comparison subjects (Chamberlain *et al.* 2006, 2007). Impaired SSRT was further correlated with reduced gray matter in orbitofrontal and right inferior frontal regions, as well as with increased gray matter in the cingulate, parietal, and striatal regions (Menzies *et al.* 2007). Since these studies focused on patients with predominantly washing/checking symptoms, further research is needed to determine if the results generalize to other OCD subgroups. Still, these findings provide some evidence for OCD as a disorder of disinhibition.

A deficit in reversal learning has also been proposed as a putative neurobehavioral marker of OCD. Reversal learning allows behavior to be flexibly altered following negative feedback (Robbins 2007). It is thought that the orbitofrontal cortex is necessary to generate outcome expectancies that allow for the computation of prediction errors ultimately used to "update" associations (Delamater 2007). Reduced activation of several cortical regions, including the lateral orbitofrontal cortex, was observed during a reversal learning task (a trial-and-error task in which feedback was given after every second response) in OCD patients and their unaffected, never-treated first-degree relatives (Chamberlain *et al.* 2008). As with SSRT, replication and further study is required to validate reversal-learning-related hypofunction as a vulnerability marker for OCD.

Difficulty with set shifting/cognitive flexibility is yet another executive function that has been considered a neurobehavioral marker, based on the notion that compulsions are often performed according to rigid rules and such symptoms may be mediated by problems shifting attentional focus (Chamberlain *et al.* 2005). OCD subjects and their unaffected first-degree relatives showed deficits in extradimensional set shifting, as measured by the Intradimensional/Extradimensional Shift Task (Chamberlain *et al.* 2006, 2007). The deficit was specific to the stage of the task in which it was necessary to shift attentional focus away from a previously relevant stimulus dimension (similar to a category shift on the Wisconsin Card Sorting Test). However, no group differences in brain activation during extradimensional set shifting were found (Chamberlain *et al.* 2008). Furthermore, the finding of an extradimensional set-shifting deficit has not been consistent (Simpson *et al.* 2006), and does not appear to be specific to OCD (e.g., reported in a Tourette syndrome sample: Watkins *et al.* 2005).

Difficulty with planning has also been reported in OCD (Delorme *et al.* 2007), but the low specificity of this executive deficit and its prevalence in other neuropsychiatric disorders make it a less attractive option to pursue.

7.3.2 Potential physiological measures

A physiological measure that holds promise as a candidate biological marker of OCD is error-related negativity (ERN). ERN is a sharp negative deflection in the event-related potential (ERP) recorded from midline frontal or central scalp electrodes that peaks about 50–150 milliseconds after the commission of an error. The ERP reflects early error-processing activity of the anterior cingulate cortex (Olvet & Hajcak 2008). Increased action monitoring as indexed by the ERN has been theorized as a putative risk factor for anxiety disorders and depression. Response monitoring tasks, such as the stop-signal task, provoke error responses that can then be used to detect an ERN response. Studies in both adults and children confirm that OCD subjects consistently produce an abnormal ERN response (Olvet & Hajcak 2008), but data on unaffected relatives of OCD probands are needed. Additionally, the exaggerated ERN response observed in OCD appears to be a trait-like marker in that it is not altered with treatment of OCD symptoms (Hajcak *et al.* 2008). Given the familial relationship between OCD and generalized anxiety disorder (GAD) (Nestadt *et al.* 2001), it is of interest that both GAD and OCD produce an exaggerated ERN response, in contrast to phobic disorders and controls (Hajcak *et al.* 2003).

Another physiological measure under consideration as a biological marker of OCD is prepulse inhibition (PPI). PPI is a robust measure of sensorimotor gating that has been validated across vertebrate species (Geyer *et al.* 2001). Sensorimotor gating refers to the process by which a neural system screens or "gates" extraneous external (sensory) and internal (cognitive, motor) information out of awareness, so that an individual can focus on the most salient stimuli (Butler *et al.* 1990). Specifically, PPI represents the reduction in the startle reflex that occurs when a startling stimulus is preceded by a barely detectable "prepulse" stimulus (Graham 1975). The prepulse thus inhibits or "gates" the startle reflex. In humans, PPI is assessed by measuring the degree to which a weak acoustic stimulus (the prepulse) suppresses the startle response (measured by eye blink) to a later acoustic stimulus (the pulse). Experimentally, PPI is elicited on the first exposure to the combination of prepulse and pulse stimuli, is not a form of conditioning, and does not exhibit habituation or extinction over multiple testing sessions (Hoffman & Ison 1980). The intrusive thoughts and images (i.e., obsessions) and repetitive acts (i.e., compulsions) that characterize OCD are thought to reflect sensorimotor gating deficits that arise from deficient central inhibitory functioning. Two preliminary studies have reported decreased PPI of the acoustic startle response in OCD patients (Swerdlow *et al.* 1993, Hoenig *et al.* 2005). Further research in OCD subjects and their first-degree relatives, along with validation with brain imaging, is needed to elucidate the utility of impaired PPI as a candidate OCD endophenotype.

7.3.3 Potential neuroimaging measures

Modern neuroimaging techniques have allowed abnormalities in white-matter brain tissue to be investigated as potential OCD endophenotypes. Using diffusion tensor imaging, a magnetic resonance imaging technique that quantifies water diffusion, Menzies and colleagues (2008) found significantly reduced fractional anisotropy in right inferior parietal white matter and significantly increased fractional anisotropy in a right medial frontal region in OCD subjects, as compared to matched healthy controls. Unaffected first-degree relatives of OCD probands exhibited similar white-matter abnormalities, which led the authors to propose that such abnormalities may be markers of increased genetic risk for OCD. As this is the first study to examine white-matter differences in relatives of OCD patients, replication is necessary.

7.4 Conclusions and future directions

The phenotype of OCD is heterogeneous, and this heterogeneity presumably underlies differences between individuals in treatment response and the variability observed in biological and genetic findings. To advance both treatment and our understanding of the etiology and pathophysiology of OCD, researchers have increasingly looked for ways to characterize more homogeneous components of OCD. These efforts have included attempts to clarify both key phenotypes and characteristic endophenotypes of OCD.

Subtypes of OCD have been proposed, based on early age of onset, tic comorbidity, and OCPD comorbidity. These categorical subtypes are relatively easy to identify and may be helpful for clinicians to note due to their distinct clinical presentations. The problem with this approach is that these categories may or may not map dichotomously onto biological features, and recruiting only one or the other subtype makes research difficult, given the relatively low prevalence of OCD and the need for large samples to power studies involving analyses of subgroups.

A dimensional approach avoids this problem of categorization, since all individuals can be scored along dimensions, which serve as quantitative measures of the phenotype. As a result, there has been great interest in deriving a multidimensional model of OCD based on symptom content. However, a comprehensive dimensional structure has not been agreed upon, and the methods for dimensionalizing the phenotype are not yet standardized amongst researchers. Symptom-based research is limited by the psychometric properties of the measurement tools, and greater attention needs to be paid to the reliability and validity of symptom assessment. New instruments, like the Dimensional YBOCS (DYBOCS) (Rosario-Campos *et al.* 2006) and the Dimensional Obsessive-Compulsive Scale (DOCS) (Abramowitz *et al.* 2010) will allow collection of symptom data in a dimensional manner. Although preliminary data suggest that these dimensions are mediated by relatively distinct neural systems, these intriguing findings require replication. Genetic studies incorporating the symptom dimensions are also under way.

Another approach to deconstructing the heterogeneity of OCD is the identification of vulnerability markers or endophenotypes. As reviewed above, a few putative endophenotypes have been proposed, although this work is in its infancy. A strength of this approach is that endophenotypes rely upon objective measurements instead of subjective ratings of symptoms. In addition, many of the proposed endophenotypes can be studied in animal models, where the technology exists to dissect cellular and molecular mechanisms. A challenge of this approach is to link the putative endophenotypes back to the clinical phenomenon in such a way that advances in knowledge about the endophenotype lead to advances in clinical care. If researchers focus too narrowly on the use of endophenotypes in genetic studies, they may overlook important biological markers that might not be useful for genetic studies but might instead predict who may or may not respond to specific treatments. The process of identifying and validating markers of OCD may also yield new treatment targets, such as neurocognitive deficits, that interfere with psychosocial functioning and quality of life. Finally, the likelihood that environmental causes (e.g., trauma, stressful life events, infection) and gene–environment interactions play an important role in the etiology of OCD may make the identification of endophenotypes more difficult than it might appear.

Integrating phenotypical and endophenotypical approaches may be fruitful in advancing the field. Phenotypical insights might suggest putative endophenotypes, and, in turn, endophenotypes may help revise our notion of phenotype. For example, the dimensional approach has helped researchers account for phenotypic heterogeneity and has led to findings of distinct neuropsychological profiles (Lawrence *et al.* 2006) and neural systems (van den Heuvel *et al.* 2009) for the various OCD symptom dimensions. In conclusion, as reviewed in this chapter, researchers are pursuing multiple avenues to overcome the problem of heterogeneity in OCD, in the hopes of making gains in conceptualization, pathophysiology, and treatment.

Acknowledgments

Supported by NIMH grants K23 MH080221 (Pinto) and R24 MH080022 (Simpson).

References

Abramowitz, J. S., Deacon, B. J., Olatunji, B. O., Wheaton, M. G., Berman, N. C., Losardo, D., Timpano, K. R., McGrath, P. B., Riemann, B. C., Adams, T., Bjorgvinsson, T., Storch, E. A. & Hale, L. R. (2010). Assessment of obsessive-compulsive symptom dimensions: development and evaluation of the Dimensional Obsessive-Compulsive Scale. *Psychological Assessment*, **22**, 180–198.

Albert, U., Picco, C., Maina, G., *et al.* (2002). [Phenomenology of patients with early and adult onset obsessive–compulsive disorder]. *Epidemiologiae Psichiatria Sociale*, **11** (2), 116–126.

Albert, U., Maina, G., Forner, F., & Bogetto, F. (2004). DSM-IV obsessive–compulsive personality disorder: prevalence in patients with anxiety disorders and in healthy comparison subjects. *Comprehensive Psychiatry*, **45**, 325–332.

Alonso, P., Menchon, J. M., Pifarre, J., *et al.* (2001). Long-term follow-up and predictors of clinical outcome in obsessive–compulsive patients treated with serotonin reuptake inhibitors and behavioral therapy. *Journal of Clinical Psychiatry*, **62**, 535–540.

Alsobrook, J. P., Leckman, J. F., Goodman, W. K., Rasmussen, S. A., & Pauls, D. L. (1999). Segregation analysis of obsessive–compulsive disorder using symptom-based factor scores. *American Journal of Medical Genetics*, **88**, 669–675.

Baer, L. (1994). Factor analysis of symptom subtypes of obsessive compulsive disorder and their relation to personality and tic disorders. *Journal of Clinical Psychiatry*, **55** (Suppl), 18–23.

Bloch, M. H., Landeros-Weisenberger, A., Rosario, M. C., Pittenger, C., & Leckman, J. F. (2008). Meta-analysis of the symptom structure of obsessive–compulsive disorder. *American Journal of Psychiatry*, **165**, 1532–1542.

Boucher, L., Palmeri, T. J., Logan, G. D., & Schall, J. D. (2007). Inhibitory control in mind and brain: An interactive race model of countermanding saccades. *Psychological Review*, **114**, 376–397.

Braun, A. R., Randolph, C., Stoetter, B., *et al.* (1995). The functional neuroanatomy of Tourette's syndrome: an FDG-PET study. II: Relationships between regional cerebral metabolism and associated behavioral and cognitive features of the illness. *Neuropsychopharmacology*, **13**, 151–168.

Butler, R. W., Braff, D. L., Rausch, J. L., *et al.* (1990). Physiological evidence of exaggerated startle response in a subgroup of Vietnam veterans with combat-related PTSD. *American Journal of Psychiatry*, **147**, 1308–1312.

Calvo, R., Lazaro, L., Castro-Fornieles, J., *et al.* (2008). Obsessive–compulsive personality disorder traits and personality dimensions in parents of children with obsessive–compulsive disorder. *European Psychiatry*, **24**, 201–206.

Cavedini, P., Erzegovesi, S., Ronchi, P., & Bellodi, L. (1997). Predictive value of obsessive-compulsive personality disorder in antiobsessional pharmacological treatment. *European Neuropsychopharmacology*, **7**, 45–49.

Chamberlain, S. R., Blackwell, A. D., Fineberg, N. A., Robbins, T. W., & Sahakian, B. J. (2005). The neuropsychology of obsessive compulsive disorder: the importance of failures in cognitive and behavioural inhibition as candidate endophenotypic markers. *Neuroscience and Biobehavioral Reviews*, **29**, 399–419.

Chamberlain, S. R., Fineberg, N. A., Blackwell, A. D., Robbins, T. W., & Sahakian, B. J. (2006). Motor inhibition and cognitive flexibility in obsessive–compulsive disorder and trichotillomania. *American Journal of Psychiatry*, **163**, 1282–1284.

Chamberlain, S. R., Fineberg, N. A., Menzies, L. A., *et al.* (2007). Impaired cognitive flexibility and motor inhibition in unaffected first-degree relatives of patients with obsessive–compulsive disorder. *American Journal of Psychiatry*, **164**, 335–338.

Chamberlain, S. R., Menzies, L., Hampshire, A., *et al.* (2008). Orbitofrontal dysfunction in patients with obsessive–compulsive disorder and their unaffected relatives. *Science*, **321**, 421–422.

Coles, M. E., Pinto, A., Mancebo, M. C., Rasmussen, S. A., & Eisen, J. L. (2008). OCD with comorbid OCPD: a subtype of OCD? *Journal of Psychiatric Research*, **42**, 289–296.

Cooper, J. (1970). The Leyton Obsessional Inventory. *Psychological Medicine*, **1**, 48–64.

Crino, R. D., & Andrews, G. (1996). Personality disorder in obsessive compulsive disorder: a controlled study. *Journal of Psychiatric Research*, **30**, 29–38.

Crosbie, J., Perusse, D., Barr, C. L., & Schachar, R. J. (2008). Validating psychiatric endophenotypes: inhibitory control and attention deficit hyperactivity disorder. *Neuroscience and Biobehavioral Reviews*, **32**, 40–55.

Cullen, B., Brown, C. H., Riddle, M. A., *et al.* (2007). Factor analysis of the Yale–Brown Obsessive Compulsive Scale in a family study of obsessive–compulsive disorder. *Depression and Anxiety*, **24**, 130–138.

Delamater, A. R. (2007). The role of the orbitofrontal cortex in sensory-specific encoding of associations in Pavlovian and instrumental conditioning. *Annals of the New York Academy of Sciences*, **1121**, 152–173.

Delorme, R., Golmard, J. L., Chabane, N., *et al.* (2005). Admixture analysis of age at onset in obsessive-compulsive disorder. *Psychological Medicine*, **35**, 237–243.

Delorme, R., Gousse, V., Roy, I., *et al.* (2007). Shared executive dysfunctions in unaffected relatives of patients with autism and obsessive–compulsive disorder. *European Psychiatry*, **22**, 32–38.

Diaferia, G., Bianchi, I., Bianchi, M. L., *et al.* (1997). Relationship between obsessive–compulsive personality disorder and obsessive–compulsive disorder. *Comprehensive Psychiatry*, **38**, 38–42.

Diniz, J. B., Rosario-Campos, M. C., Shavitt, R. G., *et al.* (2004). Impact of age at onset and duration of illness on the expression of comorbidities in obsessive–compulsive disorder. *Journal of Clinical Psychiatry*, **65**, 22–27.

Eisen, J. L., Coles, M. E., Shea, M. T., *et al.* (2006). Clarifying the convergence between obsessive compulsive personality disorder criteria and obsessive compulsive disorder. *Journal of Personality Disorders*, **20**, 294–305.

Fontenelle, L. F., Mendlowicz, M. V., Marques, C., & Versiani, M. (2003). Early- and late-onset obsessive–compulsive disorder in adult patients: an exploratory clinical and therapeutic study. *Journal of Psychiatric Research*, **37**, 127–133.

Geyer, M. A., Krebs-Thomson, K., Braff, D. L., & Swerdlow, N. R. (2001). Pharmacological studies of prepulse inhibition models of sensorimotor gating deficits in schizophrenia: a decade in review. *Psychopharmacology*, **156**, 117–154.

Gottesman, II, & Gould, T. D. (2003). The endophenotype concept in psychiatry: etymology and strategic intentions. *American Journal of Psychiatry*, **160**, 636–645.

Grados, M. A., Riddle, M. A., Samuels, J. F., *et al.* (2001). The familial phenotype of obsessive–compulsive disorder in relation to tic disorders: the Hopkins OCD Family Study. *Biological Psychiatry*, **50**, 559–565.

Graham, F. K. (1975). Presidential address, 1974. The more or less startling effects of weak prestimulation. *Psychophysiology*, **12**, 238–248.

Grant, J. E., Mancebo, M. C., Pinto, A., *et al.* (2007). Late-onset obsessive compulsive disorder: Clinical characteristics and psychiatric comorbidity. *Psychiatry Research*, **152**, 21–27.

Hajcak, G., McDonald, N., & Simons, R. F. (2003). Anxiety and error-related brain activity. *Biological Psychology*, **64**, 77–90.

Hajcak, G., Franklin, M. E., Foa, E. B., & Simons, R. F. (2008). Increased error-related brain activity in pediatric obsessive–compulsive disorder before and after treatment. *American Journal of Psychiatry*, **165**, 116–123.

Hasler, G., Pinto, A., Greenberg, B. D., *et al.* (2007). Familiality of factor analysis-derived YBOCS dimensions in OCD affected sibling pairs from the OCD Collaborative Genetics Study. *Biological Psychiatry*, **61**, 617–625.

Hoenig, K., Hochrein, A., Quednow, B. B., Maier, W., & Wagner, M. (2005). Impaired prepulse inhibition of acoustic startle in obsessive–compulsive disorder. *Biological Psychiatry*, **57**, 1153–1158.

Hoffman, H. S., & Ison, J. R. (1980). Reflex modification in the domain of startle: I. Some empirical findings and their implications for how the nervous system processes sensory input. *Psychological Review*, **87**, 175–189.

Kessler, R. C., Berglund, P., Demler, O., *et al.* (2005). Lifetime prevalence and age-of-onset distributions of DSM-IV disorders in the national comorbidity survey replication. *Archives of General Psychiatry*, **62**, 593–602.

Koran, L. M. (2000). Quality of life in obsessive–compulsive disorder. *Psychiatric Clinics of North America*, **23**, 509–517.

Lawrence, N. S., Wooderson, S., Mataix-Cols, D., *et al.* (2006). Decision making and set shifting impairments are associated with distinct symptom dimensions in obsessive–compulsive disorder. *Neuropsychology*, **20**, 409–419.

Leckman, J. F., Grice, D. E., Boardman, J., *et al.* (1997). Symptoms of obsessive–compulsive disorder. *American Journal of Psychiatry*, **154**, 911–917.

Leckman, J. F., Pauls, D. L., Zhang, H., *et al.* (2003). Obsessive–compulsive symptom dimensions in affected sibling pairs diagnosed with Gilles de la Tourette syndrome. *American Journal of Medical Genetics B: Neuropsychiatric Genetics*, **116B**, 60–68.

Lenane, M., Swedo, S. E., Leonard, H. L., *et al.* (1990). Psychiatric disorders in first degree relatives of children and adolescents with obsessive–compulsive disorder.

Journal of the American Academy of Child and Adolescent Psychiatry, **29**, 407–412.

Leonard, H. L., Lenane, M. C., Swedo, S. E., *et al.* (1992). Tics and Tourette's disorder: a 2- to 7-year follow-up of 54 obsessive–compulsive children. *American Journal of Psychiatry*, **149**, 1244–1251.

Maina, G., Albert, U., Salvi, V., Pessina, E., & Bogetto, F. (2008). Early-onset obsessive–compulsive disorder and personality disorders in adulthood. *Psychiatry Research*, **158**, 217–225.

Mataix-Cols, D., Rauch, S. L., Manzo, P. A., Jenike, M. A., & Baer, L. (1999). Use of factor-analyzed symptom dimensions to predict outcome with serotonin reuptake inhibitors and placebo in the treatment of obsessive–compulsive disorder. *American Journal of Psychiatry*, **156**, 1409–1416.

Mataix-Cols, D., Rauch, S. L., Baer, L., *et al.* (2002a). Symptom stability in adult obsessive–compulsive disorder: data from a naturalistic two-year follow-up study. *American Journal of Psychiatry*, **159**, 263–268.

Mataix-Cols, D., Marks, I. M., Greist, J. H., Kobak, K. A., & Baer, L. (2002b). Obsessive–compulsive symptom dimensions as predictors of compliance with and response to behaviour therapy: results from a controlled trial. *Psychotherapy and Psychosomatics*, **71**, 255–262.

Mataix-Cols, D., Wooderson, S., Lawrence, N., *et al.* (2004). Distinct neural correlates of washing, checking, and hoarding symptom dimensions in obsessive–compulsive disorder. *Archives of General Psychiatry*, **61**, 564–576.

Mataix-Cols, D., Rosario-Campos, M. C., & Leckman, J. F. (2005). A multidimensional model of obsessive–compulsive disorder. *American Journal of Psychiatry*, **162**, 228–238.

Menzies, L., Achard, S., Chamberlain, S. R., *et al.* (2007). Neurocognitive endophenotypes of obsessive–compulsive disorder. *Brain*, **130**, 3223–3236.

Menzies, L., Williams, G. B., Chamberlain, S. R., *et al.* (2008). White matter abnormalities in patients with obsessive–compulsive disorder and their first-degree relatives. *American Journal of Psychiatry*, **165**, 1308–1315.

Miguel, E. C., Rauch, S. L. & Jenike, M. A. (1997). Phenomenology of intentional repetitive behaviors in obsessive–compulsive disorder and Tourette's disorder. *Journal of Clinical Psychiatry*, **56**, 246–255.

Miguel, E. C., Leckman, J. F., Rauch, S., *et al.* (2005). Obsessive–compulsive disorder phenotypes: implications for genetic studies. *Molecular Psychiatry*, **10**, 258–275.

Millet, B., Kochman, F., Gallarda, T., *et al.* (2004). Phenomenological and comorbid features associated in obsessive–compulsive disorder: influence of age of onset. *Journal of Affective Disorders*, **79**, 241–246.

Murray, C., & Lopez, A. (1996). *The Global Burden of Disease: a Comprehensive Assessment of Mortality and Disability from Diseases, Injuries, and Risk Factors in 1990 and Projected to 2020*. Cambridge, MA: Harvard University Press.

Nestadt, G., Samuels, J., Riddle, M., *et al.* (2000). A family study of obsessive–compulsive disorder. *Archives of General Psychiatry*, **57**, 358–363.

Nestadt, G., Samuels, J., Riddle, M. A., *et al.* (2001). The relationship between obsessive–compulsive disorder and anxiety and affective disorders: results from the Johns Hopkins OCD Family Study. *Psychological Medicine*, **31**, 481–487.

Olvet, D. M., & Hajcak, G. (2008). The error-related negativity (ERN) and psychopathology: toward an endophenotype. *Clinical Psychology Review*, **28**, 1343–1354.

Pauls, D. L., Towbin, K. E., Leckman, J. F., Zahner, G. E., & Cohen, D. J. (1986). Gilles de la Tourette's syndrome and obsessive–compulsive disorder: evidence supporting a genetic relationship. *Archives of General Psychiatry*, **43**, 1180–1182.

Pauls, D. L., Alsobrook, J. P., Goodman, W., Rasmussen, S., & Leckman, J. F. (1995). A family study of obsessive–compulsive disorder. *American Journal of Psychiatry*, **152**, 76–84.

Pigott, T. A., L'Heureux, F., Dubbert, B., Bernstein, S., & Murphy, D. L. (1994). Obsessive compulsive disorder: comorbid conditions. *Journal of Clinical Psychiatry*, **55** (Suppl), 15–27; discussion 28–32.

Pinto, A. (2009). Understanding obsessive compulsive personality disorder and its impact on obsessive compulsive disorder. Paper presented at Obsessive Compulsive Foundation Conference, Minneapolis, MN.

Pinto, A., Mancebo, M. C., Eisen, J. L., Pagano, M. E., & Rasmussen, S. A. (2006). The Brown Longitudinal Obsessive Compulsive Study: clinical features and symptoms of the sample at intake. *Journal of Clinical Psychiatry*, **67**, 703–711.

Pinto, A., Eisen, J. L., Mancebo, M. C., *et al.* (2007). Taboo thoughts and doubt/checking: a refinement of the factor structure for obsessive compulsive disorder symptoms. *Psychiatry Research*, **151**, 255–258.

Pinto, A., Eisen, J. L., Mancebo, M. C., & Rasmussen, S. A. (2008a). Obsessive compulsive personality disorder. In J. S. Abramowitz, D. McKay, & S. Taylor, eds., *Obsessive-compulsive Disorder: Subtypes and Spectrum Conditions*. New York, NY: Elsevier.

Pinto, A., Greenberg, B. D., Grados, M. A., *et al.* (2008b). Further development of YBOCS dimensions in the OCD Collaborative Genetics Study: symptoms vs. categories. *Psychiatry Research*, **160**, 83–93.

Pinto, A., Liebowitz, M. R., Foa, E. B., & Simpson, H. B. (2009). OCPD severity as a predictor of CBT outcome for OCD. Paper presented at the Congress of the International Society for the Study of Personality Disorders, New York, NY.

Pitman, R. K. (1987). Pierre Janet on obsessive–compulsive disorder (1903): review and commentary. *Archives of General Psychiatry*, **44**, 226–232.

Preston, G. A., & Weinberger, D. R. (2005). Intermediate phenotypes in schizophrenia: a selective review. *Dialogues in Clinical Neuroscience*, **7**, 165–179.

Radomsky, A. S., & Taylor, S. (2005). Subtyping OCD: prospects and problems. *Behavior Therapy*, **36**, 371–379.

Rasmussen, S. A., & Eisen, J. L. (1988). Clinical and epidemiologic findings of significance to neuropharmacologic trials in OCD. *Psychopharmacoology Bulletin*, **24**, 466–470.

Rauch, S. L., Dougherty, D. D., Shin, L. M., *et al.* (1998). Neural correlates of factor-analyzed OCD symptom dimensions: a PET study. *CNS Spectrums*, **3**, 37–43.

Robbins, T. W. (2007). Shifting and stopping: fronto-striatal substrates, neurochemical modulation and clinical implications. *Philosophical Transactions of the Royal Society B*, **362**, 917–932.

Robins, E., & Guze, S. B. (1970). Establishment of diagnostic validity in psychiatric illness: Its application to schizophrenia. *American Journal of Psychiatry*, **126**, 983–987.

Rosario-Campos, M. C., Leckman, J. F., Mercadante, M. T., *et al.* (2001). Adults with early-onset obsessive–compulsive disorder. *American Journal of Psychiatry*, **158**, 1899–1903.

Rosario-Campos, M. C., Miguel, E. C., Quatrano, S., *et al.* (2006). The Dimensional Yale–Brown Obsessive-Compulsive Scale (DY-BOCS): an instrument for assessing obsessive–compulsive symptom dimensions. *Molecular Psychiatry*, **11**, 495–504.

Rufer, M., Grothusen, A., Mass, R., Peter, H., & Hand, I. (2005). Temporal stability of symptom dimensions in adult patients with obsessive–compulsive disorder. *Journal of Affective Disorders*, **88**, 99–102.

Samuels, J., Nestadt, G., Bienvenu, O. J., *et al.* (2000). Personality disorders and normal personality dimensions in obsessive–compulsive disorder. *British Journal of Psychiatry*, **177**, 457–462.

Samuels, J., Eaton, W. W., Bienvenu, O. J., *et al.* (2002). Prevalence and correlates of personality disorders in a community sample. *British Journal of Psychiatry*, **180**, 536–542.

Saxena, S., Maidment, K. M., Vapnik, T., *et al.* (2002). Obsessive–compulsive hoarding: symptom severity and response to multimodal treatment. *Journal of Clinical Psychiatry*, **63**, 21–27.

Saxena, S., Brody, A. L., Maidment, K. M., & Baxter, L. R. (2007). Paroxetine treatment of compulsive hoarding. *Journal of Psychiatric Research*, **41**, 481–487.

Schooler, C., Revell, A. J., Timpano, K. R., Wheaton, M., & Murphy, D. L. (2008). Predicting genetic loading from symptom patterns in obsessive–compulsive disorder: a latent variable analysis. *Depression and Anxiety*, **25**, 680–688.

Simpson, H. B., Rosen, W., Huppert, J. D., *et al.* (2006). Are there reliable neuropsychological deficits in obsessive–compulsive disorder? *Journal of Psychiatric Research*, **40**, 247–257.

Skodol, A. E., Oldham, J. M., Hyler, S. E., *et al.* (1995). Patterns of anxiety and personality disorder comorbidity. *Journal of Psychiatric Research*, **5**, 361–374.

Skoog, G., & Skoog, I. (1999). A 40-year follow-up of patients with obsessive–compulsive disorder. *Archives of General Psychiatry*, **56**, 121–127.

Sobin, C., Blundell, M. L., & Karayiorgou, M. (2000). Phenotypic differences in early- and late-onset obsessive–compulsive disorder. *Comprehensive Psychiatry*, **41**, 373–379.

Stein, D. J., Andersen, E. W., & Overo, K. F. (2007). Response of symptom dimensions in obsessive–compulsive disorder to treatment with citalopram or placebo. *Revista Brasileira de Psiquiatria*, **29**, 303–307.

Stern, E., Silbersweig, D. A., Chee, K. Y., *et al.* (2000). A functional neuroanatomy of tics in Tourette syndrome. *Archives of General Psychiatry*, **57**, 741–748.

Swedo, S. E., Rapoport, J. L., Leonard, H. L., Lenane, M. C., & Cheslow, D. (1989). Obsessive compulsive disorder in children and adolescents: Clinical and phenomenology of 70 consecutive cases. *Archives of General Psychiatry*, **46**, 335–341.

Swerdlow, N. R., Benbow, C. H., Zisook, S., Geyer, M. A., & Braff, D. L. (1993). A preliminary assessment of sensorimotor gating in patients with obsessive compulsive disorder. *Biological Psychiatry*, **33**, 298–301.

Torgersen, S., Kringlen, E., & Cramer, V. (2001). The prevalence of personality disorders in a community sample. *Archives of General Psychiatry*, **58**, 590–596.

van den Heuvel, O. A., Remijnse, P. L., Mataix-Cols, D., *et al.* (2009). The major symptom dimensions of obsessive–compulsive disorder are mediated by partially distinct neural systems. *Brain*, **132**, 853–868.

Watkins, L. H., Sahakian, B. J., Robertson, M. M., *et al.* (2005). Executive function in Tourette's syndrome and obsessive–compulsive disorder. *Psychological Medicine*, **35**, 571–582.

Wellen, D., Samuels, J., Bienvenu, O. J., *et al.* (2007). Utility of the Leyton Obsessional Inventory to distinguish OCD and OCPD. *Depression and Anxiety*, **24**, 301–306.

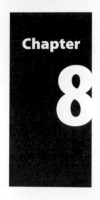

Is there a spectrum of social anxiety disorder?

Franklin Schneier, Jami Socha

8.1 Introduction

The diagnostic category of social anxiety disorder (SAD), also known as social phobia, has been well validated over the past three decades since its introduction in the DSM-III. Characterized by core features of excessive fear of embarrassment and associated avoidance of social situations, SAD can reliably be diagnosed (Mannuzza *et al.* 1995). It also can be differentiated from other anxiety disorders, and its prototypical course differs from other phobic disorders in having mean age of onset in the mid teens (later than most specific phobias and earlier than typical agoraphobia). Other common and relatively specific features include physical symptoms of blushing, sweating, or trembling (Connor *et al.* 2006a) and associated cognitive processes of self-directed attention and fears of negative evaluation (Schultz & Heimberg 2008). Family members of persons with SAD have a specific increased risk of also having the disorder (Low *et al.* 2008).

The neurobiological profile of SAD is characterized by hyper-responsivity of amygdala fear circuitry and sensitivity to fear conditioning for social threat stimuli (Stein *et al.* 2002, Lissek *et al.* 2008). There is evidence for dysregulation of serotonin, dopamine, and hypothalamic–pituitary–adrenal (HPA) axis systems (Argyropoulos *et al.* 2001), as well as differences in startle and autonomic reactivity (Cornwell *et al.* 2006). Persons with SAD respond to treatment with specific forms of cognitive–behavioral therapy and to pharmacotherapies including selective serotonin reuptake inhibitors (SSRIs), benzodiazepines, and monoamine oxidase inhibitors (MAOIs) (see Chapter 23).

A challenging issue in defining this disorder has been where to demarcate its boundary with normality. Unlike some psychiatric disorders that are characterized by features outside of usual everyday experience, such as panic attacks or hallucinations, SAD is defined by an excess of the concerns about negative evaluation that are also the currency of many normal social interactions. Differentiating SAD from normality therefore rests on the more subjective judgments of whether symptoms of SAD are "excessive and unreasonable," whether they "interfere significantly with the person's normal routine, occupational functioning, or social activities or relationships," and whether there is "marked distress about having the phobia" (American Psychiatric Association 2000). Studies have shown that varying the stringency of the definition of this threshold (e.g., by requiring moderate distress, marked distress, or distress accompanied by impairment) yields community prevalences of significant social fears ranging from 2% to 19% (Stein *et al.* 1994). Furthermore, persons with symptoms that fall short of the DSM threshold for a full diagnosis of SAD also evidence substantial impairment, based on objective assessments (Davidson *et al.* 1994, Fehm *et al.* 2008).

Some critics of psychiatry have seized upon this boundary dispute as evidence for the claim that SAD does not exist. Mental-health clinicians, on the other hand, tend not to worry about this threshold issue, because persons who are neither suffering nor impaired do not as a rule present for treatment. As researchers of SAD and social neuroscience, we find this qualitative continuity of SAD features across the diagnostic threshold to be neither a fatal flaw in the disorder's definition nor a clinically irrelevant peccadillo. Instead, it suggests a trait-like diathesis or temperament that may be essential to understanding the pathophysiology and informing the clinical treatment of SAD and related disorders.

This chapter assesses the relationship of SAD to trait phenomena of shyness, behavioral inhibition,

Anxiety Disorders: Theory, Research, and Clinical Perspectives, ed. Helen Blair Simpson, Yuval Neria, Roberto Lewis-Fernández, Franklin Schneier. Published by Cambridge University Press. © Cambridge University Press 2010.

and avoidant personality. We explore the concept that these constructs lie on a spectrum of socially anxious temperaments, and that these temperaments are essential and adaptive for group-living species. Finally, we consider evidence that the same temperamental features influence, to a variable extent, a much broader spectrum of psychopathology.

8.2 SAD and trait phenomena

Several key features of SAD are also considered defining features of personality traits and disorders, including early age of onset, chronic course, pervasive quality, and tendency to be experienced as ego-syntonic. These qualities contribute to the low rate of treatment seeking in SAD, as many persons view it as an immutable part of their personality. SAD appears to overlap "shyness," a lay term for a familiar and ubiquitous trait, reported by as many as 90% of community subjects in one survey (Zimbardo 1977). At the other extreme of severity, personality disorder researchers have characterized avoidant personality disorder, which shares with SAD the trait features of social avoidance related to anxiety (American Psychiatric Association 2000).

8.2.1 Shyness and SAD

Several studies have examined the relationship of shyness to SAD. Persons in both groups share frequent concerns about blushing, trembling, sweating, fears of negative evaluation, and avoidance of social situations (Turner et al. 1990). Most shy persons, however, do not meet criteria for SAD. For example, in a non-clinical sample of college students, SAD was diagnosed in 36% of highly shy subjects (defined by scoring in the upper 10th percentile on a shyness self-report scale) but in only 4% of moderately shy subjects (those who scored in the 40th to 60th percentile) (Stein et al. 2001a).

At the same time, a majority of SAD patients do report a history of shyness, including 76% of those with the generalized subtype, and 56% of those with the non-generalized subtype of SAD in one study (Stemberger et al. 1995). Shyness and SAD also appear to be related within families. Mothers of shy four-year-olds had an almost eight-fold increase in the rate of SAD (Cooper & Eke 1999). Thus, the existing evidence for a relationship between shyness and SAD, while limited, points to an overlap in symptomatology that differs more in severity and impairment than in quality of fears or behaviors. At higher levels of shyness, fear and avoidance of social situations are more likely to result in impairment in function that fulfills criteria for SAD.

8.2.2 Avoidant personality disorder and SAD

Avoidant personality disorder (APVD) is another trait construct that may be related to SAD. The original criteria for APVD drew upon of the work of Millon (1969), who conceptualized persons with the disorder as actively avoidant of social relationships, in contrast to the passive detachment of schizoid personality disorder. Current diagnostic criteria for APVD consist of seven items, each of which describes an element of avoidance due to fears of negative evaluation or interpersonal inadequacy (American Psychiatric Association 2000). More than two dozen studies have attempted to disentangle the relationship between APVD and SAD, but this has proven to be a difficult task, given that rates of APVD among SAD patient samples range as high as 84% (Alnaes & Torgersen 1988), with the highest rates among the more severe generalized subtype of SAD. The disorders co-occur in families (Stein et al. 1998), and they also respond to similar treatments (Turner et al. 1992), although, like SAD of greater severity, SAD with APVD may be more difficult to treat (Massion et al. 2002). Recent studies have been divided on whether SAD and APVD overlap so much that they should be considered a single category (Chambless et al. 2008, Huppert et al. 2008) or whether APVD shows some significant qualitative differences, such as a broader range of symptoms and interpersonal dysfunction (Hummelen et al. 2007). Such differences, however, may be limited to environmental rather than genetic determinants (Reichborn-Kjennerud et al. 2007). Most findings are consistent with the concept of a single continuous trait contributing to the features that are shared by these disorders.

8.2.3 Behavioral inhibition and SAD

A variety of other measurable psychological trait constructs have been closely associated with SAD, including fear of negative evaluation, avoidance of social interaction, and fear of scrutiny/performance. Traits that extend beyond the social sphere, such as neuroticism and harm avoidance, are also associated with SAD, albeit with less specificity. Among traits associated with SAD, however, behavioral inhibition to the unfamiliar has emerged as one of the most likely to be helpful in understanding the biological underpinnings specific to the disorder.

First described by Kagan and colleagues (1988) as a stable temperamental style identifiable by the second year of life, behavioral inhibition involves the tendency to withdraw in response to unfamiliar people, situations, and objects. Researchers assess the behavioral inhibition by measuring latencies to approach and vocalization in novel situations and by quantifying socially reticent behaviors in free-play situations (Fox *et al.* 2005). When behaviorally inhibited children are placed in an unfamiliar situation, they tend to cry, fret, withdraw, and/or fail to interact with others. In longitudinal studies, behavioral inhibition shows moderate stability, with 30–70% of behaviorally inhibited infants retaining the temperamental profile into childhood (Kagan *et al.* 1988, Broberg *et al.* 1990).

Although behavioral inhibition has been associated with anxiety disorders in general, and with major depression, recent longitudinal (Schwartz *et al.* 1999; Biederman *et al.* 2001; Hirshfeld-Becker *et al.* 2007) and retrospective (Hayward *et al.* 1998) studies have identified a more specific relationship with the psychopathology of SAD. Hirshfeld-Becker and colleagues (2007) found that behavioral inhibition in infancy (21 months) and childhood (four and six years) specifically predicted the onset of SAD by middle school. Schwartz and colleagues (1999) found that 34% of children originally classified as behaviorally inhibited had developed generalized social anxiety by early adolescence, significantly more than the 9% of uninhibited children who developed SAD. Similar associations of behavioral inhibition with later childhood shyness have been identified prospectively (Schmidt *et al.* 1997).

Neurobiological findings associated with behavioral inhibition show a number of parallels with findings reported in SAD, including peripheral markers showing sympathetic arousal, elevated cortisol, and increased startle (Hirshfeld-Becker *et al.* 2008). Functional magnetic resonance imaging (fMRI) studies suggest that adults with a history of behavioral inhibition (Schwartz *et al.* 2003) and young adolescents who were consistently behaviorally inhibited since childhood (Perez-Edgar *et al.* 2007) show increased amygdala activity to unfamiliar and emotional faces, respectively. This parallels findings of amygdala hyper-responsivity to harsh emotional faces in persons with SAD (Stein *et al.* 2002, Yoon *et al.* 2007). Preliminary genetic evidence suggests that presence of the short allele of the serotonin transporter may interact with environmental factors, such as low maternal social support, to increase risk for behavioral inhibition in middle childhood (Fox *et al.* 2005). In a study of children's cerebral responses

to facial expression, shyness/behavioral inhibition and presence of the short allele of the serotonin transporter were associated with altered cerebral processing of angry face stimuli (Battaglia *et al.* 2005).

An advantage of behavioral inhibition as a construct for neurobiological research is its basis in observation of behaviors, which has allowed it to be studied translationally in non-human primates. Monkeys demonstrate stable individual differences in social behaviors that appear homologous to human temperamental differences. Social inhibition has been shown to be consistent across conditions in vervet monkeys (Fairbanks *et al.* 2004a), and inhibition of approach to an unfamiliar conspecific has been associated with higher cerebrospinal levels of the serotonin metabolite 5-HIAA and higher serotonergic responsivity to fenfluramine challenge (Manuck *et al.* 2003). This temperament appears to have a heritable component that can also influence response to stressful life events. Latency to leave a mother in order to explore novel objects has been shown to be heritable in young rhesus monkeys (Williamson *et al.* 2003), as have approach behaviors in adolescent and adult vervet monkeys exposed to an unfamiliar conspecific (Fairbanks *et al.* 2004b). Higher levels of behavioral inhibition may compromise mechanisms for coping with major social stressors, such as maternal separation, leading acutely to greater cortisol elevations and the potential for longer-term social impairments (Erickson *et al.* 2005).

In summary, SAD, avoidant personality disorder, shyness, and behavioral inhibition all appear to be manifestations of a social anxiety temperamental spectrum. Shyness is a lay term representing the mildest end of this continuum; behavioral inhibition is defined more narrowly through observation of young children in a laboratory setting; SAD is a yet-narrower category, defined by distress or impairment due to social anxiety, and often characterized by emergent fears of negative evaluation; and avoidant personality disorder lies at the severe extreme, defined by broad avoidance due to social fears. Despite their varied definitions, these contructs overlap in phenomenology, genetics, neurobiology, and response to treatment. But why should this area of temperament be the focus of so many convergent constructs?

8.2.4 An evolutionary perspective

From an evolutionary perspective, the conservation of social behavioral inhibition across primate species suggests that the trait may have some adaptive value. Öhman (1986) conceived of social submissiveness as a behavioral system that may be fundamental to group-living species. Within many group-living species, dominance hierarchies manage competition for resources (Hinde 1985), and in such hierarchies, aggressive behavior of dominant individuals has the clear benefits of increasing an individual's access to resources and reproductive success, particularly when the social group is unstable. Risk taking, however, may be less beneficial in another context. In stable social groups, excessive aggression may interfere with social integration and lead to resistance from other powerful group members, whereas submissive or inhibited behavior prevents physical attack by dominant and often physically stronger individuals. This adaptive quality of behavioral inhibition may have contributed to the persistence of this trait.

Gilbert (2001) has suggested that in humans, dominance may be conferred by attractiveness more than aggression, and the social anxiety and submissive behavior associated with behavioral inhibition may function to prevent anticipated rejection or embarrassment. Carried to the extreme, however, social anxiety carries a cost of missed opportunities to advance desired relationships and social status. This perspective is consistent with the idea that trait behavioral inhibition may have adaptive functions, but its more extreme forms may lead to the misadaptation of SAD, and may also predispose to and interact with a broader range of psychopathology.

8.3 Trait social anxiety and a broader spectrum of related psychopathology

The spectrum of social anxiety temperament also appears to be related to a much broader spectrum of associated psychopathology. Identifying the relationships of trait behavioral inhibition and SAD to other psychiatric and medical disorders has implications for diagnostic nosology, clinical identification of comorbidity, and selection of treatment approaches. Awareness of such relationships can alert clinicians to explore potential comorbidities and to modify treatments to address multiple target symptoms. It can also stimulate research that crosses diagnostic boundaries to investigate more basic neurobiological and psychological constructs. The following section will critically review evidence for the relationship of trait social inhibition/anxiety and SAD to selected other psychiatric and medical disorders. The validity of these

proposed relationships will need to be confirmed by long-term prospective assessments of the relationship of behavioral inhibition to other disorders, and they may ultimately be best defined by identification of specific neurobiological or environmental commonalities. Until such knowledge becomes available, however, the delineation of a social anxiety spectrum based upon phenomenological assessments of syndromal overlap and comorbidity of SAD with other disorders may be a preliminary indicator of relevant areas of psychopathology.

8.3.1 Selective mutism

Selective mutism has been closely linked to SAD. It shares with SAD behavioral inhibition in the form of avoidance of speaking behavior, as characterized by persistent failure to speak in one or more major social situations, including school, despite the ability to comprehend spoken language and to speak. Although disparate theories have been offered for the causation of selective mutism, two of the largest descriptive studies of the disorder have suggested that it may be a variant of SAD. One study reported that 97% of 30 children with DSM-III-R selective mutism were diagnosed with social phobia or avoidant disorder of childhood (the latter has been essentially subsumed under the diagnosis of SAD in DSM-IV) (Black & Uhde 1995). The other study found that all 50 subjects in a case series of selective mutism met DSM-III-R criteria for SAD or avoidant disorder of childhood (Dummit *et al.* 1997). Rates of generalized SAD specifically have been found to be elevated in the parents of children with selective mutism (37% versus 14% in parents of control-group children) (Chavira *et al.* 2007). The possible presence of language difficulties concurrent with social anxiety may be a specific feature of selective mutism (Manassis *et al.* 2003). Pharmacological treatment with classes of medication known to be efficacious in SAD has appeared promising in small open trials (Golwyn & Sevlie 1999).

8.3.2 Autism and Asperger's syndrome

Among other childhood disorders, autism and Asperger's syndrome are less tightly linked with SAD. They do share prominent social dysfunction with SAD, and these disorders are often mentioned together when researchers have speculated about human application of animal models of social dysfunction. More than a quarter of persons with autism spectrum disorders may have SAD (Simonoff *et al.* 2008). Persons with

SAD alone, however, lack the pervasive impairment in social development and social relatedness that characterizes the autism spectrum disorders (Cath *et al.* 2008). Family studies have found an increased rate of SAD in the families of autistic spectrum probands, though the mechanism of this association remains unclear (Piven & Palmer 1999).

8.3.3 Other anxiety disorders

Other anxiety disorders – particularly other phobic disorders, panic disorder, and generalized anxiety disorder – have the highest rates of comorbidity with SAD in adults (Schneier *et al.* 1992), as well as some increased familiality and substantial overlap in the range of effective treatments and many neurobiological measures. The anxiety disorders are, of course, grouped diagnostically by the commonality of their prominent anxiety symptoms, and the phobic disorders all feature phobic avoidance. The close relationship of SAD to other anxiety disorders, though not surprising, is clinically important, and reflects shared diagnostic features and possibly shared higher-order traits, such as harm avoidance or neuroticism. SAD comorbidity among persons with other anxiety disorders may identify subgroups associated with differences in neurobiological functioning (Schneier *et al.* 2008) and differences in clinical features such as delayed treatment response (Berger *et al.* 2004).

8.3.4 Affective disorders

About a quarter of persons with major depressive disorder (MDD) also have SAD, yielding a 3.9% lifetime prevalence of the comorbid condition in the community (Kessler *et al.* 1999). Pre-existing or comorbid SAD is a well-documented risk factor for a more severe syndrome of depression with an earlier age of onset and increased number and duration of MDD episodes, suicidal ideation and attempts, alcohol dependence, and presence of the atypical subtype trait of interpersonal sensitivity (Alpert *et al.* 1997, Kessler *et al.* 1999, Parker *et al.* 1999, Nelson *et al.* 2000, Stein *et al.* 2001b, Beesdo *et al.* 2007, Dalrymple & Zimmerman 2007, Holma *et al.* 2008). In patients with a principal diagnosis of SAD, improvement in social anxiety appears to mediate improvement of depressive symptoms in cognitive–behavioral therapy (Moscovitch *et al.* 2005).

In comparison to comorbidity of SAD with MDD, comorbidity of SAD with bipolar disorder is much less common, although SAD and other anxiety disorders do co-occur with bipolar disorder at rates greater than chance (Kessler *et al.* 1999, Tamam & Ozpoyraz 2002). Perugi and colleagues (2001) have suggested that the comorbidity of SAD with bipolar disorder may have some specificity with the bipolar II subtype, especially in the presence of comorbid alcohol abuse (Perugi *et al.* 2002), and they have hypothesized that the social inhibition characterizing SAD may lie on a continuum with the disinhibition seen in bipolar II disorder (Himmelhoch 1998, Perugi *et al.* 2001).

8.3.5 Substance use disorders

Epidemiological and clinical studies have generally found SAD to be associated with increased rates of alcohol dependence, with SAD usually preceding the onset of the alcohol problem (Schneier *et al.* 2010). There is some evidence that persons with SAD are more affected by peer pressure to abuse substances. Additionally, some SAD patients experience their alcohol use as self-medication, and several models of the relationship of these disorders postulate that alcohol reduces anxiety, providing reinforcement of the drinking response. Social situations and anxiety symptoms then become conditioned cues that lead to the repeated consumption of alcohol (Morris *et al.* 2005). Thus, comorbid SAD may serve as a marker for a particular type of predisposition to alcohol abuse.

Presence of comorbid SAD can also impact the treatment of substance use disorders, for instance through refusal to participate in group modalities due to social anxiety. Studies of combined treatment for comorbid patients have had mixed results. In one study, cognitive–behavioral therapy directed at both alcoholism and social anxiety was not superior to therapy directed at alcoholism alone (Randall *et al.* 2001); paroxetine treatment of comorbid patients reduced social anxiety and altered the pattern of drinking, but did not reduce overall alcohol consumption (Book *et al.* 2008, Thomas *et al.* 2008).

8.3.6 Eating disorders

While social anxiety is not central to the conceptualizations of eating disorders, both anorexia and bulimia nervosa patients may have prominent concerns around negative evaluation of their appearance by others. In a recent study, 59% of patients with bulimia nervosa and 55% of patients with anorexia nervosa had comorbid SAD (Godart *et al.* 2000), and SAD pre-dated the eating disorder in 75% of cases. SAD features of fear of negative evaluation and attention to social comparison have been shown to be associated with eating disorder behaviors and attitudes (McClintock & Evans 2001, Gilbert & Meyer 2003).

8.3.7 Body dysmorphic disorder

Body dysmorphic disorder is characterized by preoccupation with an imagined physical anomaly, often leading to compulsive behaviors and social avoidance. For some persons with body dysmorphic disorder, fear of evaluation of their appearance by others is prominent. High rates of SAD, ranging from 20% to 50%, have been reported among patients with body dysmorphic disorder (Coles *et al.* 2006). A family-history study also found increased rates of SAD in the family of body dysmorphic disorder probands (Altamura *et al.* 2001). Recent findings, however, suggest that the longitudinal course of body dysmorphic disorder is more closely linked to obsessive–compulsive disorder than to SAD (Phillips & Stout 2006).

8.3.8 Psychotic disorders

SAD has been reported to be a pre-morbid risk factor for schizophrenia (Tien & Eaton 1992) and a comorbid disorder in as many as 36% of outpatients with schizophrenia (Pallanti *et al.* 2004). In the latter study, however, SAD was unrelated to positive or negative symptoms, which does not support its being integral to the schizophrenia syndrome. Instead, others have found that persons with schizophrenia who have comorbid SAD experience greater shame and loss of status associated with their psychotic disorder diagnosis (Birchwood *et al.* 2006). Treatment of schizophrenia with the atypical antipsychotic clozapine has been associated with an unexplained high rate of emergent SAD (Pallanti *et al.* 2000).

Taijin kyofusho (TKS) is an East Asian variant of SAD that is conceptualized as ranging from typical SAD symptoms to delusional symptoms. In addition to having features that are characteristic of SAD, such as fears of embarrassment and of showing signs of anxiety, TKS also includes several culture-specific features that may have a delusional intensity, such as a fear of offending others by making too-direct eye contact, experiencing a stiff facial expression, and emitting body odor. There has been discussion over whether to bring TKS features into future diagnostic criteria for SAD (Kinoshita *et al.* 2008).

8.3.9 Medical conditions that draw undesired attention

In Parkinson's disease, elevated rates of social anxiety symptoms have been found in some studies, with most cases reported as not purely secondary to embarrassment over Parkinsonian symptoms (Kummer *et al.* 2008). Some evidence for hypodopaminergic function in SAD has raised the question of possible shared dopaminergic mechanisms in the elevated co-occurrence of these conditions (Schneier *et al.* 2000). Other neurological and behavioral conditions with elevated rates of SAD or social anxiety symptoms include spasmodic torticollis (Gundel *et al.* 2001), essential tremor (Schneier *et al.* 2001), and stuttering (Stein *et al.* 1996). Similarly, social anxiety has been shown to be high following facial disfigurement (Newell & Marks 2000), and persons with SAD and hyperhidrosis appear to benefit most from treatment independently directed at each condition (Connor *et al.* 2006b). All these disorders draw undesired attention that may trigger social anxiety. The subset of disorders with symptoms such as tremor or sweating, which may also be *manifestations* of social anxiety, appear to have more complex interwoven relationships with SAD.

8.4 Conclusions

Social anxiety disorder is a common condition with many trait-like features. It is closely associated with trait shyness, avoidant personality disorder, and the temperament of behavioral inhibition. Social behavioral inhibition appears to be conserved as a common temperament across primate species and may have adaptive qualities. Recognition of this trait quality may be important in researching the biological and psychosocial underpinnings of SAD. Clinically, the common trait of social inhibition may influence the expression, comorbidity, and appropriate treatment of a variety of psychiatric disorders, particularly those with prominent inhibition or anxiety components. Persons with these disorders should be thoroughly assessed for features of SAD and inhibited temperament, and treatment may need to be directed at multiple targets. Future research should investigate the neurobiological and psychosocial underpinnings of the socially/behaviorally inhibited temperament and their relationships to this spectrum of psychiatric disorders.

References

Alnaes, S., & Torgersen, S. (1988). The relationship between DSM-III symptom disorders (Axis I) and personality disorders (Axis II) in an outpatient population. *Acta Psychiatrica Scandinavica*, **78**, 485–492.

Alpert, J. E., Uebelacker, L. A., McLean, N. E., *et al.* (1997). Social phobia, avoidant personality disorder and atypical depression: co-occurrence and clinical implications. *Psychological Medicine*, **27**, 627–633.

Altamura, C., Paluello, M. M., Mundo, E., Medda, S., & Mannu, P. (2001). Clinical and subclinical body dysmorphic disorder. *European Archives of Psychiatry and Clinical Neuroscience*, **251**, 105–108.

American Psychiatric Association (2000). *Diagnostic and Statistical Manual of Mental Disorders*, 4th edn, text revision (DSM-IV-TR). Washington, DC: American Psychiatric Association.

Argyropoulos, S. V., Bell, C. J., & Nutt, D. J. (2001). Brain function in social anxiety disorder. *Psychiatric Clinics of North America*, **24**, 707–772.

Battaglia, M., Ogliari, A., Zanoni, A., *et al.* (2005). Influence of the serotonin transporter promoter gene and shyness on children's cerebral responses to facial expressions. *Archives of General Psychiatry*, **62**, 85–94.

Beesdo, K., Bittner, A., Pine, D. S., *et al.* (2007). Incidence of social anxiety disorder and the consistent risk for secondary depression in the first three decades of life. *Archives of General Psychiatry*, **64**, 903–912.

Berger, P., Sachs, G., Amering, M., *et al.* (2004). Personality disorder and social anxiety predict delayed response in drug and behavioral treatment of panic disorder. *Journal of Affective Disorders*, **80**, 75–78.

Biederman, J., Hirshfeld-Becker, D. R., Rosenbaum, J. F., *et al.* (2001). Further evidence of association between behavioral inhibition and social anxiety in children. *American Journal of Psychiatry*, **158**, 1673–1679.

Birchwood, M., Trower, P., Brunet, K., *et al.* (2006). Social anxiety and the shame of psychosis: a study in first episode psychosis. *Behaviour Research and Therapy*, **45**, 1025–1027.

Black, B., & Uhde, T. (1995). Psychiatric characteristics of children with selective mutism: a pilot study. *Journal of the American Academy of Child and Adolescent Psychiatry*, **34**, 847–856.

Book, S. W., Thomas, S. E., Randall, P. K., & Randall, C. L. (2008). Paroxetine reduces social anxiety in individuals with a co-occurring alcohol use disorder. *Journal of Anxiety Disorders*, **22**, 310–318.

Broberg, A., Lamb, M., & Hwang, P. (1990). Inhibition: its stability and correlates in sixteen- to forty-month-old children. *Child Development*, **61**, 1153–1163.

Cath, D. C., Ran, N., Smit, J. H., van Balkom, A. J., & Comijs, H. C. (2008). Symptom overlap between autism spectrum disorder, generalized social anxiety disorder and obsessive–compulsive disorder in adults: a preliminary case-controlled study. *Psychopathology*, **41**, 101–110.

Chambless, D. L., Fydrich, T., & Rodebaugh, T. L. (2008). Generalized social phobia and avoidant personality disorder: meaningful distinction or useless duplication? *Depression and Anxiety*, **25**, 8–19.

Chavira, D. A., Shipon-Blum, E., Hitchcock, C., Cohan, S., & Stein, M. B. (2007). Selective mutism and social anxiety disorder: all in the family? *Journal of the American Academy of Child and Adolescent Psychiatry*, **46**, 1464–1472.

Coles, M. E., Phillips, K. A., Menard, W., *et al.* (2006). Body dysmorphic disorder and social phobia: cross-sectional and prospective data. *Depression and Anxiety*, **23**, 26–33.

Connor, K. M., Davidson, J. R., Chung, H., Yang, R., & Clary, C. M. (2006a). Multidimensional effects of sertraline in social anxiety disorder. *Depression and Anxiety*, **23**, 6–10.

Connor, K. M., Cook, J. L., & Davidson, J. R. (2006b). Botulinum toxin treatment of social anxiety disorder with hyperhidrosis: a placebo-controlled double-blind trial. *Journal of Clinical Psychiatry*, **67**, 30–36.

Cooper, P. J., & Eke, M. (1999). Childhood shyness and maternal social phobia: a community study. *British Journal of Psychiatry*, **174**, 439–443.

Cornwell, B. R., Johnson, L., Berardi, L., & Grillon, C. (2006). Anticipation of public speaking in virtual reality reveals a relationship between trait social anxiety and startle reactivity. *Biological Psychiatry*, **59**, 664–666.

Dalrymple, K. L., & Zimmerman, M. (2007). Does comorbid social anxiety disorder impact the clinical presentation of principal major depression disorder? *Journal of Affective Disorders*, **100**, 241–247.

Davidson, R. T., Hughes, D. C., George, L. K., & Blazer, D. G. (1994). The boundary of social phobia: exploring the threshold. *Archives of General Psychiatry*, **51**, 975–983.

Dummit, E. S., Klein, R. G., Tancer, N. K., *et al.* (1997). Systematic assessment of 50 children with selective mutism. *Journal of the American Academy of Child and Adolescent Psychiatry*, **36**, 653–660.

Erickson, K., Gabry, K. E., Schulkin, J., *et al.* (2005). Social withdrawal behaviors in nonhuman primates and changes in neuroendocrine and monoamine concentrations during a separation paradigm. *Developmental Psychobiology*, **46**, 331–339.

Fairbanks, L. A., Jorgensen, M. J., Huff, A., *et al.* (2004a). Adolescent impulsivity predicts adult dominance attainment in male vervet monkeys. *American Journal of Primatology*, **64**, 1–17.

Fairbanks, L. A., Newman, T. K., Bailey, J. N., *et al.* (2004b). Genetic contributions to social impulsivity and aggressiveness in vervet monkeys. *Biological Psychiatry*, **55**, 642–647.

Fehm, L., Beesdo, K., Jacobi, F., & Fiedler, A. (2008). Social anxiety disorder above and below the diagnostic threshold: prevalence, comorbidity and impairment in the general population. *Social Psychiatry and Psychiatric Epidemiology*, **43**, 257–265.

Fox, N. A., Nichols, K. E., Henderson, H. A., *et al.* (2005). Evidence for a gene–environment interaction in predicting behavioral inhibition in middle childhood. *Psychological Science*, **16**, 921–926.

Gilbert, N., & Meyer, C. (2003). Social anxiety and social comparison: differential links with restrictive and bulimic attitudes among nonclinical women. *Eating Behavior*, **4**, 257–264.

Gilbert, P. (2001). Evolution and social anxiety: the role of attraction, social competition, and social hierarchies. *Psychiatric Clinics of North America*, **24**, 723–752.

Godart, N. T., Flament, M. F., Lecrubier, Y., & Jeammet, P. (2000). Anxiety disorders in anorexia nervosa and bulimia nervosa: Comorbidity and chronology of appearance. *European Psychiatry*, **15**, 38–45.

Golwyn, D. H., & Sevlie, C. P. (1999). Phenelzine treatment of selective mutism in four prepubertal children. *Journal of Child and Adolescent Psychopharmacology*, **9**, 109–113.

Gundel, H., Wolf, A., Xidarra, V., Busch, R., & Ceballos-Baumann, A. O. (2001). Social phobia in spasmodic torticollis. *Journal of Neurology, Neurosurgery, and Psychiatry*, **71**, 499–504.

Hayward, C., Killen, J., Kraemer, K., & Taylor, C. (1998). Linking self-reported childhood behavioral inhibition to adolescent social phobia. *Journal of the American Academy of Child and Adolescent Psychiatry*, **37**, 1308–1316.

Himmelhoch, J. M. (1998). Social anxiety, hypomania and the bipolar spectrum: data, theory and clinical issues. *Journal of Affective Disorders*, **50**, 203–213.

Hinde, R. A. (1985). Expression and negotiation. In G. Zivin, ed., *The Development of Expressive Behavior*. San Diego, CA: Academic Press.

Hirshfeld-Becker, D. R., Biederman, J., Henin, A., *et al.* (2007). Behavioral inhibition in preschool children at risk is a specific predictor of middle childhood social anxiety: a five-year follow-up. *Journal of Developmental and Behavioral Pediatrics*, **28**, 225–233.

Hirshfeld-Becker, D. R., Micco, J., Henin, A., *et al.* (2008). Behavioral inhibition. *Depression and Anxiety*, **25**, 357–367.

Holma, K. M., Holma, I. A., Melartin, T. K., Rytsälä, H. J., & Isometsä, E. T. (2008). Long-term outcome of major depressive disorder in psychiatric patients is variable. *Journal of Clinical Psychiatry*, **69**, 196–205.

Hummelen, B., Wilberg, T., Pedersen, G., & Karterud, S. (2007). The relationship between avoidant personality disorder and social phobia. *Comprehensive Psychiatry*, **48**, 348–356.

Huppert, J. D., Strunk, D. R., Ledley, D. R., Davidson, J. R., & Foa, E. B. (2008). Generalized social anxiety disorder and avoidant personality disorder: structural analysis and treatment outcome. *Depression and Anxiety*, **25**, 441–448.

Kagan, J., Reznick, J. S., & Snidman, N. (1988). Biological bases of childhood shyness. *Science*, **240**, 167–171.

Kessler, R. C., Stang, P., Wittchen, H. U., Stein, M., & Walters, E. E. (1999). Lifetime co-morbidities between social phobia and mood disorders in the US National Comorbidity Survey. *Psychological Medicine*, **29**, 555–567.

Kinoshita, Y., Chen, J., Rapee, R. M., *et al.* (2008). Cross-cultural study of conviction subtype Taijin Kyofu: proposal and reliability of Nagoya–Osaka diagnostic criteria for social anxiety disorder. *Journal of Nervous and Mental Disease*, **196**, 307–313.

Kummer, A., Cardoso, F., & Teixeira, A. L. (2008). Frequency of social phobia and psychometric properties of the Liebowitz social anxiety scale in Parkinson's disease. *Movement Disorders*, **23**, 1739–1743.

Lissek, S., Levenson, J., Biggs, A. L., *et al.* (2008). Elevated fear conditioning to socially relevant unconditioned stimuli in social anxiety disorder. *American Journal of Psychiatry*, **165**, 124–32.

Low, N. C., Cui, L., & Merikangas, K. R. (2008). Specificity of familial transmission of anxiety and comorbid disorders. *Journal of Psychiatric Research*, **42**, 596–604.

Manassis, K., Fung, D., Tannock, R., *et al.* (2003). Characterizing selective mutism: is it more than social anxiety? *Depression and Anxiety*, **218**, 153–161.

Mannuzza, S., Schneier, F. R., Chapman, T. F., *et al.* (1995). Generalized social phobia. Reliability and validity. *Archives of General Psychiatry*, **52**, 230–237.

Manuck, S. B., Kaplan, J. R., Rymeski, B. A., Fairbanks, L. A., & Wilson, M. E. (2003). Approach to a social stranger is associated with low central nervous system serotonergic responsivity in female cynomolgus monkeys (Macaca fascicularis). *American Journal of Primatology*, **61**, 187–194.

Massion, A. O., Dyck, I. R., Shea, T., *et al.* (2002). Personality disorders and time to remission in generalized anxiety disorder, social phobia, and panic disorder. *Archives of General Psychiatry*, **59**, 434–440.

McClintock, J. M., & Evans, I. M. (2001). The underlying psychopathology of eating disorders and social phobia: a structural equation analysis. *Eating Behavior*, **2**, 247–261.

Millon, T., ed. (1969). *Modern Psychopathology: a Biosocial Approach to Maladaptive Learning and Functioning.* Philadelphia, PA: Saunders.

Morris, E. P., Stewart, S. H., & Ham, L. S. (2005). The relationship between social anxiety disorder and alcohol use disorders: a critical review. *Clinical Psychology Review*, **25**, 734–760.

Moscovitch, D. A., Hofmann, S. G., Suvak, M. K., & In-Albon, T. (2005). Mediation of changes in anxiety and depression during treatment of social phobia. *Journal of Clinical and Consulting Psychology*, **73**, 945–952.

Nelson, E. C., Grant, J. D., Bucholz, K. K., *et al.* (2000). Social phobia in a population-based female adolescent twin sample: co-morbidity and associated suicide-related symptoms. *Psychological Medicine*, **30**, 797–804.

Newell, R., & Marks, I. (2000). Phobic nature of social difficulty in facially disfigured people. *British Journal of Psychiatry*, **176**, 177–181.

Öhman, A. (1986). Face the beast and fear the face: animal and social fears as prototypes for evolutionary analyses of emotion. *Psychophysiology*, **23**, 123–145.

Pallanti, S., Quercioli, L., & Pazagli, A. (2000). Social anxiety and premorbid personality disorders in paranoid schizophrenic patients treated with clozapine. *CNS Spectrums*, **5** (9), 29–43.

Pallanti, S., Quercioli, L., & Hollander, E. (2004). Social anxiety in outpatients with schizophrenia: a relevant cause of disability. *American Journal of Psychiatry*, **161**, 53–58.

Parker, G., Wilhelm, K., Mitchell, P., *et al.* (1999). The influence of anxiety as a risk to early onset major depression. *Journal of Affective Disorders*, **52**, 11–17.

Perez-Edgar, K., Roberson-Nay, R., Hardin, M. G., *et al.* (2007). Attention alters neural responses to evocative faces in behaviorally inhibited adolescents. *Neuroimage*, **35**, 1538–1546.

Perugi, G., Akiskal, H. S., Toni, C., Simonini, E., & Gemignani, A. (2001). The temporal relationship between anxiety disorders and (hypo)mania: a retrospective examination of 63 panic, social phobic and obsessive–compulsive patients with comorbid bipolar disorder. *Journal of Affective Disorders*, **67**, 199–206.

Perugi, G., Frare, F., Madaro, D., Maremmani, I., & Akiskal, H. S. (2002). Alcohol abuse in social phobic patients: is there a bipolar connection? *Journal of Affective Disorders*, **68**, 33–39.

Phillips, K. A., & Stout, R. L. (2006). Associations in the longitudinal course of body dysmorphic disorder with major depression, obsessive–compulsive disorder and social phobia. *Psychiatry Research*, **40**, 360–369.

Piven, J., & Palmer, P. (1999) Psychiatric disorder and the broad autism phenotype: evidence from a family study of multiple-incidence autism families. *American Journal of Psychiatry*, **156**, 557–563.

Randall, C. L., Thomas, S., & Thevos, A. K. (2001). Concurrent alcoholism and social anxiety disorder: a first step toward developing effective treatments. *Alcoholism, Clinical and Experimental Research*, **25**, 210–220.

Reichborn-Kjennerud, T., Czajkowski, N., Torgersen, S., *et al.* (2007). The relationship between avoidant personality disorder and social phobia: a population-based twin study. *American Journal of Psychiatry*, **164**, 1631–1633.

Schmidt, L. A., Fox, N. A., Rubin, K. H., *et al.* (1997). Behavioral and neuroendocrine responses in shy children. *Developmental Psychobiology*, **30**, 127–140.

Schneier, F. R., Johnson, J., Hornig, C. D., Liebowitz, M. R., & Weissman, M. M. (1992). Social phobia. Comorbidity and morbidity in an epidemiologic sample. *Archives of General Psychiatry*, **49**, 282–288.

Schneier, F. R., Liebowitz, M. R., Abi-Dargham, A., *et al.* (2000). Low dopamine D2 receptor binding potential in social phobia. *American Journal of Psychiatry*, **157**, 457–459.

Schneier, F. R., Barnes, L. F., Albert, S. M., & Louis, E. D. (2001). Characteristics of social phobia among persons with essential tremor. *Journal of Clinical Psychiatry*, **62**, 367–372.

Schneier, F. R., Martinez, D., Abi-Dargham, A., *et al.* (2008). Striatal dopamine D2 receptor availability in OCD with and without comorbid social anxiety disorder: preliminary findings. *Depression and Anxiety*, **25**, 1–7.

Schneier, F.R., Foose, T.E., Hasin, D.S., *et al.* (2010). Social anxiety disorder and alcohol use disorder comorbidity in the National Epidemiologic Survey on Alcohol and Related Conditions. *Psychological Medicine*, **40**(6), 977–988.

Schultz, L. T., & Heimberg, R. G. (2008). Attentional focus in social anxiety disorder: Potential for interactive processes. *Clinical Psychology Review*, **8**, 1206–1221.

Schwartz, C., Snidman, N., & Kagan, J. (1999). Adolescent social anxiety as an outcome of inhibited temperament in childhood. *Journal of the American Academy of Child and Adolescent Psychiatry*, **38**, 1008–1015.

Schwartz, C.E., Wright, C.I., Shin, L.M., Kagan, J., & Rauch, S.L. (2003). Inhibited and uninhibited infants "grown up": adult amygdalar response to novelty. *Science*, **300**, 1952–1953.

Simonoff, E., Pickles, A., Charman, T., *et al.* (2008). Psychiatric disorders in children with autism spectrum disorders: prevalence, comorbidity, and associated factors in a population-derived sample. *Journal of the American Academy of Child and Adolescent Psychiatry*, **47**, 921–929.

Stein, M. B., Walker, J. R., & Forde, D. R. (1994). Setting diagnostic thresholds for social phobia: considerations from a community survey of social anxiety. *American Journal of Psychiatry*, **151**, 408–412.

Stein, M. B., Baird, A., & Walker, J. R. (1996). Social phobia in adults with stuttering. *American Journal of Psychiatry*, **153**, 278–280.

Stein, M. B., Chartier, M. J., Hazen, A. L., *et al.* (1998). A direct-interview family study of generalized social phobia. *American Journal of Psychiatry*, **155**, 90–97.

Stein, M. B., Chavira, D. A., & Jang, K. L. (2001a). Bringing up bashful baby: developmental pathways to social phobia. *Psychiatric Clinics of North America*, **24**, 661–675.

Stein, M. B., Fuetsch, M., Müller, N., *et al.* (2001b). Social anxiety disorder and the risk of depression: a prospective community study of adolescents and young adults. *Archives of General Psychiatry*, **58**, 251–256.

Stein, M. B., Goldin, P. R., Sareen, J., Zorrilla, L. T., & Brown, G. G. (2002). Increased amygdala activation to angry and contemptuous faces in generalized social phobia. *Archives of General Psychiatry*, **59**, 1027–1034.

Stemberger, R. T., Turner, S. M., Beidel, D. C., & Calhoun, K. S. (1995). Social phobia: an analysis of possible developmental factors. *Journal of Abnormal Psychology*, **104**, 526–531.

Tamam, L., & Ozpoyraz, N. (2002). Comorbidity of anxiety disorder among patients with bipolar I disorder in remission. *Psychopathology*, **35**, 203–209.

Thomas, S. E., Randall, P. K., Book, S. W., & Randall, C. L. (2008). A complex relationship between co-occurring social anxiety and alcohol use disorders: what effect does treating social anxiety have on drinking? *Alcoholism, Clinical and Experimental Research*, **32**, 77–84.

Tien, A. Y., & Eaton, W. W. (1992). Psychopathologic precursors and sociodemographic risk factors for the schizophrenia syndrome. *Archives of General Psychiatry*, **49**, 37–46.

Turner, S. M., Beidel, D. C., & Townsley, R. M. (1990). Social phobia: relationship to shyness. *Behaviour Research and Therapy*, **28**, 497–505.

Turner, S. M., Beidel, D. C., & Townsley, R. M. (1992). Social phobia: a comparison of specific and generalized subtypes and avoidant personality disorder. *Journal of Abnormal Psychology*, **101**, 326–331.

Williamson, D. E., Coleman, K., Bacanu, S. A., Devlin, B. J., Rogers, J., Ryan, N. D., & Cameron, J. L. (2003). Heritability of fearful-anxious endophenotypes in infant rhesus macaques: a preliminary report. *Biological Psychiatry*, **53**, 284–291.

Yoon, K. L., Fitzgerald, D. A., Angstadt, M., McCarron, R. A., & Phan, K. L. (2007). Amygdala reactivity to emotional faces at high and low intensity in generalized social phobia: A 4-Tesla functional MRI study. *Psychiatry Research: Neuroimaging*, **154**, 93–98.

Zimbardo, P. G. (1977). *Shyness: What It is, What to Do About It*. Reading, MA: Addison-Wesley.

Co-occurring anxiety and depression: concepts, significance, and treatment implications

Patrick J. McGrath, Jeffrey M. Miller

9.1 Introduction

Anxiety and depression frequently co-occur in the same individual, either simultaneously or sequentially. The purpose of this chapter is to review the phenomenology and neurobiology of co-occurring anxious and depressive symptoms and disorders and to describe their clinical relevance, including prognostic and treatment implications. Several clinical syndromes in which anxiety and depression co-occur are described in more detail below.

9.2 Epidemiology

9.2.1 Syndromes

The term "anxious depression" is used frequently in the literature but is not consistently defined. A syndromal *Diagnostic and Statistical Manual of Mental Disorders, Fourth Edition* (DSM-IV) depressive disorder (e.g., major depressive disorder [MDD], dysthymia, or bipolar disorder) can occur together with one or more syndromal DSM-IV anxiety disorders (e.g., panic disorder, obsessive–compulsive disorder, generalized anxiety disorder, specific phobia, social anxiety disorder, or posttraumatic stress disorder): in this chapter we refer to this as "comorbid depressive and anxiety disorders." A syndromal depressive disorder can also co-occur with *subsyndromal* anxiety symptoms that do not meet full criteria for a DSM-IV anxiety disorder: we refer to this as "depression with subsyndromal anxiety." Conversely, a syndromal anxiety disorder can co-occur with subsyndromal depressive symptoms (including depressive disorder not otherwise specified or an adjustment disorder): we refer to this as "anxiety with subsyndromal depression." Finally, subsyndromal depressive symptoms can co-occur with subsyndromal anxiety symptoms. This final category is an official diagnosis

in the *International Statistical Classification of Diseases and Related Health Problems, 10th Revision* (ICD-10), called "mixed anxiety–depression disorder" (ICD-10 MADD), which is defined as mild-to-moderate anxious and depressive symptoms with at least transient vegetative symptoms (such as changes in sleep or appetite) but of insufficient severity to meet criteria for either a depressive episode or an anxiety disorder (World Health Organization 1992). Similarly, the DSM-IV created a set of research criteria for "mixed anxiety–depressive disorder" (DSM-IV MADD) that includes subsyndromal depressive and anxious symptoms (American Psychiatric Association 1994). We note here that one of the largest studies to examine "anxious depression" has been the Sequenced Treatment Alternatives to Relieve Depression (STAR*D). This study used a definition that combines the first two definitions, including patients with syndromal depression and either syndromal or subsyndromal anxiety disorders.

9.2.2 Comorbid mood and anxiety disorders are extremely common

The prevalence of comorbid mood and anxiety disorders has been described thoroughly in the landmark National Comorbidity Survey (NCS), which surveyed a representative sample ($n = 8098$) of the United States population. A full 58% of subjects who had a diagnosis of MDD at some point in their life met criteria for at least one lifetime anxiety disorder (Kessler *et al.* 1996). Figure 9.1 shows the lifetime prevalence of specific anxiety disorders among those subjects with a lifetime diagnosis of MDD, which are all significantly higher than the prevalence of these anxiety disorders in the general population.

Conversely, the lifetime prevalence of MDD among subjects with generalized anxiety disorder (GAD) was

Anxiety Disorders: Theory, Research, and Clinical Perspectives, ed. Helen Blair Simpson, Yuval Neria, Roberto Lewis-Fernández, Franklin Schneier. Published by Cambridge University Press. © Cambridge University Press 2010.

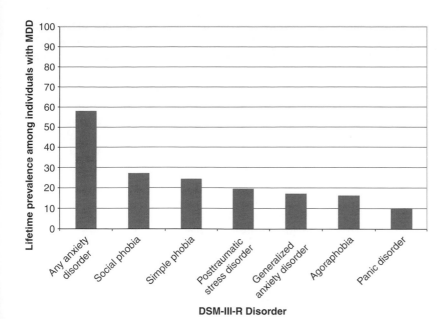

Figure 9.1. Lifetime prevalence of specific anxiety disorders among subjects with a diagnosis of major depressive disorder (MDD) at any point in their lifetime. Data from the National Comorbidity Study (Kessler *et al.* 1996).

58% (Kessler *et al.* 1999). Among subjects with panic disorder without agoraphobia, 34.7% had a lifetime diagnosis of a major depressive episode, 9.6% had dysthymia, and 14.4% had bipolar disorder type I or II (Kessler *et al.* 2006). Rates of depressive comorbidity were higher among subjects with panic disorder that included agoraphobia. Among subjects with social anxiety disorder (SAD) in the National Comorbidity Survey Replication (NCS-R), 47.2% had a lifetime diagnosis of MDD, 14.8% had dysthymia, and 13.8% had bipolar disorder (Ruscio *et al.* 2008). Rates of depressive illnesses were quite similar for subjects with obsessive–compulsive disorder in the NCS-R: 40.7% had lifetime MDD, 13.1% had lifetime dysthymia, and 23.4% had lifetime bipolar disorder (Ruscio *et al.* 2010). Obsessive–compulsive disorder (OCD) was slightly more likely to present before mood disorders in cases in which a clear temporal sequence could be established (45.6% OCD first, 40.2% mood disorder first, 14.2% onset in same year). These high rates of comorbid anxiety and depressive disorders are of great clinical significance, as will be discussed shortly.

9.2.3 Are those with "anxious depression" different than those with depression alone?

The largest clinical sample of MDD in which the phenotype of anxious depression has been studied comes from the multicenter STAR*D project (Fava *et al.* 2006). This study of treatments for MDD recruited a representative sample of treatment-seeking outpatients. Anxious depression was defined by scores above a threshold on an anxiety factor derived from the Hamilton Rating Scale for Depression (Cleary & Guy 1977). Unfortunately, this definition of anxious depression therefore encompasses two different categories of individuals, not distinguishing them from each other in their analyses: patients with comorbid MDD and syndromal anxiety disorder(s) (21% of anxious depressed subjects), as well as patients with MDD and subsyndromal anxiety (79% of anxious depressed subjects). Of 2876 patients in Level I treatment in STAR*D, 53.2% met criteria for anxious depression, defined in this way.

Anxious depression was associated with greater depression severity, a greater likelihood of having melancholic features, and a lower likelihood of having atypical features as compared to non-anxious depressed patients, providing some support for the idea that anxious depression represents a clinically meaningful phenotype. Anxious depression was additionally associated with greater severity of perceived physical impairment, diminished quality of life, greater likelihood of reporting suicidal ideation or a personal history of attempted suicide, and greater reported medical comorbidity, supporting the notion of higher functional impairment among subjects with anxious depression. Importantly, patients with anxious depression were more likely to report symptoms of a range of anxiety disorders, with 21% meeting syndromal criteria for at least one comorbid anxiety disorder.

Several demographic factors were also associated with anxious depression, including African-American or Hispanic race or ethnicity, unemployment, and lower educational attainment or income. These findings suggest that anxious depression is associated with less favorable socioeconomic status, although the direction of causality is unclear. This study also reported the effect of anxious depression on treatment outcome, which will be discussed in section 9.4.1.

9.2.4 Anxiety disorders in clinical bipolar disorder samples

The rates of comorbidity between anxiety disorders and bipolar disorders are also quite high. The Systematic Treatment Enhancement Program for Bipolar Disorder (STEP-BD), a large multicenter longitudinal study of bipolar disorders, examined anxiety disorder comorbidity, focusing on its association with longitudinal course (Otto *et al.* 2006). Of the first 1000 subjects enrolled in this study, 32% met full syndromal criteria for a current comorbid anxiety disorder, including social anxiety disorder (13.3%), generalized anxiety disorder (13.3%), panic disorder (8.5%), obsessive–compulsive disorder (6.8%), posttraumatic stress disorder (4.8%), and agoraphobia without history of panic attacks (4.1%) (prevalences were not exclusive). Based on NCS data, for most of these anxiety disorders these point prevalences were significantly higher than in the general population. In STEP-BD, active comorbid anxiety disorders were described during depressive, hypomanic/manic, and recovered phases of bipolar illness.

9.2.5 Controversies

9.2.5.1 Mixed anxiety–depression: is this a stable diagnosis?

Evidence that subsyndromal symptoms of depression and anxiety are both common and cause significant clinical impairment was the impetus behind the inclusion of a diagnosis for subjects with subsyndromal anxiety comorbid with subsyndromal depression in the ICD-10 and DSM-IV. In the DSM-IV Field Trial for Mixed Anxiety–Depression, for example, 8% of patients interviewed in primary care settings had subsyndromal anxiety and/or depressive symptoms (Zinbarg *et al.* 1994). Further, subjects in primary care samples not meeting full criteria for depressive or anxiety disorders nonetheless reported significant degrees of distress (Moras *et al.* 1996).

Some studies have called the prevalence and stability of ICD-10 MADD and DSM-IV MADD into question. A recent study examining 12-month follow-up clinical status among subjects diagnosed with ICD-10 MADD found that they had comparable rates of depressive disorders at one year to subjects initially diagnosed with MDD, and comparable rates of anxiety disorders to those initially diagnosed with an anxiety disorder (Barkow *et al.* 2004). This suggests that ICD-10 MADD may represent a phase of illness of anxiety and depressive disorders, rather than a distinct clinical entity. Similar instability was noted for the diagnosis of DSM-IV MADD in one study (Weisberg *et al.* 2005), but the diagnosis was noted to be stable at one-year follow-up among a sample of 400 psychiatric outpatients in a naturalistic study (Usall & Marquez 1999). In addition, the prevalence of DSM-IV MADD in primary care samples had been found to be quite low, estimated at 0.2–0.6% in one large study (Weisberg *et al.* 2005), and not found at all in a second small sample (Means-Christensen *et al.* 2006).

9.2.5.2 Is GAD distinct from MDD?

Similar to the case of MADD, there has been debate whether DSM-IV generalized anxiety disorder (GAD) represents a distinct clinical entity or is better conceived of as a subset of MDD, either antedating or co-occurring with the onset of depressive symptoms (Kessler *et al.* 1999). As GAD is highly comorbid with other Axis I disorders, some have questioned the extent to which GAD itself contributes directly to functional impairment (Breslau & Davis 1985). In the NCS sample, significant social and occupational functional impairment was attributable to GAD alone among subjects with comorbid GAD and MDD, supporting the validity of this diagnosis (Kessler *et al.* 1999). The study also found the highest impairment among subjects with comorbid MDD and GAD.

Among the original NCS sample, 5001 respondents participated in a 10-year follow-up survey, which provided further information regarding the temporal relationship between GAD and MDD (Kessler *et al.* 2008). The investigators noted that a diagnosis of GAD predicted the subsequent development of a major depressive episode (MDE) and vice versa. However, whereas GAD predicted a persistent MDE, MDE did not predict persistent GAD. While this finding might seem to provide support for the notion of anxiety symptoms as a prodrome in MDD, the authors argue against such an interpretation, as the time interval from GAD to the onset of an MDE extended beyond the period typical of a prodrome. It is possible, however, that anxiety symptoms could long pre-date MDE yet be part of a prodrome.

9.3 Genetic association

In this section, we examine the extent to which genetic factors contributing to anxiety and depression are shared by reviewing family, twin, and molecular association studies.

9.3.1 Family studies

A three-generation family study found that in families with familial major depression, the emergence of anxiety disorders was an early manifestation of psychopathology in the grandchildren (Weissman *et al.* 2005). This was consistent with the progression of psychiatric symptoms noted in the parents when they were the same age as the grandchildren (Wickramaratne & Weissman 1998). A similar progression from anxiety symptoms in childhood to depression in adolescence and young adulthood has been observed repeatedly in community studies. The authors argue that "[childhood] anxiety can be viewed as an age-dependent expression of the same underlying disorder," that is, major depression (Weissman *et al.* 2005). In these families with highly familial depression across three generations, the early emergence of anxiety disorder as a precursor of depression may suggest one of two possibilities. One is that highly familial depression may be more severe, at least in the sense of early onset and greater comorbidity, and more severe depression tends to be associated with an anxiety precursor. Alternatively, depression and anxiety disorders may be manifestations of a common genetic diathesis, which can be expressed in either anxiety disorder and depression, or both, at different life phases. The former possibility is supported by a study of melancholic depression in 1902 twins selected from a population-based register (Kendler 1997). In that study, melancholia, which the investigators found to be a valid and severe subtype of depression, was found to have increased comorbidity with anxiety disorders and nicotine dependence but not with alcohol dependence or bulimia. By extension, the increased comorbidity with anxiety disorders could be thought of as one dimension of that increased severity. Alternatively, twin data (discussed below) support a common genetic diathesis for generalized anxiety and major depression.

9.3.2 Twin studies

A unique series of twin studies has examined the genetic contribution to the comorbidity of MDD and GAD, that is, comorbid depressive and anxiety disorders. In the first study, 1033 pairs of twins from the Virginia Twin Registry were examined (Kendler *et al.* 1992). This study used a statistical method that assumes twin resemblance arises from three factors: (1) additive genes, contributing twice as much to monozygotic twins as to dizygotic twins; (2) shared environment, contributing equally; and (3) individually specific environment. Statistical models estimated the contribution of these three factors to the correlations of diagnoses between twin pairs. Strikingly, the genetic correlation between the disorders was almost perfect, using a variety of definitions of GAD, and no shared environmental effects were shown. This suggests a remarkable degree of overlap in genetic risk for GAD and MDD, and that individuals with the genetic risk alleles would develop either of the disorders purely as a result of unshared environmental factors. These findings were confirmed in three other large studies (Roy *et al.* 1995, Kendler 1996, Kendler *et al.* 2007). In one, a Swedish twin study, the same investigators examined bivariate twin models applied to lifetime diagnoses of major depression and generalized anxiety disorder. They again estimated the genetic correlation between the disorders at +1.00 for females but at +0.74 for males. Taken together, this impressive consistency of findings suggests that the genetic substrates for MDD and GAD are closely interrelated, although this differs by gender, with the correlations higher in women than in men. There have not been similar twin studies by other groups to provide independent validation of these data. The authors have argued that these two disorders, now in two different categories of disorder in DSM-IV, might better be placed in the same diagnostic category because of their close genetic affinity (Kendler *et al.* 2007). Others have argued that this close genetic affinity is not itself sufficient to determine nosologic arrangement of these disorders. The proposed draft revisions for DSM-5 maintain MDD and GAD as distinct entities (www.dsm5.org).

9.3.3 Molecular genetic association studies

The advent of modern molecular genetics, including the sequencing of the human genome, has made the search for the molecular genetic basis of familial association feasible for the first time. One family of proteins of great interest in this regard is the neurotrophin family, which includes growth factors with strong influence on the survival and plasticity of neurons. One of the neurotrophins, which has been shown to affect neuronal survival, is brain-derived neurotrophic factor (BDNF). An innovative study investigated the association of trait measures of anxiety with single nucleotide polymorphisms (SNPs) in the BDNF gene (Jiang *et al.* 2005). This study found an allele protective against anxiety (–281 C>A) in the *BDNF* gene promoter region and a distinct allele (Val66Met) associated with higher levels of anxiety. Importantly, the Val66Met allele was significantly more common (31%) in individuals with diagnoses of both MDD and an anxiety disorder (comorbid depressive and anxiety disorders) compared to those with only MDD (13%). This study not only suggests that the Val66Met polymorphism is associated with anxiety as a trait, but also that its presence may alter the phenotype of MDD to include more features of anxiety and a greater likelihood of frank comorbidity.

In an extension and replication of this work, this research group explored alleles of the gene coding for the enzyme catechol-O-methyltransferase (*COMT*), which is a major metabolic pathway for the metabolism of both dopamine and noradrenaline (Enoch *et al.* 2008). Subjects without a psychiatric disorder and with the lower-activity Met158 allele have previously shown greater hemodynamic responses in brain areas activated by unpleasant stimuli in a functional magnetic resonance imaging (fMRI) task, accounting for up to 38% of the variance in responses (Smolka *et al.* 2005). This allele has also been linked to higher trait anxiety levels and to the occurrence of both panic disorder and obsessive–compulsive disorder. In addition to neurophysiologic differences in response according to allelic status, this study found that subjects with greater levels of anxiety had higher frequencies of both the Met158 allele of *COMT* and the Met66 allele in *BDNF*.

This study supports the previous finding concerning *BDNF* in patients with comorbid anxiety disorders and depression, and identifies another gene, in subjects without psychiatric disorder, which may contribute to the phenotype of comorbid anxiety and depression. Taken together, the two loci identified in *BDNF* and the single locus in *COMT* may be the beginning of a genetic signature of risk for anxiety that may manifest during the course of major depression. The molecular genetics of apparently polygenic diseases like depression and the anxiety disorders has shown that the most common situation is a multiplicity of genes of small effect. These findings also suggest that when genetic polymorphisms carrying risk for different psychiatric

conditions or traits co-occur, they can predispose to the expression of phenotypes involving co-occurring depression and anxiety.

9.4 Treatment implications

9.4.1 Prognostic implications

Several (Fava *et al.* 1997, Flint & Rifat 1997, Davidson *et al.* 2002), but not all (Tollefson *et al.* 1994, Russell *et al.* 2001), short-term clinical trials of depression with anxiety symptoms using a range of antidepressant medications have shown a lower rate of response for depressed patients with high levels of concurrent anxiety symptoms, though the presence of anxiety disorders was not systematically addressed in these trials. In addition, one study has shown a slower rate of response to treatment among depressed patients with high levels of anxiety symptoms (Clayton *et al.* 1991).

A problem with these studies, and with others to be discussed, is that the instruments used to rate response, principally the Hamilton Rating Scale for Depression (HAM-D), include anxiety symptoms. The presence of higher levels of anxiety symptoms at baseline, used to diagnose depression with anxious features, means that those subjects are likely to have higher scores after treatment, as baseline scores are a strong predictor of post-treatment scores with antidepressant treatment. This leads to a confounding of outcome measurement with the categorizing variable of anxiety. This might seem easy to overcome by using the depression scale without counting the anxiety items. However, depression measures have been validated including the anxiety items, and their validity without those items is uncertain. More subtly, if anxiety leads a subject to be more likely to report distress of all kinds, then all self-rated measures, including such constructs as impaired social functioning, are liable to be inflated by this reporting bias. Absent a measure of response independent of patient self-perception of their symptoms, this factor confounds all efforts to determine the effect of anxiety on outcome.

To date, the best-powered study to explore the prognostic effect of anxiety on the outcome of treatment for depression has been the STAR*D trial, described earlier in this chapter (Fava *et al.* 2008). "Anxious depression" was defined by a cutoff score on a scale of anxiety symptoms derived from the HAM-D, yielding a phenotype that included comorbid mood and anxiety disorders as well as depression with subsyndromal anxiety. The remission rate for patients with anxious depression with citalopram treatment in STAR*D was 22.2%, compared to 33.4% for those without anxious depression, a 33.5% relative decrease; the effect was similar using response, rather than remission, as the clinical outcome measure. In addition, the authors determined that the presence of a comorbid syndromal anxiety disorder was also predictive of both decreased response and remission, independent of the anxiety subscale score, although the continuous measure appeared to account for a larger proportion of outcome variance. The durations to both remission and response were also increased by the presence of anxious features. Patients with anxious features had a greater frequency, intensity, and burden of side effects than the non-anxious group, as well as more serious adverse events. Interestingly, the anxious group had a rate of hospitalization for general medical conditions more than double that of the comparison group, which indicates one aspect of the increased severity associated with this comorbidity.

9.4.2 Association of co-occurring depression and anxiety with suicide

One crucial way in which state anxiety affects the course of depression is through its relationship to suicide. In a landmark paper, Fawcett and colleagues (1990) found that both severe symptoms of psychic anxiety and panic attacks were associated with an increased rate of suicide within one year among a sample of 954 patients with affective disorders. Similarly, comorbid anxiety disorders in the STEP-BD sample were associated with a higher likelihood of suicide attempts and suicidal ideation (Simon et al. 2007), although some of this association was explained by greater depression severity among bipolar subjects with a comorbid anxiety disorder. This association with suicide is perhaps the strongest reason to assess carefully for comorbid symptoms of anxiety or comorbid anxiety disorders among patients evaluated for depression.

9.4.3 Potential pharmacologic treatment strategies

9.4.3.1 Differential antidepressant efficacy in unipolar depression

Because all of the marketed selective serotonin reuptake inhibitor (SSRI) antidepressants have an indication for treatment of at least one anxiety disorder, many clinicians assume that any would be a reasonable choice for a patient with depression with subsyndromal anxiety, or

for MDD with a comorbid anxiety disorder. Since bupropion does not have such an indication, some have raised the question of whether bupropion shares other antidepressants' efficacy in treating the symptoms of anxiety that occur with major depression (Stahl et al. 2003, 2004, Nutt et al. 2007). A pooled analysis of 10 double-blind, randomized, placebo-controlled studies including 1275 patients with anxious depression as defined by STAR*D criteria (see section 9.2.3) was conducted to examine this question (Papakostas et al. 2008). The researchers determined response rates to bupropion and a comparator SSRI among subjects with anxious depression, and reported that the response rate was modestly, though statistically significantly, greater with SSRI treatment (65.4%) compared to bupropion treatment (54.5%). This small difference, corresponding to a number needed to treat of 17, suggests that there is only a slight advantage to SSRI treatment of anxious depression compared to bupropion treatment. In an analysis of the second-step treatment response for 727 subjects in STAR*D that compared response to a second SSRI, sertraline, a dual reuptake inhibitor (SNRI), venlafaxine, and bupropion, no advantage for remission was found for either sertraline or venlafaxine over bupropion for patients with anxious depression (Rush et al. 2008). In sum, these studies do not support a strong clinical advantage of SSRIs over bupropion in treating patients with anxious depression as defined in STAR*D.

One open-label study has suggested that mirtazapine might be especially effective in patients with MDD and comorbid GAD (Goodnick et al. 1999), possibly related to its blockade of postsynaptic alpha-2-noradrenergic receptors. Controlled studies are needed to confirm this, and the side-effect burden of mirtazapine, which prominently includes both sedation and weight gain, may make this applicable only to a small number of patients.

Some have considered the syndrome of atypical depression to be characterized by high levels of anxiety symptoms (Davidson 2007). Monoamine oxidase inhibitors (MAOIs) have demonstrated efficacy superior to tricyclic antidepressants (TCAs) in patients with atypical depression (Quitkin 2002). However, by examining baseline self-rated anxiety as a predictive variable, a study of atypical depression has shown that anxiety severity did not account for the superiority of the MAOI phenelzine over the TCA imipramine in treating patients with MDD (Quitkin et al. 1990).

One study has shown equivalent efficacy for SSRIs and TCAs in atypical depression (McGrath et al. 2000), which might suggest by extrapolation that MAOIs are superior to SSRIs for this population. However, no study has directly addressed MAOI efficacy in depression with subsyndromal anxiety, or in comorbid mood and anxiety disorders. Other antidepressants have not been systematically studied in these subgroups of patients.

9.4.3.2 Bipolar disorder

In the STEP-BD study an effect of comorbid anxiety disorders on treatment outcome in bipolar disorder was observed: the presence of at least one comorbid anxiety disorder was associated with fewer days well during 12 months of prospective observation, a lower quality of life, and a shorter time to relapse among those whose bipolar illness was in remission at some point during the study (Otto *et al.* 2006). Also, comorbid anxiety disorders negatively impacted the course of bipolar illness when they occurred, not only during depressive phases but also during periods of relative recovery; their impact on hypomanic and manic phases of illness was not examined due to smaller sample sizes. Due to concerns about the use of antidepressants in bipolar patients, clinicians should consider cognitive–behavioral therapy (CBT) for treatment of comorbid anxiety disorder in the context of bipolar disorder. Although there has been little study of its efficacy in such cases, there are evidence-based CBT protocols for all the anxiety disorders (including GAD, OCD, posttraumatic stress disorder [PTSD], and panic disorder). Similarly, benzodiazepines might be considered, at least for GAD and panic disorder, but again this has not been systematically studied.

9.4.3.3 Benzodiazepines

Clinicians routinely use benzodiazepines to treat anxiety symptoms comorbid with depression. Thus, the idea that this would be an effective augmentation to antidepressants to treat either concurrent anxiety symptoms or comorbid anxiety disorder seems appealing. While there have been several controlled studies examining benzodiazepine co-administration in patients with MDD, to our knowledge no clinical trials have been conducted using this approach for patients with co-occurring anxiety symptoms or diagnoses. In a randomized placebo-controlled study of 80 adult outpatients with major depression who were not characterized for anxious symptoms or for concurrent anxiety disorder, clonazepam or placebo was added during the first three weeks of an eight-week course of fluoxetine. Fluoxetine was dosed initially at 20 mg for six weeks and raised to 40 mg thereafter, if necessary (Smith *et al.* 1998). The

patients taking clonazepam 0.5–1.0 mg at bedtime improved significantly more during the first three weeks than those on fluoxetine alone by both the HAM-D and global measures by patient and clinician, without significant adverse effects and with only mild and transitory discontinuation effects. Whether this salutary effect might specifically benefit patients with high levels of anxiety symptoms was not examined in this trial.

In further analysis of this trial, the authors found that the clonazepam co-therapy improved not only the HAM-D total score but also the anxiety, sleep, and core depressive symptoms clusters (Londborg *et al.* 2000). They also found that treatment-emergent anxiety and sleep disturbance were significantly reduced in the co-therapy group, while there was a non-significant numerical increase in sedation and dry mouth for the co-therapy patients.

This same research group then conducted another double-blind, placebo-controlled study of similar design to examine whether continued clonazepam administration conferred benefits beyond the early treatment weeks (Smith *et al.* 2002). They found that fluoxetine/clonazepam co-therapy was superior to fluoxetine monotherapy at one week on the HAM-D but not at other time points. Co-therapy reduced insomnia but neither anxiety nor core depressive symptoms. Again, subjects with anxiety comorbidity were not examined separately. The conclusion of these two controlled studies appears to be that a benzodiazepine can be safely administered with an SSRI antidepressant, and this appears to speed symptomatic improvement, though without evidence of an ultimately higher response rate in patients not selected either for high levels of anxiety symptoms or for anxiety disorder comorbidity. Whether patients with co-occurring depression and anxiety in particular might derive a greater long-term benefit from benzodiazepine augmentation is not yet known and is deserving of future study. While patients with MDD and subsyndromal anxiety may benefit from a benzodiazepine, one might be cautious about extending this to patients with certain comorbid anxiety disorders. For example, benzodiazepines are not effective in OCD, PTSD, and specific phobia, and other treatments are thought to be preferable for GAD and SAD, at least when they are the primary disorder.

9.4.3.4 Second-generation antipsychotics

An alternative pharmacologic strategy would be to employ either typical or second-generation antipsychotics (SGA) in the treatment of either bipolar or unipolar depression with subsyndromal anxious features. Gao and colleagues (2006) recently reviewed the use of antipsychotics to treat primary and secondary anxiety symptoms or disorders. The authors discussed two large randomized trials of SGAs in bipolar depression. The first study found that both olanzapine and the combination of olanzapine and fluoxetine were more effective than placebo at reducing anxiety as assessed by the Hamilton Rating Scale for Anxiety (HAM-A), but it found no advantage for the combination over monotherapy (Tohen *et al.* 2003). In the second study, quetiapine reduced anxiety ratings compared to placebo (Calabrese *et al.* 2005), although there was no active comparator treatment. These studies provide some suggestion that comorbid anxiety during the course of bipolar depression might respond to treatment with an SGA.

While there are no randomized trials of SGA medications for the treatment of comorbid anxiety symptoms in unipolar depression, older and methodologically weaker studies have suggested that the typical antipsychotics combined with antidepressants may have some advantages in reducing anxiety symptoms over antidepressant monotherapy (Gao *et al.* 2006). In a recently published merged analysis of two large clinical trials of adjunctive aripiprazole in MDD, the authors showed a similar and significant advantage over placebo in both depressed patients with anxious features and those without anxious features (Trivedi *et al.* 2008). In contrast to the STAR*D study, which showed that patients with anxious features did worse than those without such features on a range of antidepressant treatments, this study suggests that adding aripiprazole to antidepressants, and perhaps other SGAs by extension, may provide an important option in treating such patients.

9.4.3.5 Novel and non-antidepressant therapeutic agents

A variety of other medications have been studied in anxiety disorders and may be worth investigating for the treatment of depressed patients with prominent anxious features. For example, pregabalin, structurally related to gabapentin, has been studied in GAD (Montgomery *et al.* 2006) and in SAD (Pande *et al.* 2004), although it is not approved by the US Food and Drug Administration (FDA) for either indication. In a pooled analysis of six studies, pregabalin has shown

efficacy in GAD patients with significant depressive symptomatology, though not to the threshold for MDD (Stein *et al.* 2008). There is some evidence suggesting that buspirone, which has been demonstrated to have efficacy for GAD, has some efficacy for MDD when used in high dosage (Rickels *et al.* 1991).

9.4.4 Psychotherapy for co-occurring depression and anxiety

Although there has been considerable effort in the area of psychotherapy for both MDD and anxiety disorders such as GAD, there have been no studies reported that specifically address psychotherapy for patients with comorbid conditions. As pointed out in a review of this area, CBT interventions to date have focused on either depressive or anxious symptomatology, and no psychotherapy has been developed that simultaneously addresses both (Roy-Byrne 2008). The author suggests that clinical experience indicates that CBT targeted toward rumination and catastrophization may be especially suitable for depression characterized by marked anxiety symptoms.

9.4.5 Interaction with other depression subtypes

One possible nosological connection between anxious depression and poorer response to antidepressant medication is based on recent findings from detailed analysis of the STAR*D data. In an analysis of the effect of the presence of melancholic features, the investigators found that melancholic features were associated with a 24.1% decrease in the chance of remission with citalopram monotherapy (McGrath *et al.* 2008). In addition, a significantly higher proportion of patients with melancholic features met the criterion for anxious depression from the HAM-D subscale (71.1% versus 47.7% for those without melancholic features). The study also found that all anxiety disorders examined were significantly more prevalent among those with melancholic features, suggesting that anxiety symptoms, or anxiety disorders associated with melancholia, might partly account for lower remission rates with pharmacotherapy. Using a multivariate analysis controlling for anxious features, outcome was significantly poorer for those with melancholic features on some but not all measures. These data suggest that high levels of anxiety associated with melancholic features accounted for at least some of the variance in outcome.

9.4.6 Summary of treatment implications

In summary, current evidence indicates that anxious depression, broadly defined by subsyndromal anxiety or comorbid anxiety disorders, is associated with poorer outcome with a range of antidepressant medications, and that no antidepressant has so far been shown to be significantly more effective for such patients. There are some data suggesting a minimally better outcome with an SSRI antidepressant compared to bupropion, and other data suggest that anxious depression is strongly associated with melancholic features, a depression subtype familiar to most clinicians and not usually thought to be associated with anxiety. A promising strategy that has not been explored sufficiently is the use of an SGA augmentation either of a mood stabilizer in bipolar depression or of an antidepressant in unipolar depression to achieve higher remission rates for these patients. Additionally, it may be important to consider treatment response characteristics specific to particular comorbid anxiety disorders.

9.5 The neurobiology of co-occurring depression and anxiety

9.5.1 Electrophysiologic findings

One research group compared electrical event-related potentials (ERPs) among subjects with pure anxiety disorders to ERPs among subjects with anxiety disorders comorbid with MDD or an alcohol use disorder (Enoch *et al.* 2008). Specifically, they looked at an electrical response reflective of working memory and attention called the P300 ERP. They found that individuals with a pure anxiety disorder had higher P300 amplitudes than those with an anxiety disorder comorbid with MDD or those with pure MDD, although they did not state whether these specific comparisons were statistically significant. Similarly, they noted better performance on a neuropsychological task that assays working memory and attention, the digital symbol task, in subjects with pure anxiety disorder than in subjects with comorbid anxiety disorder and MDD or subjects with pure MDD. While preliminary, these studies suggest an attentional and working memory deficit that is common to both pure depression and comorbid anxiety and depression but that is relatively rare in pure anxiety disorders.

An older study of sleep EEG profiles compared subjects with dysthymia alone to subjects with dysthymia and comorbid anxiety disorders (which were heterogeneous and included panic disorder, simple phobia, and OCD) (Akiskal *et al.* 1984). They found that subjects with dysthymia alone achieved REM sleep in a shorter amount of time and spent a greater percentage of time in REM sleep than dysthymic subjects with a comorbid anxiety disorder. These results provide a possible electrophysiologic marker of anxiety comorbidity among subjects with depressive illness that is deserving of further study using current diagnostic criteria.

9.5.2 Neurochemical findings

A recent positron emission tomography (PET) study attempted to quantify brain serotonin transporter (SERT) in vivo among subjects with and without MDD and additionally to examine the effect of current (state) anxiety on SERT levels (Reimold *et al.* 2008). No subjects in this study had a frank comorbid anxiety disorder. The authors reported that subjects with MDD had lower levels of SERT in the thalamus than healthy controls, consistent with several previous studies. Among depressed subjects, higher levels of state anxiety were associated with lower SERT levels in the midbrain, amygdala, and thalamus. While this study suffers from some methodological limitations, it suggests either an additive effect of anxiety symptoms and depression on SERT deficiency or, alternatively, that degree of state anxiety may be driving the observed SERT abnormalities in depression.

Another PET study examined the effect of anxiety symptoms on serotonin 1A (5-HT_{1A}) receptor levels among subjects with MDD, a significant minority of whom had a comorbid anxiety disorder (Sullivan *et al.* 2005). Using principal components analysis of the Hamilton Rating Scale for Depression and the Beck Depression Inventory, they identified measures of psychic, somatic, and motoric anxiety. Across multiple cortical regions, they found that somatic anxiety was negatively correlated with 5-HT_{1A} receptor levels, and that psychic anxiety was positively correlated with 5-HT_{1A} receptor levels. In addition, depressed subjects with comorbid panic disorder were found to have lower 5-HT_{1A} receptors across multiple brain regions than depressed subjects without panic disorder. This is possibly consistent with the prominent somatic anxiety that accompanies panic attacks, and also with a 5-HT_{1A} receptor PET imaging finding in subjects with pure panic disorder (Nash *et al.* 2008). This study suggests that neurobiological correlates of psychic anxiety may contrast with those of somatic anxiety, and furthermore that the neurochemical correlates of panic disorder and depression may be additive.

9.5.3 Regional cerebral glucose metabolism

A PET study compared regional cerebral glucose metabolism patterns between subjects with MDD alone, OCD alone, MDD comorbid with OCD (MDD+OCD), and healthy controls (Saxena *et al.* 2001). The authors hypothesized that patterns of glucose metabolism in the MDD+OCD group would overlap patterns in the MDD-alone and OCD-alone groups. Some of their findings were consistent with this hypothesis, including reduced hippocampal glucose metabolism among both MDD-alone and MDD+OCD groups as compared to controls. In contrast, they noted a seemingly paradoxical finding of increased thalamic metabolism in both the MDD-alone and OCD-alone groups, which was not found among the MDD+OCD group. Finally, there was a trend toward higher metabolism in the right caudate nucleus among the OCD-alone group as compared to the OCD+MDD group. These findings suggest that a simple model of additive effects of anxiety and depressive disorders is insufficient to explain the pathophysiology of comorbid states. The authors suggested that "secondary" depression may be mediated by different neural networks than "primary" depression, although they did not provide a rationale for considering the depression in the MDD+OCD group as secondary.

9.5.4 Neuroanatomical findings

At least one paper has reported associations of differential neuroanatomy among subjects with anxiety symptoms co-occurring with MDD. A structural MRI study reported that among a sample of 23 pediatric subjects age 8–17 with MDD, the ratio of amygdala to hippocampus volume was greater in subjects with co-occurring anxiety symptoms (MacMillan *et al.* 2003). Some authors have speculated that this may reflect amygdala hyperactivity related to anxiety symptoms and/or hypoactive hippocampal function related to depressive symptoms (Stahl & Wise 2008), although these hypotheses would require specific study using functional imaging techniques, and their generalizability to adult samples has not been investigated.

9.6 Conclusions and areas of future inquiry

The evidence from multiple lines of inquiry suggests that there is a biologic relationship between anxiety and depression, including a shared genetic diathesis that may manifest in either a depression or an anxiety phenotype. Among subjects with familial depression, the occurrence of either phenotype may be determined by life cycle, with an anxious phenotype more likely to be expressed in childhood and adolescence, and a depressive phenotype later. The concomitant occurrence of anxiety with depression appears to be associated with more severe symptoms and with a poorer response to pharmacologic treatment in both unipolar and bipolar depression. Many biologic findings have been associated with the concurrent expression of anxiety and depressive symptoms or comorbidity between both types of disorder, and at least some genotypic associations have been delineated that may characterize the comorbid group. Brain imaging studies suggest that comorbid anxiety and depression may exhibit some additive effects of the pathophysiology of individual depression and anxiety disorders, but this does not fully explain the patterns associated with comorbid states. No treatment has been clearly shown to be more efficacious, either for patients with MDD and subsyndromal depressive symptoms or for those with comorbid anxiety disorders. Inconsistencies in definitions of anxious depression in the literature across treatment, epidemiological, and neurobiological studies have been an obstacle in comparing and generalizing findings in this field. Further research to clarify the underlying biology of co-occurring anxiety and depression may alter current nosologic concepts and suggest avenues for more effective treatment intervention.

References

Akiskal, H. S., Lemmi, H., Dickson, H., *et al.* (1984). Chronic depressions: Part 2. Sleep EEG differentiation of primary dysthymic disorders from anxious depressions. *Journal of Affective Disorders*, **6**, 287–295.

American Psychiatric Association (1994). *Diagnostic and Statistical Manual of Mental Disorders*, 4th edn (DSM-IV). Washington DC: American Psychiatric Association.

Barkow, K., Heun, R., Wittchen, H. U., *et al.* (2004). Mixed anxiety–depression in a 1 year follow-up study: shift to other diagnoses or remission? *Journal of Affective Disorders*, **79**, 235–239.

Breslau, N., & Davis, G. C. (1985). Further evidence on the doubtful validity of generalized anxiety disorder. *Psychiatry Research*, **16**, 177–179.

Calabrese, J. R., Keck, P. E., Macfadden, W., *et al.* (2005). A randomized, double-blind, placebo-controlled trial of quetiapine in the treatment of bipolar I or II depression. *American Journal of Psychiatry*, **162**, 1351–1360.

Clayton, P. J., Grove, W. M., Coryell, W., *et al.* (1991). Follow-up and family study of anxious depression. *American Journal of Psychiatry*, **148**, 1512–1517.

Cleary, P., & Guy, W. (1977). Factor analysis of the Hamilton depression scale. *Drugs Under Experimental and Clinical Research*, **1**, 115–120.

Davidson, J. R. (2007). A history of the concept of atypical depression. *Journal of Clinical Psychiatry*, **68** (Suppl 3), 10–15.

Davidson, J. R., Meoni, P., Haudiquet, V., Cantillon, M., & Hackett, D. (2002). Achieving remission with venlafaxine and fluoxetine in major depression: its relationship to anxiety symptoms. *Depression and Anxiety*, **16**, 4–13.

Enoch, M. A., White, K. V., Waheed, J., & Goldman, D. (2008). Neurophysiological and genetic distinctions between pure and comorbid anxiety disorders. *Depression and Anxiety*, **25**, 383–392.

Fava, M., Uebelacker, L. A., Alpert, J. E., *et al.* (1997). Major depressive subtypes and treatment response. *Biological Psychiatry*, **42**, 568–576.

Fava, M., Rush, A. J., Alpert, J. E., *et al.* (2006). What clinical and symptom features and comorbid disorders characterize outpatients with anxious major depressive disorder: a replication and extension. *Canadian Journal of Psychiatry*, **51**, 823–835.

Fava, M., Rush, A. J., Alpert, J. E., *et al.* (2008). Difference in treatment outcome in outpatients with anxious versus nonanxious depression: a STAR*D report. *American Journal of Psychiatry*, **165**, 342–351.

Fawcett, J., Scheftner, W. A., Fogg, L., *et al.* (1990). Time-related predictors of suicide in major affective disorder. *American Journal of Psychiatry*, **147**, 1189–1194.

Flint, A. J., & Rifat, S. L. (1997). Anxious depression in elderly patients: response to antidepressant treatment. *American Journal of Geriatric Psychiatry*, **5**, 107–115.

Gao, K., Muzina, D., Gajwani, P., & Calabrese, J. R. (2006). Efficacy of typical and atypical antipsychotics for primary and comorbid anxiety symptoms or disorders: a review. *Journal of Clinical Psychiatry*, **67**, 1327–1340.

Goodnick, P. J., Puig, A., DeVane, C. L., & Freund, B. V. (1999). Mirtazapine in major depression with comorbid generalized anxiety disorder. *Journal of Clinical Psychiatry*, **60**, 446–448.

Jiang, X., Xu, K., Hoberman, J., *et al.* (2005). BDNF variation and mood disorders: a novel functional promoter polymorphism and Val66Met are associated with anxiety but have opposing effects. *Neuropsychopharmacology*, **30**, 1353–1361.

Kendler, K. S. (1996). Major depression and generalised anxiety disorder: same genes, (partly) different environments – revisited. *British Journal of Psychiatry Supplement*, (30), 68–75.

Kendler, K. S. (1997). The diagnostic validity of melancholic major depression in a population-based sample of female twins. *Archives of General Psychiatry*, **54**, 299–304.

Kendler, K. S., Gardner, C. O., Gatz, M., & Pedersen, N. L. (2007). The sources of co-morbidity between major depression and generalized anxiety disorder in a Swedish national twin sample. *Psychology and Medicine*, **37**, 453–462.

Kendler, K. S., Neale, M. C., Kessler, R. C., Heath, A. C., & Eaves, L. J. (1992). Major depression and generalized anxiety disorder. Same genes, (partly) different environments? *Archives of General Psychiatry*, **49**, 716–722.

Kessler, R. C., Nelson, C. B., McGonagle, K. A., *et al.* (1996). Comorbidity of DSM-III-R major depressive disorder in the general population: results from the US National Comorbidity Survey. *British Journal of Psychiatry Supplement*, (30), 17–30.

Kessler, R. C., DuPont, R. L., Berglund, P., & Wittchen, H. U. (1999). Impairment in pure and comorbid generalized anxiety disorder and major depression at 12 months in two national surveys. *American Journal of Psychiatry*, **156**, 1915–1923.

Kessler, R. C., Chiu, W. T., Jin, R., *et al.* (2006). The epidemiology of panic attacks, panic disorder, and agoraphobia in the National Comorbidity Survey Replication. *Archives of General Psychiatry*, **63**, 415–424.

Kessler, R. C., Gruber, M., Hettema, J. M., *et al.* (2008). Co-morbid major depression and generalized anxiety disorders in the National Comorbidity Survey follow-up. *Psychology and Medicine*, **38**, 365–374.

Londborg, P. D., Smith, W. T., Glaudin, V., & Painter, J. R. (2000). Short-term cotherapy with clonazepam and fluoxetine: anxiety, sleep disturbance and core symptoms of depression. *Journal of Affective Disorders*, **61**, 73–79.

MacMillan, S., Szeszko, P. R., Moore, G. J., *et al.* (2003). Increased amygdala : hippocampal volume ratios associated with severity of anxiety in pediatric major depression. *Journal of Child and Adolescent Psychopharmacology*, **13**, 65–73.

McGrath, P. J., Stewart, J. W., Janal, M. N., Petkova, E., Quitkin, F. M., & Klein, D. F. (2000). A placebo-controlled study of fluoxetine versus imipramine in the acute treatment of atypical depression. *American Journal of Psychiatry*, **157**, 344–350.

McGrath, P. J., Khan, A., Trivedi, M. H., *et al.* (2008). Response to a selective serotonin reuptake inhibitor (citalopram) in major depressive disorder with melancholic features: a STAR*D report. *Journal of Clinical Psychiatry*, **69**, 1847–1855.

Means-Christensen, A. J., Sherbourne, C. D., Roy-Byrne, P. P., *et al.* (2006). In search of mixed anxiety-depressive disorder: a primary care study. *Depression and Anxiety*, **23**, 183–189.

Montgomery, S. A., Tobias, K., Zornberg, G. L., Kasper, S., & Pande, A. C. (2006). Efficacy and safety of pregabalin in the treatment of generalized anxiety disorder: a 6-week, multicenter, randomized, double-blind, placebo-controlled comparison of pregabalin and venlafaxine. *Journal of Clinical Psychiatry*, **67**, 771–782.

Moras, K., Clar, L. A., Katon, W., *et al.* (1996). Mixed anxiety–depression. In T. A. Widiger, A. J. Frances, H. A. Pincus, *et al.*, eds., *DSM-IV Sourcebook*. Washington, DC: American Psychiatric Association.

Nash, J. R., Sargent, P. A., Rabiner, E. A., *et al.* (2008). Serotonin 5-HT$_{1A}$ receptor binding in people with panic disorder: positron emission tomography study. *British Journal of Psychiatry*, **193**, 229–234.

Nutt, D., Demyttenaere, K., Janka, Z., *et al.* (2007). The other face of depression, reduced positive affect: the role of catecholamines in causation and cure. *Journal of Psychopharmacology*, **21**, 461–471.

Otto, M. W., Simon, N. M., Wisniewski, S. R., *et al.* (2006). Prospective 12-month course of bipolar disorder in outpatients with and without comorbid anxiety disorders. *British Journal of Psychiatry*, **189**, 20–25.

Pande, A. C., Feltner, D. E., Jefferson, J. W., *et al.* (2004). Efficacy of the novel anxiolytic pregabalin in social anxiety disorder: a placebo-controlled, multicenter study. *Journal of Clinical Psychopharmacology*, **24**, 141–149.

Papakostas, G. I., Stahl, S. M., Krishen, A., *et al.* (2008). Efficacy of bupropion and the selective serotonin reuptake inhibitors in the treatment of major depressive disorder with high levels of anxiety (anxious depression): a pooled analysis of 10 studies. *Journal of Clinical Psychiatry*, **69**, 1287–1292.

Quitkin, F.M. (2002). Depression with atypical features: diagnostic validity, prevalence, and treatment. *Primary Care Companion Journal of Clinical Psychiatry*, **4**, 94–99.

Quitkin, F. M., McGrath, P. J., Stewart, J. W., *et al.* (1990). Atypical depression, panic attacks, and response to imipramine and phenelzine: a replication. *Archives of General Psychiatry*, **47**, 935–941.

Reimold, M., Batra, A., Knobel, A., *et al.* (2008). Anxiety is associated with reduced central serotonin transporter availability in unmedicated patients with unipolar major depression: a [11C]DASB PET study. *Molecular Psychiatry*, **13**, 606–613, 557.

Rickels, K., Amsterdam, J. D., Clary, C., Puzzuoli, G., & Schweizer, E. (1991). Buspirone in major depression: a controlled study. *Journal of Clinical Psychiatry*, **52**, 34–38.

Roy, M. A., Neale, M. C., Pedersen, N. L., Mathe, A. A., & Kendler, K. S. (1995). A twin study of generalized anxiety disorder and major depression. *Psychology and Medicine*, **25**, 1037–1049.

Roy-Byrne, P. (2008). Comorbid MDD and GAD: revisiting the concept of "anxious depression". *Psychiatric Times* (Suppl.), August (1), 25–30.

Ruscio, A. M., Brown, T. A., Chiu, W. T., *et al.* (2008). Social fears and social phobia in the USA: results from the National Comorbidity Survey Replication. *Psychology and Medicine*, **38**, 15–28.

Ruscio, A. M., Stein, D. J., Chiu, W. T., & Kessler, R. C. (2010). The epidemiology of obsessive–compulsive disorder in the National Comorbidity Survey Replication. *Molecular Psychiatry*, **15**, 53–63.

Rush, A. J., Wisniewski, S. R., Warden, D., *et al.* (2008) Selecting among second-step antidepressant medication monotherapies: predictive value of clinical, demographic, or first-step treatment. *Archives of General Psychiatry*, **65**, 870–880.

Russell, J. M., Koran, L. M., Rush, J., *et al.* (2001). Effect of concurrent anxiety on response to sertraline and imipramine in patients with chronic depression. *Depression and Anxiety*, **13**, 18–27.

Saxena, S., Brody, A. L., Ho, M. L., *et al.* (2001). Cerebral metabolism in major depression and obsessive–compulsive disorder occurring separately and concurrently. *Biological Psychiatry*, **50**, 159–170.

Simon, N. M., Zalta, A. K., Otto, M. W., *et al.* (2007). The association of comorbid anxiety disorders with suicide attempts and suicidal ideation in outpatients with bipolar disorder. *Journal of Psychiatric Research*, **41**, 255–264.

Smith, W. T., Londborg, P. D., Glaudin, V., & Painter, J. R. (1998). Short-term augmentation of fluoxetine with clonazepam in the treatment of depression: a double-blind study. *American Journal of Psychiatry*, **155**, 1339–1345.

Smith, W. T., Londborg, P. D., Glaudin, V., & Painter, J. R. (2002). Is extended clonazepam cotherapy of fluoxetine effective for outpatients with major depression? *Journal of Affective Disorders*, **70**, 251–259.

Smolka, M. N., Schumann, G., Wrase, J., *et al.* (2005). Catechol-O-methyltransferase val158met genotype affects processing of emotional stimuli in the amygdala and prefrontal cortex. *Journal of Neuroscience*, **25**, 836–842.

Stahl, S. M., Zhang, L., Damatarca, C., & Grady, M. (2003). Brain circuits determine destiny in depression: a novel approach to the psychopharmacology of wakefulness, fatigue, and executive dysfunction in major depressive disorder. *Journal of Clinical Psychiatry*, **64** (Suppl 14), 6–17.

Stahl, S. M., Pradko, J. F., Haight, B. R., *et al.* (2004). A review of the neuropharmacology of bupropion, a dual norepinephrine and dopamine reuptake inhibitor. *Primary Care Companion Journal of Clinical Psychiatry*, **6**, 159–166.

Stahl, S. M., & Wise, D. D. (2008). The potential role of a corticotropin-releasing factor receptor-1 antagonist in psychiatric disorders. *CNS Spectrums*, **13**, 467–483.

Stein, D. J., Baldwin, D. S., Baldinetti, F., & Mandel, F. (2008). Efficacy of pregabalin in depressive symptoms associated with generalized anxiety disorder: a pooled analysis of 6 studies. *European Neuropsychopharmacology*, **18**, 422–430.

Sullivan, G. M., Oquendo, M. A., Simpson, N., *et al.* (2005). Brain serotonin1A receptor binding in major depression is related to psychic and somatic anxiety. *Biologial Psychiatry*, **58**, 947–954.

Tohen, M., Vieta, E., Calabrese, J., *et al.* (2003). Efficacy of olanzapine and olanzapine-fluoxetine combination in the treatment of bipolar I depression. *Archives of General Psychiatry*, **60**, 1079–1088.

Tollefson, G. D., Holman, S. L., Sayler, M. E., & Potvin, J. H. (1994). Fluoxetine, placebo, and tricyclic antidepressants in major depression with and without anxious features. *Journal of Clinical Psychiatry*, **55**, 50–59.

Trivedi, M. H., Thase, M. E., Fava, M., *et al.* (2008). Adjunctive aripiprazole in major depressive disorder: analysis of efficacy and safety in patients with anxious and atypical features. *Journal of Clinical Psychiatry*, **69**, 1928–1936.

Usall, J., & Marquez, M. (1999). [Mixed anxiety and depression disorder: a naturalistic study]. *Actas Españolas de Psiquiatría*, **27**, 81–86.

Weisberg, R. B., Maki, K. M., Culpepper, L., & Keller, M. B. (2005). Is anyone really M.A.D.? The occurrence and course of mixed anxiety-depressive disorder in a sample of primary care patients. *Journal of Nervous and Mental Diseases*, **193**, 223–230.

Weissman, M. M., Wickramaratne, P., Nomura, Y., *et al.* (2005). Families at high and low risk for depression: a 3-generation study. *Archives of General Psychiatry*, **62**, 29–36.

Wickramaratne, P. J., & Weissman, M. M. (1998). Onset of psychopathology in offspring by developmental phase and parental depression. *Journal of the American Academy of Child and Adolescent Psychiatry*, **37**, 933–942.

World Health Organization (1992). *The ICD-10 Classification of Mental and Behavioural Disorders: Clinical Descriptions and Diagnostic Guidelines.* Geneva: World Health Organization.

Zinbarg, R. E., Barlow, D. H., Liebowitz, M., *et al.* (1994). The DSM-IV field trial for mixed anxiety-depression. *American Journal of Psychiatry*, **151**, 1153–1162.

Chapter 10

Understanding health anxiety

Kelli Jane K. Harding, Natalia Skritskaya, Emily R. Doherty, Brian A. Fallon

10.1 Introduction

Health anxiety, also known as illness worry, is an umbrella term that encompasses a wide range of excessive health-related concerns (e.g., rumination on having an illness, suggestibility if one reads or hears about a disease, unrealistic fear of infection), somatic perceptions (e.g., preoccupation with bodily sensations or functioning), and behaviors (e.g., repeated reassurance seeking, avoidance of medications or medical personnel). For a person with a medical illness, his/her reaction is out of proportion to what would be expected. While health anxiety is not a term found in the *Diagnostic and Statistical Manual of Mental Disorders* (DSM), it is a construct linked to various DSM-IV categories. One of those is the most severe form of health anxiety, known as hypochondriasis, in which concerns about having a serious illness persist at least six months despite medical reassurance, and these concerns cause clinically significant impairment or distress (Table 10.1) (American Psychiatric Association 2000). Health anxiety also overlaps with somatization disorder, obsessive–compulsive disorder (OCD), body dysmorphic disorder (BDD), panic disorder, and delusional disorder. This chapter discusses a conceptual framework for health anxiety, focusing on diagnostic considerations, epidemiology, etiology, measures of health anxiety, clinical considerations, practical management, treatments, and future research directions.

10.2 Conceptualization of health anxiety

Appropriate behavior when one has a medical concern or a physical symptom, such as pain or discomfort, is to seek the opinion and care of a physician. In fact, concern about illness, suffering, and death are part of the normal human experience. However, excessive health anxiety can be pathological. Central to this chapter is the question: *What is appropriate and what is excessive health vigilance?*

Individuals have varying levels of awareness of physical symptoms, attributions for the same symptoms, and intensity of healthy and pathologic health-related behaviors. Somewhere at the intersection of these variations in somatic perceptions, cognitive attributions, and health behaviors is appropriate health vigilance (Figure 10.1). People who experience bodily sensations in response to emotional distress are known as somatizers, and they may seek symptom diagnosis and resolution. Patients with health anxiety not only are concerned about unexplained bodily symptoms but also they make the conceptual leap to fearing these symptoms may be signs of serious illness. Therefore, both groups present to doctors with bothersome physical symptoms for which there is no known diagnosable disease, also known as medically unexplained symptoms.

On the continuum of health behaviors, some people have high degrees of help-seeking behaviors and are quick to seek reassurance from doctors, family members, friends, and the internet, while others avoid medical resources altogether for fear of what may be uncovered. Severely avoidant patients might try to escape all illness reminders, including visits to sick relatives or funerals, risking conflicts with family and friends. Stoic individuals with both low symptom awareness and low cognitive appraisal of bodily changes are unlikely to seek medical attention, and, similar to those with avoidant health anxiety, risk poor health outcomes by not seeking medical care until diseases are significantly advanced. Individuals with low symptom awareness and high cognitive awareness are more likely to present with general anxiety, not specifically health-related.

Clinical examples of several health anxiety subtypes – cognitive, somatizing, and behavioral – are

Anxiety Disorders: Theory, Research, and Clinical Perspectives, ed. Helen Blair Simpson, Yuval Neria, Roberto Lewis-Fernández, Franklin Schneier. Published by Cambridge University Press. © Cambridge University Press 2010.

Table 10.1. DSM-IV-TR hypochondriasis diagnostic criteria

A	Preoccupation with fears of having, or the idea that one has, a serious disease based on the person's misinterpretation of bodily symptoms.
B	The preoccupation persists despite appropriate medical evaluation and reassurance.
C	The belief in Criterion A is not of delusional intensity (as in delusional disorder, somatic type) and is not restricted to a circumscribed concern about appearance (as in body dysmorphic disorder).
D	The preoccupation causes clinically significant distress or impairment in social, occupational, or other important areas of functioning.
E	The duration of the disturbance is at least 6 months.
F	The preoccupation is not better accounted for by generalized anxiety disorder, obsessive–compulsive disorder, panic disorder, a major depressive episode, separation anxiety, or another somatoform disorder.

Specify if:

With poor insight: if, for most of the time during the current episode, the person does not recognize that the concern about having a serious illness is excessive or unreasonable.

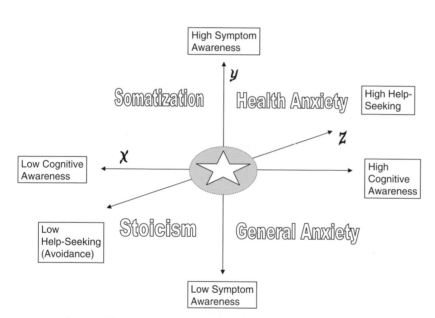

Figure 10.1 Conceptualizing medically unexplained symptoms. On the *x*-axis is cognitive awareness and anxiety (low to high), on the *y*-axis is somatic symptom amplification or awareness (low to high), on the *z*-axis is healthcare behavior (low help-seeking to high help-seeking). Appropriate health vigilance is at the intersection of these vectors (demarcated by the star and surrounding area).

presented in Table 10.2. Some patients with health anxiety are more cognitively focused on fear of disease, similar to patients with OCD, while others have more symptom awareness and bodily preoccupation, as seen in somatization disorder (Figure 10.2). These differences may speak to differing etiologies, as outlined later in this chapter. Health anxiety can also be conceptualized on a spectrum of belief intensity and associated impairment (Figure 10.3), with less severe, more transient symptoms on one end and the more severe, persistent symptoms of hypochondriasis on the other (Barsky *et al.* 1986, Asmundson *et al.* 2001). For example:

Transient health anxiety – One young man with a relative who dies of a myocardial infarction (MI) worries for weeks that he too may have an MI. During that time he is less productive at work and less social with friends. After his doctor evaluates him, he is told he has normal cardiac functioning and no significant risk factors. He feels reassured by this information and is quickly back to his usual level of functioning.

Persistent health anxiety – Another young man with a relative who dies of an MI also worries that he too may have an MI, but this young man, though given the same information by his doctor

Table 10.2. Clinical subtypes of health anxiety with case examples

Health anxiety clinical subtype	Case example
Cognitive type Health anxiety with high cognitive awareness and more pronounced fear of disease (Figure 10.2)	**Mrs. N**, a 24-year-old married woman, developed a fear of having HIV after having an extramarital affair one year ago. She reports no history of depression; she has a sister with OCD. Fearing transmission to her husband, Mrs. N has refrained from any sexual relations with her husband for about 12 months, a behavior that is leading to severe marital discord. She reports increased tearfulness, sleep disruption, and a loss of appetite. Her stress led her to start smoking again. She has been tested eleven times for HIV, all of which came back negative, but her worries persist. She states, "I've had so many tests, but within hours I begin to worry again. I don't know what to do. I know it is irrational, but I can't stop. For hours a day I'm frozen with fear. I try not to watch, but every time I see a news story about someone with HIV, I start to cry and can't stop for hours. What if the virus is hibernating in my body? I've done a lot of internet research, and I know people can have it without any symptoms. I know it sounds crazy, but I worry it's hiding somewhere in my body."
Somatizing type Health anxiety with high symptom awareness and more pronounced bodily preoccupation (Figure 10.2)	**Mr. A** is a 40-year-old history teacher and former college track star who reports a prior history of depression and family history of somatoform disorder. Mr. A reports worrying much of the day every day about having a heart attack after scanning his body for irregularities. He reports frequent shortness of breath, nausea, dizziness, tingling, and palpitations. He feels so poorly he stopped going for his daily run over the past year and gained 30 lb. "In the last month I've gone to the ER too many times to count because I felt I was having a heart attack. I've seen countless specialists, and they tell me my heart is fine, that it's all in my head or that I'm having panic attacks. But I'm sure I'm dying! Ever since my dad died of a heart attack last year I've been concerned about my health. I check my body every day to see if something doesn't feel or look right. I'm a teacher, so I try to hide my daily worries from my students; however, several times I've had to end class early because I could feel my heart pounding, and I was afraid I would have a heart attack in front of them. At night I lie awake for hours listening to my heart, waiting for it to either explode or stop completely."
Behavioral type Health anxiety with high disease conviction and avoidance (Figure 10.3)	**Ms. S** is a 33-year-old biomedical engineer who has significant worries about having undetected breast cancer that are interfering with her social and occupational functioning. Ms. S reports checking a lump she found in her armpit for the past year. Although her sister and mother repeatedly assured her it was an ingrown hair, Ms. S found she is unable to stop checking the site on her body several times a day, such that the site has swelled to an even greater degree and developed some discoloration and bruising. "During the day I check my body for cancer every time I visit the rest room. There is a lump there. It could be too late. I'm terrified of dying or becoming dependent on someone else, but I won't go to the doctor to check it. I'm sure they'll tell me I'm dying."

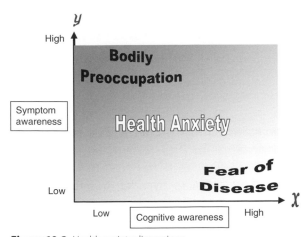

Figure 10.2 Health anxiety dimensions.

The young man remains unconvinced and visits the emergency room multiple times over several months. His persistent worry with high disease conviction interferes with his ability to complete tasks at work and socialize with friends. Ironically, his fear causes him to stop his regular gym workouts.

As exemplified above, patients with higher levels of disease conviction may be less receptive to reassurance, increasing the likelihood of functional impairment.

On the far end of the insight spectrum are somatic-related delusions, or fixed false beliefs resistant to reality testing. Delusional disorder, somatic subtype, is diagnosed when patients are rigidly convinced they have an illness and are not reassurable. For instance, a 72-year-old woman whose husband died of colon cancer believes she also has colon cancer. Despite multiple negative colonoscopies, she continues to state, "I know I have colon cancer!" When questioned if there could be any other explanations for her abdominal discomfort, she states "only the cancer."

as the young man above, is only temporarily reassured. Convinced he is in danger, he then sees a cardiologist, who also says he has normal cardiac functioning and no significant risk factors.

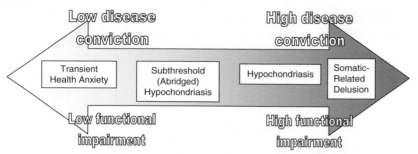

Figure 10.3 The spectrum of disease conviction and functional impairment. The spectrum of health anxiety and disease fear ranges from mild forms, or transient symptoms, to persistent and chronic forms of heightened illness concern or hypochondriasis. The further to the right on the spectrum, the greater the disease conviction, and therefore the greater the likelihood of functional impairment. On the very far end of the spectrum are somatic-related delusions seen in delusional disorder, somatic type, where patients have a fixed false belief that they have an illness.

Table 10.3. Special cases of health anxiety

Internet-related phenomenology (cyberchondria and Munchausen by internet)
Adding to the impairment that someone with health anxiety can experience is overuse of the internet, a powerful resource with limitless health information that has replaced the *Merck Manual* as the new frontier for symptom checking. With the advent of fast, new technology, patients have much to gain in terms of accessing information about medical care. However, for those who suffer from health anxiety, web resources can kindle health fears. In 2006, a study by Harris Interactive found that 136 million people go online for health information, with evidence suggesting that percentage is on the rise (Harris Poll 2006). Approximately 75–80% of all internet users have looked on the Web for health information. Of those who check, about 10% felt "frightened by the serious or graphic nature of the information they found online," 18% felt "confused by the information they found online," and 25% felt "overwhelmed" by the amount of information they encountered (Fox 2006).
"**Cyberchondria**" is a term used to describe the health anxiety and compulsive checking experienced by some individuals who engage in internet health searches. It involves spending inordinate amounts of time researching medical symptoms online. Individuals feel they are unable to stop checking, and experience disproportionate distress at the possibility of having a serious, if rare, condition or side effect. These individuals, if they have also been evaluated by a physician but were not reassured by negative test results, would likely meet criteria for hypochondriasis.
Additionally, the internet also seems to have sparked a new form of a factitious disorder – that group of disorders in which individuals intentionally wish to take on the sick role. Several case studies have been reported of "Virtual Munchausen's" or "**Munchausen by internet**" (Feldman 2000), wherein healthy individuals pose as patients on blogs and in chatrooms, alleging personal illnesses they do not have. While those with health anxiety also visit internet sites for illnesses they ultimately do not have, the difference is that individuals with factitious disorders are consciously producing their symptoms.
Mass sociogenic illness (MSI)
While health anxiety is typically observed in individuals, groups are sometimes susceptible. This phenomenon is called "mass sociogenic illness (MSI)" (Philen *et al.* 1989), "fear contagion" (de Gelder *et al.* 2004), or "epidemic hysteria" (Barsky & Deans 2006). It typically begins when someone becomes suddenly ill, alarming others in the school, workplace, or community that they were exposed to something contagious or toxic. Transmission is by line of sight, telephone, media, and healthcare professionals. MSI tends to develop in populations with some recent stress or intense pressure. Typically, no plausible cause is ever identified, and the non-specific symptoms of MSI, such as headache, dizziness, nausea, malaise, syncope, hyperventilation, are better accounted for by anxiety, stress, and acute somatization (Nemery *et al.* 1999). For instance, after several teenagers reported feeling ill following drinking Coca-Cola in Belgium in 1999, numerous similar cases were reported across the country and northern France, yet no plausible cause was ever discovered (Nemery *et al.* 2002). Symptoms tend to be time-limited and not develop into functional impairment; however, some people may continue to report health fears long after the initial scare (Morgan *et al.* 2008).

As demonstrated above, the rigidity of mindset is what distinguishes delusional disorder, somatic subtype, from hypochondriasis. Patients with hypochondriasis are briefly reassured, even if the reassurance does not last. See Table 10.3 for special cases of health anxiety.

10.2.1 Diagnostic considerations

Symptom severity and duration are the major ways health anxiety is categorized for research. The current

DSM-IV-TR criteria for hypochondriasis (Table 10.1) (American Psychiatric Association 2000) are considered by some researchers to be so narrow as to lack clinical and nosologic validity (Fink *et al.* 2004). While it is unclear how the criteria will be modified in the upcoming revision of the DSM, some have advocated that the diagnosis of "hypochondriasis" be replaced by a more inclusive category, such as "health anxiety disorder," given that the current criteria set for hypochondriasis captures only the most severe cases of health anxiety

(Gureje *et al.* 1997, Bleichardt & Hiller 2007). Missed in the current classification, for example, would be the following individuals: (a) those who fear having an illness but do not have a somatic symptom; (b) those who can be reassured by a physician's examination but only for a short interval of time; (c) those whose duration of fear does not last a full six months; (d) those who are irrationally worried about illness but do not experience clinically significant distress or functional impairment. Studies demonstrate that patients who do not quite meet full criteria for DSM-IV hypochondriasis but worry about having a serious physical illness most of the time show significant differences from controls, including higher healthcare utilization and lower quality of life (Creed & Barsky 2004, Martin & Jacobi 2006).

In addition to hypochondriasis, the differential diagnosis for someone with excessive health anxiety and fears predominantly about getting or catching a disease includes OCD or specific disease phobia. If a patient presents with worry in multiple life domains, such as financial, interpersonal, or occupational, and not just with regards to illness, then generalized anxiety disorder (GAD) may be a more appropriate diagnosis.

For patients presenting primarily with somatic concerns, somatoform diagnoses to consider include somatization, identified by unexplained symptoms in multiple organ systems; pain disorder, characterized by pain with significant psychological contributions; or BDD, with the key feature of preoccupation with an imagined or slight defect in physical appearance. BDD would not be considered a form of health anxiety, as the concern is not about illness but about appearance.

For patients who present with either bizarre health concerns or rigidly unreassurable health anxiety, a diagnosis of psychotic disorder should be considered. Possibilities include delusional disorders (as discussed above), major depressive disorder with psychotic features, and other chronic conditions such as schizophrenia. Given that health anxiety frequently co-occurs with anxiety and mood disorders, the clinician should also evaluate for the presence of anxiety disorders with prominent somatic symptoms, such as panic disorder, and mood disorders, such as major depression.

10.3 Epidemiology

Determining the prevalence of health anxiety is challenging in large part due to variability in classification. Population studies using current criteria for hypochondriasis yield surprisingly few cases, from 0.05% to 0.4%, without a clear gender difference (Looper & Kirmayer 2001, Lieb *et al.* 2002, Noyes *et al.* 2005, Martin & Jacobi

2006, Bleichardt & Hiller 2007). In medical outpatient settings, hypochondriasis rates based on DSM-III or DSM-IV and ICD-10 criteria are more prevalent than in the general population, with studies showing a point prevalence rate of 4.2% (range 0.8–8.5%) (Creed & Barsky 2004). Population studies focusing on the broader concept of illness worry or health anxiety show prevalence rates in the general population in the range of 4–10%, also affecting roughly equal proportions of men and women (Looper & Kirmayer 2001, Rief *et al.* 2001, Noyes *et al.* 2005). Thus, while hypochondriasis is rare in the community, health anxiety is relatively common.

While there are few studies looking at characteristic longitudinal courses for people with hypochondriasis, patients with more chronic health anxiety are more likely to have marked illness worry, greater baseline impairment/high healthcare utilization, and higher baseline levels of anxiety or depressive symptoms (Creed & Barsky 2004).

10.4 Etiology

Determining the underlying cause of health anxiety involves two main considerations: (1) Why are some individuals more aware of physical symptoms and pain than others? and (2) Why are some people more prone to make the cognitive connection between symptom awareness and serious disease? The answers likely involve predisposing, precipitating, and perpetuating factors.

When considering predisposing factors for health anxiety, family studies can be informative. While the genetics of health anxiety are not yet understood, by examining related disorders we can gain a sense of familial risk factors. For example, one family study of patients with hypochondriasis showed a higher than expected rate of somatization disorder among relatives (Noyes *et al.* 1997). A family study of patients with OCD and their first-degree relatives found a higher rate of hypochondriasis among the OCD patient relative probands compared to control relative probands (Bienvenu *et al.* 2000). The first study, therefore, suggests hypochondriasis is more closely related to somatization disorder than other disorders, while the second study suggests that hypochondriasis and OCD may have common genetic links. Unfortunately, the family study of hypochondriasis has been the only such investigation, and the sample size was quite small. However, if indeed people suffering from health anxiety share a similar underlying genetic profile with people suffering from OCD, the two groups may also have common neurobiological deficits, such as the impaired striatal functioning commonly found in OCD (Saxena *et al.* 1998, van den Heuvel *et al.* 2005). This is currently being investigated at the New York Psychiatric Institute. Lastly, hypochondriasis frequently coexists with panic disorder (Noyes *et al.* 1986, Abramowitz & Moore 2007), another condition that involves misinterpretation of bodily sensations and the fear that one is going to immediately die, usually of a heart attack. Health anxiety differs from panic disorder in that its presence is not necessarily associated with the short time period of an acute panic attack or the full cluster of panic symptoms; however, given its frequent comorbidity, more research in this area is needed.

One significant precipitating factor for health anxiety may be early trauma. In one study, hypochondriasis significantly correlated with reported traumatic sexual contact, violence, or major parental upheaval before age 17 (Barsky *et al.* 1994). In another study, general medical patients who met DSM-III-R criteria for hypochondriasis reported traumatic events and circumstances, such as serious illness or injury in childhood, more frequently than patients who did not meet hypochondriasis criteria (Noyes *et al.* 2002).

Other precipitants of health anxiety may include personal experience with a disease (Druss 1995). Following recovery from illness, the person may become fearful of relapse and interpret normal somatic sensations (e.g., muscle aches or stomach discomfort) as evidence of re-emerging illness. Given a known history of medical conditions, vigilance and follow-up are appropriate; however, when health anxiety escalates to levels chronically interfering with normal social and occupational functioning despite medical reassurance, it becomes pathologic. For instance, a 60-year-old woman with a history of a ruptured peptic ulcer requiring prolonged hospitalization began to decline repeated invitations to see her grandchildren because she considered her son's home "too far" from her doctor's office. Despite reassurance from her doctor that she had fully recovered, the woman also canceled multiple vacations that she had planned. She avoided ill friends and family, fearing that hearing about their illnesses would make her too anxious about her own health.

For other people, the illness of a loved one may precipitate an episode of health anxiety. For instance, a young man whose father died of lung cancer became vigilant about lung problems, constantly scanning his breathing for any irregularity. He was seen by multiple pulmonologists, who reassured him that his lungs appeared normal. Despite these evaluations, he repeatedly visited the emergency room and his student health center with concerns. His grades started to decline because of missed classes. His anxiety was perpetuated by the belief that he would eventually find a doctor to diagnose and cure his symptoms.

A factor perpetuating health anxiety, as well as somatization, is the process of somatosensory amplification, whereby a person focuses on normal bodily sensations that otherwise would go unnoticed. Barsky and colleagues (1990) found that somatosensory amplification was significantly higher in a sample of participants with hypochondriasis than in a comparison sample without hypochondriasis. How might symptom amplification occur? The human brain filters out information received from the body that is determined not important enough for conscious awareness. In the case of pain, initial studies show the brain responds similarly to imagined and experienced pain (Raij *et al.* 2005), yet how one interprets that pain has to do with how that information is cognitively processed (Lamm *et al.* 2007). People who report increased pain sensitivity show differences in activation in specific brain areas, such as the anterior cingulate and the somatosensory and prefrontal cortex (Coghill *et al.* 2003), indicating that differing neural substrates (either from genetic endowment or from later alteration) may account for different thresholds for somatic awareness.

The somatic amplification seen in health anxiety, as well as somatization and pain disorders, may also occur through a process of immune-mediated sensitization. In response to trauma or infection, the body releases proinflammatory cytokines, compounds used in cellular communication, throughout both the periphery and the central nervous system. This normal response produces non-specific illness symptoms and behaviors that make someone feel "sick," such as feeling tired, unmotivated, and depressed. In most people, when the infection or trauma resolves or heals, so do the sickness symptoms; however, for those who have a chronically activated immune system, the symptoms may persist. Re-exposure or additional trauma may cause amplification of the non-specific symptoms of disease (Dimsdale & Dantzer 2007). This theory may explain why patients with medically unexplained symptoms continuously feel lousy and doctors are unable to identify an underlying problem.

10.5 Measures of health anxiety

There are several measures used in research and clinical settings to evaluate patients with health anxiety and related conditions. One method of evaluation uses a structured diagnostic interview employing specific criteria (such as DSM-IV or ICD-10) to establish a diagnosis, e.g., the Somatoform Disorders Schedule or the Structured Diagnostic Interview for Hypochondriasis (Barsky *et al.* 1992). This method, employing the judgment of a clinician in the semi-structured evaluation, results in a categorical classification – the disorder is either present or absent. Another method of evaluation is based on a continuum of patient self-reported symptoms or attitudes about illness. The instruments listed below can contribute helpful supplementary information to a thorough clinical evaluation, which would include a careful medical history and review of past treatment records. When evaluating patients with excessive health anxiety, it is important to keep in mind that physical illnesses are occasionally overlooked or missed by the patient's treating physician, and these instruments do not rule out a serious physical condition.

10.5.1 Whiteley Index

The Whiteley Index is psychometrically well developed and is probably the most widely used instrument for assessing health anxiety and hypochondriasis. This self-report scale consists of 14 yes/no items and three subscales. It is easy and quick to administer and to score and is sensitive to symptom change in response to treatment. Although it is useful as a screening tool for excessive health anxiety and hypochondriasis, even in primary-care offices, the Whiteley self-report does not provide sufficient information on which solely to base a diagnosis. In screening, a score of eight or more positive responses is considered consistent with a probable diagnosis of hypochondriasis (Pilowsky 1967).

10.5.2 Illness Attitude Scales

Consisting of 29 items divided into nine subscales, the Illness Attitude Scales (IAS) (Kellner 1987) can assess state, trait, general hypochondriasis, and abnormal illness behavior. Unlike most of the measures in this area, the IAS also collects information on whether there has been any diagnosis of a serious medical condition accompanying reported illness attitudes. Scores of three or four on either the *hypochondriacal beliefs* or *disease phobia* subscales are highly suggestive of hypochondriasis. The scale has good sensitivity and successfully discriminates between subgroups of patients with illness behavior (Sirri *et al.* 2008).

10.5.3 Somatosensory Amplification Scale

The Somatosensory Amplification Scale (SSAS) (Barsky *et al.* 1990) is a self-report tool that was developed to assess sensitivity to mild uncomfortable body experiences. The instrument consists of 10 statements rated on a one-to-five scale, covering a range of uncomfortable bodily sensations not indicative of serious disease. While postulated to be of clinical value and to show sensitivity to treatment change (Visser & Bouman 2001), the validity (Aronson *et al.* 2001) and usefulness of the SSAS in identifying patients with hypochondriasis in comparison to the IAS and Whiteley (Speckens *et al.* 1996) has been questioned.

10.5.4 Structured Diagnostic Interview for Hypochondriasis

The Structured Diagnostic Interview for Hypochondriasis (SDIH) (Barsky *et al.* 1992), a clinically administered interview consisting of 12 questions, was developed as a module of the Structured Clinical Interview for DSM-III-R to diagnose hypochondriasis. It can also be administered independently.

10.5.5 Hypochondriasis Scale of the MMPI-2

The Hypochondriasis Scale of the MMPI-2 (Butcher *et al.* 1989) primarily focuses on physical symptoms experienced but does not assess attitudes about them. Therefore, it is of limited use in diagnosing hypochondriasis. In addition, patients with actual physical illnesses affecting multiple bodily systems would score high on the hypochondriasis scale even though they are not hypochondriacal.

10.5.6 Heightened Illness Concern – Severity Scale

Modeled after the Clinical Global Impression (CGI) Severity scale, the Heightened Illness Concern – Severity Scale (HIC-Severity) (Fallon 2001) is a clinician-rated, seven-item severity scale that is useful for classifying hypochondriacal severity over the prior two-week interval and monitoring change in response to treatment. The clearly defined clinical anchors for each of the seven items emphasize frequency of illness worries, severity of distress, and duration of worry during each episode.

10.6 Clinical considerations and practical management

Since patients with health anxiety typically present with somatic complaints, they usually seek help from non-mental-health professionals, such as primary care physicians (PCPs). These patients are often sensitive to interpersonal interactions and are slower to trust their doctor, perhaps due to negative experiences in the past, and they may not appreciate psychological explanations of their symptoms. Current medical practice demands, often limiting doctor–patient encounters to 15 minutes or less, can exacerbate the problem. For example, patients sometimes complain that they cannot trust a doctor's recommendation because it was given before they had even finished presenting their complaints.

Establishing rapport with patients suffering from health anxiety is crucial; however, there is a balance to keep in mind. Even though a well-meaning PCP might want to reassure the patient that there is nothing to worry about, repeated reassurance is usually not helpful, especially for those individuals plagued by obsessional doubt. In fact, unless accompanied by a careful evaluation, quick reassurance may make many patients feel their concerns are not being taken seriously. Those patients plagued by the pathology of doubt may be very briefly reassured by a physician's words, but any new trigger – a symptom, a clinical detail not mentioned, or a disease reminder in the media – will reinvigorate the intense anxiety and need for additional reassurance.

Illustrating this point was the public response to a 2006 London health risk announcement following the polonium poisoning of Mr. Alexander Litvinenko, a former Russian spy, in which traces of radiation were found in multiple locations he visited (Rincon 2006). After the publication of the health risk announcement, 872 callers requested reassurance, yet seven individuals could not be reassured by the Health Protection Agency staff, requiring extensive phone interventions with a psychiatrist (Morgan et al. 2008). This case demonstrates the vulnerability of people with health anxiety and their exaggerated response to public health reports. It also demonstrates that a subgroup of these anxious individuals may be particularly poorly responsive to repeated reassurance.

Practical guidelines can aid in initial management of patients with health anxiety in primary-care settings, with the main goal of minimizing unnecessary tests and treatment. Such strategies include helping patients feel their suffering is appreciated, limiting the use of medical jargon for normal variations in functioning, and scheduling regular appointments independent from symptom status. Given that their suffering is real, patients with health anxiety should be approached with empathy and acceptance, while refocusing treatment away from a "cure" and toward symptom management (Barsky & Ahern 2004).

10.7 Treatments of health anxiety

Early identification and treatment of health anxiety can help curtail unnecessary suffering. Treatment is more likely to produce an effect before the sick role becomes an entrenched pattern (Barsky et al. 2001). The earlier the intervention, the less financial loss to the individual and society, since chronic somatoform diseases, including hypochondriasis, are associated with high direct and indirect health costs (Hiller & Fichter 2004). With early intervention there is also less risk of unnecessary treatments and iatrogenic harm that comes with more interventions (Kouyanou et al. 1997). Finally, early intervention and practical management can help preserve the doctor–patient relationship and reduce the frustrations of dealing with medically unexplained symptoms for both patients and healthcare professionals.

The two treatment modalities for hypochondriasis with the most empirical support, cognitive–behavioral therapy (CBT) and selective serotonin reuptake inhibitors (SSRIs), are discussed below.

10.7.1 Psychotherapies

Among psychotherapeutic treatments for health anxiety, cognitive–behavioral approaches have been the most carefully studied (Kroenke 2007, Thomson & Page 2007). Cognitive therapy focuses on modifying dysfunctional thoughts in response to symptoms, while behavioral therapy deals with decreasing problematic behaviors and teaching new skills. Other variations include behavioral stress management, with a focus on educating individuals about behaviors that can be used to help reduce stress. A recent Cochrane meta-analysis (Thomson & Page 2007) found both cognitive therapy and behavioral stress-management treatments effective in improving symptoms of hypochondriasis along with comorbid depression and anxiety. Behavioral therapy with exposure and response prevention (ERP) was also effective in treating hypochondriasis, but ERP did not help the associated depression. Participants in

CBT, compared to the usual-medical-care group, significantly improved on measures of general functioning and physical symptoms at a 12-month follow-up. Although the overall effectiveness of CBT for hypochondriasis is supported, a better understanding of specific elements responsible for the treatment effect is needed, as well as clarification as to which treatments are most acceptable to patients.

Data for a related approach, psychoeducation, are less uniform. According to the Cochrane review, "explanatory therapy" – providing patient reassurance and education on topics such as the principles of selective attention – did not significantly improve measures of hypochondriasis and physical symptoms, although it did result in participants using significantly fewer health resources (Thomson & Page 2007). Some studies offer support for psychoeducation as a useful component of a treatment package or as an initial low-cost intervention. For example, in a study by Buwalda and colleagues (2006), six-week group psychoeducation treatments based either on the cognitive–behavioral or the problem-solving approach provided significant improvement in hypochondriacal concerns, as well as depression and trait anxiety, at six-month follow-up. At the same time, even in the sample of self-referred and relatively well-functioning participants, improvement did not reach the level of functioning found in the general community sample.

As a search for new psychotherapeutic treatments continues, attention training techniques are being investigated in light of the attention bias toward threatening health-related information in patients with hypochondriasis (Papageorgiou & Wells 1998, Bouman & Vervaeke 2006). Others look to better understand reassurance-seeking behaviors and childhood attachment with caregivers (Schmidt *et al.* 2002, Noyes *et al.* 2003, Wearden *et al.* 2006). Problem-solving approaches to address related aspects of somatization might be another potential treatment. For example, Nezu and colleagues (2007) found non-cardiac chest pain participants had less effective social problem solving than matched participants with cardiac chest pain, as well as higher depression, anxiety, and perceived stress and anger.

There are also case reports of augmenting CBT with motivational interviewing (MI) for patients with strong disease conviction, or near-delusional hypochondriasis (McKay & Bouman 2008). Adding MI to the initial stages of CBT might help engage and keep in therapy those patients with health anxieties who are reluctant to admit psychological factors are at play. Such an investigation would present additional information to the treatment paradigm for health anxiety, parallel to the MI augmentation in treatment of other mental health conditions, e.g. OCD (Simpson *et al.* 2008).

10.7.2 Medication

Selective serotonin reuptake inhibitors (SSRIs) are the current cornerstone of pharmacotherapy for individuals with severe health anxiety or hypochondriasis. Open-label trials have suggested that fluvoxamine may be effective (Fallon *et al.* 2003). Greeven and colleagues (2007) conducted a double-blind, placebo-controlled trial that supported paroxetine use in the treatment of short-term hypochondriasis, while another controlled trial confirmed the efficacy of fluoxetine compared to placebo (Fallon *et al.* 2008). Studies suggest that some patients may require the higher doses of SSRIs that are more typical of OCD treatment (Greeven *et al.* 2007, Fallon *et al.* 2008). While SSRIs appear to be efficacious in diminishing hypochondriasis, the study by Fallon and colleagues (2008) did not show a difference between placebo and drug in improvement in somatization. Interestingly, concomitant benzodiazepine use may have a negative effect on the efficacy of CBT or SSRIs for hypochondriasis (Greeven *et al.* 2007), similar to the effect observed in treatment studies of panic disorder and social anxiety disorder (Fava *et al.* 1994).

While SSRIs are considered to be the mainstay of pharmacological treatment for non-delusional hypochondriasis, other medications may play a role. A recent case report (Politi 2007) presented evidence of significant improvement in a patient with refractory hypochondriasis without comorbidity following treatment with duloxetine, suggesting that the dual serotonin/norepinephrine reuptake inhibitors may also be helpful. A previous study similarly supported duloxetine's potential utility for the treatment of health anxiety, demonstrating that patients with depression treated with duloxetine had a significant reduction in hypochondriasis (Hirschfeld *et al.* 2005). Of note, there is limited evidence that reduction of anxiety and depressive symptoms reduces health anxiety (Robbins & Kirmayer 1996, Simon *et al.* 2001); however, this is not a consistent finding, and it illustrates the challenge in differentiating hypochondrias from these disorders (Creed & Barsky 2004).

10.7.3 Combined treatment: psychotherapy and medication

With demonstrated effectiveness of medication and of CBT, the question of the comparative effectiveness of combined treatment has arisen. Although no studies have yet been published, there is a placebo-controlled, NIMH-funded clinical trial currently under way at Columbia University and Harvard University in which CBT, fluoxetine, placebo, and a combination of CBT and fluoxetine are being compared.

10.7.4 Treatment of hypochondriacal delusions

When patients have fixed delusions with no insight into the irrationality of their illness concerns, they are referred to as having delusional disorder, somatic subtype. There have been numerous case reports and small studies documenting the efficacy of typical and atypical antipsychotics in the treatment of delusional parasitosis in particular, with marked improvement in two-thirds of cases (Aw *et al.* 2005, reported on 8 patients; Pavlovsky *et al.* 2008, reported on 12 patients). There have been two small placebo-controlled trials with ON-OFF-ON design of delusional parasitosis (n = 10 or 11) using the antipsychotic medication pimozide (Hamann 1982, Ungvari 1986). On the basis of these studies and the observational works of Riding and Munro, pimozide was considered the treatment of choice in delusional parasitosis in the 1980s. There have been two significant meta-analyses of delusional parasitosis, with conclusions supporting the benefits of typical and atypical antipsychotics (Trabert 1995, Freudenmann & Lepping 2008). Insufficient evidence exists from which to determine whether SSRIs may play a role in the treatment of the psychotic end of health anxiety.

10.8 Conclusion and future directions

Health anxiety and medically unexplained symptoms are challenging both for patients and for clinicians. The good news is that there are a variety of psychological and pharmacologic approaches that are helpful in reducing excessive illness worry. The bad news is that there still is no diagnostic category that adequately encompasses the full range of patients with excessive illness concerns. The most pressing agenda, therefore, is the development of clear, empirically established diagnostic categories for patients with health anxiety.

A recent effort in this direction by Fink and colleagues (2004) was based on a study of a large sample of primary care patients, suggesting that rumination about illness plus one of five other symptoms – with a division of cases into "mild" and "severe" – would produce a better-performing, distinct diagnostic entity with greater clinical utility in primary care and less overlap with the other somatoform disorders. These five symptoms are: (1) worry about harboring or contracting a severe disease and/or intense awareness of bodily functions misinterpreted as serious disease, (2) suggestibility if one reads or hears about a disease, (3) excessive fascination with medical information, (4) unrealistic contamination fears, and (5) fear of taking prescribed medication. Currently, hypochondria is nestled in the somatoform section of DSM-IV; however, with revised criteria and further analyses, it may be found to have a more appropriate location within the anxiety disorder section (Kroenke *et al.* 2007).

Other new directions for research include advancing our understanding of genetic and neurobiological differences in those with health anxiety, and better comprehending the physiological processes, including the psychoneuroimmune pathophysiology, behind symptom amplification. Identification of clinically useful biomarkers of symptom amplification could have profound implications for how physicians and patients conceptualize medically unexplained symptoms seen in health anxiety and somatization, moving them from perceived as a primarily psychological phenomenon to a more integrated psychobiological one. Reconceptualization may reduce the stigmatization of these conditions and result in greater appreciation of a patient's genuine suffering.

Advances in empirically based treatments, such as combined treatments, can help patients return to their full lives and refocus their energies on truly healthy behaviors, such as diet and exercise. Given the reluctance of people with illness anxiety to seek mental-health services as opposed to other medical treatment, further data that can help determine the optimum level of collaboration between primary-care and mental-health professionals is needed. While advances have been made in the treatment of health worries, the treatment of somatization and somatoform pain has been a neglected area of research. Results from the pharmacologic studies reviewed above demonstrate that illness worries often improve, but somatic distress may continue unabated. Novel approaches are needed to help reduce somatic symptoms. Additionally, many people with health anxiety bypass the medical system by primarily utilizing the internet, and suffer needlessly in isolation.

While there is much to be learned, recent research in health anxiety provides much reason for optimism among both health providers and patients.

References

Abramowitz, J. S., & Moore, E. L. (2007). An experimental analysis of hypochondriasis. *Behaviour Research and Therapy*, **45**, 413–424.

American Psychiatric Association (2000). *Diagnostic and Statistical Manual of Mental Disorders*, 4th edn, text revision (DSM-IV-TR). Washington, DC: American Psychiatric Association.

Aronson, K. R., Feldman Barrett, L., & Quigley, K. S. (2001). Feeling your body or feeling badly. Evidence for the limited validity of the Somatosensory Amplification Scale as an index of somatic sensitivity. *Journal of Psychosomatic Research*, **51**, 387–394.

Asmundson, G. J. G., Taylor, S., Sevgur, S., & Cox, B. J. (2001). Health anxiety: classification and clinical features. In G. J. G. Asmundson, S. Taylor, & B. J. Cox, eds., *Health Anxiety: Clinical and Research Perspectives on Hypochondriasis and Related Conditions.* Chichester: Wiley.

Aw, D. C., Thong, J. Y., & Chan, H. L. (2005). Delusional parasitosis: case series of 8 patients and review of the literature. *Annals of the Academy of Medicine*, **34** (1), 141–142.

Barsky, A. J., & Ahern, D. K. (2004). Cognitive behavior therapy for hypochondriasis. *JAMA*, **291**, 1464–1470.

Barsky, A. J., & Deans, E. C. (2006). *Stop Being Your Symptoms and Start Being Yourself: a Six Week Mind–Body Program to Ease Your Chronic Symptoms.* New York, NY: HarperCollins.

Barsky, A. J., Wyshak, G., & Klerman, G. L. (1986). Hypochondriasis: an evaluation of the DSM-III-R criteria in medical outpatients. *Archives of General Psychiatry*, **43**, 493–500.

Barsky, A. J., Wyshak, G., & Klerman, G. L. (1990). The somatosensory amplification scale and its relationship to hypochondriasis. *Journal of Psychiatric Research*, **24**, 323–334.

Barsky, A. J., Cleary, P. D., Wyshak, G., *et al.* (1992). A structured diagnostic interview for hypochondriasis: a proposed criterion standard. *Journal of Nervous & Mental Disease*, **180**, 20–27.

Barsky, A. J., Wool, C., Barnett, M. C., & Cleary, P. D. (1994). Histories of childhood trauma in adult hypochondriacal patients. *American Journal of Psychiatry*, **151**, 397–401.

Barsky, A., Ettner, S. L., Horsky, J., & Bates, D. W. (2001). Resource utilization of patients with hypochondriacal health anxiety and somatization. *Medical Care*, **39**, 705–715.

Bienvenu, O. J., Samuels, J. F., Riddle, M. A., *et al.* (2000). The relationship of obsessive–compulsive disorder to possible spectrum disorders: from a family study. *Biological Psychiatry*, **48**, 287–293.

Bleichardt, G., & Hiller, W. (2007). Hypochondriasis and health anxiety in the German population. *British Journal of Health Psychology*, **12**, 511–523.

Bouman, T. K., & Vervaeke, G. (2006). [Training in Attention Manipulation (TAM) as a treatment for hypochondriasis: case illustrations.] (Dutch). *Gedragstherapie*, **39**, 293–305.

Butcher, J. N., Dahlstrom, W. G., Graham, J. R., Tellegen, A., & Kaemmer, B. (1989). *MMPI-2 (Minnesota Multiphasic Personality Inventory-2): Manual for administration and scoring.* Minneapolis, MN: University of Minnesota Press.

Buwalda, F. M., Bouman, T. K., & van Duijnb, M. A. J. (2006). Psychoeducation for hypochondriasis: a comparison of a cognitive–behavioral approach and a problem-solving approach. *Behaviour Research and Therapy*, **45**, 887–899.

Coghill, R. C., McHaffie, J. G., & Yen, Y. F. (2003). Neural correlates of interindividual differences in the subjective experience of pain. *Proceedings of the National Academy of Sciences of the USA*, **100**, 8538–8542.

Creed, F., & Barsky, A. J. (2004). A systematic review of the epidemiology of somatization disorder and hypochondriasis. *Journal of Psychosomatic Research*, **56**, 391–408.

de Gelder, B., Snyder, J., Greve, D., Gerard, G., & Hadjikhani, N. (2004). Fear fosters flight: a mechanism for fear contagion when perceiving emotion expressed by a whole body. *Proceedings of the National Academy of Sciences of the USA*, **101**, 16701–16706.

Dimsdale, J. E., & Dantzer, R. (2007). A biological substrate for somatoform disorders: importance of pathophysiology. *Psychosomatic Medicine*, **69**, 850–854.

Druss, R. G. (1995). *The Psychology of Illness: in Sickness and in Health.* Washington DC: American Psychiatric Press.

Fallon, B. A. (2001). Pharmacologic strategies for hypochondriasis. In V. Starcevic & D. R. Lipsett. eds., *Hypochondriasis: Modern Perspectives on an Ancient Malady.* New York, NY: Oxford Univerity Press.

Fallon, B. A., Qureshi, A. I., Schneier, F. R., *et al.* (2003). An open trial of fluvoxamine for hypochondriasis. *Psychosomatics*, **44**, 298–303.

Fallon, B. A., Petkova, E., Skritskaya, N., *et al.* (2008). A double-masked, placebo-controlled study of fluoxetine for hypochondriasis. *Journal of Clinical Psychopharmacology*, **28** (6), 638–645.

Fava, G. A., Grandi, S., Belluardo, P., *et al.* (1994). Benzodiazepines and anxiety sensitivity in panic disorder. *Progress in Neuro-Psychopharmacology and Biological Psychiatry*, **18**, 1163–1168.

Feldman, M. D. (2000). Munchausen by Internet: detecting factitious illness and crisis on the Internet. *Southern Journal of Medicine*, **93**, 669–672.

Fink, P., Ørnbøl, E., Toft, T., *et al.* (2004). A new, empirically established hypochondriasis diagnosis. *American Journal of Psychiatry*, **161** (9), 1680–1691.

Fox, S. (2006). Online health search. Last modified October 29, 2006. www.pewinternet.org/Reports/2006/Online-Health-Search-2006.aspx (accessed February 25, 2010).

Freudenmann, R. W., Lepping, P. (2008) Second-generation antipsychotics in primary and secondary delusional parasitosis: outcome and efficacy. *Journal of Clinical Psychopharmacology*, **28**, 500–508.

Greeven, A., van Balkom, A. J. L. M., Visser, S., *et al.* (2007). Cognitive behavior therapy and paroxetine in the treatment of hypochondriasis: a randomized controlled trial. *American Journal of Psychiatry*, **164**, 91–99.

Gureje, O., Ustun, T. B., & Simon, G. E. (1997). The syndrome of hypochondriasis: a cross-national study in primary care. *Psychological Medicine*, **27**, 1001–1010.

Hamann, K., & Avnstorp, C. (1982) Delusions of infestation treated by pimozide: a double-blind crossover clinical study. *Acta Dermato-Venereologica*, **62**, 55–58.

Harris Poll (2006). Number of "cyberchondriacs" – adults who have ever gone online for health information – increases to an estimated 136 million nationwide. #59 August 1, 2006. www.harrisinteractive.com/harris_poll/index.asp?PID=686 (accessed February 25, 2010).

Hiller, W., & Fichter, M. (2004). High utilizer of medical care: a crucial subgroup among somatizing patients. *Journal of Psychosomatic Research*, **56**, 437–443.

Hirschfeld, R. M., Mallinckrodt, C., Lee, T. C., & Detke, M. J. (2005). Time course of depression symptom improvement during treatment with duloxetine. *Depression and Anxiety*, **21**, 170–177.

Kellner, R. (1987). Abridged manual of the illness attitude scales (mimeographed). Albuquerque, NM: University of New Mexico Department of Psychiatry.

Kouyanou, K., Pither, C. E., & Wessely, S. (1997). Iatrogenic factors and chronic pain. *Psychosomatic Medicine*, **59**, 597–604.

Kroenke, K. (2007). Efficacy of treatment for somatoform disorders: a review of randomized controlled trials. *Psychosomatic Medicine*, **69**, 881–888.

Kroenke, K., Sharpe, M., & Sykes, R. (2007). Revising the classification of somatoform disorders: key questions and preliminary recommendations. *Psychosomatics*, **48**, 277–285.

Lamm, C., Nusbaum, H. C., Meltzoff, A. N., & Decety, J. (2007). What are you feeling? Using functional magnetic resonance imaging to assess the modulation of sensory and affective responses during empathy for pain. *PLoS ONE*, **2** (12), e1292.

Lieb, R., Zimmermann, P., Friis, R. H., Höfler, M., Tholen, S., & Wittchen, H. U. (2002). The natural course of DSM-IV somatoform disorders and syndromes among adolescents and young adults: a prospective–longitudinal community study. *European Psychiatry*, **17**, 321–331.

Looper, K. J., & Kirmayer, L. J. (2001). Hypochondriacal concerns in a community population. *Psychological Medicine*, **31**, 577–584.

Martin, A., & Jacobi, F. (2006). Features of hypochondriasis and illness worry in the general population in Germany. *Psychosomatic Medicine*, **68**, 770–777.

McKay, D., & Bouman, T. K. (2008). Enhancing cognitive–behavioral therapy for monosymptomatic hypochondriasis with motivational interviewing: three case illustrations. *Journal of Cognitive Psychotherapy*, **22**, 154–166.

Morgan, O. W., Page, L., Forrester, S., & Maguire, H. (2008). Polonium-210 poisoning in London: hypochondriasis and public health. *Prehospital and Disaster Medicine*, **23**, 96–97.

Nemery, B., Fischler, B., Boogaerts, M., & Lison, D. (1999). Dioxins, Coca-Cola, and mass sociogenic illness in Belgium. *Lancet*, **354**, 77.

Nemery, B., Fischler, B., Boogaerts, M., Lison, D., & Willems, J. (2002). The Coca-Cola incident in Belgium, June 1999. *Food and Chemical Toxicology*, **40**, 1657–1667.

Nezu, A. M., Nezu, C. M., Jain, D., *et al.* (2007). Social problem solving and noncardiac chest pain. *Psychosomatic Medicine*, **69**, 944–951.

Noyes, R., Reich, J., Clancy, J., & O'Gorman, T. W. (1986). Reduction in hypochondriasis with treatment of panic disorder. *British Journal of Psychiatry*, **149**, 631–635.

Noyes, R., Holt, C. S., Happel, R. L., Kathol, R. G., & Yagla, S. J. (1997). A family study of hypochondriasis. *Journal of Nervous and Mental Disorders*, **185**, 223–232.

Noyes, R., Stuart, S., Langbehn, D. R., *et al.* (2002). Childhood antecedents of hypochondriasis. *Psychosomatics*, **43**, 282–289.

Noyes, R., Stuart, S. P., Langbehn, D. R., *et al.* (2003). Test of an interpersonal model of hypochondriasis. *Psychosomatic Medicine*, **65**, 292–300.

Noyes, R., Carney, C. P., Hillis, S. L., Jones, L. E., & Langbehn, D. R. (2005). Prevalence and correlates of illness worry in the general population. *Psychosomatics*, **46**, 529–539.

Oosterbaan, D. B., van Balkom, A. J., van Boeijen, C. A., de Meij, T. G. J., & van Dyck, R. (2001). An open study of paroxetine in hypochondriasis. *Progress in Neuro-Psychopharmacology and Biological Psychiatry*, **25**, 1023–1033.

Papageorgiou, C., & Wells, A. (1998). Effects of attention training on hypochondriasis: a brief case series. *Psychological Medicine*, **28**, 193–200.

Pavlovsky, F., Peskin, V., Di Noto, L., & Stagnaro, J. C. (2008). [Delusion of parasitosis: report of twelve cases]. *Vertex*, **19** (79), 99–111.

Philen, R. M., Kilbourne, E. M., McKinley, T. W., & Parrish, R. G. (1989). Mass sociogenic illness by proxy: parentally reported epidemic in an elementary school. *Lancet*, **334**, 1372–1376.

Pilowsky, I. (1967). Dimensions of hypochondriasis. *British Journal of Psychiatry*, **113**, 89–93.

Politi, P. (2007). Successful treatment of refractory hypochondriasis with duloxetine. *Progress in Neuro-Psychopharmacology and Biological Psychiatry*, **31**, 1145–1146.

Raij, T. T., Numminen, J., Narvanen, S., Hiltunen, J., & Hari, R. (2005). Brain correlates of subjective reality of physically and psychologically induced pain. *Proceedings of the National Academy of Sciences of the USA*, **102**, 2147–2151.

Rief, W., Hessel, A., & Braehler, E. (2001). Somatization symptoms and hypochondriacal features in the general population. *Psychosomatic Medicine*, **63**, 595–602.

Rincon, P. (2006). Sophistication behind spy's poisoning. Last modified November 28, 2006. http://news.bbc.co.uk/1/hi/sci/tech/6190144.stm. Accessed March 26, 2009.

Robbins, J. M., & Kirmayer, L. J. (1996). Transient and persistent hypochondriacal worry in primary care. *Psychological Medicine*, **26**, 575–589.

Saxena, S., Brody, A. L., Schwartz, J. M., & Baxter, L. R. (1998). Neuroimaging and frontal–subcortical circuitry in obsessive–compulsive disorder. *British Journal of Psychiatry Supplement*, (35), 26–37.

Schmidt, S., Strauss, B., & Braehler, E. (2002). Subjective physical complaints and hypochondriacal features from an attachment theoretical perspective. *Psychology and Psychotherapy*, **75**, 313–332.

Simon GE, Gureje O, Fullerton C. (2001). Course of hypochondriasis in an international primary care study, *General Hospital Psychiatry*, **23**, 51–55.

Simpson, H. B., Zuckoff, A., Page, J. R., Franklin, M. E., & Foa, E. B. (2008). Adding motivational interviewing to exposure and ritual prevention for obsessive–compulsive disorder: An open pilot trial. *Cognitive Behaviour Therapy*, **37**, 38–49.

Sirri, L., Grandi, S., & Fava, G. A. (2008). The Illness Attitude Scales: a clinimetric index for assessing hypochondriacal fears and beliefs. *Psychotherapy and Psychosomatics*, **77**, 337–350.

Speckens, A. E. M., Van Hemert, A. M., Spinhoven, P., & Bolk, J. H. (1996). The diagnostic and prognostic significance of the Whiteley Index, the Illness Attitude Scales and the Somatosensory Amplification Scale. *Psychological Medicine*, **26**, 1085–1090.

Thomson, A., & Page, L. (2007). Psychotherapies for hypochondriasis. *Cochrane Database of Systematic Reviews*, (4), CD006520.

Trabert, W. (1995). 100 years of delusional parasitosis. *Psychopathology*, **28**, 238–246.

Ungvári G, & Vladár, K. (1986) Pimozide treatment for delusion of infestation. *Act Nerv Super (Praha)*, **28** (2), 103–107.

van den Heuvel, O. A., Veltman, D. J., Groenewegen, H. J., *et al.* (2005). Disorder-specific neuroanatomical correlates of attentional bias in OCD, PD and Hypochondriasis. *Archives of General Psychiatry*, **62**, 922–933.

Visser, S., & Bouman, T. K. (2001). The treatment of hypochondriasis: exposure plus response prevention vs. cognitive therapy. *Behavior Research and Therapy*, **39**, 423–442.

Wearden, A., Perryman, K., & Ward, V. (2006). Adult attachment, reassurance seeking and hypochondriacal concerns in college students. *Journal of Health Psychology*, **11**, 877–886.

Axis II and anxiety disorders

Matthew J. Kaplowitz, John C. Markowitz

11.1 Introduction

Since 1980, when the third edition of the *Diagnostic and Statistical Manual of Mental Disorders* (DSM-III) (American Psychiatric Association 1980) reliably defined both anxiety disorders (ADs) on Axis I and personality disorders (PDs) on Axis II, research has studied the relationships between them. This chapter addresses the complex interrelationships between ADs and PDs, including diagnostic controversies, patterns of comorbidity, and prognostic implications for treatment.

11.2 Classifying Axis II and anxiety disorders

11.2.1 Axis II

The DSM-III created five axes for diagnostic classification, including Axis I for illnesses such as ADs and Axis II for PDs. Few empirical data existed on which to base diagnostic criteria sets, so diagnoses were conceptualized as tentative hypotheses, based on the consensus of expert clinicians of various perspectives (Spitzer 2001). PDs were considered to differ fundamentally from clinical disorders by an earlier age of onset; a more chronic, less episodic course, and a more enduring, even immutable, prognosis (Frances & Cooper 1981). One rationale for creating Axis II was to encourage the diagnosis of PDs comorbid with Axis I disorders (Spitzer 2001); allowing for the simultaneous presence of more than one disorder made it possible to examine empirically the relationships between meaningfully defined ADs and PDs.

Axis II also encouraged clinicians to consider the contribution of a patient's personality to Axis I clinical syndromes (Frances 1980). The relationship between Axes I and II might have been considered analogous

to weather and climate. If Axis II PDs represented the general climate of the patient's condition, episodic Axis I disorders such as panic disorder were the weather. This scheme is consistent with a stress-diathesis model of illness, where an anxiogenic PD presents an underlying vulnerability to developing ADs. It may usefully describe certain patients.

However, the analogy becomes strained when one considers that many Axis I disorders are not episodic and may share with PDs an early age of onset and generally stable chronicity. Social anxiety disorder (SAD), also known as social phobia, often begins early in life and may appear as much like an Axis II syndrome as avoidant personality disorder (AVPD). Obsessive–compulsive disorder (OCD) shares symptomatic and course features with obsessive–compulsive personality disorder (OCPD). Indeed, over time some patients intermittently meet criteria for one, the other, or both (Maina *et al.* 2008, Eisen *et al.* 2006). Further, although PDs were once considered chronic and largely immutable, recent research has shown that many patients carefully diagnosed with borderline, avoidant, schizotypal, and obsessive–compulsive PDs remit from those criteria over time with or without treatment (Shea *et al.* 2002, Grilo *et al.* 2004, Zanarini *et al.* 2006). Thus the distinction between episodic "disease" and enduring "personality" is complex and potentially misleading.

11.2.2 DSM-IV personality disorders

In current DSM-IV nosology, "character" comprises four basic elements: cognition, affect, interpersonal functioning, and impulse control, disorders of which must be enduring, pervasive and inflexible (American Psychiatric Association 1994). Manifestations of these elements provide descriptive criteria for 11 PDs: paranoid, schizoid, schizotypal, antisocial, borderline, histrionic, narcissistic, avoidant, dependent,

Anxiety Disorders: Theory, Research, and Clinical Perspectives, ed. Helen Blair Simpson, Yuval Neria, Roberto Lewis-Fernández, Franklin Schneier. Published by Cambridge University Press. © Cambridge University Press 2010.

Table 11.1. DSM-IV personality disorders (PDs)

Cluster A (odd)	Cluster B (dramatic)	Cluster C (anxious)	Personality disorder not otherwise specified
Paranoid PD	Antisocial PD	Avoidant PD	
Schizoid PD	Borderline PD	Dependent PD	
Schizotypal PD	Histrionic PD	Obsessive–compulsive PD	
	Narcissistic PD		

obsessive–compulsive, and not otherwise specified. DSM-IV groups these eleven diagnoses in three clusters: odd, dramatic, and anxious (Table 11.1). The Axis II anxious cluster presents obvious symptomatic overlaps with Axis I ADs. The anxious cluster comprises AVPD, dependent PD, and OCPD (see DSM-IV for descriptive criteria).

11.2.3 Problems in assessing DSM-IV personality disorders

Despite nearly 30 years of research, reliably assessing PDs remains problematic for several reasons. Diagnosing a patient with a PD requires determining the presence of pervasive patterns of functioning, some of which may lie outside the patient's conscious awareness. The presence of an Axis I "state" disorder may confound diagnosis of Axis II "trait." Thus, patients suffering from anxiety or mood disorders frequently *appear* personality-disordered, but if the Axis I condition is treated to remission, the Axis II diagnosis may vanish. PDs are also more difficult than Axis I disorders to define with purely descriptive criteria and involve some meaning-based characteristics such as an unstable self or a sense of entitlement. Diagnosing panic attacks, with their obvious physical symptoms, is simpler than diagnosing paranoid PD, which is defined partly by chronic interpersonal patterns.

Empirical assessment of PDs also remains complicated. Corroborative sources may help in validating the chronicity of essentially lifelong symptoms; yet, short of prospective longitudinal studies that follow patients over time, it is questionable whether PDs can be definitively assessed. Furthermore, studies of PD prevalence rely either on self-report questionnaires or on structured clinical interviews. In either format a respondent may underendorse (or overendorse) symptom items. In live interviews, the interviewer has the discretion to judge the presentation, and some personality traits may be a subtext of the interview (e.g., bizarre behavior or appearance in schizotypal PD). This observational skill improves with training and experience; however, large-scale epidemiological studies require the use of lay interviewers, with minimal clinical experience, who must determine a PD based on a structured interview at a single sitting, sometimes over the telephone. Such large studies compensate by comparing lay interviews to self-report instruments (which, however, tend to yield false positives) and to clinical structured interviews of subsamples of those surveyed.

11.2.4 Interpreting comorbidity

While comorbidity indicates that two disorders co-occur, it does not explain what, if any, causal relationship exists between them. Studying the intersection of PDs and ADs requires interpreting potential methodological and/or etiological explanations.

Methodology can influence comorbidity rates in several ways (Table 11.2). First, since many of the descriptive criteria of different DSM disorders are similar, comorbidity may reflect the diagnostic overlaps that occur between syndromes, for example, obsessions and compulsions in OCD and OCPD or social avoidance symptoms in SAD and AVPD. If comorbidity were determined purely by overlapping criteria, comorbidity rates should follow a predictable path, raising the question of whether the comorbid disorders are simply variations of the same disorder. For example, criteria for SAD and AVPD overlap considerably, and they have consistently high comorbidity rates (see below).

Conversely, descriptive criteria can denote conceptual distinction. A criterion for one disorder may disqualify an individual for another disorder (e.g., hypomania obviates dysthymic disorder). Sometimes a criterion has different meanings for different disorders (e.g., social isolation in AVPD versus schizoid PD), and assessment must discern subtle but crucial differences (one wants but fears company, the other rejects it). Comorbidity rates may reflect inaccurate assessment.

Additionally, in some sense illness breeds comorbidity. That is, patients who cross the threshold for one

Table 11.2. Types of comorbidity

Methodologically influenced	
Diagnostic criteria	Symptom overlap between syndromes explains comorbidity
Assessment	Unreliable assessment procedures give appearance of comorbidity
Selection	Comorbidity rates affected by setting or severity of illness in sample

Etiologically determined	
Genetic	Separate disorders share a common genetic predisposition
Trait	Separate disorders share a common predisposing trait
Scarring	A chronic disorder causes "scarring," which meets criteria for a second disorder
Stress-diathesis	One disorder creates a particular vulnerability to another disorder
Traumatic	Common environmental trigger induces comorbid disorders
Coincidental	Separate disorders arise independently

PD are likely to qualify for multiple PDs and Axis I disorders. In general, comorbidity means greater severity. Patients carrying a "pure" Axis I AD diagnosis, without comorbidity, will likely have milder symptoms than patients meeting criteria for multiple diagnoses. Since comorbidity increases among the severely ill, study samples can influence the prevalence of comorbidity through selection bias (Berkson's bias). Clinic populations are sicker than general populations. Hospital inpatients will be sicker than outpatients at an AD clinic, who in turn will have more comorbidity than outpatients recruited from the community by advertisement or random digit dialing. In more clinically intense settings, one can expect higher comorbidity.

When little overlap exists between symptom criteria sets for comorbid disorders, we should expect, based on symptom criteria alone, to find low comorbidity rates. When studies show elevated comorbidity between symptomatically diverse disorders, as with paranoid PD and panic disorder (Reich & Braginsky 1994, Ozkan & Altindag 2005), we must look beyond criteria for an explanation. However, this does not require an etiological explanation. For panic disorder and paranoid PD, for example, elevated comorbidity rates might reflect methodological influences. Reich and Braginsky (1994) found paranoid PD the most common PD (54%) among patients with panic disorder, and presence of paranoia in panic patients was associated with earlier onset, longer duration of illness, and more severe interpersonal deficits. Their study

sample comprised 28 patients consecutively admitted to a university anxiety clinic; of these, 82% were agoraphobic, and 68% had more than one comorbid Axis I diagnosis. The high comorbidity and presence of agoraphobia denote greater severity of illness, and the study has limitations in its small sample size and use of a single true/false self-report measure to assess PDs. Subject selection and inaccurate assessment present more parsimonious explanations than the discovery of a "paranoid subset" of panic disorder patients (Reich & Braginsky 1994). In sum, methodological "noise" may simulate or obscure clinically relevant associations.

11.2.5 Etiologically determined comorbidity

Psychiatric syndromes lack defined etiology. The biopsychosocial model (Engel 1977) suggests that illness arises from the interplay of genetic, trait, and environmental influences. Diagnostic heterogeneity reflects the complexity of these factors.

Etiologically determined comorbidity might occur in several ways (Table 11.2). Separate disorders might share a common genetic predisposition or a common predisposing trait. For example, the same anxious behavioral trait might generate a Cluster C PD and vulnerability to trauma that later resulted in comorbid posttraumatic stress disorder (PTSD). Common genetic make-up also could generate two separate disorders: Reichborn-Kjennerud and colleagues (2007) found that, among 1427 young adult female–female twin pairs (898 monozygotic, 529 dizygotic), the same genetic factors influenced the presence of AVPD and SAD.

Alternatively, an Axis I disorder, particularly if chronic, might cause behavioral "scarring," yielding a de-facto Axis II state. Years of panic disorder, for example, might induce generalized avoidant behavior that not only meets criteria for Axis I agoraphobia or generalized anxiety disorder (GAD) but alternatively (or also) Axis II avoidant or dependent PD. Conversely, a PD might create vulnerability to particular Axis I disorders. For example, patients with AVPD might be prone to SAD or GAD. Johnson and colleagues (2006) found that presence of any DSM-III PD features between the ages of 14 and 22 were associated with elevated risk for ADs by mean age 33.

A PD might also influence an individual's susceptibility to stress. Vulnerability to a particular disorder, such as panic, could increase the likelihood of a comorbid AD. Alternatively, a common environmental stressor might induce comorbid disorders. For example, traumatic childhood abuse might predispose to both PTSD and borderline, avoidant, or another PD.

Finally, comorbidity might appear in individuals by chance, a diagnostic coincidence arising from independent genetic and/or environmental influences. To further complicate matters, psychiatric disorders have sufficient heterogeneity that all of the above interrelationships might hold for different patients with the same comorbidity: scarring for some, trauma for others, etc.

11.3 Research findings

PDs are less prevalent than ADs. As expected, prevalences for PDs vary according to the population sampled and the methodology used (4.4–15.7%).

11.3.1 Comorbidity between ADs and PDs

Limited information exists on the comorbidity between ADs and PDs in the general population. Given the complexity of identifying PDs, most large epidemiologic surveys in the United States and elsewhere either have not assessed them or have reported only the presence or absence of any PDs, not specific Axis II diagnoses. Recently, two nationwide surveys in the United States, the National Comorbidity Survey Replication (NCS-R) and the National Epidemiologic Survey on Alcohol and Related Conditions (NESARC), reported the comorbidity burden of many Axis I and Axis II disorders in the general population.

NESARC is the largest comorbidity sample to date, with an 81% response rate from a sample of 43 093 civilian non-institutionalized adults (18+ years) residing throughout the USA. The study employed the AUDADIS-IV, a structured diagnostic instrument for lay interviewers, administered in face-to-face interviews assisted by laptop computer software. A subsample of 2657 respondents was randomly re-interviewed with sections of the AUDADIS-IV to check data quality and test–retest reliability. Ten weeks later, 282 respondents were re-interviewed with the antisocial PD module and another 315 re-interviewed with other PD modules, producing fair to good reliability (k = 0.40 for histrionic PD to k = 0.67 for antisocial PD).

Survey data showed PDs were as prevalent among individuals with any AD (41.8%) as among those with any mood disorder (46.8%). As expected in a large sample size, all of the associations between PDs and current anxiety and mood disorders were statistically significant (Table 11.3). Consistent with the clinical literature, two Cluster C PDs – avoidant and dependent PDs – were more closely related to all of the ADs (OR = 5.4–37.2) than were the other PDs (OR = 2.9–13.1). In particular, AVPD was strongly associated with SAD (OR = 27.3) and panic disorder with agoraphobia (OR = 21.0).

The third Cluster C PD, OCPD, and the two Cluster B PDs studied, histrionic and antisocial, were each strongly related to panic disorder with agoraphobia, SAD, and GAD, as well as with mania. Panic disorder without agoraphobia and specific phobia were the ADs least correlated with any of the PDs (OR = 2.9–7.1). Although Cluster A PDs have shown weak associations with both ADs and mood disorders (Lenzenweger et al. 2007; Table 11.4), Grant and colleagues (2005) found associations for both paranoid and schizoid PDs with panic disorder with agoraphobia, SAD, and GAD, as well as dysthymia and mania, suggesting high comorbidity is not limited to the conceptually related PD clusters. Grant and colleagues (2005), using NESARC data, provide the most complete survey of comorbidity between specific ADs and PDs from one sample. Nevertheless, this study did not assess all ADs (omitting PTSD and OCD) or PDs (omitting schizotypal, borderline, and narcissistic). Indeed, no epidemiologic or clinical study has examined the full range of ADs and PDs.

Lenzenweger and colleagues (2007) used the NCS-R data (n = 5692) to compare comorbidity rates between ADs and the three PD clusters, as well as borderline and antisocial PD. Unlike NESARC (Grant et al. 2005), NCS-R data found PDs to be less prevalent among individuals with an AD (28.8%) than among those with a mood disorder (38.1%). Otherwise, the NCS-R comorbidity rates between ADs and PD clusters are fairly consistent with the NESARC findings, although NESARC did not assess PD clusters or all PDs within each PD cluster except Cluster C. Comorbidity for specific ADs is discussed below.

11.3.2 Panic disorder and PDs

Reported prevalences of any PD among clinical and research samples of outpatients with panic disorder range from 30% to 49% (Dyck et al. 2001, Ozkan & Altingday 2005, Milrod et al. 2007). The "anxious" cluster (Cluster C), and particularly avoidant and dependent PDs, account for much of the prevalence of PDs found among outpatients with panic disorder (Sanderson et al. 1993, Dyck et al. 2001, Ozkan & Altingday 2005, Milrod et al. 2007). Sanderson and

Table 11.3. Odds ratios of DSM-IV personality disorders (PDs) with 12-month DSM-IV anxiety disorders (ADs) in Grant *et al.* 2005

	Any PD	Cluster A		Cluster B		Cluster C		
		Paranoid PD	Schizoid PD	Antisocial PD	Histrionic PD	Avoidant PD	Dependent PD	Obsessive–compulsive PD
Any AD	5.6	7.4	5.9	3.3	6.6	11.9	12.9	4.7
Panic disorder + agoraphobia	13.4	12.4	13.1	5.7	8.1	21.0	37.2	7.4
Panic disorder– agoraphobia	4.7	5.6	4.1	3.8	4.3	5.4	6.2	3.8
Social anxiety disorder	10.0	10.4	10.0	3.4	5.6	27.3	17.2	6.4
Specific phobia	4.2	5.2	4.1	2.9	5.4	6.4	7.1	3.8
Generalized anxiety disorder	9.6	10.9	8.2	4.4	6.7	14.2	18.6	6.4

Table 11.4. Odds ratios of DSM-IV personality disorders (PDs) with 12-month DSM-IV anxiety disorders (ADs) in Lenzenweger *et al.* 2007

	Any PD	Cluster A	Cluster B	Cluster C	Antisocial PD	Borderline PD
Any AD	7.0	2.5	8.4	4.0	5.4	8.1
Panic disorder ± agoraphobia	8.0	3.1	8.3	4.2	10.8	10.0
Social anxiety disorder	9.9	2.4	6.1	6.5	4.3	7.1
Specific phobia	4.5	2.2	4.5	3.7	2.0	5.3
Generalized anxiety disorder	5.7	2.3	7.6	3.4	7.4	6.9
Posttraumatic stress disorder	5.8	2.5	7.3	3.2	9.8	5.8

colleagues (1993) found high Cluster C prevalence (17%), moderate Cluster B prevalence (7%), and no Cluster A prevalence associated with panic disorder. Ozkan & Altingday (2005) reported high rates of Clusters B (25%) and C (23.2%), and Dyck and colleagues (2001) reported high rates of AVPD (20.7%). Since panic involves avoidance and/or dependence on phobic companions, high Cluster C prevalence makes clinical sense.

Several clinical studies have shown a moderate to strong relationship with the "dramatic" cluster (Cluster B) in panic patients. Skodol and colleagues (1995) found panic disorder more strongly associated with borderline PD (OR = 8.2) and histrionic PD (OR = 4.0) than with dependent PD (OR = 3.5), AVPD (OR = 3.4), or OCPD (OR = 3.4). In the community, Lenzenweger and colleagues (2007) found respondents with panic disorder had comorbid borderline PD (11.6%) and, to a lesser degree, antisocial PD (4.4%), while Grant and colleagues (2005) found higher rates of antisocial PD

among respondents with panic disorder (12.1% without agoraphobia, 17.3% with agoraphobia).

Cluster A is most symptomatically disparate from panic disorder, and findings in clinical settings show low prevalence (0.0–7.1%) in panic patients (Ozkan & Altingday 2005, Sanderson *et al.* 1993). In the community, however, epidemiologic surveys have found higher rates of comorbid Cluster A. In fact, Lenzenweger and colleagues (2007) reported that while Cluster C (21.3%) was most comorbid among individuals with panic disorder, Cluster A (15.7%) was more prevalent than Cluster B (10.4%). Grant and colleagues (2005) also found elevated rates of paranoid PD and schizoid PD among individuals with panic disorder in the general population. These findings suggest that Cluster A PDs can be comorbid with panic disorder but that such individuals do not frequent treatment clinics. Alternatively, it is conceivable that lay interviews may have confused phobic avoidance with paranoid ideation.

Grant and colleagues (2005) also found that, in the general population, individuals with panic disorder with agoraphobia had higher PD comorbidity than individuals with panic disorder without agoraphobia (69.4% vs. 44.1%). Indeed, agoraphobia is often a later-onset consequence of panic – extreme avoidance, in effect. Agoraphobic patients therefore tend to be more compromised and sicker than panic patients without agoraphobia, and more likely to also suffer from a PD.

11.3.3 Social anxiety disorder and PDs

The study of PD comorbidity and SAD has been notable for the consistently high prevalences (28.2–89%) for AVPD among patients with SAD (Schneier *et al.* 1991, Alnaes & Torgersen 1988, Dyck *et al.* 2001, Hummelen *et al.* 2007). An extensive literature has attempted to determine whether the overlap of DSM symptom criteria for AVPD and generalized SAD explains the high comorbidity between these two disorders, which would imply that AVPD is simply a more severe and chronic variant of generalized SAD. In contrast, non-generalized SAD (e.g., fear of public speaking) might have a lower correlation with AVPD (e.g., 21% in Schneier *et al.* 1991).

Dependent PD also appears prevalent (5.8–27%) among patients with SAD (Sanderson *et al.* 1993, Dyck *et al.* 2001, Hummelen *et al.* 2007). Avoidance and dependence may be two sides of the same coin. If an avoidant individual manages to escape isolation and form a relationship, he or she will likely cling to it for dear life. This logic may similarly explain the elevated comorbidity rates for generalized SAD and dependent PD.

PDs other than dependent PD and AVPD have shown low comorbidity with SAD in both inpatient and outpatient clinical samples (0.0–7.8%, OR < 3.0: Dyck *et al.* 2001, Skodol *et al.* 1995). One recent exception occurred among outpatients in Norway who showed higher comorbidity trends for Cluster A PDs, particularly a higher prevalence of schizoid PD (50%) than AVPD (48%) (Hummelen *et al.* 2007). This finding may reflect cultural differences between the populations in Norway and the United States. It also calls to mind the fact that DSM-III separated schizoid PD from AVPD, a controversial event at the time. Researchers and clinicians recognized that individuals with these disorders might closely resemble one another (Frances 1980), with the patient's motivation for social isolation the principal distinction.

Patients with AVPD crave closeness but avoid it for fear of criticism and rejection, whereas patients with schizoid PD lack interpersonal desire. However, critics feared that this inferred distinction could not be made reliably.

Comorbidity trends for SAD in the general population differ only slightly from clinical populations. In NESARC, Cluster A was higher than in clinical studies (Grant *et al.* 2005). In the NCS-R, Cluster C was not significantly more prevalent than Cluster B (Lenzenweger *et al.* 2007). These differences between settings may reflect varying assessment procedures or the healthier samples surveyed in community studies, although the rise in Cluster A rates is again consistent with the expectation that this cluster avoids treatment more than Cluster C individuals.

11.3.4 Specific phobia and PD

The few surveys of PD comorbidity in specific phobia among clinical populations show very low comorbidity rates with any PD (0–12%; Sanderson *et al.* 1993). Skodol and colleagues (1995; $n = 200$) found specific phobia not significantly associated with any PD. Given the paucity of clinical studies and low sample sizes, comorbidity rates for PDs in patients with specific phobia remain unclear.

In the general population, individuals with specific phobia had a 0.0–38.3% prevalence of comorbid PDs, with an expectedly stronger trend among the "anxious" Cluster C (Grant *et al.* 2005, Lenzenweger *et al.* 2007). Grant and colleagues (2005) found OCPD was the PD with the highest prevalence (21.6%) among individuals with specific phobia.

11.3.5 Obsessive–compulsive disorder and PDs

Most surveys of PD comorbidity in OCD have been restricted to clinical populations. These studies consistently find elevated rates of OCPD in subjects with OCD (5.0–32.4%; Table 11.5). The other two Cluster C PDs have also shown high comorbidity with OCD: AVPD 4.6–27.0% and dependent PD 4.2–16.9%. The general population again shows a higher rate of Cluster A comorbidity than clinical samples. Although the two large US surveys (NCS-R and NESARC) did not assess OCD, a recent, large ($n = 8399$) national survey in Great Britain found that subjects with OCD were as likely to have a comorbid PD in Cluster A (50.5%) as in Cluster C (48.1%), and were half as likely to have one in Cluster B (23.4%) (Torres *et al.* 2006). Despite the study's large

Table 11.5. Prevalences (%) of DSM-IV and DSM-III personality disorders (PDs) among individuals with obsessive–compulsive disorder (OCD)

	Torres *et al.* 2006	Maina *et al.* 2008	Denys *et al.* 2004	Samuels *et al.* 2000	Matsunaga *et al.* 1998	Sanderson *et al.* 1993
Nomenclature	DSM-IV	DSM-IV	DSM-IV	DSM-IV	DSM-III-R	DSM-III
Location	UK	Italy	Netherlands	DC & MD	Japan	U. Penn, PA
Sample	General	Outpatients	Outpatients	Outpatients	Outpatients	Outpatients
n (OCD n)	8399 (108)	(148)	(420)	(72)	(75)	347 (21)
Prevalence (%)						
Any PD	73.8	—	32.0	44.3	53.3	24
Any Cluster A	50.5	—	1.4	4.4	29.4	—
Paranoid	35.3	6.8	0.2	4.3	12.0	—
Schizoid	26.4	8.1	0.0	0	5.4	—
Schizotypal	24.9	10.1	1.2	0	12.0	—
Any Cluster B	23.4	—	9.7	12.9	17.3	10
Antisocial	10.8	6.1	0.5	0	4.0	—
Borderline	12.0	13.5	5.6	5.7	8.0	—
Histrionic	—	6.1	1.5	4.2	2.7	5
Narcissistic	4.5	8.1	2.4	6.9	2.7	—
Any Cluster C	48.1	—	20.7	36.6	53.3	14
Avoidant	27.0	20.9	4.6	15.3	25.3	5
Dependent	11.7	16.9	7.6	4.2	12.0	5
OCPD	28.6	29.1	9.0	32.4	13.3	5
PD not otherwise specified	—	3.4	6.6			5

sample size, only 108 subjects had OCD, limiting the statistical power of the findings.

As with SAD and AVPD, there is an extensive literature evaluating the qualitative differences between OCD and OCPD (Coles *et al.* 2008, Eisen *et al.* 2006). A study using the Collective Longitudinal Personality Study (CLPS) data (*n* = 629) to assess the role of individual criteria in the convergence of OCD and OCPD (*n* = 53) found their overlap primarily explained by the criteria of hoarding, perfectionism, and preoccupation with details (Eisen *et al.* 2006). Coles and colleagues (2008) found that patients with comorbid OCD/OCPD, compared to patients with "pure" OCD, had significantly greater impairment, earlier age of onset of obsessive–compulsive symptoms (9.7 vs. 12.7 years), and earlier age of onset of full syndromal DSM-IV OCD (15.9 vs. 18.8 years).

At least some cases of OCD and OCPD share a common etiology. Samuels and colleagues (2000) found that 12% (*n* = 34) of first-degree relatives of OCD outpatients had OCPD, compared to 6% (*n* = 4) of first-degree relatives of a non-OCD community sample, indicating that

OCPD may share a common familial etiology with OCD. In a retrospective study of early- versus late-onset OCD, Maina and colleagues (2008) found that reported childhood-onset OCD increased the odds of developing OCPD in adulthood. This may indicate a common etiology (e.g., genetic), or it may be an example of "scarring."

11.3.6 Posttraumatic stress disorder and PDs

Prevalence rates for PDs among PTSD patients range from 0% to 76%; however, studies investigating the full range of comorbid PDs in PTSD patients (Faustman & White 1989, Southwick *et al.* 1993, Bollinger *et al.* 2000, Dunn *et al.* 2004) suffer from methodological limitations. Faustman and White's (1989) study had the highest sample size (*n* = 536), but PD assessment among Veterans Administration (VA) inpatients relied upon retrospective survey of discharge summaries. Dunn and colleagues (2004) evaluated PDs via validated structured interviews (SCID-II), but raters were graduate-level students; Golier and colleagues

(2003) used only one master's-level psychologist to evaluate PDs among 180 outpatients. Thus, prevalences for PDs among PTSD patients (0–76%) are less than reliable.

Among PD patients, 51% of borderline PD patients met criteria for comorbid PTSD, compared to 39.7% of schizotypal PD, 37.1% of AVPD, and 21.6% of OCPD patients (Yen *et al.* 2002). Among PTSD patients, 5.8–76.0% met criteria for comorbid borderline PD (Faustman & White 1989, Southwick *et al.* 1993, Dunn *et al.* 2004). Southwick and colleagues (1993), who found the highest borderline PD prevalence (76%), had limited statistical power due to small sample size (*n* = 34) in a VA inpatient and outpatient sample.

As borderline PD is also frequently associated with early-life trauma, some theorists (e.g., Herman *et al.* 1989, Gunderson & Sabo 1993) have examined the extent to which borderline PD reflects underlying PTSD. The association between trauma and PDs does not mean that PTSD is an inevitable comorbid diagnosis. Trauma may have various psychiatric consequences and may result in a PD or mood disorder rather than PTSD. When PTSD and PDs are comorbid, chronic early-onset PTSD might give rise to a PD through "scarring." For example, military personnel traumatized by combat in their late teens, when personality is still impressionable, might develop AVPD or paranoid PD. Alternatively, a PD might constitute a complex form of PTSD in response to profound trauma at an early age.

In the general population, only the NCS-R surveyed PD comorbidity among individuals with PTSD (Table 11.4) (Lenzenweger *et al.* 2007). As with clinical samples, the "dramatic" cluster (Cluster B) was more strongly related (OR = 7.3) to PTSD than Cluster A (OR = 2.5) or Cluster C (OR = 3.2). Unlike clinical samples, however, antisocial PD (OR = 9.8) had a stronger association with PTSD than borderline PD (OR = 5.8).

11.3.7 Generalized anxiety disorder and PDs

The few surveys of PD prevalence among patients with GAD suggest a close linkage: 37.7–49.0% (Sanderson *et al.* 1993, Dyck *et al.* 2001). The chronic nature of GAD symptoms may make it more trait- than state-like; however, too few studies exist to confirm this trend. In clinical studies, GAD is most frequently comorbid with the "anxious" Cluster C, particularly with AVPD and OCPD.

In community studies, as in clinical settings, PD comorbidity with GAD is high (60.6%) (Grant *et al.* 2005), but which PDs are most prevalent differs. While OCPD remained highest (33.5%), paranoid PD had similar prevalence (30.5%), and while AVPD was also common (21.9%), schizoid had near parity (19.1%). Curiously, the lowest comorbid prevalence rate in the general population was dependent PD (6.4%).

11.4 Prognostic implications: toxic versus benign comorbidity

Comorbidity on any DSM axis generally implies greater symptomatic severity and hence might be expected to have a negative prognostic effect. A recent, population-based longitudinal study (*n* = 629) found that the presence of comorbid Axis I and Axis II disorders in adolescence carried a consistently heightened risk for negative prognoses for academic, occupational, interpersonal, and psychiatric functioning at 20-year follow-up compared to diagnoses on either axis alone (Crawford *et al.* 2008). Clinicians, in fact, often assume that a comorbid PD is "toxic" to the treatment of Axis I patients, making these patients more difficult to treat and less likely to benefit from Axis I treatment (Dreessen & Arntz 1999). While several studies do report a negative influence of PDs on AD treatment outcome, especially in pharmacotherapy studies (Reich 2003, Weertman *et al.* 2005), other studies report no effect or even positive effects for Axis II comorbidity (Dreessen & Arntz 1998).

Differential treatment effects have been found in different PD–AD combinations. A recent cognitive–behavioral therapy outcome study of 39 outpatients with OCD found that presence of Cluster A or B PDs predicted significantly less improvement at 12-month follow-up than in OCD patients without these PDs, while OCD patients with Cluster C PD showed significantly better outcomes at follow-up than OCD patients without Cluster C (Hansen *et al.* 2007). Another study found a positive treatment effect for comorbid Cluster C PDs among 49 outpatients with panic disorder treated with psychodynamic psychotherapy (Milrod *et al.* 2007). However, these findings do not hold across all studies. One Cluster C PD, AVPD, is frequently cited as a predictor of poor outcome, especially in panic disorder (Chambless *et al.* 1992, Weertman *et al.* 2005) but also in generalized SAD (Feske *et al.* 1996).

There is controversy over how to interpret findings from these comorbidity studies, particularly given the problem of state effects in PD assessment procedures (Reich 2003). More severely ill Axis I patients may be incorrectly assigned a PD diagnosis, thus exaggerating the impact of PD on prognosis. Knowing whether comorbid AVPD moderates poor prognosis would be clinically useful because avoidant traits, such as heightened sensitivity to rejection in social contexts, pose interpersonal challenges to therapy not addressed in treatment protocols. However, the parsimonious explanation remains methodological: studies are too few and tend to have low sample size, limiting statistical power to find moderating effects. Unfortunately, most outcome research on ADs has ignored Axis II comorbidity altogether, but the studies cited above suggest its potentially meaningful effect on outcome. Outcome research on Axis II comorbidity deserves greater attention.

11.5 Conclusion

Available data suggest that PD comorbidity among ADs is common, except in the case of specific phobia. Some combinations are more common than others. Histrionic PD is rarely comorbid with generalized SAD, for example, whereas AVPD is commonly comorbid with SAD. While individuals with ADs have prevalent Cluster A and B comorbidity, Cluster C PDs have particularly high prevalence. In many cases, the level of comorbidity is complicated by study methodology (as in studies assessing panic disorder and paranoid PD) or simply by lack of research (e.g., PTSD and any PD except borderline). It also remains unclear when PDs are shaped by the experience of having an AD (i.e., "scarring"), when PDs act as risk factors for ADs (i.e., stress-diathesis), or when PDs (or traits) and ADs arise from common causes (i.e., genetic comorbidity and trait comorbidity).

The DSM-III multiaxial system highlighted PDs and their frequent coexistence with, and possible contribution to, other psychiatric disorders. At the time, PDs were thought to be stable, immutable, and pervasive, in contrast to Axis I disorders, which were considered more episodic. PDs created an underlying context from which – in conjunction with environmental stressors – ADs were thought to emerge. Nearly three decades of research have produced evidence that challenges these early assumptions and raises questions about diagnosis, assessment, and prognosis.

Are PDs and ADs always separate disorders, or sometimes a single disorder that manifests differently and hence qualifies for different diagnoses over time? Are PDs necessarily more chronic and pervasive than

some ADs and other Axis I disorders? Is personality pathology best conceptualized in terms of enduring traits (Frances 1980), which the present PD nosology may not adequately reflect, or are personality traits better understood as enduring, temperamental (genetic) vulnerabilities that underlie both PDs and ADs, with periodic flare-ups in the signs and symptoms that meet diagnostic criteria (Shea & Yen 2003)?

Current evidence yields more questions than answers, due in part to the complexity of assessing PDs and the labor and expense of large-scale, longitudinal studies. The field of PD research has produced a host of assessment instruments of varying sensitivities and specificities, with no one gold standard. We do not entirely understand the extent to which current anxiety states, or state effects from any comorbid condition, affect personality assessment (i.e., assessment-based comorbidity). Future research will need to disentangle state and trait. Are there descriptive features that reflect patterns of functioning 10 years prior? Can we trust individuals' memory of themselves, especially individuals with an unstable sense of self (e.g., borderline PD)?

A crucial value of comorbidity is its potentially moderating effect on treatment outcome. Outcome studies to illuminate these moderating effects of PDs on Axis I treatment are necessary to advance the clinical utility of the DSM. Only preliminary evidence exists, indicating differential treatment effects of Axis II comorbidity (Dreessen & Arnst 1998, Milrod et al. 2007). Future outcome research should routinely assess PDs and their effect on treatment response.

Acknowledgments

Supported in part by grant R01 MH079078 from the National Institute of Mental Health.

References

Alnaes, S., & Torgersen, S. (1988). The relationship between DSM-III symptom disorders (Axis I) and personality disorders (Axis II) in an outpatient population. *Acta Psychiatrica Scandinavica*, 78, 485–492.

American Psychiatric Association (1980). *Diagnostic and Statistical Manual of Mental Disorders*, 3rd edn (DSM-III). Washington, DC: American Psychiatric Association.

American Psychiatric Association (1994). *Diagnostic and Statistical Manual of Mental Disorders*, 4th edn (DSM-IV). Washington, DC: American Psychiatric Association.

Bollinger, A., Riggs, D., Blake, D., & Ruzek, J. (2000). Prevalence of personality disorders among combat veterans with posttraumatic stress disorder. *Journal of Traumatic Stress*, **13**, 255–270.

Chambless, D., Renneberg, B., Goldstein, A., & Gracely, E. D. (1992). MCMI diagnosed personality disorders among agoraphobic outpatients: Prevalence and relationship to severity of treatment outcome. *Journal of Anxiety Disorders*, **6**, 193–211.

Coles, M. E., Pinto, A., Mancebo, M. C., Rasmussen, S.A., & Eisen, J. L. (2008). OCD with comorbid OCPD: a subtype of OCD? *Journal of Psychiatric Research*, **42**, 289–296.

Crawford, T. N., Cohen, P., First, M. B., *et al.* (2008). Comorbid Axis I and Axis II disorders in early adolescence. *Archives of General Psychiatry*, **65**, 641–648.

Denys, D., Tenney, N., van Megen, H. J., de Geus, F., & Westenberg, H. G. (2004). Axis I and II comorbidity in a large sample of patients with obsessive–compulsive disorder. *Journal of Affective Disorders*, **80**, 155–162.

Dreessen, L., & Arntz, A. (1998). The impact of personality disorders on treatment outcome in anxiety disorders: best evidence synthesis. *Behaviour Research and Therapy*, **36**, 483–504.

Dreessen, L., & Arntz, A. (1999). Personality disorders have no excessively negative impact on therapist-rated therapy process in the cognitive and behavioural treatment of Axis I anxiety disorders. *Clinical Psychology and Psychotherapy*, **6**, 384–399.

Dunn, N., Yanasak, E., & Schillaci, J. (2004). Personality disorders in veterans with posttraumatic stress disorder and depression. *Journal of Trauma Stress*, **17**, 75–82.

Dyck, I. R., Phillips, K. A., Warshaw, M. G., *et al.* (2001). Patterns of personality pathology in patients with generalized anxiety disorder, panic disorder with and without agoraphobia, and social phobia. *Journal of Personality Disorders*, **15**, 60–71.

Eisen, J. L., Coles, M. E., Shea, M. T., *et al.* (2006). Clarifying the convergence between obsessive compulsive personality disorder criteria and obsessive compulsive disorder. *Journal of Personality Disorders*, **20**, 294–305.

Engel, G. L. (1977). The need for a new medical model: a challenge for biomedicine. *Science*, **196**, 129–136.

Faustman, W., & White, P. (1989). Diagnostic and psychopharmacological treatment characteristics of 536 inpatients with posttraumatic stress disorder. *Journal of Nervous & Mental Disease*, **177**, 154–159.

Feske, U., Perry, K. J., Chambless, D. L., Renneberg, B., & Goldstein, A. (1996). Avoidant personality disorder as a predictor for treatment outcome among generalized social phobics. *Journal of Personality Disorders*, **10**, 174–184.

Frances, A. (1980). The DSM-III personality disorders section: a commentary. *American Journal of Psychiatry*, **137**, 1050–1054.

Frances, A., & Cooper, A. M. (1981). Descriptive and dynamic psychiatry: a perspective on DSM-III. *American Journal of Psychiatry*, **138**, 1198–1202.

Golier, J. A., Yehuda, R., Bierer, L. M., *et al.* (2003). The relationship of borderline personality disorder to posttraumatic stress disorder and traumatic events. *American Journal of Psychiatry*, **160**, 2018–2024.

Grant, B. F., Hasin, D. S., Stinson, F. S., *et al.* (2005). Co-occurrence of 12-month mood and anxiety disorders and personality disorders in the US: results from the National Epidemiologic Survey on Alcohol and Related Conditions. *Journal of Psychiatric Research*, **39**, 1–9.

Grilo, C. M., Sanislow, C. A., Gunderson, J.G., *et al.* (2004). Two-year stability and change in schizotypal, borderline, avoidant and obsessive–compulsive personality disorders. *Journal of Consulting and Clinical Psychology*, **72**, 767–775.

Gunderson, J., & Sabo, A. (1993). The phenomenological and conceptual interface between borderline personality disorder and PTSD. *American Journal of Psychiatry*, **150**, 19–27.

Hansen, B., Vogel, P. A., Stiles, T. C., & Gotestam, K. G. (2007). Influence of co-morbid generalized anxiety disorder, panic disorder and personality disorders on the outcome of cognitive behavioural treatment of obsessive–compulsive disorder. *Cognitive Behaviour Therapy*. **36**, 145–155.

Herman, J. L., Perry, J. C., & van der Kolk, B. A. (1989). Childhood trauma in borderline personality disorder. *American Journal of Psychiatry*, **146**, 490–495.

Hummelen, B., Wilberg, T., Pedersen, G., & Karterud, S. (2007). The relationship between avoidant personality disorder and social phobia. *Comprehensive Psychiatry*, **48**, 348–356.

Johnson, J. G., Cohen, P., Kasen, S., & Brook, J. S. (2006). Personality disorders evident by early adulthood and risk for anxiety disorders during middle adulthood. *Anxiety Disorders*, **20**, 408–426.

Lenzenweger, M. F., Lane, M., & Loranger, A. W. (2007). DSM-IV personality disorders in the National Comorbidity Survey Replication (NCS-R). *Biological Psychiatry*, **62**, 553–564.

Maina, G., Albert, U., Salvi, V., Pessina, E., & Bogetto, F. (2008). Early-onset obsessive–compulsive disorder and personality disorders in adulthood. *Psychiatry Research*, **158**, 217–225.

Matsunaga, H., Kiriike, N., Miyata, A., *et al.* (1998). Personality disorders in patients with obsessive–compulsive disorder in Japan. *Acta Psychiatria Scandinavia*, **98**, 128–134.

Milrod, B., Leon, A. C., Barber, J. P., Markowitz, J. C., & Graf, E. (2007). Do comorbid personality disorders moderate psychotherapy response in panic disorder? A preliminary empirical evaluation of the APA Practice Guideline. *Journal of Clinical Psychiatry*, **68**, 885–891.

Ozkan, M., & Altindag, A. (2005). Comorbid personality disorders in subjects with panic disorder: do personality disorders increase clinical severity? *Comprehensive Psychiatry*, **46**, 20–26.

Reich, J. (2003). The effect of Axis II disorders on the outcome of treatment of anxiety and unipolar depressive disorders: a review. *Journal of Personality Disorders*, **17**, 387–405.

Reich, J., & Braginsky, Y. (1994). Paranoid personality traits in a panic disorder population: a pilot study. *Comprehensive Psychiatry*, **35**, 260–264.

Reichborn-Kjennerud, T., Czajkowski, N., Torgersen, S., *et al.* (2007). The relationship between avoidant personality disorder and social phobia: a population-based twin study. *American Journal of Psychiatry*, **164**, 1722–1728.

Samuels, J., Nestadt, G., Bienvenu, O. J., *et al.* (2000). Personality disorders and normal personality dimensions in obsessive–compulsive disorder. *British Journal of Psychiatry*, **177**, 457–462.

Sanderson, W. C, Wetzler, S., Beck, A. T., & Betz, F. (1993). Prevalence of personality disorders among patients with anxiety disorders. *Psychiatry Research*, **51**, 167–174.

Schneier, F. R., Spitzer, R. L., Gibbon, M., Fyer, A. J., & Liebowitz, M. R. (1991). The relationship of social phobia subtypes and avoidant personality disorder. *Comprehensive Psychiatry*, **32**, 496–502.

Shea, M. T., & Yen, S. (2003). Stability as a distinction between Axis I and Axis II disorders. *Journal of Personality Disorders*, **17**, 373–386.

Shea M. T., Stout R., Gunderson J. G., *et al.* (2002). Short-term diagnostic stability of schizotypal, borderline, avoidant, and obsessive–compulsive personality disorders. *American Journal of Psychiatry*, **159**, 2036–2041.

Skodol, A., Oldham, J. M., Hyler, S. E., *et al.* (1995). Patterns of anxiety and personality disorder comorbidity. *Journal of Psychiatric Research*, **29**, 361–374.

Southwick, S., Yehuda, R., & Giller, E. (1993). Personality disorders in treatment-seeking combat veterans with posttraumatic stress disorder. *American Journal of Psychiatry*, **150**, 1020–1023.

Spitzer, R. L. (2001). Values and assumptions in the development of DSM-III and DSM-III-R: an insider's perspective and a belated response to Sadler, Hulgus, and Agich's "On values in recent American psychiatric classification". *Journal of Nervous and Mental Disease*, **189**, 351–358.

Torres, A. R., Prince, M. J., Bebbington, P. E., *et al.* (2006). Obsessive–compulsive disorder: prevalence, comorbidity, impact and help-seeking in the British National Psychiatric Morbidity Survey of 2000. *American Journal of Psychiatry*, **163**, 1978–1985.

Weertman, A., Arntz, A., Schouten, E., & Dreessen, L. (2005). Influences of beliefs and personality disorders on treatment outcome in anxiety patients. *Journal of Consulting and Clinical Psychology*, **73**, 936–944.

Yen, S. R. S., Shea, T. M., Battlle, L. C., *et al.* (2002). Traumatic exposure and posttraumatic stress disorder in borderline, schizotypal, avoidant and obsessive–compulsive personality disorders: findings from the Collaborative Longitudinal Personality Disorders Study. *Journal of Nervous and Mental Diseases*, **190**, 510–518.

Zanarini, M. C., Frankenburg, F. R., Hennen, J., Reich, D. B., & Silk, K. R. (2006). Prediction of the 10-year course of borderline personality disorder. *American Journal of Psychiatry*, **163**, 827–832.

Chapter 12

"Idioms of distress" (culturally salient indicators of distress) and anxiety disorders

Devon E. Hinton, Roberto Lewis-Fernández

12.1 Introduction

"Idioms of distress" (Nichter 1981) may be defined as the ways in which members of sociocultural groups convey affliction. These idioms vary across cultures, depending on the salient metaphors and popular traditions that pattern the human biological capacity for experiencing distress, including conditions that are sufficiently severe to meet criteria for psychiatric disorder. Cultural groups, for example, may describe distress in more psychological or more somatic terms, or may cluster syndromes in different ways, connecting symptoms together that other cultures do not acknowledge as related (Good 1977). This leads to substantial diversity in culturally defined syndromes across groups.

Our common human biology, however, constrains the range of idioms of distress to a finite number of expressions. Idioms of distress focused on feared heart pathology, for example, are ubiquitous yet can differ substantially, as evidenced by the differences between the fear of "heart attacks" among Manhattan executives versus concerns over "heart distress" in Iran. The former associates stress and overwork in hypercompetitive, frequently male, professional environments with chest tightness and fear of sudden death, while the latter is predominantly an idiom used by working-class women to describe "irregular heart sensations believed to be caused by emotional or interpersonal problems, by childbirth, pregnancy or contraception, or by a variety of diseases" (Good 1977, pp. 33–34). For the clinician intent on alleviating distress, the issue is recognizing how the idiom of distress patterns the expression of the illness and how it affects the sufferer's understandings of the problem and of its treatment.

In this chapter, we describe the clinical relevance of idioms of distress for the generation and treatment of anxiety disorders, focusing mainly on those related to panic disorder and posttraumatic stress disorder (PTSD) in Southeast Asian and Latino populations, on whom our research has been based. Our review illustrates that idioms of distress are key aspects of patients' experience of anxiety disorders, and important "cogs" in the generation of anxiety in specific cultural contexts. We highlight the importance to clinical care of evaluating and addressing idioms of distress in patients with anxiety disorders.

12.2 Types of idioms of distress

Several types of idioms of distress have been proposed (Figure 12.1; Nichter 1981). Some prototypical idioms include cultural illness syndromes (e.g., an *ataque de nervios*, literally, an "attack of nerves"), a psychological or somatic complaint (e.g., of being "sad," of bodily pain), religious involvement (e.g., joining a possession cult), accusation of witchcraft assault (i.e., the assertion of having been attacked by sorcery or other supernatural mechanism), or acting-out behaviors (e.g., drinking). In each of these idioms, various elements, including folk etiologies, vulnerabilities, ethnopathological mechanisms, symptoms, and expected remedies, "run together" to form a relatively coherent whole (Good 1977, 1994).

In this chapter we review idioms of distress that are cultural illness syndromes. In Table 12.1 we describe some key ways of analyzing idioms of distress, while providing examples of cultural illness syndromes common in Latino and Southeast Asian populations. Though we focus on these cultural groups because they have been extensively studied, other idioms of distress have also been well described in relationship to anxiety disorders, such as *taijin kyofusho*, a cultural syndrome common in Japan and Korea that has considerable overlap with social anxiety disorder and body dysmorphic disorder (Kleinknecht *et al.* 1997, Kinoshita *et al.* 2008).

Anxiety Disorders: Theory, Research, and Clinical Perspectives, ed. Helen Blair Simpson, Yuval Neria, Roberto Lewis-Fernández, Franklin Schneier. Published by Cambridge University Press. © Cambridge University Press 2010.

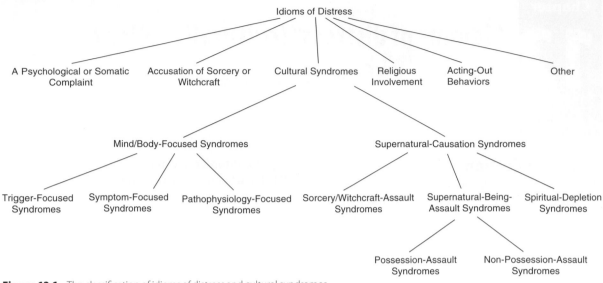

Figure 12.1. The classification of idioms of distress and cultural syndromes.

12.2.1 Examples of idioms of distress: Caribbean Latino and Cambodian cases

As illustrated in Table 12.1, when viewed phenomenologically, one important typology of idioms of distress is based on their time course. Some idioms correspond to a continuous process (often a trait-like condition); others are episodic, that is, they suddenly occur, and then end minutes or hours later. When the idiom of distress is a continuous condition, it is often thought to predispose to yet other idioms of distress.

As an example of a continuous-type idiom of distress, Latino patients may respond to life difficulties by starting to *padecer de los nervios* (literally, "to suffer from nerves"). This is also referred to as *los nervios alterados* (literally, "altered nerves"), a condition typically characterized in psychiatric terms by chronic symptoms of anxiety, depression, somatization, and/or dissociation. This condition is thought to result from the interaction of adversity and inherent vulnerability, an indigenous stress-diathesis model. A person with *nervios* is thought to be predisposed to recurrent emotional upset and anxiety and to developing other idioms of distress. If untreated and exacerbated – for example, by experiencing further adversity – chronic *nervios* is feared to lead to *locura* ("madness"), understood as a violent and potentially incurable form of insanity characterized by delirium, indiscriminate violence, and self-harm. Chronic *nervios* may also result in an episodic condition called *ataque de nervios*. *Ataques de nervios* are acute crises that may involve screaming; crying; throwing things; severe somatic symptoms, such as trembling, palpitations, and shortness of breath; and dissociative states, such as depersonalization – a syndrome most often found among Spanish speakers of the Caribbean (Guarnaccia *et al.* 2003).

To give another cultural example of a continuous idiom of distress, a Cambodian refugee patient with certain symptoms – especially frequent palpitations, startle, and poor appetite and sleep – may consider him- or herself to be "weak" (*khsaoy*) or, worse yet, to have a "weak heart" (*khsaoy beh doung*). Weakness, a chronic condition, is thought to predispose to episodic palpitations upon hearing loud noises, and possibly cardiac arrest, as well as to having "*khyâl* attacks" (Hinton *et al.* 2002). *Khyâl* attacks are episodes that last from minutes to hours and are characterized by panic-like symptoms such as dizziness, palpitations, shortness of breath, neck soreness, cold extremities, blurry vision, and tinnitus. *Khyâl* is a wind-like substance that is thought to flow alongside blood in the vessels of the body, and *khyâl* attacks are interpreted as the result of a dangerous dysregulation of the flow of *khyâl* and blood. *Khyâl* attacks are treated by various traditional methods, such as "coining," in which a coin's edge is dragged along skin that has been rubbed with a medicinal fluid, thereby restoring the normal flow of *khyâl* and blood, and releasing *khyâl* directly from the skin pores of the body.

Table 12.1. Idioms of distress: key dimensions

Syndrome name	Where found	Typical length	Typical causes of the syndrome	Cultural ideas about vulnerability	Typical symptoms	Associated psycho- and ethnophysiology	Feared consequences	Typical self-treatments
Ataque de nervios	Most common in Spanish-speaking populations of the Caribbean	From a few minutes to an hour	Hearing upsetting news; anger; interpersonal conflict; worry episodes; suffering from "*nervios*"	*Nervios*	Anger, trembling, palpitations, shortness of breath, depersonalization, acting out (throwing things, yelling), suicidal ideation or attempt	Ideas about the nervous system; need to remain "in control" despite adversity	Loss of control, leading to injury of self or others, permanent damage to the nervous system, suicide	Applying *alcoholado* (a cooling liquid) to the body; *desahogarse*, i.e., expressing one's feelings; treatments with a curer, like a "cleaning" (*limpieza*)
Padecer de los nervios	Spanish-speaking populations	Chronic condition	Chronic worry; adverse life events: trauma; poverty, family conflict, inborn predisposition	See causes	Anxiety, depressive, and somatization symptoms, in particular, trembling, headache, bodily aches, palpitations, chest tightness, GI upset	The conception of the nervous system as prone to alteration as a result of adversity	Memory loss, medical illnesses, insanity, predisposition to startle, and in the case of Caribbean patients, to *ataque de nervios*	*Alcoholado*; *desahogarse*; going to a doctor to rule out a physical ailment; using natural remedies; traditional treatments such as a "cleaning" (*limpieza*); praying; involvement in religion
Susto	Spanish-speaking populations of indigenous background	Acute condition and chronic condition	An initial fright that then results in a vulnerable state	Weakness, *nervios*	Anxiety, depression, somatic symptoms including headache, fever, bodily aches, vomiting, diarrhea	Ideas about the dislodgeable soul	Physical illness (e.g., diabetes), death, or other dire event as a result of fright	Praying; calling the soul back to the body; various traditional healing rituals
Khyâl attack	Cambodian refugees (similar syndromes based on fear of the consequences of a dysregulation of the flow of an inner wind-like substance are found in many Asian populations)	From a few minutes to hours	"Weakness," and any cause of anxiety: startle, awakening from a nightmare, a worry episode, standing up	Weakness	Anxiety symptoms, in particular, dizziness, palpitations, shortness of breath, cold extremities, blurry vision, tinnitus	The ethnophysiology of *khyâl* and blood	That *khyâl* and blood will surge upward in the body to cause various disasters: "death of the limbs"; heart arrest; asphyxia; neck-vessel rupture; blindness; deafness; syncope	"Coining," "cupping," and other methods to remove *khyâl* from the body and restore proper flow of *khyâl* and blood

Table 12.1 (cont.)

Syndrome name	Where found	Typical length	Typical causes of the syndrome	Cultural ideas about vulnerability	Typical symptoms	Associated psycho- and ethnophysiology	Feared consequences	Typical self-treatments
"Khyâl overload" (a *khyâl* attack triggered by standing that is so severe it causes collapse to the ground)	Found among Cambodian refugees	Acute episode	Triggered by standing	Weakness	All the symptoms listed under *khyâl* attack, in particular dizziness	The ethnophysiology of *khyâl* and blood	Syncope and death, and all the feared consequences listed under *khyâl* attack	All the methods listed under *khyâl* attack, and in addition, special techniques like pulling the arms and biting the ankles
"Weakness" (*khsaoy*)	Found among Cambodian patients ("weakness syndromes" are common among several other Asian populations)	Acute episode (when there is a drop in energy) and a chronic condition (a state of depletion)	Worry, poor appetite, poor sleep, frequent startle or anxiety, overwork	See causes	Anxiety symptoms, predisposition to worry, to having *khyâl* attacks, to having "weak heart"	Ideas about bodily and mental energy	Death from depletion, predisposition to dangerous conditions like weak heart	Traditional medicines to strengthen the body; religious practices to decrease worry; seeking medical help to restore appetite and sleep
"Hit by the wind" (*trúng gió*)	Vietnamese refugees	Acute episodes	Being hit by a wind at a time the weather is changing, being hit by a so-called poisonous wind (*gió*), e.g., a cool breeze on a warm day	Weakness, leading to pore dilatation, among other vulnerabilities (that weakness being caused by chronic worry, among other causes)	Pain in the area thought to be "hit by the wind," chills, dizziness, palpitations, blurry vision, tinnitus	The pathophysiology of *gió* infiltration into the body	Loss of limb use in the area hit by *gió*, heart arrest, syncope	Various methods like coining or a steam bath to remove *gió* from the body and return normal flow of blood

"Thinking too much" (*suy ngii nhieu*)	Vietnamese refugees (a similar syndrome occurs among Cambodians, called "*kut caraeun*")	An acute condition (the worry episode) that occurs chronically	Chronic worry, weakness	See causes	The rapid induction of somatic and psychological symptoms by worry	That worry depletes the bodily energy and dysregulates the flow of blood and other substances in the body; that worry will tense nerve fibers within the brain	A dangerous depletion of the body, causing heart arrest or other dire events, including dysregulation of the flow of blood and other substances; the ripping of nerve fibers in the brain, causing a permanent loss of mental powers, such as memory, and possibly insanity	Taking tonics, and performing coining and other methods, including steaming, to restore the normal flow of blood and other substances
"Weak heart" (*yeu tim*)	Vietnamese refugees (a similar syndrome occurs among Cambodian refugees, called *khsaoy beh doung*)	A chronic condition	Chronic worry, weakness	See causes	The rapid induction of somatic and/or psychological symptoms by any event, from a worry episode to a loud noise to standing; a predisposition to worry	That the person is in a dangerous state of depletion, that the heart may be disturbed by any of multiple causes, that the heart will not adequately pump blood	Heart arrest, fainting upon standing, poor circulation of blood	Taking tonics that improve the ability to eat and sleep; eating and sleeping increase bodily energy

12.3 Clinical relevance of idioms of distress

Idioms of distress matter for the provision of effective care. If a clinician does not recognize complaints as culture-specific idioms, he or she may miss information critical to both diagnosis and treatment. Below we outline several types of clinical relevance that idioms of distress may have.

12.3.1 Indicators of psychopathology

Idioms of distress may be markers or expressions of psychopathology that may be easily elicited in cross-cultural assessments, including psychopathology dimensions (e.g., anxiety, depression, or dissociation tendency) or specific disorders (e.g., PTSD and generalized anxiety disorder). These relationships can be investigated in studies that first separately assess idiom expression and the psychopathological constructs and then explore their relationship through analyses of association, such as odds ratios and correlation coefficients. Various idioms of distress have been found to have consistently strong correlations with a variety of psychiatric disorders, not a one-to-one relationship with a single DSM disorder. For example, *ataque de nervios* is associated not just with panic disorder but also with depression and other DSM disorders. This suggests that a "comorbidity approach" is a more fruitful way to study the relationship between idioms and diagnoses than to prematurely conflate the two (Lewis-Fernández *et al.* 2009a).

Several examples may help illustrate the association between idioms of distress and psychiatric disorders. One study showed that having *khyâl* attacks in the last month is highly associated with PTSD presence (OR = 6.4) and that the severity of *khyâl* attacks in the last month is correlated with PTSD severity ($r = 0.72$), explaining 52% of the variance in a Cambodian refugee sample (Hinton 2008). In addition, several somatic complaint-focused syndromes such as neck-focused panic attacks, orthostatic panic attacks (i.e., panic attacks experienced upon standing up), and gastrointestinal-focused panic attacks – which center on catastrophic cognitions about *khyâl* flow and also involve metaphoric associations and trauma associations to somatic sensations – are highly associated with PTSD presence and severity (Hinton *et al.* 2001a, 2001b, 2006a, 2007, 2008a).

Similar relationships have been found among Puerto Ricans and US Latinos between *ataque de nervios* and certain psychiatric disorders. *Ataque* has been shown in population-based studies in both adults and children to be associated consistently with anxiety and depressive disorders (Guarnaccia *et al.* 1993, 2005, 2010); in Puerto Rican children, *ataques* are also associated with disruptive disorders. In a household sample of US Latinos from various national origins, multivariate regression showed that after depressive disorders (OR = 5.7), *ataque* is the next best correlate of anxiety disorders (OR = 5.3), much higher than substance abuse (OR = 2.7) or any sociodemographic predictor (OR = 1.3–2.0). In adult psychiatric populations of Puerto Ricans and Dominicans in the USA, *ataque* is specifically linked with panic disorder, PTSD, and the dissociative disorders (the latter not investigated in community studies) (Lewis-Fernández *et al.* 2002a, 2002b).

12.3.2 Indicators of risk for destructive behaviors

Idioms of distress are in some cases highly associated with destructive behaviors such as violent anger episodes and suicidality risk. For example, episodes of *ataque* may involve the expression of intense anger and aggression, such as attacking people indiscriminately or breaking things. Moreover, there is a strong relationship between *ataque de nervios* and suicidal ideation (OR = 6.2) and attempt (OR = 8.1) (Guarnaccia *et al.* 1993). Multivariate regression with a household sample of US Latinos has confirmed this specific association. After adjusting for sociodemographic characteristics, lifetime *ataque de nervios* and traumatic exposure are each independently associated with suicidality, whereas a lifetime diagnosis of anxiety, depressive, or substance use disorder is not (Lewis-Fernández *et al.* 2009b).

12.3.3 Indicators of life distress

An idiom of distress may be a strong indicator of the general level of life distress experienced by an individual. The type of life distress that is indicated by the idiom can vary, including interpersonal distress, health-related concerns about the person's health or that of a loved one, concerns about personal safety (e.g., fear of physical or sexual assault in the living environment), and financial distress.

Let us take the example of interpersonal distress. Having a cultural syndrome may indicate that a person has interpersonal problems, such as spousal abuse, acting-out children, or conflicts with siblings.

In many cultures, interpersonal conflict is considered to be a well-defined cause of certain cultural syndromes. Among Latino patients, an episode of *ataque de nervios* often indicates a dispute involving the family (Guarnaccia *et al.* 1993), and so too, among Cambodian speakers, a *khyâl* attack. In a Puerto Rican community sample, 92% of first *ataque* experiences were directly provoked by a distressing situation; 81% occurred in the presence of others; and 67% led to the person receiving help. Contrary to usual panic disorder, most respondents report feeling better (71%) or feeling relieved (81%) after their first *ataque*. These findings suggest that first episodes of *ataque de nervios* are closely tied to the interpersonal world of the sufferer and that they result in an unburdening (*desahogarse*) of one's life problems, at least temporarily (Lewis-Fernández *et al.* 2005).

In many cultural syndromes across various groups, worry is considered a key etiologic factor, and worry episodes are often considered the cause of a continuous-type idiom of distress, predisposing to an episodic syndrome. Worry may also trigger events of the episodic syndrome directly. Escalating worries about finances or vulnerable offspring (e.g., a son in jail) may cause a predisposed Dominican patient to have an *ataque de nervios* or a Cambodian patient to have a *khyâl* attack. Through these mechanisms, worry about life distress issues is linked to cultural syndromes. The relationship between worry and idioms of distress is explored in more detail later in the chapter (section 12.3.5).

12.3.4 Indicators of psychosocial functioning

Certain idioms of distress may indicate impairment in psychosocial functioning, including work and social functioning, as well as general well-being, as assessed by quality-of-life and disability measures (for one review, see Hinton *et al.* 2007b). For instance, the complaint of "weakness" may be particularly associated with poor psychosocial functioning in Asian populations (Hinton *et al.* 2007). Likewise, US Latinos with *ataque de nervios* have over twice the odds of being disabled due to a mental health problem than Latinos without *ataque*, after adjusting for sociodemographic and clinical characteristics, including the presence of depressive, anxiety, and substance use disorders (Lewis-Fernández *et al.* 2009b). In traumatized groups, certain idioms of distress may significantly explain variance in social functioning beyond that explained by PTSD severity. For instance, *ataque* status remains independently associated with mental-health-related

disability after adjusting for traumatic exposure and the presence of anxiety disorders, including PTSD (Lewis-Fernández *et al.* 2009b).

12.3.5 Causes of distress

In addition to their function as expressions of distress, idioms of distress may paradoxically help to perpetuate the very distress they are attempting to dissipate. *Ataque de nervios*, for example, is associated with elevated rates of anxiety sensitivity (Hinton *et al.* 2008b), that is, fear of anxiety symptoms. One possible explanation is that the *ataque* is related to a person's difficulty tolerating anxiety and other strong emotions (e.g., anger). In this view, the anxiety sensitivity is primary and derives from a relative intolerance of arousal because of the fear that arousal itself will lead to dangerous consequences (e.g., loss of control, violence). The *ataque* would then arise as a secondary reaction to the fear of arousal, as a sign that the person is overwhelmed by this fear and unable to cope in other ways. Alternatively – and this is the mechanism that concerns us now – it has been hypothesized that the idiom of distress itself may help elevate anxiety sensitivity. According to this alternative, arousal symptoms (e.g., racing thoughts, shortness of breath, shakiness of the limbs) are frightening precisely because of the concern that they will precipitate an *ataque*, which may then lead to a series of bodily catastrophes – such as losing control, going insane, being unable to breathe, or having a seizure. Here the idiom acts as a primary *precipitant* of distress (Hinton *et al.* 2009). In other words, cultural constructs such as *ataque* may elevate anxiety sensitivity by providing a widely accepted ethnopathological mechanism linking the feeling of anxiety to specific bodily catastrophes (Hinton *et al.* 2008b).

A similar argument has been made regarding Cambodian cultural syndromes (Hinton *et al.* 2006b). Cambodians attribute many anxiety symptoms to a disturbance in the physiological flows of *khyâl* and blood. For example, cold extremities may be attributed to a lack of flow of *khyâl* and blood along the limbs, leading to fear that (a) the lack of flow along the limbs may cause the loss of the use of the arms and legs, that is, a stroke, and (b) the *khyâl* and blood – unable to make their normal descent – may surge upward in the body, and so cause various bodily disasters, such as pressing on the the heart and lungs, bringing about heart arrest and asphyxia, and rising into the neck, bursting the neck vessels, and entering the head, bringing about syncope. These ethnophysiological notions involving

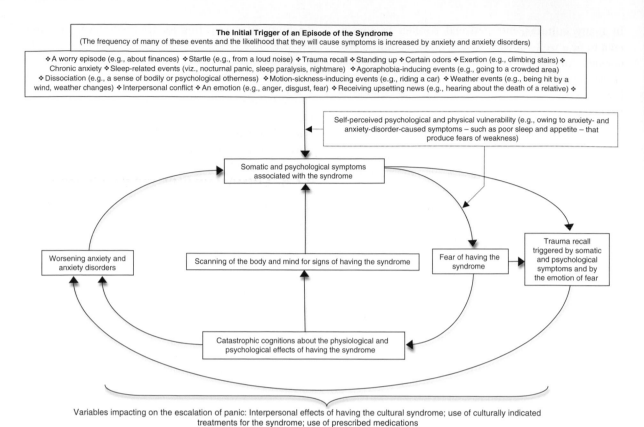

Figure 12.2. The idiom-of-distress–anxiety-disorders model: the generation of an idiom of distress and relationship to anxiety and anxiety-disorder severity.

khyâl may help elevate anxiety sensitivity by facilitating cognitive links ("cogs") between anxiety symptoms and catastrophic cognitions.

Worry may play a special role in this process. In certain cultures, worry is assigned great etiological significance; when prolonged, for example, it is thought to cause substantial harm (e.g., insanity). If an idiom of distress is culturally associated with worry, either as an expression of this emotion or as its product, the presence of the idiom may predispose to higher rates or greater severity of worry-related pathology such as generalized anxiety disorder (GAD). This is in line with research showing that fear about the negative consequences of worry increases GAD severity (Wells 2000). Research on *ataque* provides some evidence of this connection, since one possible cause of this idiom is catastrophic cognitions about recurrent worry. Interestingly, the presence of *ataque* is strongly correlated with GAD (OR = 3.9) in epidemiological studies with US Latinos (Guarnaccia *et al.* 2010). Likewise, it is possible that the predisposition to catastrophic cognitions would cause worry episodes in a culture to escalate to the level of

panic, worsening panic disorder and potentially PTSD. Figure 12.2 provides a model, based on Clark's (1986) model of the panic spiral, of how idioms of distress may perpetuate anxiety disorders.

12.3.6 Indicators of past exposure to trauma

Whether an idiom of distress can be a fairly specific indicator of traumatic exposure has not been sufficiently studied. For instance, a cultural syndrome may be present when a person has suffered great trauma and disability, even when full PTSD criteria are not met. To investigate this question, one would need to examine systematically the correlations between traumatic events and the severity of the idiom of distress in question. Research on *khyâl* attacks has started to address this issue. Linear regression analysis shows that severity of neck-related *khyâl* attacks is associated with PTSD symptom severity in Cambodian panic disorder patients, after adjusting for age and gender. This relationship is mediated by neck-related catastrophic cognitions (i.e., fears that neck symptoms will lead to terrible outcomes) as well as by neck-related flash-backs, usually involving neck sensations associated with traumatic events during the Cambodian genocide (Hinton *et al.* 2006a). Future studies should examine the relationship between traumatic exposure and *khyâl* attacks, even in the absence of PTSD.

To date, research on *ataque de nervios* in this regard has shown conflicting results. One study showed that adults with *ataque* were significantly more likely to have suffered childhood trauma than those without the syndrome (Schechter *et al.* 2000). A second study, however, showed that childhood traumatic exposure was high across Puerto Rican psychiatric outpatients regardless of *ataque* status, suggesting that, in a clinical sample, other factors in addition to childhood trauma may account for the syndrome (Lewis-Fernández *et al.* 2002a).

12.3.7 Targets for therapeutic intervention

In a cultural group, certain idioms of distress may play a key role in perpetuating distress in a way that is immediately comprehensible to a member of the group and can therefore be profitably targeted in treatment. The targeted idiom of distress may vary depending on the treatment aim. For example, if the aim is to treat symptoms of GAD, panic, or PTSD, the treatment should target those co-occurring cultural syndromes that generate fear about these types of symptoms and, in particular, should address syndrome-associated catastrophic cognitions. Illustrating this approach, in a culturally adapted CBT treatment of Cambodian refugees that targets both PTSD and orthostatic panic (associated with *khyâl* overload), improvement in PTSD is significantly mediated by improvement in orthostatic panic severity (Hinton *et al.* 2008a). In syndromes in which worry plays a key role, treatment should specifically focus on the worry topics that are signaled by the cultural syndromes, since these represent "experience-near" entry points for the intervention with clear face validity for the patient. In *ataque de nervios*, the immediate precipitant – for example, spousal disagreement or conflicts with the person's children triggered by acculturation differences – should be the first focus of psychotherapy. Evidence-based psychotherapies, such as CBT and interpersonal psychotherapy, are being adapted for diverse cultural groups and psychiatric disorders – including by incorporating information on relevant cultural syndromes – and will increasingly become available for the treatment of anxiety disorders (Hinton *et al.* 2008a, Markowitz *et al.* 2009).

12.3.8 Facilitators of empathy

In many groups, the distressed patient may consider an idiom of distress specific to that culture to be his or her most salient problem. If the clinician does not ask about this complaint and does not specifically address the syndrome-related concerns, the patient will likely not feel understood, thereby limiting therapeutic rapport and efficacy.

12.4 Clinical evaluation of a patient with an idiom of distress

The first step in including idioms of distress in treatment is to evaluate their role in the patient's clinical picture during the psychiatric evaluation. A guideline for how to conduct such an evaluation is included in Appendix I of DSM-IV-TR, the "Outline for cultural formulation" (American Psychiatric Association 2000). (For a description of how to implement the cultural formulation, see Lewis-Fernández & Díaz 2002.) As indicated in Figure 12.2, this evaluation should include several elements. The clinician should examine the interpersonal effects of having the cultural syndrome, that is, how having the syndrome impacts the patient's interpersonal dynamics. Culturally indicated treatments of the syndrome should also be explored, since these may have important effects on the trajectory of the illness. This includes treatments the patient uses during acute episodes of the illness, as well as between episodes. In addition, the clinician should examine whether the syndrome has been treated within Western medical settings, what diagnosis and treatment were offered, and the reaction of the patient and his/her social network to them. Finally, it is important to allow time for the patient to "tell the story" of the syndrome, to explain the link of associations that led to symptom expression, and to relate the heightened fears that provoked the current crisis. In Caribbean Latino ethnopsychology, this is known as allowing the person to "*desahogarse*" (unburden him/herself), and it is considered an essential aspect of any therapy.

A key task of the clinician in carrying out treatment is to try to decrease the patient's sense of vulnerability. As a result, the various events that are thought to potentially trigger episodes of the syndrome will be less feared, which will decrease the likelihood that an episode will occur. Moreover, even if the syndrome-related symptoms are experienced, the patient will be less likely to consider these as indicators of the onset of the syndrome.

The sense of vulnerability can be decreased in many ways. Medications that improve sleep, appetite, and energy cause the patient to feel less weak and vulnerable. Prescribed medications should preferably be framed as being directed at the cultural syndrome, in addition to more experience-distant conditions such as an anxiety disorder. The clinician can also give alternative medical explanations for the cause of the symptoms ascribed to the cultural syndrome and reassure the patient that they are harmless. For example, the clinician may explain that, in the context of anxiety, cold extremities usually result from harmless vasoconstriction, or that palpitations are caused by fear and that they are not dangerous, no more dangerous than those experienced upon exercising.

The key is to convince the patient that his or her symptoms are not catastrophic, rather that they are signs of a condition that is indeed in need of treatment but that will not result in imminent disaster. It is particularly important to address the syndrome-associated cognitions. These can be quite difficult to change, having resulted from a lifetime of experience and interpretation. The key is to introduce a measure of doubt about the certainty of the catastrophic outcome and then to build on it based on therapeutic success. This entails explaining, for instance, to a Latino patient with *padecer de los nervios*, that excessive worry will not *necessarily* cause permanent loss of memory or that decreased concentration is not *always* a sign of incipient insanity; to a Cambodian or Vietnamese patient with "weakness," that worry will not weaken the body to the point that cardiac arrest and death will result; and to a Cambodian patient, that cold hands and feet will not invariably lead to stroke and will not cause *khyâl* and blood to surge upward in the body with precipitous results.

In this way, the clinician acknowledges the cultural associations but introduces hope for improvement in the current situation. Interoceptive exposure and reassociation to the syndrome-related sensations (e.g., pairing dizziness to pleasurable experiences like rolling down a hill as a youth) may be helpful in this process, in order to reduce fear of the sensations. The patient should be taught methods, such as applied muscle relaxation, to decrease fear of somatic symptoms and to stop the escalating spiral of panic. Medication, such as a benzodiazepine, that can be taken upon the onset of symptoms of the episode is often extremely helpful. The clinician must reassure the patient that the syndrome in question is not serious, but that the medication can be taken at its onset to decrease the secondary fears that are provoked by the syndrome and so prevent it or decrease its severity. Whether trauma recall occurs during events of the syndrome should be determined; if so, one should determine what triggers recall of the trauma event – often somatic sensations do; for example, shortness of breath may recall a drowning experience – and have the patient describe the trauma event.

Awareness of the relationship between cultural syndromes and anxiety disorders can enhance clinicians' ability to engage patients about a variety of therapeutic approaches and to tailor evidence-based treatments to patients' cultural understandings and experiences. Future research should focus on whether these cultural adaptations lead to improved effectiveness in clinical care.

12.5 Conclusions

In this chapter we have illustrated the key role that idioms of distress may play in the presentation and generation of anxiety symptoms and disorders. Idioms of distress, which vary across cultures, are not esoteric events; rather, they are a core aspect of the experiencing of anxiety states and disorders. They may produce catastrophic cognitions about anxiety symptoms, lead the person to seek certain types of treatments and not others, and pattern the reactions of the patient's social network. Idioms of distress not only shape anxiety presentations, they also often constitute the very cogs of the disorder, shaping profoundly the experience of anxiety. To adequately evaluate and treat anxiety symptoms and disorders among persons from diverse cultural groups, clinicians must investigate (a) whether these clinical conditions are attributed to specific idioms of distress, (b) the cultural understandings of the physiology and psychology associated with having that idiom, (c) whether the idiom is stigmatized, (d) how the idiom is supposed to be treated in that context, and (e) the social and other current life problems that the idiom of distress is typically thought to indicate.

We have presented a model of how anxiety disorders and idioms of distress mutually reinforce each other, forming interacting escalating loops that link expectation, attention, catastrophic cognitions, and activation of the autonomic nervous system. Through such loops, cultural syndromes become a key aspect of the experience, meaning, and generation of anxiety (Kirmayer & Sartorius 2007). We have also suggested ways in which these cultural syndromes may be investigated, including a series of testable hypotheses about their clinical utility. We have delineated what "distress" these cultural syndromes may indicate, including interpersonal conflict, economic distress, specific forms of psychopathology, poor psychosocial functioning, and traumatization. Empirical research should continue to determine what kinds of distress an "idiom of distress" tends to indicate in a particular cultural context.

More generally, this chapter has described the complexity of idioms of distress. The data presented indicate the need to expand the DSM-IV-TR glossary of cultural-bound syndromes in order to delineate the aspects of cultural syndromes illustrated in this chapter – whether it is a chronic or acute condition, the associated catastrophic cognitions, and the typical causes according to that cultural group. An additional option is to add a specifier or other method in DSM-5 that may be used to record a cultural syndrome as linked to the specific DSM disorder associated with it in the case of the particular patient.

These changes in DSM-5 would help clinicians remain alert to the possibility that the anxiety disorder they diagnose may be understood by the affected individual to indicate the presence of a particular idiom of distress. This idiom may well be the cognitive frame, the mindset, through which the anxiety disorders and its symptoms are understood and interpreted, a cognitive frame that profoundly influences a person's experience of an anxiety disorder and its symptoms.

References

American Psychiatric Association (2000). *Diagnostic and Statistical Manual of Mental Disorders*, 4th edn, text revision (DSM-IV-TR). Washington, DC: American Psychiatric Association.

Clark, D. M. (1986). A cognitive approach to panic. *Behaviour Research and Therapy*, **24**, 461–470.

Good, B. J. (1977). The heart of what's the matter: the semantics of illness in Iran. *Culture, Medicine, and Psychiatry*, **1**, 25–58.

Good, B. J. (1994). *Medicine, Rationality, and Experience: an Anthropological Perspective*. Cambridge: Cambridge University Press.

Guarnaccia, P. J., Canino, G., Rubio-Stipec, M., & Bravo, M. (1993). The prevalence of ataques de nervios in the Puerto Rico disaster study. *Journal of Nervous and Mental Disease*, **181**, 157–165.

Guarnaccia, P. J., Lewis-Fernández, R., & Rivera Marano, M. (2003). Toward a Puerto Rican popular nosology: nervios and ataque de nervios. *Culture, Medicine, and Psychiatry*, **27**, 339–366.

Guarnaccia, P. J., Martínez, I., Ramírez, R., & Canino, G. (2005). Are ataques de nervios in Puerto Rican children associated with psychiatric disorder? *Journal of the American Academy of Child and Adolescent Psychiatry*, **44**, 1184–1192.

Guarnaccia, P. J., Lewis-Fernández, R., Martínez Pincay, I., *et al.* (2010). Ataque de nervios as a marker of social and psychiatric vulnerability: results from the NLAAS. *International Journal of Social Psychiatry*, **56**(3), 298–309.

Hinton, D. E. (2008). Key idioms of psychological distress among Cambodian refugees. International Society for Traumatic Stress Studies (ISTSS), 24th Annual Meeting: Terror and its Aftermath. Chicago, IL, November 13–15.

Hinton, D. E., Um, K., & Ba, P. (2001a). Kyol goeu ("wind overload") part I: a cultural syndrome of orthostatic panic among Khmer refugees. *Transcultural Psychiatry*, **38**, 403–432.

Hinton, D. E., Um, K., & Ba, P. (2001b). Kyol goeu ("wind overload") part II: prevalence, characteristics and mechanisms of kyol goeu and near-kyol goeu episodes of Khmer patients attending a psychiatric clinic. *Transcultural Psychiatry*, **38**, 433–460.

Hinton, D. E., Hinton, S., Um, K., Chea, A., & Sak, S. (2002). The Khmer "weak heart" syndrome: Fear of death from palpitations. *Transcultural Psychiatry*, **39**, 323–344.

Hinton, D. E., Chhean, D., Pich, V., *et al.* (2006a). Neck-focused panic attacks among Cambodian refugees: A logistic and linear regression analysis. *Journal of Anxiety Disorders*, **20**, 119–138.

Hinton, D. E., Pich, V., Safren, S. A., *et al.* (2006b). Anxiety sensitivity among Cambodian refugees with panic disorder: a factor analytic investigation. *Journal of Anxiety Disorders*, **20**, 281–295.

Hinton, D. E., Chhean, D., Fama, J. M., Pollack, M. H., & McNally, R. J. (2007a). Gastrointestinal focused panic attacks among Cambodian refugees: associated psychopathology, flashbacks, and catastrophic cognitions. *Journal of Anxiety Disorders*, **21**, 42–58.

Hinton, D. E., Sinclair, J., Chung, R. C., & Pollack, M. H. (2007b). The SF-36 among Cambodian and Vietnamese refugees: an examination of psychometric properties. *Journal of Psychopathology and Behavioral Assessment*, **29**, 38–45.

Hinton, D. E., Hofmann, S. G., Pitman, R. K., Pollack, M. H., & Barlow, D. H. (2008a). The panic attack–PTSD model: applicability to orthostatic panic among Cambodian refugee. *Cognitive Behaviour Therapy*, **27**, 101–116.

Hinton, D. E., Chong, R., Pollack, M. H., Barlow, D. H., & McNally, R. J. (2008b). Ataque de nervios: Relationship to anxiety sensitivity and dissociation predisposition. *Depression and Anxiety*, **25**, 489–495.

Hinton, D. E., Lewis-Fernández, R., Pollack, M. H. (2009). A model of the generation of ataque de nervios: The role of fear of negative affect and fear of arousal symptoms. *CNS Neuroscience & Therapeutics*, **15**, 264–275.

Kinoshita, Y., Chen, J., Rapee, R. M., *et al.* (2008). Cross-cultural study of conviction subtype Taijin Kyofu: proposal and reliability of Nagoya–Osaka diagnostic criteria for social anxiety disorder. *Journal of Nervous & Mental Disease*, **196**, 307–313.

Kirmayer, L. J., & Sartorius, M. (2007). Cultural models and somatic models. *Psychosomatic Medicine*, **69**, 832–840.

Kleinknecht, R. A., Dinnel, D. L., Kleinknecht, E. E., Hiruma, N., & Harada, N. (1997). Cultural factors in social anxiety: A comparison of social phobia symptoms. *Journal of Anxiety Disorders*, **11**, 157–177.

Lewis-Fernández, R., & Díaz, N. (2002). The cultural formulation: a method for assessing cultural factors affecting the clinical encounter. *Psychiatric Quarterly*, **73**, 271–295.

Lewis-Fernández, R., Garrido-Castillo, P., Bennasar, M. C., *et al.* (2002a). Dissociation, childhood trauma, and ataque de nervios among Puerto Rican psychiatric outpatients. *American Journal of Psychiatry*, **159**, 1603–1605.

Lewis-Fernández, R., Guarnaccia, P. J., Martínez, I. E., *et al.* (2002b). Comparative phenomenology of ataques de nervios, panic attacks, and panic disorder. *Culture, Medicine, and Psychiatry*, **26**, 199–223.

Lewis-Fernández, R., Guarnaccia, P. J., Patel, S., Lizardi, D., & Díaz, N. (2005). *Ataque de nervios*: anthropological,

epidemiological, and clinical dimensions of a cultural syndrome. In A. M. Georgiopoulos & J. F. Rosenbaum, eds., *Perspectives in Cross-Cultural Psychiatry*. Philadelphia, PA: Lippincott Williams & Wilkins, pp. 63–85.

Lewis-Fernández, R., Guarnaccia, P.J., & Ruiz, P. (2009a). Culture-bound syndromes. In B.J. Sadock, V.A. Sadock, & P. Ruiz, eds., *Kaplan and Sadock's Comprehensive Textbook of Psychiatry*, 9th edn, Vol. 2. Philadelphia, PA: Lippincott Williams & Wilkins, pp. 2519–2538.

Lewis-Fernández, R., Horvitz-Lennon, M., Blanco, C., Alegría, M., & Guarnaccia, P. J. (2009b). Significance of endorsement of psychotic symptoms by U.S. Latinos. *Journal of Nervous and Mental Disease*, **197**, 337–347.

Markowitz, J. C., Patel, S.R., Balán, I., *et al.* (2009). Toward an adaptation of interpersonal psychotherapy for depressed Hispanic patients. *Journal of Clinical Psychiatry*, **70**, 214–222.

Nichter, M. (1981). Idioms of distress: alternatives in the expression of psychosocial distress. A case from South India. *Culture, Medicine, and Psychiatry*, **5**, 379–408.

Schechter, D. S., Marshall, R., Salmán, E., *et al.* (2000). Ataque de nervios and history of childhood trauma. *Journal of Traumatic Stress*, **13**, 529–534.

Wells, A. (2000). *Emotional Disorder and Metacognitions: Innovative Cognitive Therapy*. Chichester: Wiley.

Current status of research in the genetics of anxiety disorders

Nicole R. Nugent, Myrna Weissman, Abby Fyer, Karestan C. Koenen

Our instinctive emotions are those that we have inherited from a much more dangerous world, and contain, therefore, a larger portion of fear than they should.

Bertrand Russell

13.1 Introduction

Fear and anxiety are basic emotions recognized across human cultures and among non-human animals. The evolutionary conservation of fear and anxiety across species supports the supposition that such emotions are adaptive. However, nearly one in five Americans reports problematic levels of anxiety, including diagnostic levels of panic disorder, social anxiety disorder (SAD, also known as social phobia), specific phobia, generalized anxiety disorder (GAD), posttraumatic stress disorder (PTSD), and obsessive–compulsive disorder (OCD) (Kessler *et al.* 2005). In this chapter, we provide an overview of the evidence for the role of genetic factors in the etiology of anxiety disorders. We first briefly summarize the genetic study designs used in research on anxiety disorders. Next, we review the evidence from family, twin, and molecular genetic studies for the role of genetic factors in specific anxiety disorders. We end by discussing the genetic overlap among anxiety disorders and the intermediate phenotypes that might account for the overlap.

13.2 Genetic study designs

Genetic research in anxiety disorders relies on family, twin, and molecular genetic study designs. In family studies, researchers test whether risk of having the disorder is higher among family members of individuals with the disorder (called *probands* in genetic studies) than non-relatives. If relatives of probands have a higher risk of the disorder, then it is said to "run in families" or be "familial." However, anxiety disorders may run in families for genetic or environmental reasons. Family members have both more similar genetic features and more shared environmental exposures than do non-relatives. Family studies are, therefore, often considered only the first step in genetics research.

Twin studies are needed to disentangle the role of genetic and environmental influences in the risk of developing an anxiety disorder. The twin design is used to calculate the heritability, or the proportion of the variance in an anxiety disorder explained by genetic factors. The basic twin method compares the degree of similarity within identical or monzygotic (MZ) pairs with the degree of similarity within fraternal or dizygotic (DZ) pairs. At the most basic level, twin research assumes that MZ twins share 100% of their genes and 100% of the environment, whereas DZ twins share on average 50% of their genes and 100% of the environment (see Hetherington *et al.* 1993 for a classic review of the importance of non-shared environmental influences in twins). If MZ twins are significantly more similar on a characteristic than DZ twins, then this phenotype (observed characteristic) is interpreted as being genetically influenced. The heritability estimate is derived by $2(r\text{MZ} - r\text{DZ})$, where r = the intraclass twin correlation (Plomin *et al.* 2001). For categorical phenotypes, such as an anxiety disorder diagnosis, the tetrachoric correlation, which assumes an underlying normal distribution of liability, is used to calculate heritability.

Molecular genetic studies have sought to identify variants in specific genes that increase the risk of having an anxiety disorder. Although the precise definition of a gene has changed over time (Gerstein *et al.* 2007), for the present purposes genes will be considered to be putatively functional units of deoxyribonucleic acid (DNA) sequences. Human beings are over 99% genetically identical; thus, research aimed at identifying genes that explain individual differences in risk for anxiety disorders focuses on the tiny fraction of the DNA sequences that differs among individuals. The majority of human genetic variation consists of

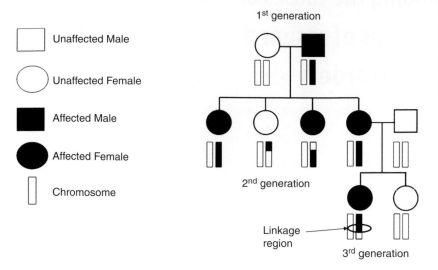

Figure 13.1. Example of a genetic pedigree chart or family tree used in linkage analysis to identify chromosomal location(s) inherited along with the disorder. *Unaffected* refers to individuals who do not have the disorder. *Affected* refers to individuals who have the disorder.

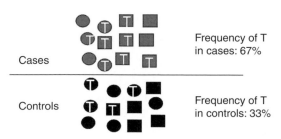

Chi-square test to test for significance (*P* value < 0.05)

Figure 13.2. Hypothetical example of case–control candidate gene association study involving a single SNP. In this case, a single base is one of two alleles, C or T. Individuals have one of three genotypes, CC, CT, or TT. Cases have a higher frequency of allele T than controls, suggesting that allele T confers increased risk of disease.

single nucleotide polymorphisms (SNPs, pronounced "snips"), which occur when a single nucleotide (A, T, C, or G) in the DNA sequence is altered. An example of a SNP is a change in the DNA sequence from CGTTGG to CGATGG. By definition, the frequency of SNPs must be at least 1% in the population; there are approximately three million SNPs in the human genome.

Molecular genetic study designs used to investigate the genetics of anxiety disorders include linkage analysis and candidate gene association studies. Linkage analysis uses data from family members to identify the location of a disease gene relative to a genetic marker or DNA sequence that has a known chromosomal location. Linkage is said to occur when the disease gene and genetic marker co-segregate or tend to be inherited together. Genome-wide linkage studies examine the entire genome for potential linkage regions. Figure 13.1 presents a simplified example of a linkage analysis. The pedigree (family tree) presented here starts with a first generation in which the father is affected (has the disorder) and the mother is unaffected (does not have the disorder). The disease gene is located somewhere on the paternal chromosome indicated by the black rectangle. Linkage analysis tracks the inheritance of DNA markers

on this paternal chromosome along with the disorder in the children in the second generation and the grandchildren in the third generation. The circled area on the first granddaughter's chromosome represents the region with strongest evidence for linkage. Typically, this would be represented by a LOD score, which is a statistical estimate of whether two loci are likely to lie near each other on a chromosome and are therefore likely to be inherited together. A LOD score of three or more is generally taken to indicate linkage.

Candidate gene association studies are more targeted than linkage studies and use extant research (i.e., linkage studies or information about the putative function of a particular gene) to guide selection of genes to test for potential associations with the disorder. The association method detects genes with small effects on risk and has been, until very recently, the method of choice for molecular genetic studies of complex disorders (Risch & Merikangas 1996). Disorders are referred to as "complex" when their etiology is thought to involve a combination of many genes and environmental factors, which is the case in all anxiety disorders. Association studies correlate a DNA marker's alleles with an outcome. Figure 13.2 presents an example of the case–control association design. Assume that each individual has either a C or a T allele. The investigator tests whether the T allele is more common among anxiety disorder cases. If it is, as in this example, further studies will be done to determine if this SNP is causally implicated in the etiology of the disorder (called the *causal variant*).

13.3 Genetics of specific disorders

13.3.1 Panic disorder

Multiple family studies and one meta-analysis support familial aggregation of panic disorder, with risk to first-degree relatives of probands ranging from 8% to 17% (Noyes *et al.* 1986, Maier *et al.* 1993, Mendlewicz *et al.* 1993, Horwath *et al.* 1995, Fyer *et al.* 1996, Hettema *et al.* 2001). Twin studies support a heritability estimate between 30% and 40% (Torgersen 1983, Kendler *et al.* 1993, 1995, 2001a, Skre *et al.* 1993, Perna *et al.* 1997, Bellodi *et al.* 1998). Even higher heritability has been shown when the age of onset was below 20 years of age (Goldstein *et al.* 1997). Figure 13.3 presents the heritability estimates for panic disorder as well as the other anxiety disorders.

Genome-wide linkage studies have reported promising regions including 7p15 (Knowles *et al.* 1998, Crowe *et al.* 2001, Logue *et al.* 2003), 13q32 (Weissman *et al.* 2000, Hamilton *et al.* 2003), 12q (Smoller *et al.* 2001a), 11p15 (Gelernter *et al.* 2001), a region of 16p (Crowe *et al.* 2001, Hamilton *et al.* 2003), 22q (Hamilton *et al.* 2003), 9q31 (Thorgeirsson *et al.* 2003), and a region of 15q (Fyer *et al.* 2006). Partly based on evidence from linkage studies, candidate gene research has identified significant associations between the cAMP responsive element modulator (*CREM*) gene and panic disorder

(Hamilton *et al.* 2004a). Infrequently, studies of panic disorder have applied both genetic linkage and gene association techniques, with support found for the adenosine 2A receptor (*ADORA2A*) gene (Hamilton *et al.* 2004b) and the gene for the tachykinin receptor 1 (*TACR1*) (Hodges *et al.* 2009). Across anxiety disorders, findings from candidate gene studies have often been mixed, with inconsistencies partly attributable to the operationalization of the phenotype. For example, genetic differences may exist as a function of subtypes of panic disorder (i.e., with or without agoraphobia), comorbid diagnoses, and symptom severity. Inconsistencies may also be attributable to unmeasured interactions between genes, to differing ethnic compositions across studies, or varying environmental factors, such as exposure to negative life events. Given the wealth of published molecular genetic studies in anxiety disorders (more than 100 studies over the past decade alone), as well as the early concerns related to inconsistencies and poor replication of findings in molecular genetics, we focus our present report on genes that have been (1) examined in at least two disorders and (2) replicated in at least one disorder. Table 13.1 summarizes molecular genetic findings that meet our criteria.

Genes in the serotonergic system have been perhaps the most widely studied genes in psychiatric genetics, partly due to the efficacy of medications known to influence serotonergic function (Gordon & Hen 2004). Initial support has been found for an association with the putative gene coding for the serotonin receptor (*5HT$_{2A}$*) (Inada *et al.* 2003, Maron *et al.* 2005) but not for the promoter region (*5-HTTLPR*) of the serotonin transporter (*SLC6A4*) (Deckert *et al.* 1997, Ishiguro *et al.* 1997, Matsushita *et al.* 1997, Strug *et al.* 2010).

Genes implicated in modulation of the autonomic nervous system, and particularly those involved in

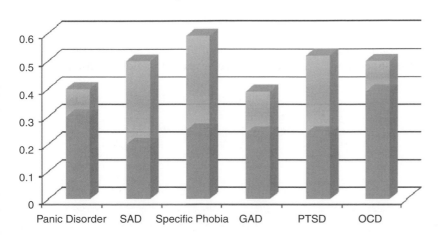

Figure 13.3. Estimated heritability of anxiety disorders. See text for a more detailed account of anxiety disorder heritability. Shading illustrates the range reported by heritability estimates.

Table 13.1. Summary of replicated findings in molecular genetic studies of anxiety disorders

Gene name and abbreviation	Location	Disorder	Studies supporting an association	Studies not supporting an association
Serotonergic system				
5-hydroxytryptamine receptor 2A ($5HT_{2A}$)	13q14–q21	Panic disorder	Inada *et al.* 2003 Maron *et al.* 2005	
		Social anxiety disorder	Stein *et al.* 1998	Lochner *et al.* 2007
		GAD	–	Fehr *et al.* 2001
		OCD	Enoch, 2003 [a] Meira-Lima *et al.* 2004 [a] Tot *et al.* 2003 Walitza *et al.* 2002 [a]	Frisch *et al.* 2000 Hemmings *et al.* 2003 Nicolini *et al.* 1996 Saiz *et al.* 2008
Serotonin transporter (*SLC6A4*)	17q11.1–q12	Panic disorder	Deckert *et al.* 1997 Ishiguro *et al.* 1997 Matsushita *et al.* 1997 Strug *et al.* 2008 [a]	
		Social anxiety disorder	Furmark *et al.* 2004 [a] Stein *et al.* 2006 [a]	
		GAD	Ohara *et al.* 1999 You *et al.* 2005	
		PTSD	Kilpatrick *et al.* 2007 [a] Lee *et al.* 2005	
		OCD	Baca-Garcia *et al.* 2007 Bengel *et al.* 1999 Hu *et al.* 2006 McDougle *et al.* 1998 Ohara *et al.* 1999 Saiz *et al.* 2008	Billett *et al.* 1997 Camarena *et al.* 2001a Cavallini *et al.* 2002 Chabane *et al.* 2004 Di Bella *et al.* 2002 Frisch *et al.* 2000 Kim *et al.* 2005 Kinnear *et al.* 2000 Meira-Lima *et al.* 2004 Walitza *et al.* 2004
Modulation of monoamine metabolism				
Catechol-O-methyl-transferase (*COMT*)	22q11.2	Panic disorder	*Domschke et al.* 2007 [a] Freitag *et al.* 2006	
		Specific phobia	McGrath *et al.* 2004	
		OCD	Alsobrook *et al.* 2001 [a] Karayiorgou *et al.* 1997 [a] Karayiorgou *et al.* 1999 [a] Niehaus *et al.* 2001 Schindler *et al.* 2000	*Azzam & Mathews 2003* Erdal *et al.* 2003 Meira-Lima *et al.* 2004 Ohara *et al.* 1998
Monoamine oxidase A (*MAOA*)	Xp11.4-p11.23	Panic disorder	Deckert *et al.* 1999 Maron *et al.* 2005 Samochowiec *et al.* 2004	Tadic *et al.* 2003 [a]
		Specific phobia	Samochowiec *et al.* 2004 [a]	
		GAD	Samochowiec *et al.* 2004 Tadic *et al.* 2003	
		OCD	Camarena *et al.* 2001b [a] Karayiorgou *et al.* 1999 [a]	Hemmings *et al.* 2003

Table 13.1 (cont.).

Gene name and abbreviation	Location	Disorder	Studies supporting an association	Studies not supporting an association
Dopaminergic system				
Dopamine receptor D$_4$ (*DRD4*)	11p15	Panic disorder	Maron *et al.* 2005	Hamilton *et al.* 2000
		Social anxiety disorder	–	Kennedy *et al.* 2001
		OCD	Billett *et al.* 1998 Camarena *et al.* 2007 Hemmings *et al.* 2004 [a] Millet *et al.* 2003	Frisch *et al.* 2000 Hemmings *et al.* 2003
Dopamine receptor D$_2$ (*DRD2*)	11q23	Social anxiety disorder	–	Kennedy *et al.* 2001
		PTSD	Comings *et al.* 1991 Comings *et al.* 1996 Young, *et al.* 2002 [a]	Gelernter *et al.* 1999
		OCD	Denys *et al.* 2006 [a] Nicolini *et al.* 1996 [a]	Billett *et al.* 1998
Dopamine transporter (*DAT1*)	5p15.3	Panic disorder	–	Hamilton *et al.* 2000
		Social anxiety disorder	Rowe *et al.* 1998	Kennedy *et al.* 2001
		GAD	Rowe *et al.* 1998	
		PTSD	Segman *et al.* 2002	
Regulator of G-protein signaling				
Regulator of G-protein signaling 2 (*RGS2*)	1q31	Panic disorder	Leygraf *et al.* 2006	
		GAD	Koenen *et al.* 2009	

The table presents only findings related to genes that (1) have been examined in at least two disorders, and (2) have been replicated in at least one disorder.
Meta-analyses are shown in italics.
[a] indicates that an association was identified in a subset of participants (see text for details).

sympathetic nervous system function, have also been examined in anxiety research. The monoamine oxidase A (*MAOA*) gene, which codes for an enzyme that degrades amines such as serotonin, has been associated with panic disorder (Deckert *et al.* 1999, Samochowiec *et al.* 2004, Maron *et al.* 2005), although this association was not supported in an examination of patients with panic disorder, depression, and GAD (Tadic *et al.* 2003). Stratification for gender and ethnicity in a meta-analysis of the catechol-O-methyl-transferase (*COMT*) gene suggested an association of panic disorder with *COMT* in Caucasian and Asian females (Domschke *et al.* 2007). A recent study identified a significant interaction between *COMT* and serotonin receptor 1A (*5-HT$_{1A}$*) (Freitag *et al.* 2006).

Candidate gene examinations of the dopaminergic system have looked at genes shown to influence dopamine receptors and transport. Investigations of dopamine receptor D$_4$ (*DRD4*) in panic disorder have been mixed (Hamilton *et al.* 2000, Maron *et al.* 2005). Studies have found little support for the role of the dopamine transporter (*DAT*) gene in panic disorder (Hamilton *et al.* 2000).

More recently, regulators of G-protein signaling have been investigated regarding anxiety-related phenotypes including panic disorder. Leygraf and colleagues (2006) found that polymorphisms in *RGS2* were associated with panic disorder, with the strongest association being observed for a haplotype containing SNPs *rs4606* and *rs3767488*.

13.3.2 Social anxiety disorder

Family studies suggest that risk of SAD to first-degree relatives of SAD probands ranges from 16% to 26% (Smoller 2008). Heritability estimates for SAD range from 20% to 50% (Kendler *et al.* 2001b, Middledorp *et al.* 2005, Distel *et al.* 2008), with greater family aggregation in severe levels of social anxiety disorder (Stein *et al.* 1998a).

To date, a single genome-wide linkage study has been conducted, with evidence for markers on chromosome 16 (62cM, 71cM) (Gelernter *et al.* 2004). Most gene association examinations of social anxiety have targeted functional genes of the serotonergic system. Although a small sample of social anxiety patients did not support an association between $5\text{-}HT_{2A}$ and social anxiety (Stein *et al.* 1998b), a recent investigation reported a possible role for the $5\text{-}HT_{2A}$ $T102C$ polymorphism in the development of SAD (Lochner *et al.* 2007). *SLC6A4* variant *5-HTTLPR* (s) was associated with increased symptom severity as well as amygdala activity in SAD patients (Furmark *et al.* 2004). The *5-HTTLPR* genotype evidenced a trend ($p = 0.051$) toward the prediction of selective serotonin reuptake inhibitor (SSRI) efficacy in SAD patients (Stein *et al.* 2006).

Examinations of the dopaminergic system have failed to identify a consistent association with SAD. Whereas linkage studies of *DRD2, DRD3, DRD4,* and *DAT* identified no significant linkage with SAD (Kennedy *et al.* 2001), an early investigation of children with internalizing disorders reported an association between social anxiety symptoms and dopamine transporter *SLC6A3 (DAT1)* 3" polymorphism (Rowe *et al.* 1998).

13.3.3 Specific phobia

Family studies have demonstrated that specific phobias are familial, with risk to first-degree relatives of probands as high as 31% (Fyer *et al.* 1990, 1993, Stein *et al.* 1998a, Smoller 2008). Heritability estimates for specific phobias range from 25% to 59% (Kendler *et al.* 1999, 2001b). Longitudinal twin research supports a "developmentally dynamic" hypothesis of the heritability for intensity of specific fears (Kendler *et al.* 2008). More specifically, the effect of one set of genetic factors found to influence early phobias during childhood declined with age, with new sets of genetic risk factors becoming prominent over the course of development. Examinations of children have reported slightly stronger effects for heritability and have supported a role for family environment (Lichtenstein & Annas 2000, Bolton *et al.* 2006).

To date, few molecular genetic studies have been conducted related to specific phobia. Gelernter and colleagues (2003) examined specific phobia in a family study of panic disorder, reporting that 14 of 19 families had two or more family members affected by specific phobia. Chromosome 14q13.3 was identified as a promising region. Phobic anxiety was reported to be associated with *COMT* (McGrath *et al.* 2004), and a trend was reported for *MAOA* in females with specific phobia relative to controls (Samochowiec *et al.* 2004).

13.3.4 Generalized anxiety disorder

Early family studies reported significantly greater risk for GAD in first-degree relatives of GAD probands, with risk to first-degree relatives ranging from 9% to 20% (Smoller 2008) and relative risk ratios ranging from 4.7 to 6.7 (Noyes *et al.* 1987, Mendlewicz *et al.* 1993). However, a more recent investigation reported odds ratios of 1.4–1.8 in first-degree relatives of probands, with differences across studies potentially attributable to differences in recruitment (Newman & Bland 2006). Consistent with this possibility, recent research has found that probands recruited from clinic settings evidence greater familial aggregation than GAD probands recruited from the community (Low *et al.* 2008). Compared with studies of all first-degree relatives, higher risk ratios have been reported in studies restricted to proband offspring (Newman & Bland 2006), particularly when both parents meet criteria for GAD (Johnson *et al.* 2008). A meta-analysis of family and twin studies of anxiety disorder estimated GAD heritability to be 32% (Hettema *et al.* 2001).

Molecular genetic studies have reported support for significant associations between GAD and *SLC6A4* (Ohara *et al.* 1999, You *et al.* 2005). *MAOA* has been associated with GAD in females relative to controls (Samochowiec *et al.* 2004) and GAD relative to panic disorder or major depression (Tadic *et al.* 2003). One study reported an association between GAD and *DAT1* in an examination of children with internalizing disorders (Rowe *et al.* 1998). Finally, *RGS2* has recently been associated with GAD in an epidemiologic sample (Koenen *et al.* 2009).

13.3.5 Posttraumatic stress disorder

Compared with other anxiety disorders, relatively few family studies of PTSD have been conducted. Family studies of PTSD are challenging, in that the disorder cannot be assessed in relatives who have not experienced a traumatic event. However, researchers have consistently found increased risk of PTSD among offspring of PTSD probands compared to trauma-exposed controls who did not develop PTSD. For example, logistic regression analyses revealed that parent PTSD was the strongest predictor of PTSD in adult children of Holocaust survivors, even after controlling for gender and parental Holocaust exposure (Yehuda *et al.* 2001). Cambodian refugee children whose mother and father both had PTSD were five times more likely to receive the diagnosis than refugee children whose parents did not have PTSD; levels of war trauma exposure did not differ between groups (Sack *et al.* 1995). Twin studies estimate the heritability of PTSD to range from 30% to 35% in both veteran and civilian samples (True *et al.* 1993, Stein *et al.* 2002).

To date, no linkage studies of PTSD have been conducted, and only 12 candidate gene association studies of PTSD have been published. Studies have only recently examined serotonergic-system genes in PTSD, with a significant association reported between *SLC6A4* polymorphisms and PTSD, although control participants were not necessarily trauma-exposed (Lee *et al.* 2005). Illustrating the importance of environmental factors in gene expression, Kilpatrick and colleagues (2007) found a significant association between an *SLC6A4* genotype and PTSD in adults with high stress exposure (defined as high hurricane exposure and low social support) but not low stress exposure.

Molecular studies in PTSD have focused on the dopaminergic system, as both animal and human studies have implicated this neurotransmitter in the etiology of PTSD. Whereas initial investigations found a positive association with *DRD2* (Comings *et al.* 1991, 1996), findings were not replicated in an investigation that did not assess for trauma exposure in the control group (Gelernter *et al.* 1999). A subsequent investigation of combat veterans reported a positive association between *DRD2A1* and PTSD only in the subset of PTSD cases who engaged in harmful drinking (Young *et al.* 2002). An examination of *DAT1* identified a positive association with chronic PTSD relative to trauma-exposed healthy controls (Segman *et al.* 2002).

13.3.6 Obsessive–compulsive disorder

Numerous family studies have been conducted on OCD. Prevalence estimates of OCD in first-degree relatives range from approximately 9% to 25%, with increased risk found in early-onset cases of OCD (Lenane *et al.* 1990, Bellodi *et al.* 1992, Pauls *et al.* 1995, do Rosario-Campos *et al.* 2005, Chacon *et al.* 2007, Nestadt *et al.* 2000). Research with youth with OCD reported rates of OCD among relatives of probands with early-onset OCD to be 25.2 times higher than rates for non-relatives matched for age, gender, and area of residence (do Rosario-Campos *et al.* 2005), although an adult investigation of OCD patients reported no relationship between familial aggregation and best-estimate ratings for age of onset (Fyer *et al.* 2005). A meta-analysis of early studies supported increased occurrence in first-degree relatives, reporting an odds ratio of 4.0 in relatives of probands versus relatives of controls (Hettema *et al.* 2001). Heritability estimates from twin studies range from 45% to 65% in children and from 39% to 50% in adults (van Grootheest *et al.* 2005, 2007).

To date, two genome-wide linkage studies have been conducted for OCD. Hanna and colleagues (2002) examined seven probands with childhood age of onset ranging from three to fourteen. Analyses suggested possible linkage for a region on the telomere of chromosome 9p, with weaker support found for linkage on chromosomes 2q, 6q, 16q, 17q, and 19q. Evidence for linkage at chromosomal region 9p24 was replicated by a subsequent linkage study (Willour *et al.* 2004). Interestingly, 9p24 contains the gene putatively encoding for the glutamate transporter *SLC1A1*, which has been associated with OCD in subsequent candidate gene studies (Arnold *et al.* 2006, Dickel *et al.* 2006, Stewart *et al.* 2007). However, a linkage investigation of a larger sample of OCD families failed to replicate these findings, reporting evidence for linkage on chromosomes 3q, 7p, 1q, 15q, and 6q instead (Shugart *et al.* 2006).

Based on the serotonergic hypothesis of OCD, most molecular genetic studies have focused on functional variants believed to influence the serotonin system. Linkage analysis has reported increased transmission of a variant of the *SLC6A4* gene to OCD-affected offspring (McDougle *et al.* 1998). Although five association studies have reported an association between OCD and *SLC6A4* (Bengel *et al.* 1999, Ohara *et al.* 1999, Hu *et al.* 2006, Baca-Garcia *et al.* 2007, Saiz *et al.* 2008), 10 separate investigations did not support this association (Billett *et al.* 1997, Frisch *et al.* 2000, Kinnear *et al.* 2000, Camarena *et al.* 2001a, Cavallini *et al.* 2002, Di Bella *et al.* 2002, Chabane *et al.* 2004, Meira-Lima *et al.* 2004, Walitza *et al.* 2004, Kim *et al.* 2005). Serotonin receptor studies have been similarly mixed. Although four investigations reported no association between OCD and $5\text{-}HT_{2A}$ alleles (Nicolini *et al.* 1996, Frisch *et al.* 2000, Hemmings *et al.* 2003, Saiz *et al.* 2008), examinations of subsets of participants have identified associations between $5\text{-}HT_{2A}$ and OCD in females (Enoch *et al.* 2003), in early-onset OCD (Walitza *et al.* 2002), in adult probands relative to controls (Meira-Lima *et al.* 2004), and in patients with severe OCD (Tot *et al.* 2003).

Examinations of *COMT* and OCD have produced mixed findings, with one study reporting an association between *COMT* homozygosity and OCD (Schindler *et al.* 2000), another study supporting increased *COMT* heterozygosity in OCD (Niehaus *et al.* 2001), and three other studies citing no relationship between *COMT* and OCD (Ohara *et al.* 1998, Erdal *et al.* 2003, Meira-Lima *et al.* 2004). Whereas Karayiorgou and colleagues (1997, 1999) found increased *COMT Met158* allele in males with OCD using both population- and family-based association designs, Alsobrook and colleagues (2001) reported increased *COMT Met158* in females with OCD but not in males. A meta-analysis of *COMT* in OCD concluded that there was little support for an association between *COMT* and OCD, even with gender stratification (Azzam & Mathews 2003). *MAOA* polymorphisms have also been examined in OCD, with two investigations supporting sexually dimorphic associations (Karayiorgou *et al.* 1999, Camarena *et al.* 2001b) and a third reporting no relationship (Hemmings *et al.* 2003).

An association between OCD and *DRD4* was reported in three investigations (Billett *et al.* 1998, Millet *et al.* 2003, Camarena *et al.* 2007), but was not replicated in two other studies (Frisch *et al.* 2000, Hemmings *et al.* 2003). One study reported lower frequency of *DRD4* VNTR 7-repeat allele in early-onset OCD (Hemmings *et al.* 2004). Two investigations of *DRD2* in OCD produced null findings (Billett *et al.* 1998, Nicolini *et al.* 1996), although the study by Nicolini and colleagues noted an association with the subset of patients exhibiting vocal tics, and a recent investigation reported differences in *DRD2* in male OCD patients relative to male controls (Denys *et al.* 2006).

13.4 Genetic overlap among anxiety disorders and intermediary phenotypes

Anxiety disorders are highly comorbid with each other, and twin studies suggest this may be partly explained by overlapping genetic influences. Hettema and colleagues (2005) found two genetic factors to be common across anxiety disorders. The first factor showed highest loadings on GAD, panic disorder, agoraphobia, and SAD, whereas specific phobias were found to load most highly on a second genetic factor. Neither PTSD nor OCD were examined in this investigation; however, another study reported that genetic influences common to GAD and panic disorder symptoms overlap with those for PTSD (Chantarujikapong *et al.* 2001). Anxiety disorder research has also examined co-occurring overlap of anxiety disorders with medical concerns. For example, emerging from genetic linkage research, evidence was found for "chromosome 13 syndrome" (later referenced as "PD syndrome") involving panic disorder as well as kidney or bladder problems, headaches, thyroid problems, and/or mitral valve prolapse (Weissman *et al.* 2000, 2004, Hamilton *et al.* 2003). A recent investigation replicated and extended these findings, reporting that participants with panic disorder and/or SAD as well as their first-degree relatives were markedly more likely to report chromosome 13 syndrome medical concerns than comparison participants (Talati *et al.* 2008). Evidence of shared genetic liability among anxiety disorders has led investigators to study intermediary phenotypes thought to represent underlying vulnerability to multiple anxiety disorders; these include neuroticism, behavioral inhibition, and anxiety sensitivity.

Neuroticism, a stable tendency to experience negative emotional states, has been consistently associated with anxiety symptoms and diagnoses (Jardine *et al.* 1984, Kirk *et al.* 2000, Hettema *et al.* 2004, 2006a). Overlap between genetic factors that influence neuroticism and anxiety disorders is substantial but incomplete (Hettema *et al.* 2006a). A large twin study of over 9000 twins examined genetic correlations between neuroticism and internalizing disorders, with evidence for correlations with neuroticism of 0.82 for SAD, 0.77 for GAD, 0.74 for situational phobia, 0.69 for panic disorder, 0.67 for agoraphobia, and 0.58 for animal phobia (Hettema *et al.* 2006a). Shifman and colleagues (2008) conducted a whole-genome association study of neuroticism, with inconsistent support for the phosphodiesterase D_4 (*PDE4D*) gene and no loci found to consistently account for more than 1% of the variance. Hence, it is likely that numerous genes confer small amounts of risk for anxiety disorders. Research modeling genetic covariation of neuroticism and internalizing disorders (including SAD, agoraphobia, and panic disorder) supported a role for glutamate decarboxylase (*GAD1*) in neuroticism (Hettema *et al.* 2006b). Meta-analytic examinations of neuroticism and *5-HTTLPR* have produced conflicting findings (Munafo *et al.* 2005, Schinka 2005). Neuroticism was associated with *COMT* in a sample of college students (Stein *et al.* 2005). Although studies of neuroticism and brain-derived neurotrophin factor (*BDNF*) alone have not identified significant associations (Willis-Owen *et al.* 2005), *BDNF* polymorphisms have been shown to interact with the dopamine transporter gene (Hunnerkopf *et al.* 2007). Studies using healthy volunteers have identified significant associations between neuroticism and *DRD4* (Tochigi *et al.* 2006) and, in males only, *DRD2* (Wacker *et al.* 2006).

Behavioral inhibition, or withdrawal from novelty (Kagan *et al.* 1989), has been characterized as a behavioral expression of neuroticism (Turner *et al.* 1996). Behavioral inhibition shows estimated heritability exceeding that of the anxiety disorders themselves, with estimates as high as 90% (Matheny 1989, Robinson *et al.* 1992, Plomin *et al.* 1993, DiLalla *et al.* 1994, Goldsmith & Lemery 2000, Eley *et al.* 2003). Behavioral inhibition is a familial and developmental risk factor for panic disorder and SAD (Mannasis *et al.* 1995, Battaglia *et al.* 1997, Schwartz *et al.* 1999, Rosenbaum *et al.* 2000, Biederman *et al.* 2001). Based on evidence from mouse models, early research in behavioral inhibition involved family-based association analyses of four genes, finding a modest association between behavioral inhibition and the glutamic acid decarboxylase gene, which encodes an enzyme involved in GABA synthesis (Smoller *et al.* 2001b). Behavioral inhibition has been associated with *RGS2* markers, which were also associated with activity in the amygdala and the insular cortex (Smoller *et al.* 2008a). Behaviorally inhibited temperament was also highly associated with the corticotropin-releasing hormone gene, *CRH* (Smoller *et al.* 2003, 2005). Studies of childhood and early adolescent shyness/behavioral inhibition have been associated with *SLC6A4* (Jorm *et al.* 2000, Arbelle *et al.* 2003).

Anxiety sensitivity (AS), a fear of anxiety-related sensations, has also served as a quantitative endophenotype in anxiety disorder research. Family and twin studies of AS suggest that AS is heritable (Stein *et al.* 1999, van Beek & Griez 2003), particularly in women (Jang *et al.* 1999, Taylor *et al.* 2008). More recently, Stein and colleagues (2008) conducted a genotype-by-environment investigation of AS, reporting an interaction between childhood maltreatment and the *5-HTTLPR* genotype. Individuals with two short-version alleles of *5-HTTLPR* and high levels of maltreatment reported significantly greater AS than comparison participants. Of note, neuroticism did not evidence a gene–environment interaction between *5-HTTLPR* and level of childhood maltreatment.

13.5 Conclusions

Although anxiety disorders are substantially heritable (Figure 13.3), knowledge of the molecular genetics of these disorders is still very limited. Investigations of panic disorder, specific phobias, SAD, and OCD have produced some evidence of linkage to specific regions, but results of candidate gene association studies have been inconsistent. Moreover, there have been no linkage studies of GAD or PTSD, and few candidate gene association studies have been replicated in independent samples. Historically, candidate genes were selected on the basis of neurobiologic alterations observed in respective disorders; however, this approach has been criticized for reliance on existing models of disorders and for the low probability of selecting the relevant variants out of the millions of potential candidates.

The challenge of selecting strong candidate genes is one of the motivating factors behind the development of genome-wide association studies (GWAS). Rather than hypothesizing genetic association for a specific candidate gene, such studies take a more agnostic approach and compare the entire genomes of cases to controls. (For more information on GWAS studies in psychiatric disorders, see the excellent editorial by Craddock *et al.* 2008.) As of this writing, no GWAS studies of specific anxiety disorders have been published, although investigators have examined intermediary phenotypes such as neuroticism (Craddock *et al.* 2008). For this reason, no anxiety disorder, except possibly OCD, is being included in the Psychiatric GWAS Consortium (https:// pgc.unc.edu/faqs.html), which aims to conduct higher-level statistical analyses of published GWAS studies.

Two exciting yet mostly unexplored areas in anxiety disorder research are gene–environment interaction and epigenetic studies. Gene–environment interaction studies test whether gene–phenotype associations vary with level of exposure to an environmental pathogen or protective factor. Given the well-documented role of certain environmental factors (e.g., stressful life events, social support) in the etiology of anxiety disorders, gene–environmental interaction studies may be a potentially fruitful area of future research (Poulton *et al.* 2008). Epigenetic research examines the dynamic heritable changes in the *function*, but not the sequence, of a gene. Both animal and human samples point to the potential importance of epigenetic phenomena in the development of anxiety disorders (Seckl & Meaney 2006, Skinner *et al.* 2008, Yehuda *et al.* 2008).

Readers interested in learning more about genetic research on specific anxiety disorders should consult relevant recent reviews spanning panic and phobic anxiety disorders (Smoller *et al.* 2008b), OCD (Hemmings & Stein 2006, Pauls 2008), PTSD (Koenen 2007, Koenen *et al.* 2008, Nugent *et al.* 2008), and GAD (Gregory *et al.* 2008).

Acknowledgments

Dr. Koenen is supported by US-NIMH K08 MH070627 and R01 MH078928. Dr. Nugent is supported by US-NIMH T32 MH078788 and K01 MH087240.

References

Alsobrook, J. P., Zohar, A. H., Leboyer, M., *et al.* (2001). Association between the COMT locus and obsessive–compulsive disorder in females but not in males. *American Journal of Medical Genetics*, **114**, 116–120.

Arbelle, S., Benjamin, J., Golin, M., *et al.* (2003). Relation of shyness in grade school children to the genotype for the long form of the serotonin transporter promoter region polymorphism. *American Journal of Psychiatry*, **160**, 671–676.

Arnold, P., Sicard, T., Burroughs, E., Richter, M., & Kennedy, J. (2006). Glutamate transporter gene SLC1A1 associated with obsessive–compulsive disorder. *Archives of General Psychiatry*, **63**, 769–776.

Azzam, A., & Mathews, C. (2003). Meta-analysis of the association between the catecholamine-O-methyl-transferase gene and obsessive–compulsive disorder. *American Journal of Medical Genetics B: Neuropsychiatric Genetics*, **123B**, 64–69.

Baca-Garcia, E., Vaquero-Lorenzo, C., Diaz-Hernandez, M., *et al.* (2007). Association between obsessive–compulsive disorder and a variable number of tandem repeats polymorphism in intron 2 of the serotonin transporter gene. *Progress in Neuro-Psychopharmacology and Biological Psychiatry*, **31**, 416–420.

Battaglia, M., Bajo, S, Strambi, LF, *et al.* (1997). Physiological and behavioral responses to minor stressors in offspring of patients with panic disorder. *Journal of Psychiatric Research*, **31**, 365–376.

Bellodi, L., Scuito, G., Guiseppina, D., & Ronchi, P. (1992). Psychiatric disroders in the families of patients with obsessive–compulsive disorder. *Psychiatry Research*, **42**, 111–120.

Bellodi, L., Perna, G., Caldirola, D., *et al.* (1998). CO2-induced panic attacks: a twin study. *American Journal of Psychiatry*, **155**, 1184–1188.

Bengel, D., Greenberg, B. D., Cora-Locatelli, G., *et al.* (1999). Association of the serotonin transporter promoter regulatory region polymorphism and obsessive-compulsive disorder. *Molecular Psychiatry*, **4**, 463–466.

Biederman, J., Hirshfeld-Becker, D. R., Rosenbaum, J. F., *et al.* (2001). Further evidence of association between behavioral inhibition and social anxiety in children. *American Journal of Psychiatry*, **158**, 1673–1679.

Billett, E. A., Richter, M. A., King, N., *et al.* (1997). Obsessive compulsive disorder, response to serotonin reuptake inhibiters and the serotonin transporter gene. *Molecular Psychiatry*, **2**, 403–406.

Billett, E. A., Richter, M., Sam, F., *et al.* (1998). Investigation of dopamine system genes in obsessive–compulsive disorder. *Psychiatric Genetics*, **8**, 163–169.

Bolton, D., Eley, T. C., O'Connor, T. G., *et al.* (2006). Prevalence and genetic and environmental influences on anxiety disorders in 6-year-old twins. *Psychological Medicine*, **36**, 335–344.

Camarena, B., Rinetti, G., Cruz, C., *et al.* (2001a). Association study of the serotonin transporter gene polymorphism in obsessive–compulsive disorder. *International Journal of Neuropsychopharmacology*, **4**, 269–272.

Camarena, B., Rinetti, G., Cruz, C., *et al.* (2001b). Additional evidence that genetic variation of MAO-A gene supports a gender subtype in obsessive–compulsive disorder. *American Journal of Medical Genetics*, **105**, 279–282.

Camarena, B., Loyzaga, C., Aguilar, A., Weissbecker, K. & Nicolini, H. (2007). Association study between the dopamine D4 gene and obsessive–compulsive disorder. *European Neuropsychopharmacology*, **17**, 406–409.

Cavallini, M., Di Bella, D., Siliprandi, F., Malchiodi, F., & Bellodi, L. (2002). Exploratory factor analysis of obsessive–compulsive patients and association with 5-HTTLPR polymorphism. *American Journal of Medical Genetics*, **114**, 347–353.

Chabane, N., Millet, B., Delorme, R., *et al.* (2004). Lack of evidence for association between serotonin transporter gene (5-HTTLPR) and obsessive–compulsive disorder by case control and family association study in humans. *Neuroscience Letters*, **363**, 154–156.

Chacon, P., Rosario-Campos, M. C., Pauls, D. L., *et al.* (2007). Obsessive–compulsive symptoms in sibling pairs concordant for obsessive–compulsive disorder. *American Journal of Medical Genetics B: Neuropsychiatric Genetics*, **144B**, 551–555.

Chantarujikapong, S. I., Scherrer, J. F., Xian, H., *et al.* (2001). A twin study of generalized anxiety disorder symptoms, panic disorder symptoms and post-traumatic stress disorder in men. *Psychiatry Research*, **103**, 133–145.

Comings, D. E., Comings, B. G., Muhleman, D., *et al.* (1991). The dopamine D2 receptor locus as a modifying gene in neuropsychiatric disorders. *JAMA*, **266**, 1793–1800.

Comings, D. E., Muhleman, D., & Gysin, R. (1996). Dopamine D2 receptor (DRD2) gene and susceptibility to posttraumatic stress disorder: A study and replication. *Biological Psychiatry*, **40**, 368–372.

Craddock, N., O'Donovan, M. C., & Owen, M. J. (2008). Genome-wide association studies in psychiatry: lessons from early studies of non-psychiatric and psychiatric phenotypes. *Molecular Psychiatry*, **13**, 649–653.

Crowe, R. R., Goedken, R., Samuelson, S., *et al.* (2001). Genomewide survey of panic disorder. *American Journal of Medical Genetics*, **105**, 105–109.

Deckert, J., Catalano, M., & Heils, A. (1997). Functional promoter polymorphism of the human serotonin transporter: lack of association with panic disorder. *Psychiatric Genetics*, **7**, 45–47.

Deckert, J., Catalano, M., Syagailo, Y., *et al.* (1999). Excess of high activity monoamine oxidase A gene promoter alleles in female patients with panic disorder. *Human Molecular Genetics*, **8**, 621–624.

Denys, D., Van Nieuwerburgh, F., Deforce, D., & Westenberg, H. (2006). Association between the dopamine D2 receptor TaqI A2 allele and low activity COMT allele with obsessive–compulsive disorder in males. *European Neuropsychopharmacology*, **16**, 446–450.

Di Bella, D., Cavallini, M. C., & Bellodi, L. (2002). No association between obsessive–compulsive disorder and the 5-HT1Dβ receptor gene. *American Journal of Psychiatry*, **159**, 1783–1785.

Dickel, D. E., Veenstra-VanderWeele, J., Cox, N. J., *et al.* (2006). Association testing of the positional and functional candidate gene SLC1A1/EAAC1 in early-onset obsessive–compulsive disorder. *Archives of General Psychiatry*, **63**, 778–785.

DiLalla, L., Kagan, J., & Reznick, J. (1994). Genetic etiology of behavioral inhibition among 2-year-old children. *Infant Behavior Development*, **17**, 405–412.

Distel, M. A., Vink, J. M., & Willemsen, G. (2008). Heritability of self-reported phobic fear. *Behavior Genetics*, **38**, 24–33.

do Rosario-Campos, M., Leckman, J., Curi, M., *et al.* (2005). A family study of early onset obsessive–compulsive disorder. *American Journal of Medical Genetics B: Neuropsychiatric Genetics*, **136B**, 92–97.

Domschke, K., Deckert, J., O'Donovan, M. C., & Glatt, S. J. (2007). Meta-analysis of COMT val158met in panic disorder: Ethnic heterogeneity and gender specificity. *American Journal of Medical Genetics B: Neuropsychiatric Genetics*, **144B**, 667–673.

Eley, T. C., Bolton, D., O'Connor, T. G., *et al.* (2003). A twin study of anxiey-related behaviors in pre-school children. *Journal of Child Psychology and Psychiatry*, **44**, 945–960.

Enoch, M. A., Xu, K., Ferro, E., Harris, C. R., & Goldman, D. (2003). Genetic origins of anxiety in women: a role for a functional COMT polymorphism. *Psychiatric Genetics*, **13**, 33–41.

Erdal, M., Tot, S., Yazici, K., *et al.* (2003). Lack of association of catechol-o-methyltransferase gene polymorphism in obsessive–compulsive disorder. *Depression and Anxiety*, **18**, 41–45.

Fehr, C., Schleicher, A., Szegedi, A., *et al.* (2001). Serotonergic polymorphisms in patients suffering from alcoholism, anxiety disorders, and narcolepsy. *Progress in Neuro-Psychopharmacology and Biological Psychiatry*, **25**, 965–982.

Freitag, C. M., Domschke, K., Rothe, C., *et al.* (2006). Interaction of serotonergic and noradrenergic gene variants in panic disorder. *Psychiatric Genetics*, **16**, 59–65.

Frisch, A., Michaelovsky, E., Rockah, R., *et al.* (2000). Association between obsessive–compulsive disorder and polymorphisms of genes encoding components of the serotonergic and dopaminergic pathways. *European Neuropsychopharmacology*, **10**, 205–209.

Furmark, T., Tillfors, M., Garpenstrand, H., *et al.* (2004). Serotonin transporter polymorphism related to amygdala excitability and symptom severity in patients with social phobia. *Neuroscience Letters*, **362**, 189–192.

Fyer, A., Mannuzza, S., Gallops, M., *et al.* (1990). Familial transmission of simple phobias and fears. A preliminary report. *Archives of General Psychiatry*, **47**, 252–256.

Fyer, A., Mannuzza, S., Chapman, T., Liebowitz, M., & Klein, D. (1993). A direct interview family study of social phobia. *Archives of General Psychiatry*, **50**, 286–293.

Fyer, A., Mannuzza, S., Chapman, T., *et al.* (1996). Panic disorder and social phobia: effects of comorbidity on familial transmission. *Anxiety*, **2**, 173–178.

Fyer, A., Lipsitz, J., Mannuzza, S., Aronowitz, B., & Chapman, T. (2005). A direct interview family study of obsessive–compulsive disorder. I. *Psychological Medicine*, **35**, 1611–1621.

Fyer, A., Hamilton, S., Durner, M., *et al.* (2006). A third-pass genome scan in panic disorder: evidence for multiple susceptibility loci. *Biological Psychiatry*, **60**, 388–401.

Gelernter, J., Southwick, S., Goodson, S., *et al.* (1999). No association between D2 dopamine receptor (DRD2) 'A' system alleles, or DRD2 haplotypes, and posttraumatic stress disorder. *Biological Psychiatry*, **45**, 620–625.

Gelernter, J., Bonvicini, K., Page, G., *et al.* (2001). Linkage genome scan for loci predisposing to panic disorder or agoraphobia. *American Journal of Medical Genetics*, **105**, 548–557.

Gelernter, J., Page, G. P., Bonvicini, K., *et al.* (2003). A chromosome 14 risk locus for simple phobia: Results from a genomewide linkage scan. *Molecular Psychiatry*, **8**, 71–82.

Gelernter, J., Page, G., Stein, M., & Woods, S. (2004). Genome-wide linkage scan for loci predisposing to social phobia: evidence for a chromosome 16 risk locus. *American Journal of Psychiatry*, **161**, 59–66.

Gerstein, M., Bruce, C., Rozowsky, J., *et al.* (2007) What is a gene, post-ENCODE? History and updated definition. *Genome Research*, **17**, 669–681.

Goldsmith, H., & Lemery, K. (2000). Linking temperamental anxiety symptoms: a behavior-genetic perspective. *Biological Psychiatry*, **48**, 1199–1209.

Goldstein, R., Wickramante, P., Horwath, E., & Weissman, M. (1997). Familial aggregation and pheonmenology of "early"-onset (at or before age 20 years) panic disorder. *Archives of General Psychiatry*, **54**, 271–278.

Gordon, J. A., & Hen, R. (2004). The serotonergic system and anxiety. *NeuroMolecular Medicine*, **5**, 27–40.

Gregory, A., Lau, J. Y. F., & Eley, T. C. (2008). Finding gene–environment interactions for generalised anxiety disorder. *European Archives of Psychiatry and Clinical Neuroscience*, **258**, 69–75.

Hamilton, S., Haghighi, F., Heiman, G., *et al.* (2000). Investigation of dopamine receptor (DRD4) and dopamine transporter (DAT) polymorphisms for genetic linkage or association to panic disorder. *American Journal of Medical Genetics*, **96**, 324–330.

Hamilton, S., Fyer, A., Durner, M., *et al.* (2003). Further genetic evidence for a panic disorder syndrome mapping to chromosome 13q. *Proceedings from the National Academy of Sciences of the USA*, **100**, 2550–2555.

Hamilton, S., Slager, S. L., Mayo, D., *et al.* (2004a). Investigation of polymorphisms in the CREM gene in panic disorder. *American Journal of Medical Genetics B: Neuropsychiatric Genetics*, **126B**, 111–115.

Hamilton, S. P., Slager, S. L., de Leon, A. B., *et al.* (2004b). Evidence for genetic linkage between a polymorphism in the adenosine 2A receptor and panic disorder. *Neuropsychopharmacology*, **29**, 558–565.

Hanna, G. L., Veenstra-VanderWeele, J., Cox, N. J., *et al.* (2002). Genome-wide linkage analysis of families with obsessive–compulsive disorder ascertained through pediatric probands. *American Journal of Medical Genetics*, **114**, 541–552.

Hemmings, S., & Stein, D. (2006). The current status of association studies in obsessive–compulsive disorder. *Psychiatric Clinics of North America*, **29**, 411–444.

Hemmings, S., Kinnear, C., Niehaus, D., *et al.* (2003). Investigating the role of dopaminergic and serotonergic candidate genes in obsessive–compulsive disorder. *European Neuropsychopharmacology*, **13**, 93–98.

Hemmings, S., Kinnear, C., Lochner, C., *et al.* (2004). Early- versus late-onset obsessive–compulsive disorder: investigating genetic and clinical correlates. *Psychiatric Annals*, **128**, 175–182.

Hetherington, E., Reiss, D., & Plomin, R. (1993) *Separate Social Worlds of Siblings: the Impact of Nonshared Envionment on Development*. Hillsdale, NJ: Lawrence Erlbaum Associates.

Hettema, J. M., Neale, M. C., & Kendler, K. S. (2001). A review and meta-analysis of the genetic epidemiology of anxiety disorders. *American Journal of Psychiatry*, **158**, 1568–1578.

Hettema, J. M., Prescott, C. A., & Kendler, K. S. (2004). Genetic and environmental sources of covariation between generalized anxiety disorder and neuroticism. *American Journal of Psychiatry*, **161**, 1581–1587.

Hettema, J. M., Prescott, C. A., Myers, J. M., Neale, M. C., & Kendler, K. S. (2005). The structure of genetic and environmental risk ractors for anxiety disorders in men and women. *Archives of General Psychiatry*, **62**, 182–189.

Hettema, J. M., Neale, M. C., Myers, J. M., Prescott, C. A., & Kendler, K. S. (2006a). A population-based twin study of the relationship between neuroticism and internalizing disorders. *American Journal of Psychiatry*, **163**, 857–864.

Hettema, J. M., An, S. S., Neale, M. C., *et al.* (2006b). Association between glutamic acid decarboxylase genes and anxiety disorders, major depression, and neuroticism. *Molecular Psychiatry*, **11**, 794.

Hodges, L., Weissman, M., Haghighi, F., *et al.* (2009). Association and linkage analysis of candidate genes GRP, GRPR, CRHR1, and TACR1 in panic disorder. *American Journal of Medical Genetics B: Neuropsychiatric Genetics*, **150B**, 65–73.

Horwath, E., Wolk, S., Goldstein, R., *et al.* (1995). Is the comorbidity between social phobia and panic disorder due to familial cotransmission or other factors. *Archives of General Psychiatry*, **52**, 574–582.

Hu, X. Z., Lipsky, R., Zhu, G., *et al.* (2006). Serotonin transporter promoter gain-of-function genotypes are linked to obsessive–compulsive disorder. *American Journal of Human Genetics*, **78**, 815–826.

Hunnerkopf, R., Strobel, A., Gutknecht, L., Brocke, B., & Lesch, K. P. (2007). Interaction between BDNF Val66Met and dopamine transporter gene variation influences anxiety-related traits. *Neuropsychopharmacology*, **32**, 2552–2560.

Inada, Y., Yoneda, H., Koh, J., *et al.* (2003). Positive association between panic disorder and polymorphism of the serotonin 2A receptor gene. *Psychiatry Research*, **118**, 25–31.

Ishiguro, H., Arinami, T., Yamada, K., *et al.* (1997). An association study between a transcriptional polymorphism in the serotonin transporter gene and panic disorder in a Japanese population. *Psychiatry and Clinical Neurosciences*, **51**, 333–335.

Jang, K. L., Stein, M. B., Taylor, S., & Livesley, W. J. (1999). Gender differences in the etiology of anxiety sensitivity: a twin study. *Journal of Gender Specific Medicine*, **2**, 39–44.

Jardine, R., Martin, N., & Henderson, A. (1984). Genetic covariation between neuroticism and the symptoms of anxiety and depression. *Genetic Epidemiology*, **1**, 89–107.

Johnson, J., Cohen, P., Kasen, S., & Brook, J. (2008). Parental concordance and offspring risk for anxiety, conduct, depressive, and substance use disorders. *Psychopathology*, **41**, 124–128.

Jorm, A., Prior, M., Sanson, A., *et al.* (2000). Association of a functional polymorphism of the serotonin transporter gene with anxiety-related temperament and behavior problems in children: A longitudinal study from infancy to the mid-teens. *Molecular Psychiatry*, **5**, 542–547.

Kagan, J., Reznick, J., & Gibbons, J. (1989). Inhibited and uninhibited types of children. *Child Development*, **60**, 838–845.

Karayiorgou, M., Alternus, M., Galke, B., *et al.* (1997). Genotype determining low catechol-O-methyl-transferase activity as a risk factor for obsessive–compulsive disorder. *Proceedings of the National Academy of Sciences of the USA*, **94**, 4572–4575.

Karayiorgou, M., Sobin, C., Blundell, M., *et al.* (1999). Family-based association studies support a sexually dimorphic effect of COMT and MAOA on genetic susceptibility to obsessive–compulsive disorder. *Biological Psychiatry*, **45**, 1178–1189.

Kendler, K., Neale, M., Kessler, R., Heath, A., & Eaves, L. (1993). Panic disorder in women: A population-based twin study. *Psychological Medicine*, **23**, 397–406.

Kendler, K., Walters, E., Truett, K. R., *et al.* (1995). A twin family study of self-report symptoms of panic, phobia, and somatization. *Behavior Genetics*, **25**, 499–515.

Kendler, K. S., Karkowski, L. M., & Prescott, C. A. (1999). Fears and phobias: reliability and heritability. *Psychological Medicine*, **29**, 539–553.

Kendler, K. S., Gardner, C. O., & Prescott, C. A. (2001a). Panic syndromes in a population-based sample of male and female twins. *Psychological Medicine*, **31**, 989–1000.

Kendler, K. S., Myers, J., Prescott, C. A., & Neale, M. C. (2001b). The genetic epidemiology of irrational fears and phobias in men. *Archives of General Psychiatry*, **58**, 257–265.

Kendler, K., Gardner, C. O., Annas, P., *et al.* (2008). A longitudinal twin study of fears from middle childhood to early adulthood: evidence for a developmentally dynamic genome. *Archives of General Psychiatry*, **65**, 421–429.

Kennedy, J. L., Neves-Pereira, M., King, N., *et al.* (2001). Dopamine system genes not linked to social phobia. *Psychiatric Genetics*, **11**, 213–217.

Kessler, R., Chiu, W., Demler, O., Merikangas, K., & Walters, E. (2005). Prevalence, severity, and comorbidity of 12-month DSM-IV disorders in the National Comorbidity Survey Replication. *Archives of General Psychiatry*, **25**, 617–627.

Kilpatrick, D. G., Koenen, K. C., Ruggiero, K. J., *et al.* (2007). The serotonin transporter genotype and social support and moderation of posttraumatic stress disorder and depression in hurricane-exposed adults. *American Journal of Psychiatry*, **164**, 1693–1699.

Kim, S., Lee, H., & Kim, C. (2005). Obsessive–compulsive disorder, factor-analyzed symptom dimensions and serotonin transporter polymorphism. *Neuropsychobiology*, **52**, 176–182.

Kinnear, C., Niehaus, D., Moolman-Smook, J., *et al.* (2000). Obsessive–compulsive disorder and the promoter region polymorphism (5-HTTLPR) in the serotonin transporter gene (SLC6A4): a negative association study in the Afrikaner population. *International Journal of Neuropsychopharmacology*, **3**, 327–331.

Kirk, K., Birley, A., Statham, D., Haddon, B., *et al.* (2000). Anxiety and depression in twin and sib pairs extremely discordant and concordant for neuroticism: prodromus to a linkage study. *Twin Research and Human Genetics*, **3**, 299–309.

Knowles, J., Fyer, A., Vieland, V., *et al.* (1998). Results of a genome-wide genetic screen for panic disorder. *American Journal of Medical Genetics*, **81**, 139–147.

Koenen, K. C. (2007). Genetics of posttraumatic stress disorder: review and recommendations for future studies. *Journal of Traumatic Stress Studies*, **20**, 737–750.

Koenen, K. C., Nugent, N. R., & Amstadter, A. B. (2008). Gene–environment interaction in posttraumatic stress disorder: review, strategy and new directions for future research. *European Archives of Psychiatry and Clinical Neuroscience*, **258**, 82–96.

Koenen, K. C., Amstadter, A. B., Ruggiero, K. J., *et al.* (2009). *RGS2* and generalized anxiety disorder in an epidemiologic sample of hurricane-exposed adults. *Depression and Anxiety*, **26**, 309–315.

Lee, H. J., Lee, M. S., Kang, R. H., *et al.* (2005). Influence of the serotonin transporter promoter gene polymorphism on susceptibility to posttraumatic stress disorder. *Depression and Anxiety*, **21**, 135–139.

Lenane, M. C., Swedo, S. E., Leonard, H., *et al.* (1990). Psychiatric disorders in first degree relatives of children and adolescents with obsessive compulsive disorder. *Journal of the American Academy of Child and Adolescent Psychiatry*, **29**, 407–412.

Leygraf, A., Hohoff, C., Freitag, C., *et al.* (2006). Rgs 2 gene polymorphisms as modulators of anxiety in humans? *Journal of Neural Transmission*, **113**, 1921–1925.

Lichtenstein, P., & Annas, P. (2000). Heritability and prevalence of specific fears and phobias in childhood. *Journal of Child Psychology and Psychiatry and Allied Disciplines*, **41**, 927–937.

Lochner, C., Hemmings, S., Seedat, S., *et al.* (2007). Genetics and personality traits in patients with social anxiety disorder: a case–control study in South Africa. *European Neuropsychopharmacology*, **17**, 321–327.

Logue, M., Vieland, V., Goedken, R., & Crowe, R. R. (2003). Bayesian analysis of a previously published genome screen for panic disorder reveals new and compelling evidence for linkage to chromosome 7. *American Journal of Medical Genetics B: Neuropsychiatric Genetics*, **121B**, 95–99.

Low, N. C. P., Cui, L., & Merikangas, K. R. (2008). Community versus clinic sampling: Effect on the familial aggregation of anxiety disorders. *Biological Psychiatry*, **63**, 884–890.

Maier, W., Lichtermann, D., Minges, J., Oehrlein, A., & Franke, P. (1993). A controlled family study in panic disorder. *Journal of Psychiatric Research*, **27**, 79–87.

Mannasis, K., Bradley, S, Goldberg, S, Hood, J, Swinson, R. (1995). Behavioural inhibition, attachment and anxiety in children of mothers with anxiety disorders. *Canadian Journal of Psychiatry*, **40**, 87–92.

Maron, E., Nikopensius, T., Koks, S., *et al.* (2005). Association study of 90 candidate gene polymorphisms in panic disorder. *Psychiatric Genetics*, **15**, 17–24.

Matheny, A. (1989). Children's behavioral inhibition over age and across situations: genetic similarity for a trait during change. *Journal of Personality*, **57**, 215–235.

Matsushita, S., Muramatsu, T., Kimura, M., *et al.* (1997). Serotonin transporter gene regulatory region polymorphism and panic disorder. *Molecular Psychiatry*, **2**, 390–392.

McDougle, C. J., Epperson, C. N., Price, L. H., & Gelernter, J. (1998). Evidence for linkage disequilibrium between serotonin transporter protein gene (SLC6A4) and obsessive compulsive disorder. *Molecular Psychiatry*, **3**, 270–273.

McGrath, M., Kawachi, I., Ascherio, A., *et al.* (2004). Association between catechol-O-methyltransferase and phobic anxiety. *American Journal of Psychiatry*, **161**, 1703–1705.

Meira-Lima, I., Shavitt, R., Miguita, K., *et al.* (2004). Association analysis of the catechol-omethyltransferase (COMT), serotonin transporter (5-HTT) and serotonin 2A receptor (5HT2A) gene polymorphisms with obsessive–compulsive disorder. *Genes, Brain, and Behavior*, **3**, 75–79.

Mendlewicz, J., Papadimitriou, G., & Wilmotte, J. (1993). Family study of panic disorder: comparison with generalized anxiety disorder, major depression and normal subjects. *Psychiatric Genetics*, **3**, 73–78.

Middledorp, C., Birley, A., Cath, D. G., *et al.* (2005). Familial clustering of major depression and anxiety disorders in Australian and Dutch twins and siblings. *Twin Research and Human Genetics*, **8**, 609–615.

Millet, B., Chabane, N., Delorme, R., *et al.* (2003). Association between the dopamine receptor D4 (DRD4) gene and obsessive–compulsive disorder. *American Journal of Medical Genetics B: Neuropsychiatric Genetics*, **116B**, 55–59.

Munafo, M., Clark, T., & Flint, J. (2005). Does measurement instrument moderate the association between the serotonin transporter gene and anxiety-related personality traits? A meta-analysis. *Molecular Psychiatry*, **10**, 415–419.

Nestadt, G., Samuels, J., Riddle, M., *et al.* (2000). A family study of obsessive–compulsive disorder. *Archives of General Psychiatry*, **57**, 358–363.

Newman, S., & Bland, R. (2006). A population-based family study of DSM-III generalized anxiety disorder. *Psychological Medicine*, **36**, 1275–1281.

Nicolini, H., Cruz, C., Camarena, B., *et al.* (1996). DRD2, DRD3, and 5HT2A receptor genes polymorphisms in obsessive–compulsive disorder. *Molecular Psychiatry*, **1**, 461–465.

Niehaus, D., Kinnear, C., Corfield, V., *et al.* (2001). Association between a catechol-o-methyltransferase polymorphism and obsessive–compulsive disorder in the Afrikaner population. *Journal of Affect Disorders*, **65**, 61–65.

Noyes, R., Crowe, R. R., Harris, E., *et al.* (1986). Relationship between panic disorder and agoraphobia: a family study. *Archives of General Psychiatry*, **43**, 227–232.

Noyes, R., Clarkson, C., Crowe, R., Yates, W., & McChesney, C. (1987). A family study of generalized anxiety disorder. *American Journal of Psychiatry*, **144**, 1019–1024.

Nugent, N. R., Amstadter, A. B., & Koenen, K. C. (2008). Genetics of post-traumatic stress disorder: informing clinical conceptualizations and promoting future research. *American Journal of Medical Genetics C: Seminars in Medical Genetics*, **148C**, 127–132.

Ohara, K., Nagai, M., Suzuki, Y., Ochiai, M., & Ohara, K. (1998). No association between anxiety disorders and catechol-O-methyltransferase polymorphism. *Psychiatry Research*, **80**, 145–148.

Ohara, K., Suzuki, Y., Ochiai, M., *et al.* (1999). A variable-number-tandem-repeat of the serotonin transporter gene and anxiety disorders. *Progress in Neuro-Psychopharmacology and Biological Psychiatry*, **23**, 55–65.

Pauls, D. (2008). The genetics of obsessive–compulsive disorder: a review of the evidence. *American Journal of Medical Genetics C: Seminars in Medical Genetics*, **148C**, 133–139.

Pauls, D., Alsobrook, J. P., Goodman, W., Rasmussen, S., & Leckman, J. F. (1995). A family study of obsessive–

compulsive disorder. *American Journal of Psychiatry*, **152**, 76–84.

Perna, G., Caldirola, D., Arancio, C., & Bellodi, L. (1997). Panic attacks: a twin study. *Psychiatry Research*, **66**, 69–71.

Plomin, R., Emde, R., Bruaungart, J., *et al.* (1993). Genetic change and continuity from fourteen to twenty months: the MacArthur Longitudinal Twin Study. *Child Development*, **64**, 1354–1376.

Plomin, R., DeFries, J. C., McClearn, G. E., & McGuffin, P. (2001). *Behavioral Genetics*. New York, NY: Worth.

Poulton, R., Andrews, G., & Millichamp, J. (2008). Gene–environment interaction and the anxiety disorders. *European Archives of Psychiatry and Clinical Neuroscience*, **258**, 65–68.

Risch, N. J., & Merikangas, K. (1996). The future of genetic studies of complex human diseases. *Science*, **273**, 1516–1517.

Robinson, J., Kagan, J., Reznick, J., & Corley, P. A. (1992). The heritability of inhibited and uninhibited behavior: a twin study. *Development and Psychopathology*, **28**, 1030–1037.

Rosenbaum, J., Biederman, J., Hirshfeld-Becker, D. R., *et al.* (2000). A controlled study of behavioral inhibition in children of parents with panic disorder and depression. *American Journal of Psychiatry*, **157**, 2002–2010.

Rowe, D., Stever, C., Gard, J., *et al.* (1998). The relation of the dopamine transporter gene (DAT1) to symptoms of internalizing disorders in children. *Behavior Genetics*, **28**, 215–225.

Sack, W. H., Clarke, G. N., & Seeley, J. (1995). Posttraumatic stress disorder across two generations of Cambodian refugees. *Journal of the American Academy of Child and Adolescent Psychiatry*, **34**, 1160–1166.

Saiz, P. A., Garcia-Portilla, M. P., Arango, C., *et al.* (2008). Association study between obsessive–compulsive disorder and serotonergic candidate genes. *Progress in Neuro-Psychopharmacology and Biological Psychiatry*, **32**, 765–770.

Samochowiec, J., Hajduk, A., Samochowiec, A., *et al.* (2004). Association studies of MAO-A, COMT, and 5-HTT genes polymorphisms in patients with anxiety disorders of the phobic spectrum. *Psychiatry Research*, **128**, 21–26.

Schindler, K., Richter, M. A., Kennedy, J. L., Pato, M., & Pato, C. (2000). Association between homozygosity at the COMT gene locus and obsessive compulsive disorder. *American Journal of Medical Genetics*, **96**, 721–724.

Schinka, J. A. (2005). Measurement scale does moderate the association between the serotonin transporter gene and trait anxiety: comments on Munafo *et al. Molecular Psychiatry*, **10**, 892–893.

Schwartz, C., Snidman, N., & Kagan, J. (1999). Adolescent social anxiety as an outcome of inhibited temperament in childhood. *Journal of the American Academy of Child and Adolescent Psychiatry*, **38**, 1008–1015.

Seckl, J., & Meaney, M. (2006). Glucocorticoid "programming" and PTSD risk. *Annals of the New York Academy of Sciences*, **1071**, 351–378.

Segman, R. H., Cooper-Kazaz, R., Macciardi, F., *et al.* (2002). Association between the dopamine transporter gene and posttraumatic stress disorder. *Molecular Psychiatry*, **7**, 903–907.

Shifman, S., Bhomra, A., & Smiley, S. (2008). A whole genome association study of neuroticism using DNA pooling. *Molecular Psychiatry*, **13**, 302–312.

Shugart, Y., Samuels, J., Willour, V., *et al.* (2006). Genomewide linkage scan for obsessive–compulsive disorder: evidence for susceptibility loci on chromosomes 3q, 7p, 1q, 15q, and 6q. *Molecular Psychiatry*, **11**, 763–770.

Skinner, M., Anway, M. D., Savenkova, M. I., Gore, A. C., & Crews, D. (2008). Transgenerational epigenetic programming of the brain transcriptome and anxiety behavior. *PloS ONE*, **3** (11), e3745.

Skre, I., Onstad, S., Torgesen, S., Lygren, S., & Kringlen, E. (1993). A twin study of DSM-III-R anxiety disorders. *Acta Psychiatrica Scandinavica*, **88**, 85–92.

Smoller, J. W. (2008). Genetics of mood and anxiety disorders. In J. W. Smoller, B. R. Sheidley, & M. T. Tsuang, eds., *Psychiatric Genetics: Applications in Clinical Practice*. Washington, DC: American Psychiatric Publishing, pp. 131–176.

Smoller, J., Acerno, J., Rosenbaum, J., *et al.* (2001a). Targeted genome screen of panic disorder and anxiety disorder proneness using homology to murine QTL regions. *American Journal of Medical Genetics*, **105**, 195–206.

Smoller, J., Rosenbaum, J. F., Biederman, J., *et al.* (2001b). Genetic association analysis of behavioral inhibition using candidate loci from mouse models. *American Journal of Medical Genetics B: Neuropsychiatric Genetics*, **105B**, 226–235.

Smoller, J., Rosenbaum, J. F., Biederman, J., *et al.* (2003). Association of a genetic marker at the corticotropin-releasing hormone locus with behavioral inhibition. *Biological Psychiatry*, **54**, 1376–1381.

Smoller, J., Yamaki, L. H., Fagerness, J. A., *et al.* (2005). The corticotropin releasing hormone gene and behavioral inhibition in children at risk for panic disorder. *Biological Psychiatry*, **57**, 1485–1492.

Smoller, J., Paulus, M. P., Fagerness, J. A., *et al.* (2008a). Influence of RGS2 on anxiety-related temperament, personality, and brain function. *Archives of General Psychiatry*, **65**, 298–308.

Smoller, J., Gardner-Schuster, E., & Covino, J. (2008b). The genetic basis of panic and phobic anxiety disorders. *American Journal of Medical Genetics C: Seminars in Medical Genetics*, **148C**, 118–126.

Stein, M., Chartier, M., Hazen, A., *et al.* (1998a). A direct-interview family study of generalized social phobia. *American Journal of Psychiatry*, **155**, 90–97.

Stein, M. B., Chartier, M. J., Kozak, M. V., King, N., & Kennedy, J. L. (1998b). Genetic linkage to the serotonin transporter protein and 5HT2A receptor genes excluded in generalized social phobia. *Psychiatry Research*, **81**, 283–291.

Stein, M. B., Jang, K. J., & Livesley, J. (1999). Heritability of anxiety sensitivity: a twin study. *American Journal of Psychiatry*, **156**, 246–251.

Stein, M. B., Jang, K. J., Taylor, S., Vernon, P. A., & Livesley, W. J. (2002). Genetic and environmental influences on trauma exposure and posttraumatic stress disorder: a twin study. *American Journal of Psychiatry*, **159**, 1675–1681.

Stein, M., Fallin, M., Schork, N., J, & Gelernter, J. (2005). COMT polymorphisms and anxiety-related personality traits. *Neuropsychopharmacology*, **30**, 2092–2102.

Stein, M. B., Seedat, S., & Gelernter, J. (2006). Serotonin transporter gene promoter polymorphism predicts SSRI response in generalized social anxiety disorder. *Psychopharmacology*, **187**, 68–72.

Stein, M. B., Schork, N., J, & Gelernter, J. (2008). Gene-by-environment (serotonin transporter and childhood maltreatment) interaction for anxiety sensitivity, an intermediate phenotype for anxiety disorders. *Neuropsychopharmacology*, **33**, 312–319.

Stewart, S., Fagerness, J. A., Platko, J., *et al.* (2007). Association of the SLCA1 glutamate transporter gene and obsessive–compulsive disorder. *American Journal of Medical Genetics B: Neuropsychiatric Genetics*, **144B**, 1027–1033.

Strug, L., Suresh, R., Fyer, A., *et al.* (2010). Panic disorder is associated with the serotonin transporter gene (SLC6A4) but not the promoter region (5-HTTLPR). *Molecular Psychiatry*, **15**, 166–176.

Tadic, A., Rujescu, D., Szegedi, A., *et al.* (2003). Association of a MAOA gene variant with generalized anxiety disorder, but not with panic disorder or major depression. *American Journal of Medical Genetics B: Neuropsychiatric Genetics*, **117**, 1–6.

Talati, A., Ponniah, K., Strug, L., *et al.* (2008). Panic disorder, social anxiety disorder, and a possible medical syndrome previously linked to chromosome 13. *Biological Psychiatry*, **63**, 594–601.

Taylor, S., Jang, K. L., Stewart, S. H., & Stein, M. B. (2008). Etiology of the dimensions of anxiety sensitivity: a behavioral-genetic analysis. *Journal of Anxiety Disorders*, **22**, 899–914.

Thorgeirsson, T. E., Oskarsson, H., Desnica, N., *et al.* (2003). Anxiety with panic disorder linked to chromosome 9q in Iceland. *American Journal of Human Genetics*, **72**, 1221–1230.

Tochigi, M., Hibino, H., Otowa, T., *et al.* (2006). Association between dopamine D4 receptor (DRD4) exon III polymorphism and neuroticism in the Japanese population. *Neuroscience Letters*, **398**, 333–336.

Torgersen, S. (1983). Genetic factors in anxiety disorders. *Archives of General Psychiatry*, **40**, 1085–1089.

Tot, S., Erdal, M., Yazici, K., Yazici, A., & Metin, O. (2003). T102C and -1438 G/A polymorphisms of the 5-HT2A receptor gene in Turkish patients with obsessive–compulsive disorder. *European Psychiatry*, **18**, 249–254.

True, W. J., Rice, J., Eisen, S. A., *et al.* (1993). A twin study of genetic and environmental contributions to liability for posttraumatic stress symptoms. *Archives of General Psychiatry*, **50**, 257–264.

Turner, S., Bieidel, D., & Wolff, P. (1996). Is behavioral inhibition related to the anxiety disorders? *Clinical Psychology Review*, **16**, 157–172.

van Beek, N., & Griez, E. (2003). Anxiety sensitivity in first-degree relatives of patients with panic disorder. *Behavior Research and Therapy*, **41**, 949–957.

van Grootheest, D., Bartels, M., Cath, D., *et al.* (2007). Genetic and environmental contributions underlying stability in childhood obsessive–compulsive behavior. *Biological Psychiatry*, **61**, 308–315.

van Grootheest, D., Cath, D., Beekman, A., & Boomsma, D. (2005). Twin studies on obsessive–compulsive disorder: A review. *Twin Research Human Genetics*, **8**, 450–458.

Wacker, J., Reuter, M., Hennig, J., & Stemmler, G. (2006). Sexually dimorphic link between dopamine D2 receptor gene and neuroticism–anxiety. *Neuroreport*, **16**, 611–614.

Walitza, S., Wewetzer, C., Warnke, A., *et al.* (2002). 5-HT2A promoter polymorphism -1438G/A in children and adolescents with obsessive–compulsive disorders. *Molecular Psychiatry*, **7**, 1054–1057.

Walitza, S., Wewetzer, C., Gerlach, M., *et al.* (2004). Transmission disequilibrium studies in children and adolescents with obsessive–compulsive disorders pertaining to polymorphisms of genes of the serotonergic pathway. *Journal of Neural Transmission*, **111**, 817–825.

Weissman, M., Fyer, A., Haghighi, F., *et al.* (2000). Potential panic disorder syndrome: Clinical and genetic linkage evidence. *American Journal of Medical Genetics*, **96**, 24–35.

Weissman, M., Gross, R., Fyer, A., *et al.* (2004). Interstitial cystitis and panic disorder: a potential genetic syndrome. *Archives of General Psychiatry*, **61**, 273–279.

Willis-Owen, S. A. G., Fullerton, J., Surtees, P. G., *et al.* (2005). The Val66Met coding variant of the brain-derived neurotrophic factor (BDNF) gene does not contribute toward variation in the personality trait neuroticism. *Biological Psychiatry*, **58**, 738–742.

Willour, V., Yao Shugart, Y., Samuels, J., *et al.* (2004). Replication study supports evidence for linkage to 9p24 in obsessive–compulsive disorder. *American Journal of Human Genetics*, **75**, 508–513.

Yehuda, R., Halligan, S. L., & Bierer, L. M. (2001). Relationship of parental trauma exposure and PTSD to PTSD, depressive and anxiety disorders in offspring. *Journal of Psychiatric Research*, **35**, 261–270.

Yehuda, R., Bell, A., Bierer, L., & Schmeidler, J. (2008). Maternal, not paternal, PTSD is related to increased risk for PTSD in offspring of Holocaust survivors. *Journal of Psychiatric Research*, **42**, 1104–1111.

You, J.-S., Hu, S.-Y., Chen, B., & Zhang, H. G. (2005). Serotonin transporter and tryptophan hydroxylase gene polymorphisms in Chinese patients with generalized anxiety disorder. *Psychiatric Genetics*, **15**, 7–11.

Young, B. R., Lawford, B. R., Noble, E. P., *et al.* (2002). Harmful drinking in military veterans with posttraumatic stress disorder: association with the D2 dopamine receptor A1 allele. *Alcohol & Alcoholism*, **37**, 451–456.

Animal models of anxiety disorders: behavioral and genetic approaches

Jesse W. Richardson-Jones, E. David Leonardo, Rene Hen, Susanne E. Ahmari

14.1 Introduction

Animal models are key to our understanding of many human diseases, and psychiatric disorders are no exception. Animal models have provided insight into the neurotransmitter systems and brain circuitry underlying psychiatric illness, enabled the screening of potential psychiatric medications for efficacy, and guided the search for new pharmacotherapies. However, modeling complex psychiatric disorders in animals presents distinct challenges.

Modeling psychiatric disorders in animals is difficult due to the complexity of human thoughts, emotions, and behavior; the heterogeneity of many psychiatric disorders; and the requirement of self-report of internal state for diagnosis. According to the DSM-IV, most psychiatric diagnoses are made when a patient displays a certain number of diagnostic criteria (e.g., five out of nine criteria must be met to make a diagnosis of major depressive disorder) (American Psychiatric Association 2000). However, patients with the same diagnosis can differ significantly in specific symptoms, perhaps implying differences in the underlying etiology of their disorders and explaining the heterogeneity of response to pharmacotherapy (Fava *et al.* 2008). Many symptoms are identified by the patient's report of internal state (e.g., obsessive obtrusive thoughts). This leads to questions of how we best can model in animals disorders that are, by definition, both heterogeneous and dependent on report of internal state.

Rather than attempting to model a psychiatric disorder in its entirety, most neuroscientists focus on individual aspects or dimensions of a disorder (Gottesman & Gould 2003, Frazer & Morilak 2005, Lapiz-Bluhm *et al.* 2008) and use physical manifestations and measurable behaviors when modeling a particular aspect. Detailing the diverse approaches to developing animal models is beyond the scope of this chapter and has been

reviewed elsewhere (Arguello & Gogos 2006); instead, in this chapter we review methods for validating animal models of psychiatric disorders and discuss specific models of anxiety in mice. Finally, we outline some of the genetic technologies used in the mouse to address gene function, with a focus on our laboratory's use of genetically modified mice to probe the role of serotonin-1A (5-HT$_{1A}$) receptors in anxiety-like behaviors.

14.2 Types of validity

Inferences from experiments with animal models have the potential to impact clinical practice; therefore, stringently validating such models is of utmost importance. The strengths and weaknesses of a model can be conceptualized as different types of *validity*. Three important types of validity are reviewed below: *face*, *construct*, and *predictive* validity (Bloom & Kupfer 1995).

The theory of *face validity* is conceptually simple to understand. An animal model of a human psychiatric disorder can be judged by whether it "resembles" aspects of the human disorder, such as a particular symptom or set of symptoms (McKinney 1984). For example, one rodent model of depression measures the physiological and behavioral effects of chronic stress (Willner 1997). One measured outcome is the deterioration of an animal's overall coat state and a lack of grooming when its coat is soiled. Some depressed patients display decreased personal hygiene and self-care, so these measures contribute to the face validity of the chronic stress model. In general, face validity is strengthened by the number of similarities between the model and the disorder (Willner & Mitchell 2002). Thus, other outcomes of chronic stress that resemble symptoms of human depression, such as decreased feeding accompanied by weight loss or disrupted circadian rhythms, will increase the model's face validity for depression.

Anxiety Disorders: Theory, Research, and Clinical Perspectives, ed. Helen Blair Simpson, Yuval Neria, Roberto Lewis-Fernández, Franklin Schneier. Published by Cambridge University Press. © Cambridge University Press 2010.

Another method for evaluating the validity of an animal model requires defining a process hypothesized to underlie the human psychiatric disorder and measuring how well the model captures this process. This is called *construct validity* (Bloom & Kupfer 1995). For example, researchers modeling dependency and addiction often use the construct of impulsivity (Perry & Carroll 2008). The hypothesis is that the process of becoming dependent on a substance requires a switch from impulsively taking a drug to compulsively taking the drug, with initial levels of impulsivity thought to predict this switch and thus predict the risk of dependence (Belin *et al.* 2008). Impulsive behavior can be modeled in rodents by training them to wait a specific amount of time to perform a certain behavior (such as poking their nose through a hole) to receive a reward. In this task, mice or rats can be separated into those with high or low impulsivity. Those with high impulsivity quickly poke their noses through the hole; those with low impulsivity can wait for a reward. Interestingly, those with high impulsivity poke their noses through the hole repeatedly even when trained that this will result in no reward, also demonstrating construct validity for compulsivity (Robbins 2002). Construct validity is strengthened by knowledge about neural circuitry in humans. For example, if a clinical study of patients with substance dependence shows abnormal activity in a circuit involving the nucleus accumbens, the construct validity of impulsive nose poking will be increased if highly impulsive animals show increased activity in a similar circuit.

A third method for evaluating animal models focuses on the predictability of a response to a treatment intervention. If a model reliably responds to an intervention in a way similar to known outcomes in a patient population, it demonstrates *predictive validity* (Bloom & Kupfer 1995). Commonly, predictive validity in psychiatric animal models is based on pharmacotherapy. The forced swim test is a classic example of a model with strong predictive pharmacological validity. In this task, a rodent is exposed to inescapable swimming stress; 24 hours later, the animal is injected acutely with an antidepressant compound, placed back into the water, and monitored again to determine the amount of time it spends swimming. All drugs that treat depression in humans increase swimming in the forced swim test, while drug treatments for other disorders do not (Lucki 1997). Predictive validity is strengthened when a model not only responds positively to a given intervention ("true positive" effects), but also fails to respond to

interventions that are not effective in human patients ("true negative" effects) (Willner & Mitchell 2002). Thus, the validity of the forced swim test is strengthened by the that fact that swimming is not increased by non-antidepressant drugs.

The relative importance of each separate type of validity is debated in the field (van der Staay 2006), and many animal models possess some validity in each of the dimensions outlined here. For example, although the forced swim test clearly demonstrates predictive validity as described, it also demonstrates face validity. "Depressed" mice (as defined by the pharmacological response) "give up" their attempts at swimming more readily, which can be compared to the despair and helplessness seen in depressed patients. An important caveat to remember when assessing the separate types of validity is that each alone has shortcomings. Face validity can be both overly stringent (in requiring that most or all of a set of symptoms be modeled) and also overly subjective and anthropomorphic, focusing only on what a model "looks like"; construct validity can allow modeling that is overly broad, as a particular construct may underlie many related or unrelated disorders; strict predictive validity can constrain a model to what is already known about a disorder, and may select against treatments with novel mechanisms of action. Thus, good models of psychiatric disorders should be based on one or more forms of validity but should also be constantly re-evaluated as more information about the disorder and the model becomes available. Moreover, it is important to keep in mind that no single animal model of a psychiatric disorder will ever be sufficient to address all aspects of the human disorder.

14.3 Animal models of anxiety disorders

Anxiety is a normal and adaptive state of autonomic arousal and behavioral defense in response to threat, which can become pathological when it increases in scope, magnitude, or duration (Nesse 1999). As defined in the DSM-IV, there are six major anxiety disorders in adults: specific phobia, characterized by intense fear elicited by a specific trigger; panic disorder, characterized by intense and debilitating (but relatively transient) bouts of anxiety; generalized anxiety disorder, characterized by excessive and pervading worry; social anxiety disorder, characterized by avoidance and fear of social situations; posttraumatic stress disorder, characterized by anxiety and fear precipitated by reminders of a previously experienced traumatic event; and obsessive–compulsive disorder, characterized by anxiety-producing obsessions and related compulsions which tend to reduce anxiety. Behavioral tests used to model anxiety-like behavior in animals often do not distinguish between the various forms of anxiety disorders; this is likely exacerbated by the fact that some of the criteria that differentiate anxiety disorders are not easily assayed in animals (Andreatini *et al.* 2001).

As anxiety disorders have many well-documented drug therapies (Nemeroff 2003), predictive pharmacological validity is widely considered to be required when developing mouse models of anxiety. Therefore, while most animal models of anxiety do have construct and face validity, strong models are classically validated with acutely acting anxiolytics such as benzodiazepines. Some researchers argue against the use of benzodiazepines to validate all models of anxiety, in part because only some anxiety disorders respond well to these drugs (Rodgers 1997). Selective serotonin reuptake inhibitors (SSRIs), which are currently the first-line treatment for most anxiety disorders (Haller *et al.* 2004), are effective in some of the models discussed below as well.

Demonstrating specific predictive validity for animal models of anxiety is also complicated by the fact that SSRIs treat both anxiety disorders and depressive disorders, despite these drugs being commonly referred to as "antidepressants." The fact that both types of illnesses respond to the same class of medications is not surprising, considering the significant comorbidity between anxiety and depression, significant overlap in symptom dimensions, and overlap in the circuitry and neurochemistry affected (Ressler & Nemeroff 2000, Nemeroff 2002). Although an argument can be made that some behavioral models address pure "anxiety," and other models are more valid for purely depressive-like behavior (Ohl *et al.* 2001), in reality it is perhaps more accurate to describe these models as addressing affective disorders in general, with relevance to both anxiety and depression. This complexity does not prevent us from validating animal models of anxiety disorders, and it may actually permit investigation of some of the overlap between anxiety and depression.

Finally, it is important to delineate the extent to which animal models of anxiety can truly model *disorders* of anxiety in humans. An individual with an anxiety disorder has both high levels of anxiety relative to other people and impaired functioning in daily life. Although higher or lower levels of anxiety-like behavior can be determined in animal models, impairment

of daily functioning is largely meaningless in a laboratory animal. While this represents a significant challenge to modeling pathological anxiety, it does not preclude modeling anxiety in animals, as will be discussed below.

14.4 Behavioral models of anxiety

Existing models of anxiety-like behavior in rodents can be roughly separated by whether the behavior assayed is learned or innate (Millan 2003). A large body of literature about learned anxiety-related behavior revolves mostly around forms of fear conditioning (classical conditioning to an aversive stimulus). Controversy exists in the field regarding whether innate or learned anxiety-like behaviors more closely model anxiety in humans (Kalueff & Murphy 2007). Indeed, while some human anxiety disorders, such as posttraumatic stress disorder, likely incorporate learned components, other disorders, such as generalized anxiety disorder, have no clearly learned etiology. In general, animal models that require learning in addition to expression of defensive or anxiety-like behavior are difficult to interpret; for example, an increase in the expression of learned fear may arise from either a difference in memory or a difference in fear or anxiety levels (Maren 2001). To simplify the discussion, we will focus here on models that measure largely innate behaviors; fear conditioning is discussed in more depth elsewhere (Chapter 16).

A key feature of human anxiety is defensive behavior in response to a real or perceived threat. This can be mapped onto the animal construct of defensive behavior or approach/avoidance conflict (Blanchard *et al.* 2001a). Anxiety is often characterized by the internal tensions between two conflicting desires, for example, the desire to explore a novel situation (in the example of social anxiety disorder, a party) and the inhibiting fear of encountering unknown stressors in novel environments (i.e., meeting new people). Many behavioral models of anxiety in rodents use the construct of approach/avoidance behavior or defensive behavior in response to novelty or an aversive stimulus (Blanchard *et al.* 2001b). Practically, this involves observing an animal's behavior in an environment consisting of sections that are hypothesized to be "safer" and other sections that are more "dangerous." Examples include environmental exploration-based paradigms such as the elevated plus maze (Lister 1987), the open field test, the light/dark choice test (Belzung *et al.* 1987); feeding-based tasks such as the novelty-suppressed feeding and novelty-induced hypophagia tasks (Bodnoff *et al.* 1989, Dulawa & Hen 2005); and tasks that

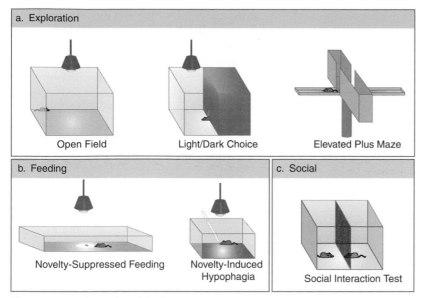

Figure 14.1. Behavioral models of anxiety.
(a) The open field, light/dark choice test, and elevated plus maze are all behavioral models of anxiety based on the conflict between exploration and avoidance of a novel environment. The aversive, or "anxiogenic," areas in these tests are: (1) the exposed center of the arena in the open field, (2) the brightly lit half of the arena in the light/dark chioce, and (3) the open, elevated platforms in the elevated plus maze. In these tests, anxiety-like behavior is scored based on the amount of total exploration and the exploration of the aversive areas in the testing arena.
(b) The novelty-suppressed feeding and novelty-induced hypophagia tests are behavioral models of anxiety based on the conflict between the desire to consume food and aversion to a bright, novel cage (in the novelty-induced hypophagia test) or to a large, bright, novel arena (in the novelty-suppressed feeding test). Anxiety-like behavior in the novelty-suppressed feeding test is assessed by measuring the latency of the mouse to consume a food pellet in the middle of the brightly lit arena following food restriction. The novelty-induced hypophagia test is slightly different, measuring the amount of sweetened condensed milk consumed in the novel environment, following home-cage training sessions that teach the animal to drink this palatable substance.
(c) The social interaction test measures an animal's response to a novel or familiar rodent, and scores its anxiety-like behavior based on time spent in social exploration versus time spent performing defensive behaviors such as freezing.

measure social behaviors, such as the social interaction test (File 1980) (Figure 14.1).

Approach/avoidance tasks have, by definition, relatively high levels of construct validity; some, like the social interaction test, even have face validity for certain anxiety disorders. All of these tasks also have predictive pharmacological validity, since the anxiety-like measures in all of them are decreased by acute administration of the anxiolytic benzodiazepines (Belzung *et al.* 1987, Lister 1987). Some anxiety-like tasks, such as the feeding-based tasks and the open field test (under certain conditions) also respond to chronic treatment with SSRIs. Fittingly, few anxiety-related measures in these tests are decreased by acute treatment with SSRIs, greatly increasing the predictive pharmacological validity of such models, since human anxiety is also insensitive to acute treatment with these drugs (Borsini *et al.* 2002).

Finally, it is instructive to examine the learned helplessness paradigm, a behavioral model most associated with depression. This task is an interesting example of the complexities involved in modeling affective disorders. Briefly, it involves giving a rodent repeated foot shocks, then measuring (1) its latency to escape from the shock environment when an exit is provided, and/or (2) the amount of time it spends in defensive behaviors such as freezing, and/or (3) other measures, such as anhedonia (Weiss *et al.* 1981). Learned helplessness is often described as an animal model of depression, since facets of this model have both face and construct validity for depression (Porter *et al.* 1986). However, it also has high predictive validity for both anxiety and depression, since administration of either chronic antidepressant compounds (of multiple classes) or acute benzodiazepine prevents the increase in escape latency caused by inescapable shock (Drugan *et al.* 1984, Gambarana *et al.* 2001). From a pharmacological validity standpoint, restriction of this model's relevance to only depression (or only anxiety) therefore seems unfounded. This complexity underscores the fact that depression and anxiety are linked disorders and also highlights the necessity of examining multiple dimensions of validity when evaluating models of psychiatric disorders.

The examples discussed above are by no means an exhaustive list of tests used to model anxiety disorders in animals. Other tests (both related and unrelated to the ones described) are commonly performed by researchers as models of anxiety, and the search for better (i.e., more valid) models is ongoing. However, the tests outlined are some of the most robust and widely used models, and understanding these models of anxiety in rodents provides an essential foundation for investigating the effects of candidate genes on anxiety.

14.5 Genetic technologies

Having reliable and validated behavioral models of anxiety disorders enables neuroscientists to test specific genetic hypotheses about these disorders. The known targets of current drug therapies, combined with specific genetic association studies, have provided clues about the neural substrates of anxiety disorders. For example, both the efficacy of SSRIs in treating anxiety and the genetic association of serotonin transporter polymorphisms with depression and anxiety have implicated the serotonergic system in the etiology and treatment of these disorders (Serretti *et al.* 2006). However, determining the identity and location of serotonin receptors involved in anxiety regulation is often impossible in humans. Directly testing hypotheses regarding the role of particular genes in anxiety is possible through the use of genetically modified mice.

For neuroscientists, mice offer the advantages of a relatively complex brain, with much circuitry similar to humans, combined with a short generation length (approximately 12 weeks) and an easily modified genome compared to other rodents (Jacob & Kwitek 2002). In 1989, Capecchi, Martins, and Smithies began exploiting these characteristics by creating the first mouse that lacked a specific gene throughout its life in all areas of the body (called a *knockout* mouse). Over the last 20 years, a number of genetic technologies in mice have been developed that advance this technology and allow for even more specific gene manipulations in vivo.

Currently, two main types of genetically modified mice are used in our laboratory: (1) *knockout mice* or *knock-in mice* and (2) *transgenic mice*. Below we review both technologies and discuss their strengths and weaknesses for determining the role of specific genes in an intact animal. Finally, we detail the ways in which a combination of the two technologies can address temporal- and region-specific gene function.

To understand the technologies described below, it is necessary to understand that a gene encoding a particular protein consists of two parts: (1) the *promoter region*, which dictates the place and time that the protein is expressed in an animal, and (2) the *coding region*, which contains the DNA representing the protein of interest. By making changes in either the promoter or the coding region, or both, our laboratory is able to directly control the time and place when particular proteins are expressed in mice.

14.5.1 Knockout and knock-in mice

A classical knockout or knock-in mouse is made by changing a specific gene in the mouse's genome. If the change turns off that gene, the mouse is called a knockout mouse. If new pieces of DNA are inserted into an existing gene in the mouse's genome, it is called a knock-in mouse (Figure 14.2a) (Melton 1994). These terms can be challenging to keep straight because, as we will discuss, knock-in technology can also be used to make a knockout mouse as well as other types of genetically modified mice.

Figure 14.2a depicts simple knockout and knock-in strategies. The first panel shows a simple knockout mouse, where the coding region has been removed from a gene, turning the gene off. Because the gene is turned off in all tissues for the animal's whole life, it is called a *constitutive* knockout. While constitutive knockout mice have furthered our understanding of gene function, this approach has several limitations. First, the specific tissue where the gene is important cannot be identified. Since genes often serve different functions in different regions of an animal, removing a gene everywhere can cause unexpected effects. For example, many genes expressed in the brain also play vital roles in the heart or kidneys; knockouts of these genes can cause complications ranging from difficulty in interpreting behavioral phenotypes to lethality. Additionally, constitutive knockouts do not allow for discrimination of different roles for a gene at different points in an animal's life cycle. In extreme cases, lacking a gene results in embryonic lethality, and the knockout mouse yields no information about adult gene function. The problem of temporal control is particularly important in the study of anxiety disorders, many of which likely have a developmental origin (Leonardo & Hen 2008). To get around these limitations, we can make changes to a gene that allow for regulation in subsets of areas at specific times using knock-in technology or transgenic mouse technology (detailed below).

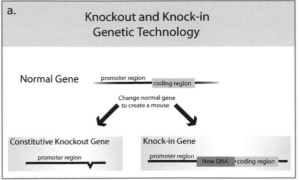

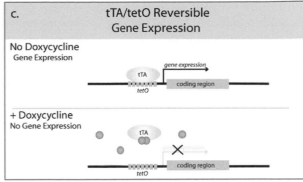

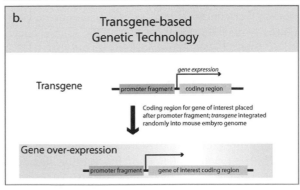

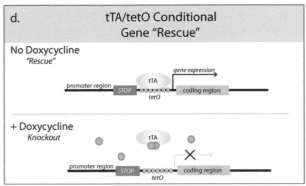

Figure 14.2. Genetic technology used to study the role of genes in behaviour.

(a) *Knockout* and *knock-in* technologies involve changing an existing gene in a mouse's genome. The change may excise the coding region for a gene (making a constitutive knockout mouse) or insert a new piece of DNA (making a knock-in mouse).

(b) *Transgenic* technology involves placing the coding sequence for a gene of interest under the transcriptional control of a well-characterized promoter fragment, creating a small, synthetic gene. The promoter fragment then controls the time and place of expression of the gene of interest. For example, this strategy may be used to "over-express" a gene of interest in a certain region of the mouse.

(c) The tTA/tetO system allows for conditional expression of a gene of interest with tetO sites placed before its coding sequence. The tTA activator protein binds tetO sites and causes gene expression; addition of the antibiotic doxycycline prevents tTA from binding to tetO sites and halts transcription.

(d) The tTA/tetO system can be used to conditionally "rescue" expression of a gene of interest. In this example, a transcriptional "STOP" sequence and tetO DNA binding sites have been knocked-in to the endogenous DNA, yielding a conditional knockout of the gene of interest. Addition of a tTA activator protein to this modified gene yields a "rescue" of the gene of interest in cells expressing the tTA protein. Gene expression governed by tTA can be blocked by administration of the drug doxycycline.

These are called *conditional* genetic strategies, because the gene can be turned on or off in more specific ways.

14.5.2 Transgenic mice

Transgenic mice differ from knockout or knock-in mice by the nature of the changes to their genome. Whereas knockout and knock-in mice have one of their own genes specifically changed, transgenic mice have DNA for a small, synthetic gene that is not their own (*transgenes*) inserted randomly into their genome (Gordon *et al.* 1980).

As shown in Figure 14.2b, a typical transgene is synthesized to consist of two parts: (1) a piece of DNA containing a well-characterized promoter fragment (which directs gene expression in a particular area) and (2) the coding sequence of another gene of interest that one wants to control. The promoter fragment directs the time and place of expression of the gene of interest. To make a transgenic mouse, the DNA of the chosen promoter fragment and the coding region of the gene of interest – together, the transgene – is introduced randomly into mouse embryo DNA. The resulting mouse contains one or many copies of the transgene in all its cells (Hickman-Davis & Davis 2006).

A simple application of this system leads to expression of a gene of interest at very high levels ("over-expression") in a specific area to address the gene's function (Figure 14.2b). In one example of this approach, researchers made a transgenic mouse with very high expression of the *TrkB* gene (which expresses the receptor for an important growth factor) in the brain, driven by the brain-specific Thy-1 promoter. These mice displayed decreased anxiety-like behavior (as assessed in the elevated plus maze) and improved spatial learning, implicating normal *TrkB* expression in these behaviors (Koponen *et al.* 2004). The power of the transgenic system becomes even more apparent when combined with a conditional gene expression system commonly used in our laboratory and described in detail below: the tetracycline-inducible tTA/tetO system.

14.5.3 The tTA/tetO system

One widely used conditional gene expression system is the tTA/tetO system, which allows us to turn genes on or off in specific areas. It consists of two parts: (1) a binding protein called tTA (tetracycline-dependent transcriptional activator) that activates gene expression and (2) a DNA sequence that this protein binds to, called tetO (Gossen & Bujard 1992). This tetO sequence is placed directly in front of the gene of interest, using either a knock-in approach, to target a gene already in the mouse, or a transgenic approach, for a gene not normally expressed by the mouse. A mouse with tetO sites in front of one gene is then bred to a mouse expressing tTA; this yields mice with both the tTA activation protein and the gene containing the tetO DNA sequence (Figure 14.2c). Anywhere the tTA activation protein is expressed, it binds to tetO DNA and activates gene expression.

A particular advantage of this system is that gene expression is reversible. tTA can form a complex with the drug tetracycline (or its brain-permeable analog, doxycycline). When it forms this complex, it cannot bind to tetO DNA. Gene expression is therefore turned off (Figure 14.2c). Removal of tetracycline or doxycycline allows gene expression to occur once more. Thus, genes can be turned on and off simply by feeding mice doxycycline or taking it away. This tTA/tetO system can be used to conditionally "rescue" gene expression in a knockout mouse, as will be discussed below (Figure 14.2d).

14.6 Our laboratory's approach: using transgenic mice to address the role of the 5-HT$_{1A}$ receptor in affective disorders

Several lines of evidence from human studies have implicated the 5-HT$_{1A}$ receptor in affective disorders. Human imaging data have reliably shown receptor binding levels to be decreased in depression (Drevets *et al.* 2007). Recently, a putatively functional polymorphism in the promoter region of the 5-HT$_{1A}$ genes has also been associated with depression and response to antidepressants (Le Francois *et al.* 2008). Moreover, this receptor is the direct target of the anxiolytic drug buspirone (Sramek *et al.* 2002).

Studies of 5-HT$_{1A}$ knockout mice (constitutively lacking all 5-HT$_{1A}$ receptors) have likewise suggested a role for this receptor in anxiety and have hinted at a role in depression and the response to antidepressants. Three separate labs have shown that 5-HT$_{1A}$ knockout mice display increased anxiety-like behavior in approach/avoidance paradigms, and one study has also shown that these mice show increased fear behavior in a fear-conditioning paradigm (Heisler *et al.* 1998, Parks *et al.* 1998, Ramboz *et al.* 1998, Klemenhagen *et al.* 2006). Lastly, one report has shown that 5-HT$_{1A}$ knockout mice do not respond to the SSRI fluoxetine either behaviorally or with increased growth of new neurons, a known effect of SSRIs in some mice (Santarelli *et al.* 2003). Together, these data suggest that 5-HT$_{1A}$ likely participates in circuitry that is important for the expression of anxiety and depression.

However, interpretation of the existing literature is complicated by the biology of the 5-HT$_{1A}$ receptor. This receptor is localized in the cell body and dendrites of both serotonergic neurons in the raphe nuclei and in non-serotonergic neurons that receive input from serotonergic axons in various regions in the rest of the brain (e.g., the hippocampus, prefrontal cortex, and amygdala). In the raphe, the 5-HT$_{1A}$ receptor acts as an inhibitory autoreceptor, regulating levels of its own neurotransmitter (Blier *et al.* 1998). In other parts of the brain, the 5-HT$_{1A}$ receptor acts as an inhibitory heteroreceptor, mediating some of the effects of released serotonin. Because 5-HT$_{1A}$ autoreceptors in the raphe set overall serotonergic tone in the brain through negative feedback regulation, these receptors have been hypothesized to contribute to the delayed therapeutic action of antidepressant drugs by limiting the initial increase in serotonin in the brain (Gardier *et al.* 1996). Constitutive knockout mice are not useful for determining the likely complex roles of 5-HT$_{1A}$ auto- and heteroreceptors in anxiety-like behaviors, since they lack the receptor all over the brain for the entire life of the animal. Our laboratory has therefore employed advanced genetic techniques to examine different 5-HT$_{1A}$ receptor populations.

14.6.1 Using tTA/tetO to "rescue" gene expression

Following the initial findings of increased anxiety in constitutive 5-HT$_{1A}$ knockout mice in our lab and others, two separate questions about the phenotype remained unanswered: (1) whether the increased anxiety in 5-HT$_{1A}$ knockout mice was a result of lacking the receptor in development or adulthood, and (2) whether 5-HT$_{1A}$ autoreceptors or heteroreceptors were responsible for the phenotype.

To summarize terminology from the above sections that is essential to understand our experimental approach to address these questions, a constitutive knockout mouse can be created by two methods: (1) deleting the part of the gene that codes for its protein (simplest case, shown in Figure 14.2a) or (2) "knocking-in" a piece of DNA that prevents transcription (a STOP sequence). A conditional knockout can be made by inserting not only the STOP sequence but also pieces of a conditional system, such as the tTA/tetO system (shown in Figure 14.2d).

To address whether 5-HT$_{1A}$ heteroreceptors might be responsible for anxiety-like behavior, we used a combination of these methods to create a conditional knockout. Specifically, by inserting pieces of DNA into the 5-HT$_{1A}$ gene that prevent normal gene expression from occurring (the STOP sequence), we created a 5-HT$_{1A}$ knockout mouse (Figure 14.2d). However, this knockout was conditional, as we also inserted tetO DNA binding sites into the 5-HT$_{1A}$ gene. Receptor expression was then "rescued" by the addition of a tTA transgene, expressed here under the control of a promoter specifying expression in the forebrain. This leads to expression ("rescue") of 5-HT$_{1A}$ receptors only in the forebrain, mimicking the normal expression of 5-HT$_{1A}$ heteroreceptors, which allows us to examine the behavioral phenotype of a mouse that has only 5-HT$_{1A}$ heteroreceptors and not autoreceptors. Moreover, because tTA-mediated transcription is stopped when we feed the mouse doxycycline, this system allows completely inducible "rescue" or conditional knockout of 5-HT$_{1A}$ heteroreceptors (Stark *et al.* 2007).

Using this system, our lab demonstrated that the increased anxiety observed in the constitutive 5-HT$_{1A}$ knockout mouse could be reversed by "rescuing" 5-HT$_{1A}$ heteroreceptor expression in the forebrain early in postnatal development (Gross *et al.* 2002). Moreover, normal anxiety-like behavior was not affected by stopping 5-HT$_{1A}$ heteroreceptor expression in adulthood (by adding doxycycline), implying that 5-HT$_{1A}$ receptors are not necessary in adulthood for the maintenance of normal anxiety-like behavior. However, waiting to initiate expression of 5-HT$_{1A}$ receptors until the third to fourth postnatal week resulted in animals that still

behaved like constitutive 5-HT$_{1A}$ knockouts (i.e., displayed increased anxiety-like behavior) (Figure 14.3). Together, these data suggested that the anxiety phenotype of constitutive 5-HT$_{1A}$ knockout mice was due to stable changes that occurred in postnatal development as a result of lacking the 5-HT$_{1A}$ heteroreceptors. Moreover, it suggests that 5-HT$_{1A}$ heteroreceptors act during postnatal development to establish stable anxiety-related circuitry that persists into adulthood regardless of adult receptor expression.

Although this transgenic system proved useful in elucidating the developmental role of the 5-HT$_{1A}$ receptor in anxiety, several caveats to the approach are clear. First, control of 5-HT$_{1A}$ expression relies on the promoter of another gene, which is a problem shared by all tTA/tetO "rescue" designs. While such a strategy might roughly recapitulate normal expression patterns and levels, it cannot faithfully capture all aspects of normal gene expression. For example, our system yields 5-HT$_{1A}$ receptor expression in the striatum, a brain region where the receptor is not normally expressed. Such expression is called *ectopic*, and it complicates the interpretation of the phenotype observed in these mice. Second, the exact timing of receptor requirement is limited by the time constraints inherent to protein manufacture and degradation. The half-life of 5-HT$_{1A}$ receptor disappearance in this system was determined to be approximately two weeks, which prevented determination of an exact time window during which receptor expression was acting in developing neural circuits to affect anxiety. These caveats have encouraged the continued refinement of transgenic technology in our lab and others.

Despite its drawbacks, our 5-HT$_{1A}$ tTA-based rescue system exemplifies the power of using transgenic approaches to ask basic questions about contributions of particular genes to the development and maintenance of anxiety disorders. This work suggests a specific time window – between approximately the second and fifth postnatal weeks – for serotonin-mediated maturation of anxiety circuitry in mice. With this information, subsequent work in the lab has focused on identifying the circuit-level changes and intracellular signaling cascades that are important during this time. Comparing the human and mouse developmental time courses of maturation in particular brain regions can also help focus the studies of human anxiety disorders to the most appropriate developmental time points. The ultimate goal of such research is to use a better understanding of the biology of developmental anxiety

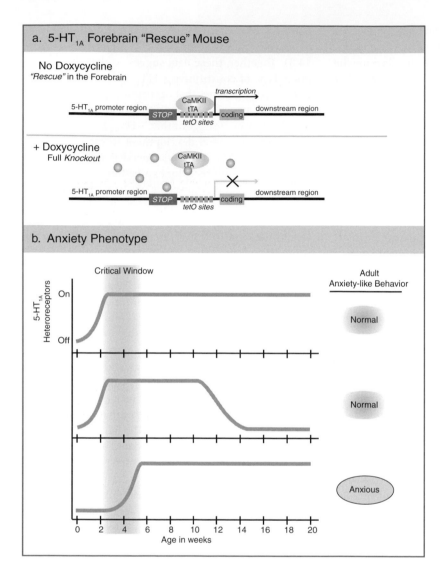

Figure 14.3. Using genetic mouse technology to address the spatial and temporal requirement for 5-HT$_{1A}$ receptors in anxiety-like behavior.

(a) The tTA/tetO system was used to create a mouse with 5-HT$_{1A}$ receptors expressed only in the forebrain (i.e., a "rescue" for 5-HT$_{1A}$ heteroreceptors). In the presence of doxycycline, the mouse lacks all 5-HT$_{1A}$ receptors (a knockout). In the absence of doxycycline, tTA causes expression of 5-HT$_{1A}$ receptors. The tTA transgene expression is governed by CaMKII promoter fragments only in the forebrain, so 5-HT$_{1A}$ receptors are "rescued" only in the forebrain.

(b) The time course of 5-HT$_{1A}$ heteroreceptor involvement in anxiety-like behavior was investigated. In the absence of doxycycline, tTA turned 5-HT$_{1A}$ receptors "on" by the second postnatal week, yielding a mouse with normal anxiety-like behavior in adulthood. Cessation of 5-HT$_{1A}$ receptor expression (with the addition of doxycycline) beginning at 12 weeks of age did not disrupt normal anxiety-like behavior. Finally, delay of 5-HT$_{1A}$ "rescue" until the fourth postnatal week was not sufficient to establish normal anxiety-like behavior in adulthood; these mice looked anxious, despite having receptors fully "on" at the time of testing. These experiments suggest that there is a critical window in the second through fourth postnatal weeks during which 5-HT$_{1A}$ heteroreceptors are necessary to help establish normal anxiety-like behavior.

programming to inform the design of more effective treatments for human anxiety disorders.

14.7 Conclusions

This overview provides a framework for interpreting experimental results from studies using animal models of anxiety and provides an overview of current state-of-the-art transgenic approaches used to dissect the neural circuitry underlying anxiety disorders. The caveats regarding interpretation of results from animal models of anxiety similarly apply to animal models of other psychiatric disorders. Likewise, the transgenic methodologies described here can be applied to genes other than the 5-HT$_{1A}$ receptor in order to determine their impact on psychiatric disorder pathophysiology.

The first section of this chapter demonstrates the importance of understanding the validity of a particular animal model, which assists in determining its clinical relevance in the context of careful interpretation. While most currently used models of anxiety are based on the construct of approach/avoidance behavior in response to a potentially threatening stimulus, it is likely that other constructs will soon be used to develop new models either of anxiety as a whole or of components of specific anxiety disorders. In addition, new paradigms will likely be developed to test and monitor anxiety-like behavior. To ensure that these models and paradigms are relevant to clinical disorders, it is important to stringently assess their validity by considering the criteria discussed here.

We have also reviewed how state-of-the-art transgenic technology can be used to make animal models that allow us to consider the contribution of particular genes to anxiety-like behaviors. Our laboratory's studies of the 5-HT$_{1A}$ receptor provide an illustrative example of the strengths and weaknesses inherent in using these genetic technologies to investigate the pathophysiology of anxiety. One major strength of this approach is that it permits investigation of the impact of gene expression during different developmental time points. Our laboratory is currently trying to improve temporal resolution in these experiments by narrowing the time window during which 5-HT$_{1A}$ receptors act in development to establish anxiety-related brain circuitry. In addition, this technology can be adapted to look at the impact of gene expression in different specific areas of the brain; this avoids the problems with ectopic expression of the receptor that are often present in the tTA/tetO system. Our lab is approaching this by developing other genetic inducible systems to more specifically target different 5-HT$_{1A}$ receptor populations (e.g., in the hippocampus or the raphe). Though transgenic studies are only one approach to investigating the impact of developmental and region-specific gene expression on the establishment of anxiety circuitry and development of anxiety-like behavior (Lo Iacono & Gross 2008), they represent a powerful method for modulating circuitry through manipulations of candidate genes.

We have focused on the 5-HT$_{1A}$ receptor in our review, but the methods discussed here can be applied to the study of other genes, both within the serotonin receptor family and outside it. For example, several lines of evidence implicate the 5-HT$_{1B}$ receptor, which has some functional characteristics similar to 5-HT$_{1A}$ receptors, in obsessive–compulsive disorder (Moret & Briley 2000, Zohar et al. 2004). We expect that some of the same methods employed to study the 5-HT$_{1A}$ receptor can be applied to study the role of the 5-HT$_{1B}$ receptor in the development of psychiatric pathophysiology. In sum, the behavioral and genetic approaches outlined here hold great potential to investigate the roles of different genes in the pathophysiology underlying many different psychiatric disorders. The genetic approaches being currently developed are constantly evolving to address ever more complex and interesting questions regarding the etiology and treatment of diverse psychiatric disorders.

References

American Psychiatric Association (2000). *Diagnostic and Statistical Manual of Mental Disorders*, 4th edn, text revision (DSM-IV-TR). Washington, DC: American Psychiatric Association.

Andreatini, R., Blanchard, C., Blanchard, R., *et al.* (2001). The brain decade in debate: II. Panic or anxiety? From animal models to a neurobiological basis. *Brazilian Journal of Medical and Biological Research*, **34**, 145–154.

Arguello, P. A., & Gogos, J. A. (2006). Modeling madness in mice: one piece at a time. *Neuron*, **52**, 179–196.

Belin, D., Mar, A. C., Dalley, J. W., Robbins, T. W., & Everitt, B. J. (2008). High impulsivity predicts the switch to compulsive cocaine-taking. *Science*, **320**, 1352–1355.

Belzung, C., Misslin, R., Vogel, E., Dodd, R. H., & Chapouthier, G. (1987). Anxiogenic effects of methyl-beta-carboline-3-carboxylate in a light/dark choice situation. *Pharmacology, Biochemistry, and Behavior*, **28**, 29–33.

Blanchard, D. C., Hynd, A. L., Minke, K. A., Minemoto, T., & Blanchard, R. J. (2001a). Human defensive behaviors to threat scenarios show parallels to fear- and anxiety-related defense patterns of non-human mammals. *Neuroscience and Biobehavioral Reviews*, **25**, 761–770.

Blanchard, D. C., Griebel, G., & Blanchard, R. J. (2001b). Mouse defensive behaviors: pharmacological and behavioral assays for anxiety and panic. *Neuroscience and Biobehavioral Reviews*, **25**, 205–218.

Blier, P., Pineyro, G., el Mansari, M., Bergeron, R., & de Montigny, C. (1998). Role of somatodendritic 5-HT autoreceptors in modulating 5-HT neurotransmission. *Annals of the New York Academy of Sciences*, **861**, 204–216.

Bloom, F. E. & Kupfer, D. J., eds. (1995). *Psychopharmacology: the Fourth Generation of Progress*. New York, NY: Raven Press.

Bodnoff, S. R., Suranyi-Cadotte, B., Quirion, R., & Meaney, M. J. (1989). A comparison of the effects of diazepam versus several typical and atypical anti-depressant drugs in an animal model of anxiety. *Psychopharmacology (Berlin)*, **97**, 277–279.

Borsini, F., Podhorna, J., & Marazziti, D. (2002). Do animal models of anxiety predict anxiolytic-like effects of antidepressants? *Psychopharmacology (Berlin)*, **163**, 121–141.

Drevets, W. C., Thase, M. E., Moses-Kolko, E. L., *et al.* (2007). Serotonin-1A receptor imaging in recurrent depression: replication and literature review. *Nuclear Medicine and Biology*, **34**, 865–877.

Drugan, R. C., Ryan, S. M., Minor, T. R., & Maier, S. F. (1984). Librium prevents the analgesia and shuttlebox escape deficit typically observed following inescapable shock. *Pharmacology Biochemistry and Behavior*, **21**, 749–754.

Dulawa, S. C., & Hen, R. (2005). Recent advances in animal models of chronic antidepressant effects: the novelty-induced hypophagia test. *Neuroscience and Biobehavioral Reviews*, **29**, 771–783.

Fava, M., Rush, A. J., Alpert, J. E., *et al.* (2008). Difference in treatment outcome in outpatients with anxious versus nonanxious depression: a STAR*D report. *American Journal of Psychiatry*, **165**, 342–351.

File, S. E. (1980). The use of social interaction as a method for detecting anxiolytic activity of chlordiazepoxide-like drugs. *Journal of Neuroscience Methods*, **2**, 219–238.

Frazer, A., & Morilak, D. A. (2005). What should animal models of depression model? *Neuroscience and Biobehavioral Reviews*, **29**, 515–523.

Gambarana, C., Scheggi, S., Tagliamonte, A., Tolu, P., & De Montis, M. G. (2001). Animal models for the study of antidepressant activity. *Brain Research. Brain Research Protocols*, **7**, 11–20.

Gardier, A. M., Malagie, I., Trillat, A. C., Jacquot, C., & Artigas, F. (1996). Role of 5-HT1A autoreceptors in the mechanism of action of serotoninergic antidepressant drugs: recent findings from in vivo microdialysis studies. *Fundamental and Clinical Pharmacology*, **10**, 16–27.

Gordon, J. W., Scangos, G. A., Plotkin, D. J., Barbosa, J. A., & Ruddle, F. H. (1980). Genetic transformation of mouse embryos by microinjection of purified DNA. *Proceedingss of the National Academy of Sciences of the USA*, **77**, 7380–7384.

Gossen, M., & Bujard, H. (1992). Tight control of gene expression in mammalian cells by tetracycline-responsive promoters. *Proceedings of the National Academy of Sciences of the USA*, **89**, 5547–5551.

Gottesman, I. I., & Gould, T. D. (2003). The endophenotype concept in psychiatry: etymology and strategic intentions. *American Journal of Psychiatry*, **160**, 636–645.

Gross, C., Zhuang, X., Stark, K., *et al.* (2002). Serotonin1A receptor acts during development to establish normal anxiety-like behaviour in the adult. *Nature*, **416**, 396–400.

Haller, J., Halasz, J., & Majercsik, E. (2004). Psychosocial conditions and the efficacy of clinically available anxiolytics. *Current Drug Targets*, **5**, 655–664.

Heisler, L. K., Chu, H. M., Brennan, T. J., *et al.* (1998). Elevated anxiety and antidepressant-like responses in serotonin 5-HT1A receptor mutant mice. *Proceedings of the National Academy of Sciences of the USA*, **95**, 15049–15054.

Hickman-Davis, J. M., & Davis, I. C. (2006). Transgenic mice. *Paediatric Respiratory Reviews*, **7**, 49–53.

Jacob, H. J., & Kwitek, A. E. (2002). Rat genetics: attaching physiology and pharmacology to the genome. *Nature Reviews Genetics*, **3**, 33–42.

Kalueff, A. V., & Murphy, D. L. (2007). The importance of cognitive phenotypes in experimental modeling of animal anxiety and depression. *Neural Plasticity*, **2007**, 52087.

Klemenhagen, K. C., Gordon, J. A., David, D. J., Hen, R., & Gross, C. T. (2006). Increased fear response to contextual cues in mice lacking the 5-HT1A receptor. *Neuropsychopharmacology*, **31**, 101–111.

Koponen, E., Voikar, V., Riekki, R., *et al.* (2004). Transgenic mice overexpressing the full-length neurotrophin receptor trkB exhibit increased activation of the trkB-PLCgamma pathway, reduced anxiety, and facilitated learning. *Molecular and Cellular Neuroscience*, **26**, 166–181.

Lapiz-Bluhm, M. D., Bondi, C. O., Doyen, J., *et al.* (2008). Behavioural assays to model cognitive and affective dimensions of depression and anxiety in rats. *Journal of Neuroendocrinology*, **20**, 1115–1137.

Le Francois, B., Czesak, M., Steubl, D., & Albert, P. R. (2008). Transcriptional regulation at a HTR1A polymorphism associated with mental illness. *Neuropharmacology*, **55**, 977–85.

Leonardo, E. D., & Hen, R. (2008). Anxiety as a developmental disorder. *Neuropsychopharmacology*, **33**, 134–140.

Lister, R. G. (1987). The use of a plus-maze to measure anxiety in the mouse. *Psychopharmacology (Berlin)*, **92**, 180–185.

Lo Iacono, L., & Gross, C. (2008). Alpha-Ca2+/calmodulin-dependent protein kinase II contributes to the developmental programming of anxiety in serotonin receptor 1A knock-out mice. *Journal of Neuroscience*, **28**, 6250–6257.

Lucki, I. (1997). The forced swimming test as a model for core and component behavioral effects of antidepressant drugs. *Behavioural Pharmacology*, **8**, 523–532.

Maren, S. (2001). Neurobiology of Pavlovian fear conditioning. *Annual Review of Neuroscience*, **24**, 897–931.

McKinney, W. T. (1984). Animal models of depression: an overview. *Psychiatric Development*, **2**, 77–96.

Melton, D. W. (1994). Gene targeting in the mouse. *Bioessays*, **16**, 633–638.

Millan, M. J. (2003). The neurobiology and control of anxious states. *Progress in Neurobiology*, **70**, 83–244.

Moret, C., & Briley, M. (2000). The possible role of 5-HT(1B/D) receptors in psychiatric disorders and their potential as a target for therapy. *European Journal of Pharmacology*, **404**, 1–12.

Nemeroff, C. B. (2002). Comorbidity of mood and anxiety disorders: the rule, not the exception? *American Journal of Psychiatry*, **159**, 3–4.

Nemeroff, C. B. (2003). Anxiolytics: past, present, and future agents. *Journal of Clinical Psychiatry*, **64** (Suppl. 3), 3–6.

Nesse, R. M. (1999). Proximate and evolutionary studies of anxiety, stress and depression: synergy at the interface. *Neuroscience and Biobehavioral Reviews*, **23**, 895–903.

Ohl, F., Toschi, N., Wigger, A., Henniger, M. S., & Landgraf, R. (2001). Dimensions of emotionality in a rat model of innate anxiety. *Behavioral Neuroscience*, **115**, 429–436.

Parks, C. L., Robinson, P. S., Sibille, E., Shenk, T., & Toth, M. (1998). Increased anxiety of mice lacking the serotonin1A receptor. *Proceedings of the National Academy of Sciences of the USA*, **95**, 10734–10739.

Perry, J. L., & Carroll, M. E. (2008). The role of impulsive behavior in drug abuse. *Psychopharmacology (Berlin)*, **200**, 1–26.

Porter, R., Bock, G., Clark, S., & Ciba Foundation (1986). *Antidepressants and Receptor Function*. Chichester; New York, NY: Wiley.

Ramboz, S., Oosting, R., Amara, D. A., *et al.* (1998). Serotonin receptor 1A knockout: an animal model of anxiety-related disorder. *Proceedings of the National Academy of Sciences of the USA*, **95**, 14476–14481.

Ressler, K. J., & Nemeroff, C. B. (2000). Role of serotonergic and noradrenergic systems in the pathophysiology of depression and anxiety disorders. *Depression and Anxiety*, **12** (Suppl. 1), 2–19.

Robbins, T. W. (2002). The 5-choice serial reaction time task: behavioural pharmacology and functional neurochemistry. *Psychopharmacology (Berlin)*, **163**, 362–380.

Rodgers, R. J. (1997). Animal models of "anxiety": where next? *Behavioural Pharmacology*, **8**, 477–496; discussion 497–504.

Santarelli, L., Saxe, M., Gross, C., *et al.* (2003). Requirement of hippocampal neurogenesis for the behavioral effects of antidepressants. *Science*, **301**, 805–809.

Serretti, A., Calati, R., Mandelli, L., & De Ronchi, D. (2006). Serotonin transporter gene variants and behavior: a comprehensive review. *Current Drug Targets*, **7**, 1659–1669.

Sramek, J. J., Zarotsky, V., & Cutler, N. R. (2002). Generalised anxiety disorder: treatment options. *Drugs*, **62**, 1635–1648.

Stark, K. L., Gross, C., Richardson-Jones, J., Zhuang, X., & Hen, R. (2007). A novel conditional knockout strategy applied to serotonin receptors. *Handbook of Experimental Pharmacology*, **178**, 347–363.

van der Staay, F. J. (2006). Animal models of behavioral dysfunctions: basic concepts and classifications, and an evaluation strategy. *Brain Research Reviews*, **52**, 131–159.

Weiss, J. M., Goodman, P. A., Losito, B. G., *et al.* (1981). Behavioral depression produced by an uncontrollable stressor: relationship to norepinephrine, dopamine, and serotonin levels in various regions of rat brain. *Brain Research Reviews*, **3**, 167–205.

Willner, P. (1997). Validity, reliability and utility of the chronic mild stress model of depression: a 10-year review and evaluation. *Psychopharmacology (Berlin)*, **134**, 319–329.

Willner, P., & Mitchell, P. J. (2002). The validity of animal models of predisposition to depression. *Behavioural Pharmacology*, **13**, 169–188.

Zohar, J., Kennedy, J. L., Hollander, E., & Koran, L. M. (2004). Serotonin-1D hypothesis of obsessive–compulsive disorder: an update. *Journal of Clinical Psychiatry*, **65** (Suppl. 14), 18–21.

Chapter 15

Role of the cortex in the regulation of anxiety states

Noelia V. Weisstaub, Caitlin McOmish, James Hanks, Jay A. Gingrich

15.1 Defining fear and anxiety

In evolutionary terms, anxiety is considered to be a conserved behavioral response to a warning signal or a threat (Fuchs & Flugge 2004). This behavior predisposes the individual to recognize potential dangers and to prepare to deal with the threat, allowing the individual to take measures to reduce exposure to danger. In this sense, an anxious state is similar to fear, differentiating itself only in that the latter manifests as an acute response to an immediate threat (Fuchs & Flugge 2004). Both, however, serve the purpose of decreasing an individual's exposure to danger. Thus, under most circumstances, anxiety is an adaptive response to chronic danger and often engages coping mechanisms that help the organism continue with behaviors necessary for survival while minimizing its exposure to danger. This response is generally mild and is associated with recruitment of several physiological systems: motor, sensory, endocrine, immune, cardiovascular, and neuronal.

Pathological anxiety, however, is characterized by a disproportionate response to a mild or non-existent threat (Lesch *et al.* 2003). In humans, the various anxiety disorders classified by the *Diagnostic and Statistical Manual* (DSM) all have a common underlying core of pathological processes, including a persistent and increased response to potential threat or a reduced threshold for treating a situation as threatening (Stein & Bienvenu 2004).

From a neurobiological standpoint, normal anxiety is an emotional state subserved by neuronal circuits, including the amygdala and the prefrontal cortex, while pathological anxiety may be viewed as maladaptive responsiveness of the same circuitry. The first attempt to identify the circuitry involved in emotional responses was undertaken by Papez in 1937. He suggested the existence of a "looped" circuit projecting from the hippocampus to the mammillary bodies, then to the anterior nucleus of the thalamus, from there to the anterior cingulate cortex, and finally back to the hippocampus (Papez 1995). These interconnected structures became known as the circuit of Papez. The modern version of Papez's circuit is now also thought to include more areas of the cortex as well as the amygdala, hippocampus, medial preoptic area, hypothalamus ventral striatum, and periaqueductal gray (PAG).

15.2 Neuroanatomy of fear and anxiety

The most widely studied behavioral model of fear is "classical fear conditioning," as it may be assessed across many different species, including humans. The circuitry underlying this process is well known and includes the amygdala as the crucial node, as well as the cortex, thalamus, and striatum. Although often referred to and considered as a single unit, the amygdala comprises several nuclei, which perform different functions. Of particular relevance to the current discussion, the basolateral nucleus of the amygdala (BLA) plays a key role as the input area for environmental cues, which elicit conditioned fear behaviors. The BLA receives environmental information from the thalamus, hippocampus, and cortex (Davis 2004); it then projects to additional nuclei of the amygdala as well as other brain regions, forming a complex network that subserves different aspects of the anxiety response. Cue-related information is transmitted via two different pathways, a fast subcortical path from dorsal thalamus and a slower regulatory cortical pathway. Context-related information is transmitted to the lateral amygdala and from there to the BLA via the hippocampus and the cortex. The BLA projects to the central nucleus of the amygdala (CeA) and to another nucleus, the bed nucleus of the stria terminalis (BNST),

Anxiety Disorders: Theory, Research, and Clinical Perspectives, ed. Helen Blair Simpson, Yuval Neria, Roberto Lewis-Fernández, Franklin Schneier. Published by Cambridge University Press. © Cambridge University Press 2010.

which is part of the extended amygdala formation. The projection areas of the CeA and BNST overlap to some extent, but they differ in their function. The CeA mediates many of the autonomic and somatic changes observed in fear, while the BNST is involved in the behavioral expression of anxiety (Davis 2006). Under conditions in which the perceived danger is not highly predictable, a sustained state of defensive behavior is required (e.g., hiding in the corner of a brightly lit arena as opposed to fleeing from a larger animal, or freezing in response to a tone associated with an aversive stimulus). Above all, it is clear that the amygdala plays an important role in the processing and expression of anxiety states.

15.3 Role of the cortex in humans

Over the last two decades there has been an increased interest in understanding the role of cortical areas in controlling anxiety, particularly due to the modulatory role that the cortex has over subcortical structures. One of the main functions of the frontal cortices, and especially the prefrontal cortex (PFC), is to enable preferential processing of task-relevant over task-irrelevant stimuli (Miller & Cohen 2001, Egner 2008). When complex stimuli arrive simultaneously, the PFC resolves the conflict between "important" stimuli and those irrelevant to the task at hand by establishing the proper mapping of inputs, internal states, and outputs. This is especially true in situations where the stimuli are ambiguous or the relevant stimulus is weaker than the task-irrelevant stimuli (Miller & Cohen 2001). This type of modulation of lower brain structures by higher regions is known as "top-down" control.

Conflicting signals can be divided in two basic categories: emotional and non-emotional. Cortical control of anxiety appears to be especially important in the presence of emotional stimuli. Emotional cues, like those that signal potential danger, are more salient than neutral cues and can effectively interfere with ongoing cognitive processing (Tipples & Sharma 2000, Etkin et al. 2006). Thus, without modulation by the PFC, emotional stimuli might direct the response of the organism, even in cases where responding to the emotionally salient stimulus is maladaptive.

Both the ventromedial prefrontal cortex (vmPFC) (including the anterior cingulate cortex [ACC] and orbitofrontal cortex [OFC]) and the hippocampus govern amygdalar activity by top-down control. Moreover, the lateral prefrontal cortex (lPFC) has also been implicated in top-down control of the amygdala and emotional stimuli. This is generally considered an example of "higher functioning" allowing for contextual information, previous experience, and self-regulation to modulate the response during potentially dangerous situations (Hariri et al. 2003, Bishop et al. 2004, Etkin et al. 2006, Mathew et al. 2008). The function of these areas of the cortex in such situations would thus be to modulate more primitive brain structures, such as the nuclei of the amygdala, by regulating their sensitivity to the stimuli and enabling appropriate context-dependent responses.

A growing number of brain imaging studies using functional magnetic resonance imaging (fMRI) have shown that healthy volunteers show activation of the amygdala when presented with fearful faces. Activity in the medial prefrontal cortex (mPFC) also appears to modulate amygdalar responses. Activation of the rostral ACC negatively correlates with activity in the amygdala, confirming a strong loop between these two structures in controlling emotional responses (Hariri et al. 2003, Vuilleumier 2005, Egner 2008). Based on these results, it is clear that the involvement of the cortex has clinical relevance and should be considered a key target of research into clinical treatment of anxiety disorders.

Studies in patients with differing forms of anxiety disorders have shown decreased activation of vmPFC and hyperactivation of the amygdala. For example, patients with posttraumatic stress disorder (PTSD) showed increased reactivity of the amygdala and a decreased response in the vmPFC during tasks designed to provoke an anxiety response (Rauch et al. 2006, Ressler & Mayberg 2007, Mathew et al. 2008). Likewise, during presentation of masked fearful faces, youths with generalized anxiety disorder (GAD) showed increased activation of the amygdala that positively correlated with the severity of their anxiety (Monk et al. 2008). Moreover, significant activation of the vmPFC is observed during extinction of fear responses, supporting a modulatory role for the vmPFC (Phelps et al. 2004, Milad et al. 2007). Lending further support to these findings, direct electrical stimulation of the rostral and ventral mPFC decreases amygdalar activation in rodents (Rosenkranz & Grace 2002, Quirk et al. 2003).

Recently, the insular cortex has gained attention as an area involved in the control of anxiety. The insular cortex plays a central role in interoception (Critchley *et al.* 2004) and is important for self awareness, serving as a link between cognitive and affective process and the current somatic state (Paulus & Stein 2006). The insular cortex has bidirectional connections with the amygdala, nucleus accumbens, and OFC. Therefore, it is well placed to receive information about the salience of stimuli and the effects that these stimuli might have upon the individual (Paulus & Stein 2006). Put simply, the role of the insular cortex is to sense how an external stimulus might affect the state of the body. Since the insular cortex mediates the processing of aversive stimuli, alterations in this capacity link the insular cortex with anxiety states. Paulus and Stein (2006) hypothesized that people who are prone to anxiety have an altered interoceptive prediction signal, and that this is the initial problem that leads to the cognitive, affective, and behavioral effects observed in anxiety disorders.

Human brain imaging studies have found insular abnormalities in anxiety patients. Patients with panic disorders display decreased $GABA_A$/benzodiazepine sites in the insular cortex (Cameron *et al.* 2007), while phobic patients show an increase in insular activity during the presentation of fearful faces (Wright *et al.* 2003). In addition, patients with obsessive–compulsive disorder have shown activation of the insular cortex during an affective switching task (Remijnse *et al.* 2006). In healthy volunteers, activity in the insular cortex is modulated by the expectation associated with an aversive stimulus (Nitschke *et al.* 2006, Sarinopoulos *et al.* 2006). In a conditioned fear experiment, increased activation of the insular and cingulate cortex was observed during cue and presentation (Marschner *et al.* 2008). In accordance with a role for the insular cortex in regulating anxiety states, administration of a selective serotonin reuptake inhibitor (SSRI) antidepressant reduced the activation of the amygdala and the insular cortex during emotional processing (Arce *et al.* 2008), which is also consistent with the role of SSRIs in decreasing anxiety in both healthy and anxious individuals.

Overall, the data suggest that the insula, together with other areas of PFC, such as the ACC, are important during anticipation of aversive stimuli and the expression of anxiety states. The involvement of cortical regions is further supported by the complexity of the nature of the anxiety response (Paulus & Stein 2006). Whether the anxiety response concerned is "normal" or pathological, it involves the coordinated activation of different systems, including cortical structures that are able to initiate and maintain complex representations.

15.4 Role of the cortex in animal models

Although most of the data regarding the role of the cortex in anxiety disorders have come from human imaging studies, there is a growing literature relating cortical areas with anxiety in animals. Particularly, the infralimbic (IL) region of the vmPFC in rats has been heavily implicated in extinction and the retrieval of extinction memories (Quirk *et al.* 2000, Quirk & Mueller 2008), a phenomenon that plays a fundamental role in anxiety disorders such as PTSD.

The mechanism by which the cortex modulates extinction is not fully elucidated, but there is consensus that its actions are due at least in part to its ability to modulate amygdalar responses. More specifically, the IL region projects to a small group of inhibitory cells called intercalated cells (ITC) (Quirk & Mueller 2008), which are situated between the BLA and the central nucleus of the amygdala. By activating these cells, the IL region might inhibit amygdalar output. Other areas of the cortex have also been implicated in the regulation of fear responses: for example, the entorhinal cortex, which projects to the ITC (Quirk & Mueller 2008), has been implicated in extinction of inhibitory avoidance (Bevilaqua *et al.* 2006).

Although many cortical regions seem to be involved in regulation of extinction, others are directly involved in regulation of fear responses. The prelimbic (PL) area of the vmPFC is necessary for fear expression: pharmacological inhibition of this region reduces conditioned fear (Corcoran & Quirk 2007). Interestingly, during fear conditioning, neurons of the PL and IL (which correspond to subsections of the vmPFC in humans) show opposite response patterns (Gilmartin & McEchron 2005): bursting in PL neurons correlates with acquisition of fear conditioning (Laviolette *et al.* 2005), while bursting in IL neurons correlates with the extinction of this behavior (Burgos-Robles *et al.* 2007). This prefrontal system is also involved in reducing fear responses in cases in which the stressor is controllable (Baratta *et al.* 2007). In other words, in cases where the stressor is controllable, the PFC is recruited and modulates the response of the animal, suggesting that IL and PL regions might be key areas modulating anxiety responses in normal conditions, and therefore that they might be good targets for manipulating pathological states.

15.5 The serotonergic system and its role in anxiety

15.5.1 Overview of the serotonin system

Pharmacological and genetic manipulations in animal models have demonstrated the relevance of numerous neurotransmitter systems in regulating anxiety responses, including glutamate, gamma-aminobutyric acid (GABA), adenosine, cannabinoids, noradrenaline, dopamine, serotonin (5-HT), and various neuropeptides (for review see Millan 2003). Long-term dysregulation of these systems contributes to the development of anxiety disorders; however, the number of pathways and their interconnections illustrates the complexity of anxiety-related circuitry, and identification of specific modulators of various anxiety pathways has been the focus of intense study.

Serotonin plays an important role in the regulation of emotions, including anxiety, fear, and depression. The serotonergic cell bodies are located in the raphe nuclei of the brainstem, and although they represent a very small proportion of the total number of cells in the brain (1/1 000 000), their highly ramified axons innervate all regions of the central nervous system (Tork 1990, Jacobs & Azmitia 1992). However, in the majority of cases, synaptic connections are not formed, and the cells release serotonin in a paracrine manner (Jacobs & Azmitia 1992). Electrophysiologically, serotonergic cells are characterized by a slow regular tonic activity (Jacobs & Azmitia 1992). The combination of these characteristics means that changes in the firing activity of serotonin cells lead to modulation of a large population of target cells in the forebrain (Celada et al. 2004). Following exposure to stressors, research has shown that neuronal activity is increased in animal models (Grahn et al. 1999, Holmes 2008) and that there is an increase in extracellular fluid concentration of serotonin in the vicinity of the raphe as well as in projection areas, including the mPFC, amygdala, and hippocampus (Holmes 2008). What is more, modulation of raphe firing can affect the release of serotonin and the behavioral expression of fear (Forster et al. 2006).

Serotonin exerts its effects through a complex system that includes multiple transporters and a wealth of receptors. There are 14 different serotonergic receptors divided into seven families according to their ligand recognition profiles, signal transduction mechanisms, and structural characteristics (Humphrey et al. 1993, Hoyer et al. 1994, Hoyer & Martin 1996). Several of these receptors have been implicated in the regulation of anxiety states, including the 5-HT$_{1A}$, 5-HT$_{1B}$, 5-HT$_{2A}$, 5-HT$_{2C}$, 5-HT$_4$, and the serotonin transporter. Based on their localization, different serotonin receptors have been proposed to modulate distinct aspects of anxiety responses. Detailed analyses of the function of the different receptors have been described previously (Holmes 2008), and here we concentrate on their involvement in the cortical modulation of anxiety responses.

15.5.2 The serotonin transporter (SERT)

One of the most widely studied targets of serotonin is the highly selective serotonin transporter (5HTT/SERT). The SERT is important in determining the magnitude and duration of the serotonin response during a stressful situation as it is the main pathway for removal of serotonin from the synaptic space. It also has an important role in regulating volume transmission of serotonin (a diffuse, long-acting signal, contrasting with the spatial and temporal restriction of "fast" synaptic transmission) (Torres & Amara 2007, Holmes 2008). Imaging studies have shown a correlation between SERT genotype and amygdalar activation in response to presentation of fearful faces, where the level of response correlated with the effect of the polymorphism. Carriers of the short (s) allele express lower levels of transporter and have greater activation of the amygdala than long (l) carriers (Hariri et al. 2002). There is also a role for SERT at the circuit level. Investigators have found that carriers of the s allele show uncoupling of a cingulate–amygdala feedback circuit that is present in l carriers and an inverse correlation between coupling and anxiety traits, suggesting that level of activity of SERT has a role in the development of essential circuits underlying anxiety responses (Pezawas et al. 2005).

Research has also shown that SERT function is subject to modulation by environmental factors in a genotype dependent manner. To elaborate, variation in the SERT gene (*5HTT*) has been linked to altered serotonergic function following stressful early life events in humans and in animal models (Murphy et al. 2001, Bennett et al. 2002). Caspi and colleagues (2003) demonstrated that people who carry one or two copies of the short functional allele in the promoter region of the SERT displayed more depressive behaviors subsequent to stressful life events. In the absence of stressful life events, however, genotype and affective symptomatology were not correlated. These effects have also been modeled in rhesus monkeys, who carry an allelic variation within the SERT gene comparable to that in humans: behavioral performance on many tasks (including peer interaction, emotional behavior, and stress reactivity) following maternal separation is subject to a genotype-by-environment interaction (Higley et al. 1991, Bennett et al. 2002, Champoux et al. 2002). Thus, the SERT may modulate how our brains respond to environmental exposures.

It must be noted, however, that a more recent meta-analysis has found no evidence of an influence of SERT genotype upon depression, nor any evidence of a genotype-by-environment interaction (Risch et al. 2009). The experimental and statistical approach varied substantially between studies and highlights the need to clarify this issue more definitively.

Genetic deletion of the gene coding for the SERT resulted in increased anxiety-like behaviors in rodents (Holmes et al. 2002, 2003a, Lira et al. 2003, Ansorge et al. 2004, Zhao et al. 2006, Carroll et al. 2007, Fox et al. 2007, Kalueff et al. 2007) accompanied by changes in stress responsiveness and depression-like behavior (Holmes et al. 2003b, Lira et al. 2003, Ansorge et al. 2004, Holmes 2008). It is worth noting that the genetic deletion of the SERT produces a phenotype opposed to the one observed under chronic pharmacologic treatment in adult animals and humans. The key difference is that genetic deletion of the SERT leads to the absence of functional SERT during critical stages of brain development (Ansorge et al. 2004, 2007).

Although the SERT is the most studied, other serotonin receptors have also been proposed to modulate distinct aspects of anxiety responses based on their neural expression pattern. Some appear to be more relevant to the cortical modulation of anxiety responses. Of these, data supporting a role for the 5-HT$_{1A}$ and 5-HT$_{2A}$ receptors in anxiety are reviewed below.

15.5.3 The 5-HT$_{1A}$ receptor

5-HT$_{1A}$ receptors (5-HT$_{1A}$Rs) have been the focus of intense study in relation to anxiety and depressive states. They are involved in the regulation of serotonin release and in mediating 5-HT effects in corticolimbic circuits. 5-HT$_{1A}$Rs are expressed in the hippocampus, amygdala, and PFC both pre- and postsynaptically. Mice lacking the 5-HT$_{1A}$R show increased anxiety in various (hippocampal-dependent) tests (Parks

et al. 1998, Ramboz et al. 1998, Gross et al. 2000, Klemenhagen et al. 2006, Tsetsenis et al. 2007), pointing to a likely role of hippocampal 5-HT$_{1A}$R in the mediation of anxiety-like behaviors. However, it is clear that other populations of 5-HT$_{1A}$R are also important. In the BLA, 5-HT$_{1A}$R activation modulates amygdalar projection neurons and GABAergic interneurons (Cheng et al. 1998, Koyama et al. 1999, Stein et al. 2000, Koyama et al. 2002), indicating that the net role of serotonin in this key area of the anxiety circuit depends upon the balance between activation of 5-HT$_{1A}$R in excitatory and inhibitory neurons. Other studies have shown that modulation of 5-HT$_{1A}$R in the amygdala affects the anxiety-related endocrine response of the animal (Krysiak et al. 2000, Li et al. 2006).

5-HT$_{1A}$Rs are also densely expressed in the mPFC (Pompeiano et al. 1992). More specifically, they are expressed in cell bodies, basal dendrites, and the axon hillock of pyramidal cells, as well as in GABAergic interneurons (Azmitia et al. 1996, Amargos-Bosch et al. 2004, Santana et al. 2004). In these regions, activation of 5-HT$_{1A}$Rs produces an inhibitory response, probably due to activation of a K$^+$ current (Araneda & Andrade 1991). Consistent with this, application of 5-HT$_{1A}$ agonists directly into the mPFC inhibits the spontaneous and glutamate-mediated firing of major projection neurons (Araneda & Andrade 1991, Cai et al. 2002), and 5-HT$_{1A}$R knockout mice display increased neuronal excitability in the mPFC due to changes in the glutamate–GABA balance (Bruening et al. 2006).

Serotonergic modulation of cortical function relies heavily upon activation of the dorsal and medial raphe nucleus and subsequent stimulation of the different receptor subtypes. Interestingly, this cortico–raphe connection is bidirectional, allowing for indirect cortical control of its own activity. Activation of 5-HT$_{1A}$R in the mPFC produces a decrease in dorsal raphe nucleus (DRN) firing and subsequent reduction of cortical 5-HT release (Celada et al. 2001, Amargos-Bosch et al. 2004). This regulation can have important behavioral consequences. Maier and Watkins (2005) reported that the mPFC–DRN pathway determines whether stress is perceived as mild or uncontrollable and, consequently, the level to which the serotonergic system is activated. In a series of studies they have shown that the mPFC controls the activation of the DRN during the presentation of stressful stimuli. In the absence of cortical control, otherwise mildly stressful stimuli can produce a response that is indistinguishable from a non-controllable one (Amat et al. 2005, Amat et al. 2006, Baratta et al. 2007). This distinction, determined by cortical regulation of "controllable" versus "uncontrollable" anxiety, is further supported by work demonstrating that activation of the mPFC during the presentation of an uncontrollable stressor prevents the behavioral, endocrine, and autonomic effects of the stressor (Amat et al. 2008). The decreased binding to 5-HT$_{1A}$R observed in the mPFC following stress (Crayton et al. 1996, Nash et al. 2008) could therefore be a compensatory mechanism acting to increase cortical activity and reverse an exaggerated and detrimental stress response. In sum, the role of the 5HT$_{1A}$R in anxiety appears to include direct modulation of serotonin levels by a presynaptic mechanism as well as a complex postsynaptic action in the modulation of anxiety responses.

15.5.4 The 5-HT$_{2A}$ receptor

Another important serotonergic receptor in the cortex is the 5-HT$_{2A}$ receptor (5HT$_{2A}$R). The expression pattern of 5HT$_{2A}$Rs overlaps many of the brain regions involved in modulating emotionality, suggesting a principal role for this receptor in mediating the effects of 5-HT on anxiety-related behaviors. In the adult nervous system, 5HT$_{2A}$Rs are found on somatodendritic regions of cells in the cortex, hippocampus, striatum, amygdala, olfactory system, basal ganglia, hypothalamus, brainstem, pons, and spinal cord. In the cortex, 5HT$_{2A}$R expression is laminar, with the highest density in the pyramidal neurons of layer V. In these neurons, 5HT$_{2A}$Rs are expressed primarily in the proximal part of the apical dendrite, including dendritic shafts and spines, but can be detected throughout the entire dendritic tree. 5HT$_{2A}$Rs are also expressed in medium-sized GABAergic interneurons throughout the cortex (Jakab & Goldman-Rakic 1998, Cornea-Hebert et al. 1999, Miner et al. 2003).

The apical dendrite is thought to be a "hot spot" for receptor effects, suggesting an influential role for 5HT$_{2A}$Rs, particularly in cortical layer V. Studies conducted in vitro and in vivo provide evidence that activation of cortical 5-HT$_{2A}$R modulates multiple neurotransmitter systems including glutamatergic, GABAergic, dopaminergic, and serotonergic systems (Vollenweider et al. 1999, Martin-Ruiz et al. 2001, Amargos-Bosch et al. 2005, Bortolozzi et al. 2005). In-vitro electrophysiological studies, primarily in rodent brain slices (Marek & Aghajanian 1998), have shown that activation of 5HT$_{2A}$Rs in the PFC exerts a facilitatory action on cortical pyramidal neurons by increasing glutamate release, suggesting that the main role of cortical 5-HT$_{2A}$R is as a modulator of the excitability of PFC networks (Beique et al. 2007). These experiments were confirmed by in-vivo studies in rodents, which showed that activation of 5-HT$_{2A}$R produces a net excitatory effect over glutamatergic activity in the mPFC (Celada et al. 2004, 2008). Historically, researchers believed thalamocortical projections mediated the changes induced by activation of 5-HT$_{2A}$R (Marek & Aghajanian 1999, Marek et al. 2001). However, new evidence suggests that activation of cortical 5-HT$_{2A}$R and subsequent changes in glutamate release are due to cortico-cortical circuits (Puig et al. 2003, Lambe & Aghajanian 2006, Celada et al. 2008).

In addition, cortical 5-HT$_{2A}$Rs modulate other neurotransmitter systems. Due to the strong connection between the mPFC and the dorsal raphe, activation of 5-HT$_{2A}$ receptors on cell bodies in the cortex modulates activity in the raphe and the release of 5-HT onto the mPFC, indicating that it is an important modulator of the distal feedback of serotonergic activity (Martin-Ruiz et al. 2001, Bortolozzi et al. 2003, Celada et al. 2004). Cortical 5-HT$_{2A}$Rs are also known to affect dopaminergic transmission by modulating the firing pattern of dopaminergic cells in the ventral tegmental area (Pehek et al. 2001, Bortolozzi 2005). Both the serotonergic and the dopaminergic modulation are thought to be mediated by 5-HT$_{2A}$Rs acting postsynaptically on glutamatergic neurons, influencing glutamate transmission. Research has shown, however, that 5-HT$_{2A}$Rs are expressed in a specific subpopulation of GABAergic cells (Santana et al. 2004). For these cells, activation of 5-HT$_{2A}$Rs will increase GABAergic transmission and play an inhibitory role in the modulation of cortical microcircuits.

Pharmacologically, there is also evidence for a role of 5-HT$_{2A}$Rs in the modulation of anxiety. Some highly specific 5-HT$_{2A}$ antagonists available have been shown in mice, rats, and monkeys to have an anxiolytic profile (Griebel et al. 1997). These pharmacological data have been confirmed in a genetic model. Mice lacking the 5-HT$_{2A}$R (2AKO) were assessed using anxiety-related tests (open field, light/dark box, elevated plus maze, and novelty-suppressed feeding). Each presents a conflict situation, in which the animal's innate tendency to explore novelty is put in opposition to its instinct to find safety in dark, unexposed locations. In each test, 2AKO mice showed a decreased level of behavioral inhibition. The design used to generate the 2AKO mice allowed the restoration of 5-HT$_{2A}$ expression in a region-specific manner, and animals whose expression

173

of 5-HT$_{2A}$ was restored in the cortex showed normalization of conflict anxiety. Thus, the anxiolytic phenotype appears to be a direct consequence of the absence of cortical 5-HT$_{2A}$R signaling. Perhaps most interestingly, these mice showed no differences in depression-related behaviors or fear-conditioned learning, allowing dissociation of the anxiety-related behavior from some of its common comorbid phenotypes (Weisstaub *et al.* 2006).

In humans, genetic studies have been inconclusive regarding the effect of different *htr2a* gene polymorphisms on affective disorders (Golimbet *et al.* 2004, Norton & Owen 2005, Tochigi *et al.* 2005, Serretti *et al.* 2007, Unschuld *et al.* 2007). However, imaging studies have shown changes in 5-HT$_{2A}$R levels in depression patients and in suicide victims, supporting changes in expression levels of 5-HT$_{2A}$R in affective disorders (Arango *et al.* 1997, Meyer *et al.* 2003, Bhagwagar *et al.* 2006). Furthermore, in healthy volunteers research has shown that the level of 5-HT$_{2A}$R binding in frontotemporal regions correlates with risk for affective disorders (Frokjaer *et al.* 2008). Thus, though the genetic evidence is not clear, human imaging studies suggest that 5HT$_{2A}$R function, particularly in the cortex, is important for modulating affect. Whether changes in cortical 5-HT$_{2A}$R expression play a causal role in pathological emotional responses remains to be seen.

There are several possibilities as to how 5-HT$_{2A}$ receptors in the cortex might modulate anxiety expression. Since the fear response and endocrine responses in these mice are normal, alterations in the PAG or the amygdala are unlikely (though these regions may exist outside of the circuit that involves the BNST). We may therefore conjecture that the decreases in cortical 2A receptor expression that result in an apparent decrease in anxiety may not be related directly to fear expression, but rather to the evaluation of its context. Extensive connections exist between the cortex and the hippocampus, a brain region strongly implicated in context-dependent behavior. Normal contextual fear conditioning in the 5HT$_{2A}$R knockout mice suggests that the hippocampus, or at least the amygdalar–hippocampal fear circuitry, is unaffected in these mice. However, this does not rule out the possibility that the connections between the cortex and the hippocampus are dysregulated.

The lack of 5HT$_{2A}$R in pyramidal cells would likely result in decreased excitability of the cells and thus reduce the cortical control over other areas. Most of the literature, especially in humans, suggests that the role of the cortex is to inhibit the activation of lower areas involved in anxiety and fear response. Thus, decreased activity in cortical 5HT$_{2A}$R-expressing pyramidal neurons, whose role would be to inhibit activation of lower areas, would result in increased activity in subcortical regions implicated in anxiety and fear responses. That said, we should keep in mind that the effects observed in humans focused upon interactions between the cortex and amygdala. We know, based on our results, that the fear response of these mice is normal, indicating that cortico–amygdalar connection is also normal. The fact that the anxiolytic phenotype observed in these mice was limited to unconditioned anxiety-related behaviors might indicate that the circuit affected involved areas other than the amygdala, or that they are a result of dysregulated cortico-cortical circuitry.

Alternatively the "anxiolytic" phenotype may be the result of cognitive deficits, in the sense of incorrect evaluation of the environment. In this case, decreased activation of cortical cells projecting to other areas would result in the interpretation that the environment is neither novel nor dangerous, possibly reflecting a deficit in risk assessment, a function that has been associated with the OFC. Another possibility is that the observed behaviors may be indicative of deficits in decision making. Based on the existing data it is not currently possible to dissociate these two hypotheses, and important follow-up studies will address more specifically the contribution of cortical 5-HT$_{2A}$R to decision-making processes and risk assessment.

15.6 Conclusions

Regulation of affect is a complex phenomenon involving many components, from autonomic response to cognitive control. It is natural, then, that serotonin appears to play multiple roles at different levels in the brain in order to achieve the complex behavioral outcome. In particular, serotonin seems to have an important role in modulating cortical function by its combined action through multiple receptors in different but interconnected cortical areas.

The complex and important role that the serotonergic system plays in emotional regulation is also unambiguous. Serotonergic modulation occurs via interaction with a wealth of receptors with complementary and sometimes opposite effects acting at different levels in the circuitry underlying anxiety. Historically, the main areas studied as targets for serotonergic modulation have been the hippocampus and the amygdala, as they are major nodes implicated in emotional regulation (Frokjaer *et al.* 2008). Recently, however, the role of the cortex in regulation of emotion, and in particular anxiety states, has become increasingly evident in light of convincing human data. As a result, there has been a growing awareness of the importance of understanding the role of serotonin in the cortex.

The role of the serotonergic system in the control of emotional responses is intricate, with the net result of complex actions over different receptor types driving the modulation of subcortical regions. Despite this complexity, animal models are starting to give us the tools to specifically dissect the role of different components of the serotonergic system, and to begin to understand the role of the cortex in regulating anxiety states.

References

Amargos-Bosch, M., Bortolozzi, A., Puig, M. V., *et al.* (2004). Co-expression and in vivo interaction of serotonin1A and serotonin2A receptors in pyramidal neurons of prefrontal cortex. *Cerebral Cortex*, **14**, 281–299.

Amargos-Bosch, M., Artigas, F., & Adell, A. (2005). Effects of acute olanzapine after sustained fluoxetine on extracellular monoamine levels in the rat medial prefrontal cortex. *European Journal of Pharmacology*, **516**, 235–238.

Amat, J., Baratta, M. V., Paul, E., *et al.* (2005). Medial prefrontal cortex determines how stressor controllability affects behavior and dorsal raphe nucleus. *Nature Neuroscience*, **8**, 365–371.

Amat, J., Paul, E., Zarza, C., Watkins, L. R., & Maier, S. F. (2006). Previous experience with behavioral control over stress blocks the behavioral and dorsal raphe nucleus activating effects of later uncontrollable stress: role of the ventral medial prefrontal cortex. *Journal of Neuroscience*, **26**, 13264–13272.

Amat, J., Paul, E., Watkins, L. R., & Maier, S. F. (2008). Activation of the ventral medial prefrontal cortex during an uncontrollable stressor reproduces both the immediate and long-term protective effects of behavioral control. *Neuroscience*, **154**, 1178–1186.

Ansorge, M. S., Zhou, M., Lira, A., Hen, R., & Gingrich, J. A. (2004). Early-life blockade of the 5-HT transporter alters emotional behavior in adult mice. *Science*, **306**, 879–881.

Ansorge, M. S., Hen, R., & Gingrich, J. A. (2007). Neurodevelopmental origins of depressive disorders. *Current Opinion in Pharmacology*, **7**, 8–17.

Araneda, R., & Andrade, R. (1991). 5-Hydroxytryptamine 2 and 5-hydroxytryptamine 1A receptors mediate opposing responses on membrane excitability in rat association cortex. *Neuroscience*, **40**, 399–412.

Arango, V., Underwood, M. D., & Mann, J. J. (1997). Postmortem findings in suicide victims. Implications for in vivo imaging studies. *Annals of the New York Academy of Sciences*, **836**, 269–287.

Arce, E., Simmons, A. N., Lovero, K. L., Stein, M. B., & Paulus, M. P. (2008). Escitalopram effects on insula and amygdala BOLD activation during emotional processing. *Psychopharmacology (Berlin)*, **196**, 661–672.

Azmitia, E. C., Gannon, P. J., Kheck, N. M., & Whitaker-Azmitia, P. M. (1996). Cellular localization of the 5-HT1A receptor in primate brain neurons and glial cells. *Neuropsychopharmacology*, **14**, 35–46.

Baratta, M. V., Christianson, J. P., Gomez, D. M., *et al.* (2007). Controllable versus uncontrollable stressors bi-directionally modulate conditioned but not innate fear. *Neuroscience*, **146**, 1495–1503.

Beique, J. C., Imad, M., Mladenovic, L., Gingrich, J. A., & Andrade, R. (2007). Mechanism of the 5-hydroxytryptamine 2A receptor-mediated facilitation of synaptic activity in prefrontal cortex. *Proceedingss of the National Academy of Sciences of the USA*, **104**, 9870–9875.

Bennett, A. J., Lesch, K. P., Heils, A., *et al.* (2002). Early experience and serotonin transporter gene variation interact to influence primate CNS function. *Molecular Psychiatry*, **7**, 118–122.

Bevilaqua, L. R., Bonini, J. S., Rossato, J. I., *et al.* (2006). The entorhinal cortex plays a role in extinction. *Neurobiology of Learning and Memory*, **85**, 192–197.

Bhagwagar, Z., Hinz, R., Taylor, M., *et al.* (2006). Increased 5-HT2A receptor binding in euthymic, medication-free patients recovered from depression: a positron emission study with [11C]MDL 100,907. *American Journal of Psychiatry*, **163**, 1580–1587.

Bishop, S., Duncan, J., Brett, M., & Lawrence, A. D. (2004). Prefrontal cortical function and anxiety: controlling attention to threat-related stimuli. *Nature Neuroscience*, **7**, 184–188.

Bortolozzi, A., Amargos-Bosch, M., *et al.* (2003) In vivo modulation of 5-hydroxytryptamine release in mouse prefrontal cortex by local 5-HT(2A) receptors: effect of antipsychotic drugs. *European Journal of Neuroscience*, **18**, 1235–1246.

Bortolozzi, A., Diaz-Mataix, L., Scorza, M. C., Celada, P., & Artigas, F. (2005). The activation of 5-HT receptors in prefrontal cortex enhances dopaminergic activity. *Journal of Neurochemistry*, **95**, 1597–1607.

Bruening, S., Oh, E., Hetzenauer, A., *et al.* (2006). The anxiety-like phenotype of 5-HT receptor null mice is associated with genetic background-specific perturbations in the prefrontal cortex GABA-glutamate system. *Journal of Neurochemistry*, **99**, 892–899.

Burgos-Robles, A., Vidal-Gonzalez, I., Santini, E., & Quirk, G. J. (2007). Consolidation of fear extinction requires

NMDA receptor-dependent bursting in the ventromedial prefrontal cortex. *Neuron*, **53**, 871–880.

Cai, X., Gu, Z., Zhong, P., Ren, Y., & Yan, Z. (2002). Serotonin 5-HT1A receptors regulate AMPA receptor channels through inhibiting Ca2+/calmodulin-dependent kinase II in prefrontal cortical pyramidal neurons. *Journal of Biological Chemistry*, **277**, 36553–36562.

Cameron, O. G., Huang, G. C., Nichols, T., *et al.* (2007) Reduced gamma-aminobutyric acidA-benzodiazepine binding sites in insular cortex of individuals with panic disorder. *Archives of General Psychiatry*, **64**, 793–800.

Carroll, J. C., Boyce-Rustay, J. M., Millstein, R., *et al.* (2007). Effects of mild early life stress on abnormal emotion-related behaviors in 5-HTT knockout mice. *Behavior Genetics*, **37**, 214–222.

Caspi, A., Sugden, K,. Moffitt, T. E., *et al.* (2003). Influence of life stress on depression: moderation by a polymorphism in the 5-HTT gene. *Science*, **301**, 386–389.

Celada, P., Puig, M. V., Casanovas, J. M., Guillazo, G., & Artigas, F. (2001). Control of dorsal raphe serotonergic neurons by the medial prefrontal cortex: involvement of serotonin-1A, GABAA, and glutamate receptors. *Journal of Neuroscience*, **21**, 9917–9929.

Celada, P., Puig, M., Amargos-Bosch, M., Adell, A., & Artigas, F. (2004). The therapeutic role of 5-HT1A and 5-HT2A receptors in depression. *Journal of Psychiatry and Neuroscience*, **29**, 252–265.

Celada, P., Puig, M. V., Diaz-Mataix, L., & Artigas, F. (2008). The hallucinogen DOI reduces low-frequency oscillations in rat prefrontal cortex: reversal by antipsychotic drugs. *Biological Psychiatry*, **64**, 392–400.

Champoux, M., Bennett, A., Shannon, C., *et al.* (2002). Serotonin transporter gene polymorphism, differential early rearing, and behavior in rhesus monkey neonates. *Molecular Psychiatry*, **7**, 1058–1063.

Cheng, L. L., Wang, S. J., & Gean, P. W. (1998). Serotonin depresses excitatory synaptic transmission and depolarization-evoked Ca2+ influx in rat basolateral amygdala via 5-HT1A receptors. *European Journal of Neuroscience*, **10**, 2163–2172.

Corcoran, K. A., & Quirk, G. J. (2007). Activity in prelimbic cortex is necessary for the expression of learned, but not innate, fears. *Journal of Neuroscience*, **27**, 840–844.

Cornea-Hebert, V., Riad, M., Wu, C., Singh, S. K., & Descarries, L. (1999). Cellular and subcellular distribution of the serotonin 5-HT2A receptor in the central nervous system of adult rat. *Journal of Computational Neurology*, **409**, 187–209.

Crayton, J. W., Joshi, I., Gulati, A., Arora, R. C., & Wolf, W. A. (1996). Effect of corticosterone on serotonin and catecholamine receptors and uptake sites in rat frontal cortex. *Brain Research*, **728**, 260–262.

Critchley, H. D., Wiens, S., Rotshtein, P., Ohman, A., & Dolan, R. J. (2004). Neural systems supporting interoceptive awareness. *Nature Neuroscience*, 7, 189–195.

Davis, M. (2004). Functional neuroanatomy of anxiety and fear. In D. S. Charney & E. J. Nestler, eds., *Neurobiology of Mental Illness*. Oxford: Oxford University Press.

Davis, M. (2006). Neural systems involved in fear and anxiety measured with fear-potentiated startle. *American Psychologist*, **61**, 741–756.

Egner, T. (2008). Multiple conflict-driven control mechanisms in the human brain. *Trends in Cognitive Science*, **12**, 374–380.

Etkin, A., Egner, T., Peraza, D. M., Kandel, E. R., & Hirsch, J. (2006). Resolving emotional conflict: a role for the rostral anterior cingulate cortex in modulating activity in the amygdala. *Neuron*, **51**, 871–882.

Forster, G. L., Feng, N., Watt, M. J., *et al.* (2006). Corticotropin-releasing factor in the dorsal raphe elicits temporally distinct serotonergic responses in the limbic system in relation to fear behavior. *Neuroscience*, **141**, 1047–1055.

Fox, M. A., Andrews, A. M., Wendland, J. R., *et al.* (2007). A pharmacological analysis of mice with a targeted disruption of the serotonin transporter. *Psychopharmacology (Berlin)*, **195**, 147–166.

Frokjaer, V. G., Mortensen, E. L., Nielsen, F. Å., *et al.* (2008). Frontolimbic serotonin 2A receptor binding in healthy subjects is associated with personality risk factors for affective disorder. *Biological Psychiatry*, **63**, 569–576.

Fuchs, E., & Flugge, G. (2004). Animal models of anxiety disorders. In D. S. Charney & E. J. Nestler, eds., *Neurobiology of Mental Illness*. Oxford: Oxford University Press.

Gilmartin, M. R., & McEchron, M. D. (2005). Single neurons in the medial prefrontal cortex of the rat exhibit tonic and phasic coding during trace fear conditioning. *Behavioral Neuroscience*, **119**, 1496–1510.

Golimbet, V. E., Alfimova, M. V., & Mitiushina, N. G. (2004) [Polymorphism of the serotonin 2A receptor gene (5HTR2A) and personality traits]. *Molecular Biology (Mosk)*, **38**, 404–412.

Grahn, R. E., Will, M. J., Hammack, S. E., *et al.* (1999). Activation of serotonin-immunoreactive cells in the dorsal raphe nucleus in rats exposed to an uncontrollable stressor. *Brain Research*, **826**, 35–43.

Griebel, G., Perrault, G., & Sanger, D. J. (1997). A comparative study of the effects of selective and non-selective 5-HT2 receptor subtype antagonists in rat and mouse models of anxiety. *Neuropharmacology*, **36**, 793–802.

Gross, C., Santarelli, L., Brunner, D., Zhuang, X., & Hen, R. (2000). Altered fear circuits in 5-HT1A receptor KO mice. *Biological Psychiatry*, **48**, 1157–1163.

Hariri, A. R., Mattay, V. S., Tessitore, A., *et al.* (2002). Serotonin transporter genetic variation and the response of the human amygdala. *Science*, **297**, 400–403.

Hariri, A. R., Mattay, V. S., Tessitore, A., Fera, F., & Weinberger, D. R. (2003). Neocortical modulation of the amygdala response to fearful stimuli. *Biological Psychiatry*, **53**, 494–501.

Higley, J. D., Suomi, S. J., & Linnoila, M. (1991). CSF monoamine metabolite concentrations vary according to age, rearing, and sex, and are influenced by the stressor of social separation in rhesus monkeys. *Psychopharmacology (Berlin)*, **103**, 551–556.

Holmes, A. (2008). Genetic variation in cortico-amygdala serotonin function and risk for stress-related disease. *Neuroscience and Biobehavioral Reviews*, **32**, 1293–1314.

Holmes, A., Yang, R. J., Murphy, D. L., & Crawley, J. N. (2002). Evaluation of antidepressant-related behavioral responses in mice lacking the serotonin transporter. *Neuropsychopharmacology*, **27**, 914–923.

Holmes, A., Lit, Q., Murphy, D. L., Gold, E., & Crawley, J. N. (2003a). Abnormal anxiety-related behavior in serotonin transporter null mutant mice: the influence of genetic background. *Genes, Brain, and Behavior*, **2**, 365–380.

Holmes, A., Murphy, D. L., & Crawley, J. N. (2003b). Abnormal behavioral phenotypes of serotonin transporter knockout mice: parallels with human anxiety and depression. *Biological Psychiatry*, **54**, 953–959.

Hoyer, D., & Martin, G. R. (1996). Classification and nomenclature of 5-HT receptors: a comment on current issues. *Behavioural Brain Research*, **73**, 263–268.

Hoyer, D., Clarke, D. E., Fozard, J. R., *et al.* (1994). International Union of Pharmacology classification of receptors for 5-hydroxytryptamine (serotonin). *Pharmacological Reviews*, **46**, 157–203.

Humphrey, P. P., Hartig, P., & Hoyer, D. (1993). A proposed new nomenclature for 5-HT receptors. *Trends in Pharmacological Sciences*, **14**, 233–236.

Jacobs, B. L., & Azmitia, E. C. (1992). Structure and function of the brain serotonin system. *Physiological Reviews*, **72**, 165–229.

Jakab, R. L., & Goldman-Rakic, P. S. (1998). 5-Hydroxytryptamine2A serotonin receptors in the primate cerebral cortex: possible site of action of hallucinogenic and antipsychotic drugs in pyramidal cell apical dendrites. *Proceedings of the National Academy of Sciences of the USA*, **95**, 735–740.

Kalueff, A. V., Fox, M. A., Gallagher, P. S., & Murphy, D. L. (2007). Hypolocomotion, anxiety and serotonin syndrome-like behavior contribute to the complex phenotype of serotonin transporter knockout mice. *Genes, Brain, and Behavior*, **6**, 389–400.

Klemenhagen, K. C., Gordon, J. A., David, D. J., Hen, R., & Gross, C. T. (2006). Increased fear response to contextual cues in mice lacking the 5-HT1A receptor. *Neuropsychopharmacology*, **31**, 101–111.

Koyama, S., Kubo, C., Rhee, J. S., & Akaike, N. (1999). Presynaptic serotonergic inhibition of GABAergic synaptic transmission in mechanically dissociated rat basolateral amygdala neurons. *Journal of Physiology*, **518**, 525–538.

Koyama, S., Matsumoto, N., Murakami, N., *et al.* (2002). Role of presynaptic 5-HT1A and 5-HT3 receptors in modulation of synaptic GABA transmission in dissociated rat basolateral amygdala neurons. *Life Sciences*, **72**, 375–387.

Krysiak, R., Obuchowicz, E., & Herman, Z. S. (2000) Conditioned fear-induced changes in neuropeptide Y-like immunoreactivity in rats: the effect of diazepam and buspirone. *Neuropeptides*, **34**, 148–157.

Lambe, E. K., & Aghajanian, G. K. (2006). Hallucinogen-induced UP states in the brain slice of rat prefrontal cortex: role of glutamate spillover and NR2B-NMDA receptors. *Neuropsychopharmacology*, **31**, 1682–1689.

Laviolette. S. R., Lipski, W. J., & Grace, A. A. (2005). A subpopulation of neurons in the medial prefrontal cortex encodes emotional learning with burst and frequency codes through a dopamine D4 receptor-dependent basolateral amygdala input. *Journal of Neuroscience*, **25**, 6066–6075.

Lesch, K. P., Zeng, Y., Reif, A., & Gutknecht, L. (2003). Anxiety-related traits in mice with modified genes of the serotonergic pathway. *European Journal of Pharmacology*, **480**, 185–204.

Li, X., Inoue, T., Abekawa, T., Weng, S., *et al.* (2006). 5-HT1A receptor agonist affects fear conditioning through stimulations of the postsynaptic 5-HT1A receptors in the hippocampus and amygdala. *European Journal of Pharmacology*, **532**, 74–80.

Lira, A,. Zhou, M., Castanon, N., *et al.* (2003). Altered depression-related behaviors and functional changes in the dorsal raphe nucleus of serotonin transporter-deficient mice. *Biological Psychiatry*, **54**, 960–971.

Maier, S. F., & Watkins, L. R. (2005). Stressor controllability and learned helplessness: the roles of the dorsal raphe nucleus, serotonin, and corticotropin-releasing factor. *Neuroscience and Biobehavioral Reviews*, **29**, 829–841.

Marek, G. J., & Aghajanian, G. K. (1998). 5-Hydroxytryptamine-induced excitatory postsynaptic currents in neocortical layer V pyramidal cells: suppression by mu-opiate receptor activation. *Neuroscience*, **86**, 485–497.

Marek, G. J., & Aghajanian, G. K. (1999). 5-HT2A receptor or alpha1-adrenoceptor activation induces excitatory postsynaptic currents in layer V pyramidal cells of the medial prefrontal cortex. *European Journal of Pharmacology*, **367**, 197–206.

Marek, G. J., Wright, R. A., Gewirtz, J. C., & Schoepp, D. D. (2001). A major role for thalamocortical afferents in serotonergic hallucinogen receptor function in the rat neocortex. *Neuroscience*, **105**, 379–392.

Marschner, A., Kalisch, R., Vervliet, B., Vansteenwegen, D., & Buchel, C. (2008). Dissociable roles for the hippo-campus and the amygdala in human cued versus context fear conditioning. *Journal of Neuroscience*, **28**, 9030–9036.

Martin-Ruiz, R., Puig, M. V., Celada, P., *et al.* (2001) Control of serotonergic function in medial prefrontal cortex by serotonin-2A receptors through a glutamate-dependent mechanism. *Journal of Neuroscience*, **21**, 9856–9866.

Mathew, S. J., Price, R. B., & Charney, D. S. (2008). Recent advances in the neurobiology of anxiety disorders: implications for novel therapeutics. *American Journal of Medical Genetics C: Seminars in Medical Genetics*, **148C**, 89–98.

Meyer, J. H., McMain, S., Kennedy, S. H., *et al.* (2003). Dysfunctional attitudes and 5-HT2 receptors during depression and self-harm. *American Journal of Psychiatry*, **160**, 90–99.

Milad, M. R., Wright, C. I., Orr, S. P., *et al.* (2007). Recall of fear extinction in humans activates the ventromedial prefrontal cortex and hippocampus in concert. *Biological Psychiatry*, **62**, 446–454.

Millan, M. J. (2003). The neurobiology and control of anxious states. *Progress in Neurobiology*, **70**, 83–244.

Miller, E. K., & Cohen, J. D. (2001). An integrative theory of prefrontal cortex function. *Annual Review of Neuroscience*, **24**, 167–202.

Miner, L. A., Backstrom, J. R., Sanders-Bush, E., & Sesack, S. R. (2003). Ultrastructural localization of serotonin2A receptors in the middle layers of the rat prelimbic prefrontal cortex. *Neuroscience*, **116**, 107–117.

Monk, C. S., Telzer, E. H., Mogg, K., *et al.* (2008). Amygdala and ventrolateral prefrontal cortex activation to masked angry faces in children and adolescents with generalized anxiety disorder. *Archives of General Psychiatry*, **65**, 568–576.

Murphy, D. L., Li, Q., Engel, S., *et al.* (2001). Genetic perspectives on the serotonin transporter. *Brain Research Bulletin*, **56**, 487–494.

Nash, J. R., Sargent, P. A., Rabiner, E. A., *et al.* (2008). Serotonin 5-HT1A receptor binding in people with panic disorder: positron emission tomography study. *British Journal of Psychiatry*, **193**, 229–234.

Nitschke, J. B., Sarinopoulos, I., Mackiewicz, K. L., Schaefer, H. S., & Davidson, R. J. (2006). Functional neuroanatomy of aversion and its anticipation. *Neuroimage*, **29**, 106–116.

Norton, N., & Owen, M. J. (2005). HTR2A: association and expression studies in neuropsychiatric genetics. *Annals of Medicine*, **37**, 121–129.

Papez, J. W. (1995). A proposed mechanism of emotion. 1937. *Journal of Neuropsychiatry and Clinical Neuroscience*, **7**, 103–112.

Parks, C. L., Robinson, P. S., Sibille, E., Shenk, T., & Toth, M. (1998). Increased anxiety of mice lacking the serotonin1A receptor. *Proceedings of the National Academy of Sciences of the USA*, **95**, 10734–10739.

Paulus, M. P., & Stein, M. B. (2006). An insular view of anxiety. *Biological Psychiatry*, **60**, 383–387.

Pehek, E. A., McFarlane, H. G., Maguschak, K., Price, B., & Pluto, C. P. (2001). M100,907, a selective 5-HT2A antagonist, attenuates dopamine release in the rat medial prefrontal cortex. *Brain Research*, **888**, 51–59.

Pezawas, L., Meyer-Lindenberg, A., Drabant, E. M., *et al.* (2005). 5-HTTLPR polymorphism impacts human cingulate-amygdala interactions: a genetic susceptibility mechanism for depression. *Nature Neuroscience*, **8**, 828–834.

Phelps, E. A., Delgado, M. R., Nearing, K. I., & LeDoux, J. E. (2004). Extinction learning in humans: role of the amygdala and vmPFC. *Neuron*, **43**, 897–905.

Pompeiano, M., Palacios, J. M., & Mengod, G. (1992). Distribution and cellular localization of mRNA coding for 5-HT1A receptor in the rat brain: correlation with receptor binding. *Journal of Neuroscience*, **12**, 440–453.

Puig, M. V., Celada, P., Diaz-Mataix, L., & Artigas, F. (2003). In vivo modulation of the activity of pyramidal neurons in the rat medial prefrontal cortex by 5-HT2A receptors: relationship to thalamocortical afferents. *Cerebral Cortex*, **13**, 870–882.

Quirk, G. J., & Mueller, D. (2008). Neural mechanisms of extinction learning and retrieval. *Neuropsychopharmacology*, **33**, 56–72.

Quirk, G. J., Russo, G. K., Barron, J. L., & Lebron, K. (2000). The role of ventromedial prefrontal cortex in the recovery of extinguished fear. *Journal of Neuroscience*, **20**, 6225–6231.

Quirk, G. J., Likhtik, E., Pelletier, J. G., & Pare, D. (2003). Stimulation of medial prefrontal cortex decreases the responsiveness of central amygdala output neurons. *Journal of Neuroscience*, **23**, 8800–8807.

Ramboz, S., Oosting, R., Amara, D. A., *et al.* (1998). Serotonin receptor 1A knockout: an animal model of anxiety-related disorder. *Proceedings of the National Academy of Sciences of the USA*, **95**, 14476–14481.

Rauch, S. L., Shin, L. M., & Phelps, E. A. (2006). Neurocircuitry models of posttraumatic stress disorder and extinction: human neuroimaging research: past, present, and future. *Biological Psychiatry*, **60**, 376–382.

Remijnse, P. L., Nielen, M. M., van Balkom, A. J., *et al.* (2006). Reduced orbitofrontal-striatal activity on a reversal learning task in obsessive–compulsive disorder. *Archives of General Psychiatry*, **63**, 1225–1236.

Ressler, K. J., & Mayberg, H. S. (2007). Targeting abnormal neural circuits in mood and anxiety disorders: from the laboratory to the clinic. *Nature Neuroscience*, **10**, 1116–1124.

Risch, N., Herrell, R., Lehner, T., *et al.* (2009). Interaction between the serotonin transporter gene (5-HTTLPR), stressful life events, and risk of depression: a meta-analysis. *JAMA*, **301**, 2462–2471.

Rosenkranz, J. A., & Grace, A. A. (2002). Cellular mechanisms of infralimbic and prelimbic prefrontal cortical inhibition and dopaminergic modulation of basolateral amygdala neurons in vivo. *Journal of Neuroscience*, **22**, 324–337.

Santana, N., Bortolozzi, A., Serrats, J., Mengod, G., & Artigas, F. (2004). Expression of serotonin1A and serotonin2A receptors in pyramidal and GABAergic neurons of the rat prefrontal cortex. *Cerebral Cortex*, **14**, 1100–1109.

Sarinopoulos, I., Dixon, G. E., Short, S. J., Davidson, R. J., & Nitschke, J. B. (2006). Brain mechanisms of expectation associated with insula and amygdala response to aversive taste: implications for placebo. *Brain, Behavior, and Immunity*, **20**, 120–132.

Serretti, A., Drago, A., & De Ronchi, D. (2007). HTR2A gene variants and psychiatric disorders: a review of current literature and selection of SNPs for future studies. *Current Medicinal Chemistry*, **14**, 2053–2069.

Stein, C., Davidowa, H., & Albrecht, D. (2000). 5-HT1A receptor-mediated inhibition and 5-HT2 as well as 5-HT3 receptor-mediated excitation in different subdivisions of the rat amygdala. *Synapse*, **38**, 328–337.

Stein, M. & Bienvenu, J. (2004). Diagnostic classification of anxiety disorders: DSM-5 and beyond. In D. S. Charney & E. J. Nestler, eds., *Neurobiology of Mental Illness*. Oxford: Oxford University Press.

Tipples, J., & Sharma, D. (2000). Orienting to exogenous cues and attentional bias to affective pictures reflect separate processes. *British Journal of Psychology*, **91**, 87–97.

Tochigi, M., Umekage, T., Kato, C., *et al.* (2005). Serotonin 2A receptor gene polymorphism and personality traits: no evidence for significant association. *Psychiatric Genetics*, **15**, 67–69.

Tork, I. (1990), Anatomy of the serotonergic system. *Annals of the New York Academy of Sciences*, **600**, 9–34.

Torres, G. E., & Amara, S. G. (2007). Glutamate and monoamine transporters: new visions of form and function. *Current Opinion in Neurobiology*, **17**, 304–312.

Tsetsenis, T., Ma, X. H., Lo Iacono, L., Beck, S. G., & Gross, C. (2007). Suppression of conditioning to ambiguous cues by pharmacogenetic inhibition of the dentate gyrus. *Nature Neuroscience*, **10**, 896–902.

Unschuld, P. G., Ising, M., Erhardt, A., *et al.* (2007). Polymorphisms in the serotonin receptor gene HTR2A are associated with quantitative traits in panic disorder. *American Journal of Medical Genetics B: Neuropsychiatric Genetics*, **144B**, 424–429.

Vollenweider, F. X., Vontobel, P., Hell, D., & Leenders, K. L. (1999). 5-HT modulation of dopamine release in basal ganglia in psilocybin-induced psychosis in man: a PET study with 11Craclopride. *Neuropsychopharmacology*, **20**, 424–433.

Vuilleumier, P. (2005). How brains beware: neural mechanisms of emotional attention. *Trends in Cognitive Science*, **9**, 585–594.

Weisstaub, N. V., Zhou, M., Lira, A., *et al.* (2006). Cortical 5-HT2A receptor signaling modulates anxiety-like behaviors in mice. *Science*, **313**, 536–540.

Wright, C. I., Martis, B., McMullin, K., Shin, L. M., & Rauch, S. L. (2003). Amygdala and insular responses to emotionally valenced human faces in small animal specific phobia. *Biological Psychiatry*, **54**, 1067–1076.

Zhao, S., Edwards, J., Carroll, J., Wiedholz, L., *et al.* (2006). Insertion mutation at the C-terminus of the serotonin transporter disrupts brain serotonin function and emotion-related behaviors in mice. *Neuroscience*, **140**, 321–334.

Chapter 16

Learned fear and innate anxiety in rodents and their relevance to human anxiety disorders

Joshua A. Gordon, Avishek Adhikari

16.1 Introduction

Any effort to understand the causes of anxiety disorders must begin with an important conceptual assumption: anxiety disorders arise from a disturbance of *brain function*. This notion raises the tantalizing possibility that we might understand what goes wrong in the brain during maladaptive anxiety states and, by extension, develop treatments aimed at reversing (or overcoming) this dysfunction.

Arguably one of the best ways of going about understanding a disease state and testing potential treatments is to develop an accurate animal model. Especially in regard to diseases that affect the brain, animal models offer the best chance of careful, in-depth analysis of pathophysiology (what goes wrong) and reproducible, safe tests of potential treatments. The principal issue to resolve is how to develop animal models of relevance to human disorders. This is especially problematic with psychiatric disorders such as anxiety disorders. How can one tell if a mouse is anxious?

It turns out, however, that observing and quantifying anxiety-like behavior in a mouse is not as difficult as one might think. The mechanisms of normative anxiety – the behavioral and physiological characteristics of normal defensive behaviors – are actually quite well conserved across species (see Chapter 6). This is evident from even a cursory consideration of anxiety-related behaviors in humans and mice. In humans, anxiety is typically manifested as worries about potentially threatening events and avoidance of places or situations that make these events more likely to occur. Thus, a dark alley evokes concerns that one might be accosted by a criminal and is avoided when possible. In mice, while it is not possible to measure worry, measuring avoidance is very simple. Given a choice between two rooms in a given apparatus, for example, a mouse will avoid a room in which it has previously received a

shock: the mouse has learned to be afraid of that room. Similarly, given a choice between a bright room and a dark room, a mouse will avoid the bright room: mice are innately afraid of bright lights, perhaps because light makes them more visible to potential predators.

Of course, the repertoire of defensive behaviors in humans and animals extends beyond simple avoidance. Consider for a moment how a person responds to a potentially threatening environment, such as the aforementioned dark alley. One can walk away from it, or approach it cautiously, alert to additional signs of danger. If there is some reason to go down that alley, say, to visit a chic night club at the other end, one ventures in slowly and quietly, alert for sudden movement or unusual objects. Students of animal behavior might describe this as "approach/avoidance behavior." See something move, or hear a loud shout, and one might turn and run – an "escape" response. Confronted with an unmistakably threatening stimulus – such as a gun, aimed and ready to shoot – and one freezes on the spot. Animals engage in exactly the same progression of defensive behaviors. When faced with an environment suggestive of a potential threat, rodents engage in approach/avoidance behavior. An actual threat (such as the presence of a predator) evokes an escape response, and an immediate threat (such as a predator about to strike) evokes freezing behavior. The animal literature tends to classify approach/avoidance and other responses to potential threats as "anxiety" and freezing and other responses to immediate threats as "fear." How these concepts of "anxiety" and "fear" map onto human anxiety disorders is unclear.

Defensive fear and anxiety behaviors have been extensively studied in rodents, using behavioral paradigms that test such behaviors in response to both learned and innately threatening stimuli. For reasons that are not necessarily clear, "fear"-like responses to immediate threats have typically been studied in the context of

Anxiety Disorders: Theory, Research, and Clinical Perspectives, ed. Helen Blair Simpson, Yuval Neria, Roberto Lewis-Fernández, Franklin Schneier. Published by Cambridge University Press. © Cambridge University Press 2010.

learning – that is, animals are taught that particular stimuli signal threats. These learned fear stimuli then evoke a pattern of behavior consistent with the immediate presence of danger. In contrast, "anxiety"-like responses to potential threats have typically been studied in the context of innate responses to non-learned stimuli.

This chapter reviews these studies of learned fear and innate anxiety, detailing the latest advances in the understanding of neurobiological mechanisms and their implications for treatment. The advantages of studying fear and anxiety in rodent models is made plain in terms of the rich mechanistic detail they provide. Consideration also is given to data from human studies, in order to examine the relevance of these animal models of normative defensive behaviors to the pathological anxious behaviors seen in patients with anxiety disorders.

16.2 Once burned, twice shy: the amygdala at the center of a fear circuit

Once burned, twice shy, goes the adage that accurately describes learned fear behaviors. Animals and people alike tend to avoid places and situations in which they have had painful or aversive experiences. This can be adaptive – it is the rare child who will touch a hot stove twice – or maladaptive, for example, when a panic attack at work forces the agoraphobic to quit his job. A principal advantage of learned fear is that it can be easily modeled in rodents, an approach which has been exploited by numerous groups to identify the neural circuits responsible for the learning, expression, and regulation of fear responses (Davis 1997, LeDoux 2003, Quirk & Beer 2006). All learned fear paradigms involve the same basic elements: a standardized, neutral stimulus (for example, a particular tone); a directly threatening stimulus (such as a mild shock); and a behavioral or physiological measure of the fear response (such as freezing behavior or increase in heart rate). For example, in the oft-studied paradigm of conditioned freezing to tone, a rat or mouse is presented simultaneously with both a neutral tone and a mild electrical shock (Figure 16.1A). The animal rapidly learns that the tone predicts a shock, a process known as classical conditioning. Subsequent playback of the same tone evokes a freezing response, in which the animal stops exploring its cage and remains motionless while the sound is being played.

Indeed, playback of the fear-conditioned tone induces a host of behavioral and physiological fear

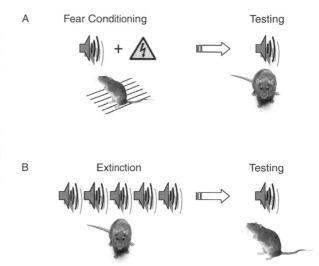

Figure 16.1. Conditioning and extinction of learned fear.
(A) Conditioning of learned fear. Pairing a neutral tone and a shock (left) results in the animal learning that the tone predicts the shock. Subsequent exposure to the tone evokes defensive behaviors such as freezing (right).
(B) Extinction. Repeated exposure to the fear-conditioned tone teaches the animal that the tone no longer predicts shock (left). Subsequent re-exposure to the tone fails to elicit defensive behaviors (right).

behaviors that can be measured in rodents, revealing a network of activated brain regions responsible for each (Davis 1992). Increased heart and respiratory rate, dilated pupils, decreased responses to pain, facial expressions of fear, increased startle responses, defecation and urination, and stimulation of corticosteroid release have all been documented in rodents exposed to fear-conditioned stimuli. Specific brain regions, such as the hypothalamus and various brainstem nuclei, serve as the foot soldiers responsible for specific fear responses. The activation of the lateral hypothalamus leads to increased activity in the sympathetic nervous system, as well as tachycardia and pupilary dilation. Activation of the midbrain central gray leads to freezing behavior. The roles of each of these regions were established through a combination of lesion and electrical stimulation studies: lesioning a specific region abolishes, and stimulating the region mimics the fear response for which that region is responsible.

If these varied brain regions are the foot soldiers of the fear response, then the central nucleus of the amygdala is the general (Figure 16.2). Neurons in this nucleus send their axons to each and every one of the brain regions responsible for the various fear reactions. Lesions of the central nucleus prevent all of the various fear reactions to conditioned stimuli, and stimulating

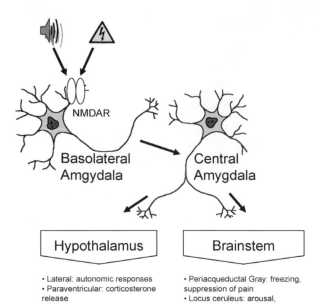

Figure 16.2. Fear-conditioning circuit. Shock and tone information is integrated in the basolateral amygdala, which, through NMDA receptor (NMDAR) activation, learns the association. The basolateral amygdala then activates the central nucleus, which in turn activates downstream regions in the hypothalamus and brainstem that are responsible for different elements of the fear response.

the central nucleus mimics a variety of these responses (Davis 1992). Thus, the central nucleus serves to trigger the myriad fear-related behavioral and physiological responses to conditioned stimuli by activating specific brain areas in the hypothalamus and brainstem.

Yet how is the central nucleus itself activated by fear stimuli? This circuit, too, has been worked out through careful study in the rodent brain. Sensory stimuli (such as the neutral tone and the mild shock) are relayed through thalamic and cortical sensory areas to the basolateral nucleus of the amygdala, which in turn projects to and activates the central nucleus (LeDoux 2000). It is in the basolateral nucleus that the requisite learning takes place; neurons here learn that the tone predicts the shock and signal the central nucleus to activate a set of defensive behaviors (e.g., freezing). Basolateral neurons learn this association by virtue of the properties of a particular receptor for the neurotransmitter glutamate: the NMDA-type glutamate receptor, so named because it can also be activated by the glutamate analog N-methyl-D-aspartic acid. In response to simultaneous activation of the postsynaptic neuron and its presynaptic inputs, the NMDA

receptor allows calcium to enter the postsynaptic neuron; calcium then initiates a cascade of intracellular events that results in a change in the strength of the incoming synapses. Blocking NMDA receptors in the basolateral nucleus of the amygdala prevents the acquisition of conditioned fear (Miserendino *et al.* 1990, Fanselow & Kim 1994, Walker & Davis 2002). This finding leads to a model of fear conditioning in which the simultaneous activation of sensory inputs carrying tone and shock information activate NMDA receptors in the basolateral nucleus, resulting in a strengthening of the synapses that signal the previously neutral tone. Following this plasticity-dependent strengthening, the now fear-conditioned tone is better able to activate basolateral neurons, which in turn activate the central nucleus, triggering a fear response.

16.2.1 Extinction: the neural substrates of overcoming fear learning involve cortical regulation of the amygdala

Once learned, the fear association can be long lasting – up to the lifetime of the animal. Yet it can also be squelched through an additional learning process, called extinction. Through re-exposure to the conditioned stimulus, this time without the reinforcing shock, the animal learns that the stimulus no longer predicts an incoming shock. The stimulus subsequently fails to elicit the fear-conditioned response (Figure 16.1B). The extinction process has two distinct components: the initial learning or pure "extinction" phase, and a subsequent "consolidation" phase in which the extinction memory is preserved for the long term. Take an animal trained to associate a tone with a shock and expose it to the same tone without any shock multiple times the following day: the animal will gradually stop responding to the tone (the fear response has been "extinguished"). Put the same animal back in the same environment 24 hours later and again expose it to the tone: it will still fail to respond (because the extinction memory has been "consolidated") (Quirk & Mueller 2008). Extinction and its consolidation resemble psychological treatments of anxiety disorders, many of which rely on repeated exposures to anxiety-provoking stimuli (see below).

Both extinction and consolidation are also dependent on NMDA receptors, suggesting that they utilize the same neural plasticity mechanisms as the initial fear conditioning. Nonetheless, the two processes are distinguished by separable neurobiological substrates. Infuse NMDA receptor antagonists into the basolateral amygdala during extinction training, and the animal will fail to learn that the stimulus no longer predicts danger (Falls *et al.* 1992). Infuse NMDA receptor antagonists into the medial prefrontal cortex (mPFC) during the extinction training, and the animal will initially extinguish its fear response but will fail to retain the extinction memory: 24 hours later the animal will again respond to the tone with a full-blown fear response (Burgos-Robles *et al.* 2007). The mPFC, located on the medial wall of the frontal cortex, is a brain region implicated in cognitive control of behavior and directly connected with the amygdala, hypothalamus, and other limbic structures. It is therefore perfectly situated to perform a regulatory role in the fear circuit, dampening fear expression by inhibiting amygdala output, a role supported by numerous additional studies of its role in defensive behaviors (Quirk & Beer 2006, Quirk & Mueller 2008).

16.2.2 Fear conditioning and extinction as models of anxiety disorders and their treatment

Fear conditioning has some superficial similarities to several forms of human anxiety disorders. Most obvious are the specific phobias, in which a specific stimulus (blood, spiders, snakes, airplanes, heights, etc.) is assigned an inappropriately threatening value, evoking extreme defensive behaviors. One can easily posit that in patients with specific phobias, the phobic stimulus activates the central nucleus of the amygdala, which in turn activates brain regions responsible for autonomic and behavioral signs of anxiety. While it is not clear that fear conditioning plays an important role in the development of most cases of specific phobias, heightened amygdala responses to phobic stimuli have been demonstrated in several studies (Schienle *et al.* 2005, Etkin & Wager 2007, Straube *et al.* 2007).

Fear conditioning plays a more obvious role in anxiety disorders that involve generalization of a fear response, such as panic disorder with agoraphobia and posttraumatic stress disorder (PTSD). In panic disorder, patients often describe their illness as beginning with an attack of extreme anxiety that comes out of the blue. Over time, however, many patients begin to associate their attacks with the places or situations in which they occur. A patient who has a panic attack at work, for example, may then experience heightened anxiety whenever she goes to work; indeed, the anxiety may be so severe that she avoids going to work altogether. It is as if this patient were a victim of a fear-conditioning experiment, with the worksite as the tone, and the panic attack as the shock. Unfortunately, unlike the limited shocks delivered to the rodents discussed above, panic attacks may continue to occur in patients with the disorder, resulting in an ever-widening circle of places and situations that the patient avoids. The end result is agoraphobia, in which the severely affected patient cannot even leave his or her home for fear of experiencing a panic attack.

Similarly, PTSD patients start out avoiding situations and places that remind them of their traumatic experience. Fear evoked in closely related situations or places results in further generalization so that severely affected patients are subject to anxiety in a variety of situations, greatly limiting their ability to function. An analogous process can be observed in fear-conditioned rodents. Pairing a fear-conditioned stimulus with an additional neutral stimulus – such as a second novel tone – can result in so-called "second order conditioning," such that the animal develops fear responses to the second tone despite the fact that it was never directly paired with shock (Gewirtz & Davis 1998). Studies of neural activity in patients with either panic disorder or PTSD have also shown hyperactivity in the amygdala, underscoring the similarities between these disorders and models of fear conditioning, although in humans amygdala activation also occurs with emotional stimuli that are not fear-inducing.

Where does extinction fit in? One intriguing possibility is that the same mechanisms that govern mPFC-mediated long-term extinction of fear-conditioning processes might underlie successful treatments of these related forms of anxiety. Indeed, the premise that the mPFC and the amygdala oppose each other in the generation of defensive behaviors is an attractive one, as the mainstay of psychotherapeutic approaches to anxiety involves enhancing cognitive control over anxiety symptoms in the context of repeated exposure to feared stimuli (Garakani *et al.* 2006, Quirk & Beer 2006, Berkowitz *et al.* 2007). Accordingly, several studies have shown that successfully treating some anxiety disorders results in increased mPFC activity and/or decreased amygdala activity, strongly suggesting that at least part of the therapeutic response involves harnessing the same sorts of mechanisms involved in extinction of learned fear (Roffman *et al.* 2005, Rauch *et al.* 2006, Etkin & Wager 2007).

16.2.3 Using neurobiological understanding of learned fear to develop novel therapeutic approaches

The recognition that at least some forms of anxiety disorders and their treatment rely on mechanisms similar to those identified in fear-conditioning models raised the seductive possibility that the neurobiological understanding might inform the development of new treatment strategies. One approach of increasing prominence (and promise) is to exploit the neural plasticity mechanism involved in extinction learning. As noted above, NMDA receptors in the amygdala and mPFC are required for extinction learning to result in long-term suppression of learned fear responses. This requirement was discovered by blocking NMDA receptors with an antagonist. The converse experiment also works: augmenting NMDA receptors, using the allosteric modulator D-cycloserine, enhances extinction (Walker *et al.* 2002). Normally, a few unreinforced exposures to the fear-conditioned tone do not result in full-blown extinction of the fear response in rodents. Administration of D-cycloserine augments the otherwise minimally effective regimen, resulting in complete and long-lasting extinction of the fear response.

Would such an approach also work in patients with anxiety disorders? Ressler and colleagues (2004) tested this idea by utilizing a standardized, virtual-reality-based exposure therapy that had been shown to be successful in acrophobia (fear of heights). This treatment paradigm is thought to work through an extinction-like mechanism: expose patients to ever-increasing virtual heights using standard anxiety-reduction techniques, and they slowly learn that heights do not pose any real danger. Patients typically require seven sessions of such therapy to experience significant reductions in discomfort and avoidance of heights. To test the effects of augmenting NMDA receptor activity with D-cycloserine, the authors combined a minimally effective regimen of two exposure therapy sessions with two single doses of the drug, given at the time of the therapy. The shorter therapy plus drug regimen was as effective as the more time-consuming therapy-alone regimen, perhaps the best example to date of a successfully translational neuroscience finding applied to psychiatry. Studies of the effectiveness of D-cycloserine augmentation of extinction therapies in other anxiety disorders relevant to fear conditioning have also yielded promising findings (Hofmann *et al.* 2006, Guastella *et al.* 2007, 2008, Kushner *et al.* 2007, Storch *et al.* 2007, Norberg *et al.* 2008, Wilhelm *et al.* 2008).

16.3 What you already know can hurt you: innate anxiety paradigms reveal additional components of a defensive behavior circuit

While learned fear paradigms have indeed taught us a lot about anxiety, not all fear responses are learned. Think of the dark alley mentioned in the introduction to this chapter. Darkness increases one's anxiety level even without prior learning. Human fear of the dark is *innate*. Innate fears tend to be species-specific. Laboratory-bred monkeys with no experience of snakes nonetheless exhibit avoidance, escape, and even freezing responses when presented with a rubber snake, much less a real one. Rodents are innately fearful of bright lights, as anyone who has had a mouse infestation and a penchant for midnight snacks has indubitably discovered when turning on the kitchen light. Turn on a light suddenly, and a rodent will escape to the dark; if escape is impossible, it will freeze. Given a choice of a bright or dark room, a rodent will spend most of its time exploring the dark room.

Several behavioral paradigms have been developed over the years to measure anxiety-related behaviors in rodents (Figure 16.3). These anxiety tests explore the conflict underlying approach/avoidance behaviors displayed by rodents placed in a novel environment. When exposed to a new place, rodents have a drive to explore the environment, an adaptive trait considering that, in their natural habitat, rodents depend on foraging to find food. However, a novel environment is also potentially threatening, for it may be a site where it is more exposed to predators. Rodents therefore take a cautious approach to exploring novel settings, exhibiting approach/avoidance behaviors and physiological signs of arousal. Moreover, rodents tend to spend more time in the safer (e.g., less exposed) areas of the new environment, an easily measured trait that has been exploited in several laboratory tests of innate anxiety (Whishaw *et al.* 2006). In the open field test, for example, a large, well-illuminated circular arena is surrounded by high walls; mice and rats tend to avoid the brightly lit center and spend most of their time near the walls (Crawley 1985, Belzung & Griebel 2001, Prut & Belzung 2003). The fraction of time spent in the periphery versus the center of the field is used as a behavioral measure of anxiety. A similar preference for closed dark spaces is seen

A. Elevated plus maze

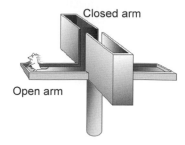

Closed arm

Open arm

B. Open Field

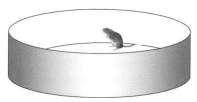

Figure 16.3. Two tests of innate anxiety: (A) the elevated plus maze; (B) the open field.

in the elevated plus maze test, in which rodents prefer either of two enclosed arms to two open ones, and the light/dark test, in which they spend most of their time in the dark half of a two-chambered environment (Montgomery 1955, Pellow et al. 1985, Rodgers 1997, Belzung & Griebel 2001). Findings such as elevated plasma levels of the stress-related hormone corticosterone support the notion that these tests are indeed anxiogenic (Pellow et al. 1985, Cruz et al. 1994).

Not all tests of anxiety rely on physical aspects of the environment to induce defensive behaviors. In the social interaction test, a paradigm used as a model of social anxiety, a similar approach/avoidance conflict occurs (File & Seth 2003). In this test the dependent variable is the time two rats spend in social interaction (sniffing, grooming, etc.). The conflict in this test is between the drive to interact socially and the risk of being harmed by the other animal. More anxious rodents will spend less time interacting with others. Although the nature of the stimuli in this test is different from that in the elevated plus maze and the open field, all these tests fundamentally exploit approach/avoidance conflicts to measure anxiety-related behavior.

Interestingly, there are suggestions of both similarities and differences in the neurobiology underlying these different tests of innate anxiety. In general, animals that perform on the anxious end of the scale on one test often tend to perform on the anxious end of the scale on other tests. However, rigorous mathematical analysis of these tendencies – called factor analysis – suggests that there are several independent factors contributing to anxiety in the tests (Griebel et al. 1996, Ramos et al. 1997, Aguilar et al. 2002). Thus, any given animal might avoid the open arms of the plus maze, for example, and subsequently fail to avoid a novel animal in the social interaction test. Such findings raise the possibility that there are different kinds of innate anxiety, just as there are different kinds of anxiety disorders in humans.

The principal advantage of these tests is that they explore innate behaviors. Thus, they are thought to explore ethologically relevant sources of anxiety and may reflect a different neural circuitry than learned behaviors. Given that many human anxiety disorders are not fully explained by learned responses to fearful stimuli, understanding the neural circuitry of innate anxiety in animals (and how it differs from the neural circuitry of learned fear paradigms) may be of some use in understanding anxiety disorders. Moreover, these tests of anxiety have been exploited both to screen for novel pharmacological compounds, as described below, and to screen genetically altered mice for anxiety-related phenotypes (see Chapter 14).

16.3.1 The effects of anxiolytic and anxiogenic drugs on innate anxiety tests in rodents

Although innate tests appear to accurately model aspects of normal and pathological anxiety in humans, such tests would not be very useful if they lacked pharmacological validity. That is, drugs that reduce or increase anxiety in humans ought to have similar effects in laboratory tests of rodent behavior. As the most commonly used anxiolytic drugs in humans are benzodiazepines (such as diazepam) and selective serotonin reuptake inhibitors (SSRIs) (such as fluoxetine), these two classes of drugs have been used extensively to validate rodent conflict anxiety tasks. Benzodiazepines reduce anxiety in virtually all tests of innate anxiety. In the open field these drugs increase time spent in the aversive center (Britton & Britton 1981, Crawley 1985, Pellow & File 1986, Schmitt & Hiemke 1998, Siemiatkowski et al. 2000), in the social interaction test they increase interaction time (de Angelis & File 1979, File & Hyde 1979), in the elevated plus maze they increase time spent on the exposed arms (Cruz et al. 1994, Pellow & File 1986), and in the light/dark test they increase time spent exploring the bright compartment (Bourin & Hascoet 2003).

The effects of SSRIs are much more complex (Gordon & Hen 2004). It is noteworthy that SSRIs are anxiogenic in humans when given acutely (Grillon et al. 2007) and anxiolytic during chronic treatments (Gorman et al. 2002). The effects of both acute and chronic SSRI treatment have been tested in animal models of anxiety. In the open field, chronic but not acute fluoxetine has been found to be anxiolytic (Dulawa et al. 2004), although others have failed to see such effects (Durand et al. 1999). In the social interaction test, acute treatment with SSRIs appears to be anxiogenic (To & Bagdy 1999, Dekeyne et al. 2000, Bagdy et al. 2001). The effects of chronic treatment with the SSRI fluoxetine in the social interaction test are unclear, as it has been reported both to be anxiogenic (Kantor et al. 2001) and to have no effect (To & Bagdy 1999). The effects of SSRI treatments in the elevated plus maze are similarly inconclusive. Generally, acute treatment with SSRIs is anxiogenic (Drapier et al. 2007, Griebel et al. 1994), in agreement with human studies. The effect of chronic SSRIs in the elevated plus maze, however, is unclear, as some studies show increased anxiety (Griebel et al. 1999, Silva & Brandao 2000) while other reports show decreased anxiety (Griebel et al. 1994, Durand et al. 1999, Kurt et al. 2000). The one consistent finding from these studies is that acute SSRI administration is anxiogenic, as it seems to be in anxiety-disorder patients.

The inconsistent effects of chronic SSRIs in tests of innate anxiety are troubling, given that these drugs are typically effective in many patients with anxiety disorders. However, not all patients (and not all disorders) benefit from even chronic SSRI administration. Furthermore, the inconsistency in the animal literature may be the result of methodological differences between laboratories in what is a relatively young field of research. While the SSRI data at present do not firmly support the validity of these tests as models of human anxiety disorders, it is perhaps too early to draw a final conclusion.

16.3.2 Towards a neural circuitry of innate anxiety

The validity of learned fear models has been confirmed in part by neuroanatomical approaches in both animals and humans, suggesting a fear circuit centered on the amygdala that is hyperactive in normal and pathological fear states (see above). Does the neuroanatomy of innate anxiety shed light on the issue of relevance to the human condition?

Studies of the neuroanatomical basis of innate anxiety tests suggest a network of sites, closely aligned with but somewhat separate from the learned fear network. In contrast to the clear effects of amygdala lesions and manipulations on fear conditioning, most lesion studies suggest that the amygdala is not required for innate anxiety (Moller et al. 1997, Kjelstrup et al. 2002, Kondo & Sakuma 2005). Instead, lesions of a related network of sites, including the ventral hippocampus, the mPFC, and the bed nucleus of the stria terminalis, disrupt anxiety-like behavior in these tests. Lesions of these regions result in effects that are similar to those of benzodiazepines in several of these tests, reducing open-arm and bright-chamber avoidance and increasing social interaction, among other effects (Treit et al. 1998, Gonzalez et al. 2000, Lacroix et al. 2000, Kjelstrup et al. 2002, Shah & Treit 2003, Bannerman et al. 2004). The ventral hippocampus, mPFC, and bed nucleus are components of the limbic system, a circuit long known to be involved in the generation of emotional behaviors; each also is tightly connected with the amygdala. Moreover, these areas also send efferent output to many of the same downstream regions as the central nucleus of the amygdala, such as the hypothalamus and brainstem. They are therefore well situated to generate and/or modulate anxiety-related behaviors, either independent from or in concert with the amygdala.

The distinction between amygdala-dependent and amygdala-independent anxiety responses has been perhaps most clearly demonstrated in an interesting paradigm that can be used to test defensive responses to both learned and innate stimuli – the potentiated startle paradigm. In the learned version, usually called fear-potentiated startle, the effect of a learned fear stimulus on the strength of animal's startle response is measured. Normally, a rat will startle to a loud noise by jumping up in the air; the force the rat uses to make the jump is a reliable measure of this "startle response." The rat's baseline startle response is measured, and then the rat is trained to associate a stimulus (such as a tone) with a shock, in much the same manner as discussed above. The tone is then presented immediately before the startle stimulus, and the strength of the rat's startle response is again measured. The startle response is much larger when the startle stimulus is given along with the learned tone, as opposed to when the startle stimulus is given alone. The strength of this increase is *fear-potentiated startle* (Campeau & Davis 1995).

In the innate version of this paradigm, no training is given, but the startle response of rodents is measured in the presence or absence of bright light. Rats will naturally startle more in the light, and the strength of the increase in startle response with light is called *light-enhanced startle*. Intriguingly, fear-potentiated startle, a learned behavior, requires the amygdala, but light-enhanced startle, which is innate, does not (Walker & Davis 1997a). Rather, it requires the bed nucleus, a region implicated in other innate forms of anxiety as noted above (Walker & Davis 1997b). The dependence of light-enhanced startle on other brain regions involved in innate anxiety (such as the ventral hippocampus and mPFC) has not yet been tested. Notably, lesions of the bed nucleus have no effect on fear-potentiated startle (Hitchcock & Davis 1991), completing the double dissociation and supporting the separability of the two anxiety-related circuits.

16.4 Separable but not separate: a unified limbic circuit of anxiety

While the aforementioned lesion studies have shown that the amygdala is not required for normal anxiety-like behavior in innate anxiety tests, there is considerable evidence that it nonetheless plays an accessory role. Infusing drugs (typically inhibitory agents such as GABA receptor agonists and benzodiazepines) into an otherwise intact amygdala has profound effects in several of these tasks, including the elevated plus maze, open field, and social anxiety tests (Green & Vale 1992, McNamara & Skeleton 1993, Zangrossi Junior & Graeff 1994, Pesold & Treit 1995, Sanders & Shekhar 1995).

Neuroanatomical data support the notion that the various structures implicated in innate forms of anxiety are part of the same circuit as the amygdala. For example, both the ventral hippocampus and the mPFC project to many of the same brainstem structures involved in producing defensive behaviors, such as the periaqueductal gray (Burwell *et al.* 1995, Vertes 2004), as does the central nucleus of the amygdala (Veening *et al.* 1984). Moreover, the bed nucleus, mPFC, and ventral hippocampus each project directly to the amygdala itself (Alheid *et al.* 1995, Burwell & Witter 2002, Vertes 2004), suggesting that the separable innate anxiety and learned fear pathways are capable of interacting. Importantly, both the mPFC and the ventral hippocampus receive highly processed contextual information from association cortices and rhinal cortices (Hoover & Vertes 2007). This suggests that the mPFC and the ventral hippocampus are in an ideal position to evaluate threats in the environment and activate

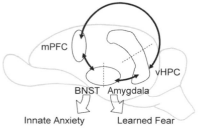

Figure 16.4. A putative unitary anxiety circuit. Information processing by the medial prefrontal cortex (mPFC) and ventral hippocampus (vHPC) guide the amygdala and bed nucleus of the stria terminalis (BNST). The former is primarily responsible for learned fear behaviors, the latter for innate anxiety.

downstream structures (such as the brainstem) to induce defensive responses.

Studies of neural activity also confirm the notion that the hippocampus, mPFC, and amygdala work together in both innate anxiety and learned fear. For example, although the hippocampus is not required for normal freezing responses to fear-conditioned tones, neural activity in the hippocampus nonetheless synchronizes with activity in the amygdala during presentation of the tone (Seidenbecher *et al.* 2003). We have recently found similar synchronization between the hippocampus and the mPFC in mice exposed to the elevated plus maze and a novel open field (Adhikari *et al.* 2010).

These findings suggest that the mPFC, hippocampus, amygdala, and bed nucleus are indeed part of a functional circuit involved in the generation and modulation of defensive behaviors (Figure 16.4). While certain elements of the circuit play particularly important roles in certain forms of anxiety (bed nucleus for light-enhanced startle, an innate response; amygdala for fear conditioning to tone, a learned response), it is likely that under normal circumstances the circuit operates together to compare and evaluate threats in the environment and to generate the appropriate specific defensive responses.

16.5 Future directions: relevance of the extended anxiety circuit to anxiety disorders in humans

Considerable questions remain with regard to the relevance of this combined circuit to human anxiety disorders. As noted above, the key elements of the learned fear pathway – chiefly the amygdala and mPFC – have been clearly implicated in anxiety disorders through neuroimaging studies. Moreover, knowledge about the mechanisms underlying learned fear – particularly the requirement for NMDA-receptor-mediated plasticity in extinction of learned fear – has led directly to novel treatment approaches. Are the brain regions required for innate anxiety involved in human anxiety disorders? Will further investigation of the patterns of neural activity responsible for innate anxiety lead to novel therapeutic targets and strategies?

Anxiety disorders clearly have learned and non-learned components, suggesting that both types of animal models are of potential relevance. The generalization seen in panic disorder and PTSD – where patients "learn" to avoid situations and places that trigger anxiety symptoms – seems to be a phenomenon akin to learned fear. Simple phobias may arise from learning, such as the child who becomes afraid of dogs after getting bitten. However, there are also examples of phobias without any evidence of prior threatening exposure, suggesting direct relevance of models of innate anxiety. Finally, generalized anxiety disorder (GAD) offers perhaps the most compelling case for the relevance of innate anxiety, in that patients worry about numerous aspects of their lives without any logical rationale or previous experience. To the extent that such patients are overly anxious in response to typical threats, they are akin to the genetically altered mouse which responds to elevated plus maze with increased open-arm avoidance: they are biased towards a stronger defensive reaction.

Moving beyond such phenomenological comparisons to hard data demonstrating the relevance of innate anxiety to human disorders will require further study. Neuroimagers might focus on neglected components of the extended anxiety circuit. For example, the anterior hippocampus (the human analog of the rodent ventral hippocampus) is located quite close to the amygdala, suggesting the possibility that abnormal amygdala activity occurs in concert with abnormal hippocampal activity. Functional connectivity between the mPFC and the amygdala has been a focus of neuroimaging studies; might the increased functional activity we have reported between the mPFC and the hippocampus also be seen in anxiety-disorder patients? Focusing on patients with disorders less readily explained through learning, such as those with specific phobias without prior exposure or those with GAD, might be particularly helpful in further exploring the relevance of animal models of innate anxiety. Studies that take into account multiple animal models of anxiety have

the potential to identify additional critical elements of abnormal brain function that lead to pathological anxiety. If such efforts succeed, they promise to enhance our understanding and treatment of anxiety disorders in all their various forms.

Acknowledgments

Some of the work referred to in this chapter was supported by grants from the NIMH (R01 MH081968 and K08 MH096823 to J.A.G.).

References

Adhikari, A., Topiwala, M.A., Gordon, J.A. (2010). Synchronized activity between the ventral hippocampus and the medial prefrontal cortex during anxiety. *Neuron*, **65**, 257–269.

Aguilar, R., Gil, L., Flint, J., *et al.* (2002). Learned fear, emotional reactivity and fear of heights: a factor analytic map from a large F2 intercross of Roman rat strains. *Brain Research Bulletin*, **57**, 17–26.

Alheid, G. F., de Olmos, J. S., & Beltramino, C. A. (1995). Amygdala and extended amygdala. In G. Paxinos, ed., *The Rat Nervous System*. New York, NY: Academic Press.

Bagdy, G., Graf, M., Anheuer, Z. E., Modos, E. A., & Kantor, S. (2001). Anxiety-like effects induced by acute fluoxetine, sertraline or m-CPP treatment are reversed by pretreatment with the 5-HT2C receptor antagonist SB-242084 but not the 5-HT1A receptor antagonist WAY-100635. *International Journal of Neuropsychopharmacology*, **4**, 399–408.

Bannerman, D. M., Rawlins, J. N., McHugh, S. B., *et al.* (2004). Regional dissociations within the hippocampus: memory and anxiety. *Neuroscience and Biobehavioral Review*, **28**, 273–283.

Belzung, C., & Griebel, G. (2001). Measuring normal and pathological anxiety-like behaviour in mice: a review. *Behavioral Brain Research*, **125**, 141–149.

Berkowitz, R. L., Coplan, J. D., Reddy, D. P., & Gorman, J. M. (2007). The human dimension: how the prefrontal cortex modulates the subcortical fear response. *Reviews in the Neurosciences*, **18**, 191–207.

Bourin, M., & Hascoet, M. (2003). The mouse light/dark box test. *European Journal of Pharmacology*, **463**, 55–65.

Britton, D. R., & Britton, K. T. (1981). A sensitive open field measure of anxiolytic drug activity. *Pharmacology, Biochemistry, and Behavior*, **15**, 577–582.

Burgos-Robles, A., Vidal-Gonzalez, I., Santini, E., & Quirk, G. J. (2007). Consolidation of fear extinction requires NMDA receptor-dependent bursting in the ventromedial prefrontal cortex. *Neuron*, **53**, 871–880.

Burwell, R. D., & Witter, M. P. (2002). Basic anatomy of the parahippocampal region in monkeys and rats. In M. P. Witter & F. G. Wouterlood, eds., *The Parahippocampal*

Region: Organization and Role in Cognitive Function. Oxford: Oxford University Press.

Burwell, R. D., Witter, M. P., & Amaral, D. G. (1995). Perirhinal and postrhinal cortices of the rat: a review of the neuroanatomical literature and comparison with findings from the monkey brain. *Hippocampus*, **5**, 390–408.

Campeau, S., & Davis, M. (1995). Involvement of the central nucleus and basolateral complex of the amygdala in fear conditioning measured with fear-potentiated startle in rats trained concurrently with auditory and visual conditioned stimuli. *Journal of Neuroscience*, **15**, 2301–2311.

Crawley, J. N. (1985). Exploratory behavior models of anxiety in mice. *Neuroscience and Biobehavioral Reviews*, **9**, 37–44.

Cruz, A. P., Frei, F., & Graeff, F. G. (1994). Ethopharmacological analysis of rat behavior on the elevated plus-maze. *Pharmacology, Biochemistry, and Behavior*, **49**, 171–176.

Davis, M. (1992). The role of the amygdala in fear and anxiety. *Annual Review of Neuroscience*, **15**, 353–375.

Davis, M. (1997). Neurobiology of fear responses: the role of the amygdala. *Journal of Neuropsychiatry and Clinical Neuroscience*, **9**, 382–402.

de Angelis, L., & File, S. E. (1979). Acute and chronic effects of three benzodiazepines in the social interaction anxiety test in mice. *Psychopharmacology (Berlin)*, **64**, 127–129.

Dekeyne, A., Brocco, M., Adhumeau, A., Gobert, A., & Millan, M. J. (2000). The selective serotonin (5-HT)1A receptor ligand, S15535, displays anxiolytic-like effects in the social interaction and vogel models and suppresses dialysate levels of 5-HT in the dorsal hippocampus of freely-moving rats: a comparison with other anxiolytic agents. *Psychopharmacology (Berlin)*, **152**, 55–66.

Drapier, D., Bentue-Ferrer, D., Laviolle, B., *et al.* (2007). Effects of acute fluoxetine, paroxetine and desipramine on rats tested on the elevated plus-maze. *Behavioral Brain Research*, **176**, 202–209.

Dulawa, S. C., Holick, K. A., Gundersen, B., & Hen, R. (2004). Effects of chronic fluoxetine in animal models of anxiety and depression. *Neuropsychopharmacology*, **29**, 1321–1330.

Durand, M., Berton, O., Aguerre, S., *et al.* (1999). Effects of repeated fluoxetine on anxiety-related behaviours, central serotonergic systems, and the corticotropic axis in SHR and WKY rats. *Neuropharmacology*, **38**, 893–907.

Etkin, A., & Wager, T. D. (2007). Functional neuroimaging of anxiety: a meta-analysis of emotional processing in PTSD, social anxiety disorder, and specific phobia. *American Journal of Psychiatry*, **164**, 1476–1488.

Falls, W. A., Miserendino, M. J., & Davis, M. (1992). Extinction of fear-potentiated startle: blockade by infusion of an NMDA antagonist into the amygdala. *Journal of Neuroscience*, **12**, 854–863.

Fanselow, M. S., & Kim, J. J. (1994). Acquisition of contextual pavlovian fear conditioning is blocked by application of an NMDA receptor antagonist D,L-2-amino-5-phosphonovaleric acid to the basolateral amygdala. *Behavioral Neuroscience*, **108**(1), 210–212.

File, S. E., & Hyde, J. R. (1979). A test of anxiety that distinguishes between the actions of benzodiazepines and those of other minor tranquilisers and of stimulants. *Pharmacology, Biochemistry, and Behavior*, **11**, 65–69.

File, S. E., & Seth, P. (2003). A review of 25 years of the social interaction test. *European Journal of Pharmacology*, **463**, 35–53.

Garakani, A., Mathew, S. J., & Charney, D. S. (2006). Neurobiology of anxiety disorders and implications for treatment. *Mount Sinai Journal of Medicine*, **73**, 941–949.

Gewirtz, J. C., & Davis, M. (1998). Application of Pavlovian higher-order conditioning to the analysis of the neural substrates of fear conditioning. *Neuropharmacology*, **37**, 453–459.

Gonzalez, L. E., Rujano, M., Tucci, S., *et al.* (2000). Medial prefrontal transection enhances social interaction. I: Behavioral studies. *Brain Research*, **887**, 7–15.

Gordon, J. A., & Hen, R. (2004). The serotonergic system and anxiety. *Neuromolecular Medicine*, **5**, 27–40.

Gorman, J. M., Kent, J. M., & Coplan, J. D. (2002). Current and emerging therapeutics of anxiety and stress disorders. In K. L. Davis, D. S. Charney, J. T. Coyle, & C. Nemeroff, eds., *Neuropsychopharmacology: the Fifth Generation of Progress*. Philadelphia, PA: Lippincott Williams & Wilkins.

Green, S., & Vale, A. L. (1992). Role of amygdaloid nuclei in the anxiolytic effects of benzodiazepines in rats. *Behavioral Pharmacology*, **3**, 261–264.

Griebel, G., Moreau, J. L., Jenck, F., Misslin, R., & Martin, J. R. (1994). Acute and chronic treatment with 5-HT reuptake inhibitors differentially modulate emotional responses in anxiety models in rodents. *Psychopharmacology (Berlin)*, **113**, 463–470.

Griebel, G., Blanchard, D. C., & Blanchard, R. J. (1996). Evidence that the behaviors in the mouse defense test battery relate to different emotional states: a factor analytic study. *Physiology and Behavior*, **60**, 1255–1260.

Griebel, G., Cohen, C., Perrault, G., & Sanger, D. J. (1999). Behavioral effects of acute and chronic fluoxetine in Wistar-Kyoto rats. *Physiology and Behavior*, **67**, 315–320.

Grillon, C., Levenson, J., & Pine, D. S. (2007). A single dose of the selective serotonin reuptake inhibitor citalopram exacerbates anxiety in humans: a fear-potentiated startle study. *Neuropsychopharmacology*, **32**, 225–231.

Guastella, A. J., Dadds, M. R., Lovibond, P. F., Mitchell, P., & Richardson, R. (2007). A randomized controlled trial of the effect of d-cycloserine on exposure therapy for spider fear. *Journal of Psychiatric Research*, **41**, 466–471.

Guastella, A. J., Richardson, R., Lovibond, P. F., *et al.* (2008). A randomized controlled trial of D-cycloserine enhancement of exposure therapy for social anxiety disorder. *Biological Psychiatry*, **63**, 544–549.

Hitchcock, J. M., & Davis, M. (1991). Efferent pathway of the amygdala involved in conditioned fear as measured with the fear-potentiated startle paradigm. *Behavioral Neuroscience*, **105**, 826–842.

Hofmann, S. G., Meuret, A. E., Smits, J. A., *et al.* (2006). Augmentation of exposure therapy with d-cycloserine for social anxiety disorder. *Archives of General Psychiatry*, **63**, 298–304.

Hoover, W. B., & Vertes, R. P. (2007). Anatomical analysis of afferent projections to the medial prefrontal cortex in the rat. *Brain Structure and Function*, **212**, 149–179.

Kantor, S., Graf, M., Anheuer, Z. E., & Bagdy, G. (2001). Rapid desensitization of 5-HT1A receptors in Fawn-Hooded rats after chronic fluoxetine treatment. *European Neuropsychopharmacology*, **11**, 15–24.

Kjelstrup, K. G., Tuvnes, F. A., Steffenach, H. A., *et al.* (2002). Reduced fear expression after lesions of the ventral hippocampus. *Proceedings of the National Academy of Sciences of the USA*, **99**, 10825–10830.

Kondo, Y., & Sakuma, Y. (2005). The medial amygdala controls the coital access of female rats: a possible involvement of emotional responsiveness. *Japanese Journal of Physiology*, **55**, 345–353.

Kurt, M., Arik, A. C., & Celik, S. (2000). The effects of sertraline and fluoxetine on anxiety in the elevated plus-maze test in mice. *Journal of Basic Clinical Physiology and Pharmacology*, **11**, 173–180.

Kushner, M. G., Kim, S. W., Donahue, C., *et al.* (2007). D-cycloserine augmented exposure therapy for obsessive–compulsive disorder. *Biological Psychiatry*, **62**, 835–838.

Lacroix, L., Spinelli, S., Heidbreder, C. A., & Feldon, J. (2000). Differential role of the medial and lateral prefrontal cortices in fear and anxiety. *Behavioral Neuroscience*, **114**, 1119–1130.

LeDoux, J. (2000). Emotion circuits in the brain. *Annual Review of Neuroscience*, **23**, 155–184.

LeDoux, J. (2003). The emotional brain, fear, and the amygdala. *Cellular and Molecular Neurobiology*, **23**, 727–738.

McNamara, R. K., & Skeleton, R. W. (1993). Effects of intracranial infusions of chlordiazepoxide on spatial learning in the Morris water maze. I. Neuroanatomical specificity. *Behavioral Brain Research*, **59**, 175–191.

Miserendino, M. J., Sananes, C. B., Melia, K. R., & Davis, M. (1990). Blocking of acquisition but not expression of conditioned fear-potentiated startle by NMDA antagonists in the amygdala. *Nature*, **345**, 716–718.

Moller, C., Wiklund, L., Sommer, W., Thorsell, A., & Heilig, M. (1997). Decreased experimental anxiety and voluntary ethanol consumption in rats following central but not basolateral amygdala lesions. *Brain Research*, **760**, 94–101.

Montgomery, K. C. (1955). The relation between fear induced by novel stimulation and exploratory behavior. *Journal of Computational Physiology and Psychology*, **48**, 254–260.

Norberg, M. M., Krystal, J. H., & Tolin, D. F. (2008). A meta-analysis of d-cycloserine and the facilitation of fear extinction and exposure therapy. *Biological Psychiatry*, **63**, 1118–1126.

Pellow, S., & File, S. E. (1986). Anxiolytic and anxiogenic drug effects on exploratory activity in an elevated plus-maze: a novel test of anxiety in the rat. *Pharmacology, Biochemistry and Behavior*, **24**, 525–529.

Pellow, S., Chopin, P., File, S. E., & Briley, M. (1985). Validation of open:closed arm entries in an elevated plus-maze as a measure of anxiety in the rat. *Journal of Neuroscience Methods*, **14**, 149–167.

Pesold, C., & Treit, D. (1995). The central and basolateral amygdala differentially mediate the anxiolytic effects of benzodiazepines. *Brain Research*, **671**, 213–221.

Prut, L., & Belzung, C. (2003). The open field as a paradigm to measure the effects of drugs on anxiety-like behaviors: a review. *European Journal of Pharmacology*, **463**, 3–33.

Quirk, G. J., & Beer, J. S. (2006). Prefrontal involvement in the regulation of emotion: convergence of rat and human studies. *Current Opinion in Neurobiology*, **16**, 723–727.

Quirk, G. J., & Mueller, D. (2008). Neural mechanisms of extinction learning and retrieval. *Neuropsychopharmacology*, **33**, 56–72.

Ramos, A., Berton, O., Mormede, P., & Chaouloff, F. (1997). A multiple-test study of anxiety-related behaviours in six inbred rat strains. *Behavioural Brain Research*, **85**, 57–69.

Rauch, S. L., Shin, L. M., & Phelps, E. A. (2006). Neurocircuitry models of posttraumatic stress disorder and extinction: human neuroimaging research: past, present, and future. *Biological Psychiatry*, **60**, 376–382.

Ressler, K. J., Rothbaum, B. O., Tannenbaum, L., *et al.* (2004). Cognitive enhancers as adjuncts to psychotherapy: use of d-cycloserine in phobic individuals to facilitate extinction of fear. *Archives General Psychiatry*, **61**, 1136–1144.

Rodgers, R. J. (1997). Animal models of "anxiety": where next? *Behavioral Pharmacology*, **8**, 477–496; discussion 497–504.

Roffman, J. L., Marci, C. D., Glick, D. M., Dougherty, D. D., & Rauch, S. L. (2005). Neuroimaging and the functional neuroanatomy of psychotherapy. *Psychological Medicine*, **35**, 1385–1398.

Sanders, S. K., & Shekhar, A. (1995). Anxiolytic effects of chlordiazepoxide blocked by injection of GABAA and benzodiazepine receptor antagonists in the region of the anterior basolateral amygdala of rats. *Biological Psychiatry*, **37**, 473–476.

Schienle, A., Schafer, A., Walter, B., Stark, R., & Vaitl, D. (2005). Brain activation of spider phobics towards disorder-relevant, generally disgust- and fear-inducing pictures. *Neuroscience Letters*, **388**, 1–6.

Schmitt, U., & Hiemke, C. (1998). Combination of open field and elevated plus-maze: a suitable test battery to assess strain as well as treatment differences in rat behavior. *Progress in Neuropsychopharmacology and Biological Psychiatry*, **22**, 1197–1215.

Seidenbecher, T., Laxmi, T. R., Stork, O., & Pape, H. C. (2003). Amygdalar and hippocampal theta rhythm synchronization during fear memory retrieval. *Science*, **301**, 846–850.

Shah, A. A., & Treit, D. (2003). Excitotoxic lesions of the medial prefrontal cortex attenuate fear responses in the elevated-plus maze, social interaction and shock probe burying tests. *Brain Research*, **969**, 183–194.

Siemiatkowski, M., Sienkiewicz-Jarosz, H., Czlonkowska, A. I., Bidzinski, A., & Plaznik, A. (2000). Effects of buspirone, diazepam, and zolpidem on open field behavior, and brain [3H]muscimol binding after buspirone pretreatment. *Pharmacology, Biochemistry and Behavior*, **66**, 645–651.

Silva, R. C., & Brandao, M. L. (2000). Acute and chronic effects of gepirone and fluoxetine in rats tested in the elevated plus-maze: an ethological analysis. *Pharmacology, Biochemistry and Behavior*, **65**, 209–216.

Storch, E. A., Merlo, L. J., Bengtson, M., *et al.* (2007). D-cycloserine does not enhance exposure-response prevention therapy in obsessive–compulsive disorder. *International Clinical Psychopharmacology*, **22**, 230–237.

Straube, T., Mentzel, H. J., & Miltner, W. H. (2007). Waiting for spiders: brain activation during anticipatory anxiety in spider phobics. *Neuroimage*, **37**, 1427–1436.

To, C. T., & Bagdy, G. (1999). Anxiogenic effect of central CCK administration is attenuated by chronic fluoxetine or ipsapirone treatment. *Neuropharmacology*, **38**, 279–282.

Treit, D., Aujla, H., & Menard, J. (1998). Does the bed nucleus of the stria terminalis mediate fear behaviors? *Behavioral Neuroscience*, **112**, 379–386.

Veening, J. G., Swanson, L. W., & Sawchenko, P. E. (1984). The organization of projections from the central nucleus of the amygdala to brainstem sites involved in central autonomic regulation: a combined retrograde transport-immunohistochemical study. *Brain Research*, **303**, 337–357.

Vertes, R. P. (2004). Differential projections of the infralimbic and prelimbic cortex in the rat. *Synapse*, **51**, 32–58.

Walker, D. L., & Davis, M. (1997a). Anxiogenic effects of high illumination levels assessed with the acoustic startle response in rats. *Biological Psychiatry*, **42**, 461–471.

Walker, D. L., & Davis, M. (1997b). Double dissociation between the involvement of the bed nucleus of the stria terminalis and the central nucleus of the amygdala in startle increases produced by conditioned versus unconditioned fear. *Journal of Neuroscience*, **17**, 9375–9383.

Walker, D. L., & Davis, M. (2002). The role of amygdala glutamate receptors in fear learning, fear-potentiated startle, and extinction. *Pharmacology, Biochemistry and Behavior*, **71**, 379–392.

Walker, D. L., Ressler, K. J., Lu, K. T., & Davis, M. (2002). Facilitation of conditioned fear extinction by systemic administration or intra-amygdala infusions of d-cycloserine as assessed with fear-potentiated startle in rats. *Journal of Neuroscience*, **22**, 2343–2351.

Whishaw, I. Q., Gharbawie, O. A., Clark, B. J., & Lehmann, H. (2006). The exploratory behavior of rats in an open environment optimizes security. *Behavioral Brain Research*, **171**, 230–239.

Wilhelm, S., Buhlmann, U., Tolin, D. F., *et al.* (2008). Augmentation of behavior therapy with d-cycloserine for obsessive–compulsive disorder. *American Journal of Psychiatry*, **165**, 335–341; quiz 409.

Zangrossi Junior, H., & Graeff, F. G. (1994). Behavioral effects of intra-amygdala injections of GABA and 5-HT acting drugs in the elevated plus-maze. *Brazilian Journal of Medical and Biological Research*, **27**, 2453–2456.

Brain systems underlying anxiety disorders: a view from neuroimaging

Amit Etkin, Tor D. Wager

17.1 Introduction

In this chapter, a central idea we explore is that clinical anxiety involves changes in brain systems that are involved in the generation and regulation of normal emotion. In particular, a common element of anxiety disorders may be an abnormally elevated threat response, which appears to involve brain systems implicated in "fear" responses and "fear learning" in animals and healthy humans. However, some anxiety disorders, such as posttraumatic stress disorder (PTSD), generalized anxiety disorder (GAD), and panic disorder, appear to involve a more generalized dysregulation of negative affect. Interestingly, "fear-like" and "anxiety-like" behaviors in animal models may be different, and their brain substrates dissociable. Thus, a brain-based model of anxiety must also consider brain systems involved in negative affective states that extend beyond what has traditionally been labeled as "fear." In this chapter, we will review the neural basis of anxiety in healthy and clinical populations, with a primary focus on functional neuroimaging studies in humans.

17.2 The "neural reference space" for emotion

"Emotion" – comprising a collection of specific thoughts, feelings, and action tendencies – is thought to emerge from one of two broad, interacting routes: (1) reactivity to a simple stimulus (such as seeing a spider) or (2) appraisal of one or more stimuli in a particular situational context. The neural reference space for emotion is thus, unsurprisingly, complex. A number of consistently activated regions from a recent meta-analysis of 163 studies are shown in Figure 17.1A. These include the amygdala; insula; ventral striatum and pallidum; periaqueducal gray (PAG); hypothalamus; medial prefrontal (mPFC),

inferior frontal (IFC), and temporal cortices; and cerebellum – in short, many of the regions implicated in animal and human studies of emotional experience and emotional learning.

It is difficult to describe a particular region or set of regions with a simple label, such as "appraisal," or even "fear." Thus, instead we adopted a "bottom-up" approach to understanding how these regions assemble into functional networks by grouping them based on their patterns of co-activation. That is, if the studies that activated the right IFC were the same studies that activated the left IFC and the dorso-medial PFC (dmPFC), these regions were grouped into a functional network. The hope is that these networks may then be related to psychological concepts such as "appraisal" and "anxiety" or map onto physiological processes or action tendencies. Moreover, because our semantic labels may not correspond cleanly with specific brain systems, understanding the organization of brain systems in emotion is also a key step towards reformulation of psychological categories to better reflect brain processes.

Our analyses identified a number of networks, shown in Figure 17.1. Figure 17.1A shows an "unfolded" map of the key brain regions in two dimensions. Each dot is a brain region, and the different colors of the dots indicate the functional groups to which they belong. The closer two dots are, the more highly co-activated they are across studies. Lines connecting the dots indicate statistically significant co-activation of the pair of connected regions. These functional groups of regions provide a rudimentary organizational framework for understanding specific components of emotional processing. Shown in yellow and magenta in Figure 17.1A is a network involving occipital sensory and association and posterior cingulate cortices, which monitor and analyze the sensory environment. These networks provide input into amygdala and other "core" limbic

Anxiety Disorders: Theory, Research, and Clinical Perspectives, ed. Helen Blair Simpson, Yuval Neria, Roberto Lewis-Fernández, Franklin Schneier. Published by Cambridge University Press. © Cambridge University Press 2010.

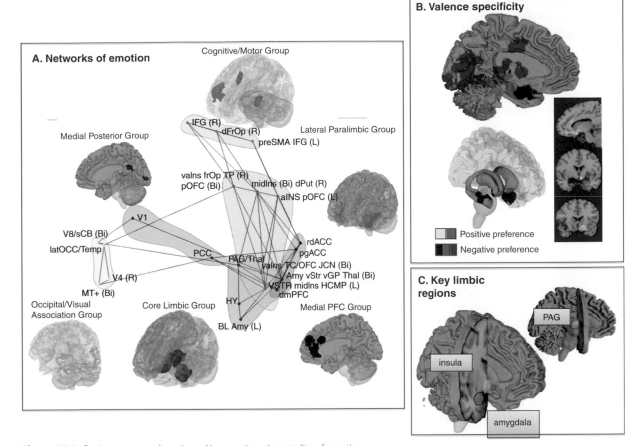

Figure 17.1. Regions commonly activated in neuroimaging studies of emotion.

(A) Grouping of regions identified by a meta-analysis of 163 studies based on patterns of co-activation reveals multiple, interacting networks of brain regions involved in a diverse set of emotion-related functions (adapted from Kober *et al.* 2008). Each point on the two-dimensional network graph identifies a brain region. The closer together the points are on the graph, the more strongly co-activated the regions tend to be. However, because the graph is a compressed two-dimensional representation of a more complex matrix of co-activations, the point location provides only a rough guideline. The lines show pairs of regions that were significantly co-activated, correcting for multiple comparisons and excluding links that were mediated by any other single region. The colors identify groups of regions that co-activated together based on cluster analyses (see Kober *et al.* 2008 for more details).

(B) Comparison of regions preferentially involved in the experience of positive versus negative emotion from the meta-analysis in (A), as reconstructed from analyses in Wager *et al.* (2008a). Hot colors indicate a relative positive emotion preference, and cool colors indicate a negative emotion preference.

(C) An outline of "core limbic" regions identified in the emotion meta-analysis, including the insula in green, the amygdala in red, and the periaqueductal gray (PAG) in burgundy.

regions (red in Figure 17.1A) and paralimbic regions (green). An interconnected network of frontal regions (aqua) whose member regions are commonly activated in tasks involving cognitive control is connected to the paralimbic network. This frontal network provides a way for items to be held in the conscious "workspace" of working memory and to influence core limbic regions. Finally, the mPFC group (blue) is closely functionally related to the core limbic regions, suggesting that the mPFC is therefore in a position to govern, and be governed by, the core limbic regions.

17.3 Brain substrates of negative reactivity and regulation

17.3.1 Fear conditioning as a core model of negative emotional reactivity

Animal studies of fear learning have provided a solid and detailed body of evidence for understanding a particular type of negative emotional reactivity – learned "fear-like" responses to cues that have been paired with aversive events in a conditioning procedure.

The behavioral expression of fear involves a pathway from the basolateral amygdala (BLA) to the central nucleus in the superior portion of the amygdala, which projects to the PAG and hypothalamus (Paxinos 2003). Stimulation of the PAG produces coordinated patterns of physiological and behavioral changes consistent with a whole-organism response mode (Bandler & Shipley 1994, Behbehani 1995). Its projections to the orbitofrontal cortex (OFC) and mPFC, the mediodorsal thalamic "association" nucleus, and neuromodulatory systems, such as the noradrenergic system, govern arousal and regulate behavior.

Substantial evidence corroborates the role of the human amygdalar complex in negative emotion-related reactivity, including numerous studies that have demonstrated conditioned responses in the amgydala to threat cues (Buchel & Dolan 2000, Etkin & Wager 2007, LaBar et al. 1998). While the amygdala appears to be a critical region for Pavlovian fear learning and an important component of fear responses, amygdala activity is by no means isomorphic with feelings of fear or anxiety. Amygdala activation is more commonly observed in response to perceiving stimuli that signal uncertainty or threat than in studies that elicit negative emotion (Phan et al. 2002, Wager et al. 2008a). It is reliably elicited by stimuli presented outside of conscious awareness (Etkin et al. 2004, Whalen et al. 2004) and that typically have no measurable impact on self-reported fear or anxiety. One way to think of amygdala activation is as a marker for vigilance for threat cues or for stimuli with behavioral relevance in the environment, which can be affected by anxiety. In our study, BLA activation to unconsciously presented fearful faces was greatest for those with the highest baseline anxiety (Etkin et al. 2004), suggesting that threat perception and learning mechanisms in the amygdala are particularly dominant in anxious individuals.

The insula is another region that is consistently responsive to negative affective states in humans, including conditioned fear cues (Etkin & Wager 2007). It is not directly involved in Pavlovian fear conditioning in animal models, but it is critical for learning and consolidating other types of anxiety-related behaviors, such as conditioned taste aversion (Eisenberg et al. 2003), highlighting the differential importance of various brain circuitry depending on the particular type of learning and emotional behavior. The insula is heavily interconnected with the amygdala, hypothalamus, and PAG (Paxinos 2003). Whereas the amygdala is particularly important for learning the affective value of isolated sensory cues, the insula is important for representing somatic and visceral information from the body. Its activation during a task in which subjects have to attend to their heartbeats, for example, was greater in individuals with greater interoceptive sensitivity and in those with higher levels of anxiety (Critchley et al. 2004). In humans, the amygdala and insula are also very commonly co-activated (Kober et al. 2008) (Figure 17.1), suggesting a prominent role for the insula in the representation of negative affective states. Thus, while the Pavlovian conditioning model has been tremendously useful in understanding fear elicited by simple cues, a broader set of systems is likely relevant for the range of negative affect involved in human anxiety.

17.3.2 Networks that support negative reactivity and regulation

The "core" limbic circuitry involved in negative emotional reactivity discussed above is probably an important component of anxiety in humans. However, other cortical and subcortical networks interact with this circuitry and can amplify, elaborate, or inhibit activity associated with behavioral and experiential aspects of negative emotion. Two large-scale networks that also can modulate fear and anxiety are shown at the right of Figure 17.2. One of these is a network of regions involved in executive working memory (aqua, top) that is broadly engaged when maintaining and manipulating information in the mind's conscious workspace (Courtney et al. 1997, D'Esposito et al. 2000, Wager & Smith 2003). Another network, shown in yellow in Figure 17.2, involves the vmPFC, hippocampus, and posterior cingulate cortex (PCC). Both of these networks are thought to work in concert to provide context-based control over the generation and regulation of negative emotion.

17.4 The executive working memory system

Executive control is critical for goal-directed cognition, including controlling the focus of attention. In Gross's influential theory of emotion regulation (Gross 1998), the earliest mechanism for regulating emotion when confronted with an adverse situation is to avoid attending to emotional, or "hot," elements of a scene. Another key "leverage point" is cognitive reappraisal, or the generation of positive meaning in response to adverse events. The "cognitive control" network in Figure 17.1 (aqua) shows the subset of the executive

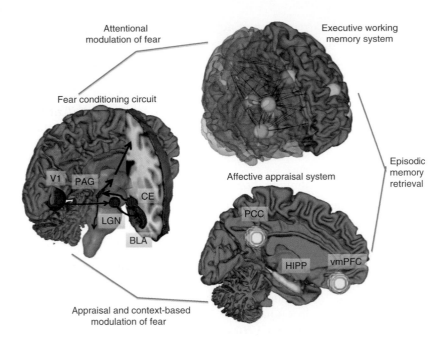

Figure 17.2. Schematic representation of two cortical networks that interact with and modulate activity in "core limbic" regions involved in fear and anxiety. Pathways related to fear conditioning are shown at the left, including a route from the primary visual cortex (V1) through the lateral geniculate nucleus (LGN) to the basolateral amygdala (BLA), and fear expression from the central nucleus of the amygdala (CE) to the brainstem through the periaqueductal gray (PAG). One modulatory network, the "executive/working memory system," includes dorsomedial and lateral prefrontal regions implicated in a range of cognitive functions. The "affective appraisal system," by contrast, involves cortical midline structures, as well as the medial temporal lobe. This network is involved in diverse functions involving memory retrieval, learning and representation of context information, and representations of the "self" and related internal contexts.

working memory system engaged most consistently during emotional processing. Numerous studies have now linked activity in multiple regions within the executive system to the cognitive reappraisal and suppression of emotion (Ochsner & Gross 2005). In a recent study of reappraisal of negative emotions elicited by aversive pictures, we found that multiple regions of the dorsomedial, superior and inferior lateral prefrontal, parietal, and temporal cortices were activated during reappraisal, and that their activity predicted greater success at reducing negative emotion (Wager *et al.* 2008b). Many of these regions correspond closely to regions reported in meta-analyses of executive working memory (Wager & Smith 2003) and controlled selection of semantic information and motor responses (Nee *et al.* 2007).

The amygdala is the emotion-related region most consistently downregulated during reappraisal (Ochsner & Gross 2005, 2008). In our recent study (Wager *et al.* 2008b), reappraisal success was positively and independently correlated with both reduced amygdala responses to aversive pictures and greater responses in the nucleus accumbens and ventral striatum. In analyzing frontal "cognitive control" regions that predicted these subcortical responses, we focused on the ventrolateral prefrontal cortex (VLPFC), which is particularly important for controlled information-selection processes. The VLPFC was positively correlated with both amygdala and accumbens activation,

suggesting a prefrontal role in both the generation and regulation of emotion. Our interpretation was that viewing the pictures requires two kinds of appraisals. Most of the aversive pictures in the standardized set we used do not elicit automatic negative reactions. Rather, they require cognitive interpretation to generate a negative response. For example, a picture of a crying elderly woman requires filling in some critical background details before it is aversive: the woman may appear to be sick, or she may be sad because a loved one has died. When participants were asked to reappraise the pictures, they were asked to generate a second, more positive appraisal: the woman is crying because her grandson has just been accepted to college and has a bright future. The idea is that of controlled information selection and memory retrieval, a process of cognitive contextualization. This cognitive control network can both increase and decrease negative emotion. Bilateral VLPFC is activated by both positive and negative emotion-induction tasks, often in tandem with subcortical activation (Kober *et al.* 2008).

A role for the executive attention system in fear conditioning has not been intensively explored, in part because fear conditioning is a very simple process at a cognitive level of analysis. However, Delgado and colleagues (2008) reported lateral PFC activity during the cognitive regulation of conditioned fear responses. The implication is that conditioned fear, like other types of negative emotional responses, can be regulated by the executive control system.

17.5 The affective appraisal network

The group of regions that we have termed the "affective appraisal network" includes the rostral mPFC, including both dorsal (dmPFC) and ventral (vmPFC) subdivisions, the hippocampus, and the posterior cingulate cortex (PCC). These regions are shown in yellow in Figure 17.2. This triad of regions, along with the inferior parietal cortex, has received much attention recently because of its role in a number of self-evaluation-related processes. The vmPFC is activated robustly even with relatively minimal manipulations of attention to the self or internal state (Northoff *et al.* 2006), and the PCC has a similar profile of activation and is often co-activated with vmPFC (Buckner & Carroll 2007, Kober *et al.* 2008). These regions have some of the highest levels of resting metabolism in the brain (Raichle *et al.* 2001). What is striking about these areas, however, is that they are robustly *deactivated* in a wide variety of cognitive tasks (Gusnard & Raichle 2001). These features have led to the labeling of the vmPFC and PCC, along with other temporal areas, as the "default mode network" (Raichle *et al.* 2001).

Interestingly, there is one kind of difficult cognitive task that reliably *increases* activity in the default mode network, the hippocampus, and medial temporal lobes: long-term memory retrieval. Recently, Buckner and Carroll (2007) have highlighted the striking similarity in activation patterns across the default mode network when no explicit task is performed: these similarities include long-term memory-related activations, prospection or prediction of future states, and processes of self-evaluation and representing others' knowledge. Thus, an integrative view of the human vmPFC and interconnected areas is that they comprise a system for retrieving information from memory about the current situation, combining it with information about the internal state of the body, and prospection about the implications of the context for the future self. This process is precisely what is captured by the term "emotional appraisal," which refers to the integration of the environmental context with an assessment of one's internal needs, goals, and capabilities.

17.5.1 Dissociable roles for the dmPFC and vmPFC in reactivity and regulation

If the mPFC is important for context-based appraisal, it should be important for both the generation and regulation of negative emotions, and ample evidence suggests that this is the case. Recent neuroimaging and animal evidence converges to suggest that the dorsal regions are most involved in generating negative appraisals, whereas the most ventral regions may play a preferential role in generating positive appraisals that reduce anxiety and negative emotion. In our meta-analysis (Wager *et al.* 2008a) and others (Kringelbach & Rolls 2004), vmPFC and medial OFC show a preference for positive emotional experiences, whereas the dmPFC shows a preference for negative experiences. This vmPFC region does not appear in the overall network analysis shown in Figure 17.1 because its activation was not consistent enough across all types of emotion.

The distinction between dorsal and ventral regions of the mPFC also is seen in animal studies of fear learning and human studies of more complex behaviors (Quirk *et al.* 2000, Milad & Quirk 2002, Milad *et al.* 2004, Vertes 2004, Gabbott *et al.* 2005). In humans, vmPFC activity is correlated with extinction memory during delayed extinction tests (Phelps *et al.* 2004, Kalisch *et al.* 2006). The dmPFC shows increased responses to conditioned cues, whereas the vmPFC shows deactivation (Phelps *et al.* 2004, Delgado *et al.* 2008). These studies suggest that dorsal portions of mPFC are important for generating fear responses, or more generally for generating negative appraisals, and ventral regions are important for representing contextual information that reduces fear expression. Combined with findings from human studies implicating mPFC in the controlled retrieval of information from memory, the overall impression is that the mPFC region is involved in the integration of sensory, interoceptive, and mnemonic information into an overall representation of the self in context.

The link between mPFC, episodic memory, and context processing may help explain the role of mPFC in fear learning and extinction. If mPFC and the hippocampus together form part of a memory-guided appraisal system, then simple forms of fear learning should not require mPFC or hippocampus. This appears to be the case. The hippocampus's role in fear learning is limited to consolidation of contextual fear (Kim *et al.* 1993, Maren *et al.* 1997), and the mPFC is not critical for fear learning or immediate fear extinction. However, in more complex learning situations the mPFC may be necessary.

Some aspects of extinction memory also appear to require the "context-based appraisal" mPFC–hippocampal circuit as well. Extinction learning, for example, is impaired by hippocampal inactivation (Corcoran *et al.* 2005). Expressing extinction behavior in the correct context also requires an intact hippocampus (Corcoran *et al.* 2005). In humans, extinction recall co-activates both vmPFC and hippocampus (Kalisch *et al.* 2006, Milad *et al.* 2007). Studies have implicated the mPFC in the generation and regulation of emotion in contexts beyond fear learning and extinction as well. In our recent emotion regulation study (Wager *et al.* 2008b), vmPFC activity was associated with increases in nucleus accumbens, which in turn predicted successful reduction of negative emotion.

Another example that extends the role of mPFC beyond the study of fear conditioning is a recent series of papers on emotional conflict. Etkin and colleagues (2006) showed subjects images of fearful or happy facial expressions and asked them to identify the emotion. Written across the faces were the words "fear" or "happy," which were either of the same emotion type as the facial expression (congruent) or a different type (incongruent). This paradigm can shed light on the brain mechanisms involved in processing affective valence and those used to ignore competing affect-related information. Emotion identification was poorer in the incongruent condition, and dmPFC activation was higher. In addition, incongruent trials produced a regulatory effect on processing in the next trial, reducing dmPFC activity to subsequent incongruent trials. This type of trial-to-trial regulation has been taken as an indication that conflict increases control mechanisms, which then reduce conflict in subsequent trials (Gratton *et al.* 1992, Botvinick *et al.* 1999, Kerns *et al.* 2004, Egner & Hirsch 2005a, 2005b). Importantly, this type of emotion regulation, unlike the reappraisal process described earlier, occurs spontaneously and without the explicit awareness of subjects, hence an "implicit" form of emotion regulation. Together, the results implicate dmPFC in processing affective conflict. A follow-up study found that activation in the nearby dorsal cingulate was common to the monitoring or evaluation of both emotional and non-emotional conflict (Egner *et al.* 2008), suggesting a broader role for dmPFC in processing competing types of information. Along these lines, activation of the dorsomedial PFC or dorsal ACC is seen during interpretation of affective ambiguity (Simmons *et al.* 2006).

More ventral areas of the mPFC, by contrast, were *more* active on incongruent trials that followed incongruent trials, suggesting a role in implementing the control processes that reduce affective ambiguity and conflict. Activation in the vmPFC during the regulation of conflict was associated with simultaneous and coordinated reduction in amygdalar activity – a relationship that predicted the behavioral success of emotion regulation.

17.6 Clinical neuroimaging studies of anxiety disorders: a meta-analytic framework

The number of functional neuroimaging studies of negative emotion in clinical anxiety disorders has grown at a rapid pace, now reaching a point at which a quantitative meta-analytic review is feasible. Much of the clinical neuroimaging literature, particularly in its earlier periods, reports studies of small groups of subjects, with significant sample heterogeneity between studies and methodologies. This has led to inconsistencies of findings across studies, even for the brain regions most heavily hypothesized to be important for anxiety. One advantage of a meta-analysis is that it allows for a quantitative summary of the findings by accounting for cross-study variability. In addition, robust meta-analytic findings can help define the regions of greatest interest and support specific hypotheses for future studies so that these studies can approach their questions in the most direct and nuanced manner possible.

In a recent meta-analysis (Etkin & Wager 2007), we compared negative emotional processing in post-traumatic stress disorder (PTSD), social anxiety disorder (SAD), and specific phobia, as well as experimentally induced anxiety to discrete cues in healthy individuals through fear conditioning. These disorders were chosen as they were the only anxiety disorders for which a sufficient number of relatively homogeneous publications were available to allow for a reliable meta-analysis. The studies included for each disorder were a combination of (1) symptom-provocation studies, in which scripts, images, or sounds were used to evoke disorder-specific anxiety symptoms, and (2) studies using generally negative, but not disorder-specific, emotional stimuli. The latter were most often pictures of aversive scenes or emotional facial expressions.

Common to all three anxiety disorders was consistent hyperactivation of the amygdala and insula in patients, compared to matched controls, as shown in Figure 17.3. A similar pattern of activation was noted during fear conditioning, suggesting that amygdala and

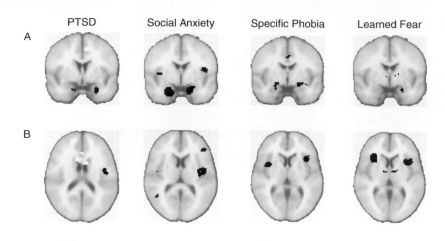

Figure 17.3. Clusters in which significant hyperactivation or hypoactivation was found in patients with posttraumatic stress disorder (PTSD), social anxiety disorder, and specific phobia relative to comparison subjects, and in healthy subjects undergoing fear conditioning. Notable is the common hyperactivation in the amygdala and insula. Adapted from Etkin and Wager (2007). Only PTSD was characterized by hypoactivation of the medial prefrontal cortex (part of the "affective appraisal system").

insula hyperactivation in patients shares common features with fear conditioning. This finding is important because it identifies a core phenotype for at least these three anxiety disorders and supports an understanding of anxiety derived from animal fear-conditioning studies. Moreover, it helps to settle debate in the literature about whether, as hypothesized, amygdalar hyperactivity is a hallmark of at least some common forms of clinical anxiety. In our meta-analysis there was also a small cluster of hypoactivation in the dorsal part of the amygdala in PTSD specifically, which was spatially distinct from the more ventral cluster showing hyperactivity. Finally, it brings the insula, which had not been a central part of previous neural circuitry conceptualizations of anxiety, into prominence alongside the amygdala.

In addition to the shared findings across disorders, there are also important differences between disorders. Most strikingly, PTSD was characterized by extensive hypoactivation in the mPFC, including the pre-SMA region, which forms part of the executive working memory system, and the rostral cingulate and vmPFC regions associated with context-based control of emotion (Figure 17.4). Hypoactivation of the vmPFC proper is significant, given the increasingly well-documented relationship between this region and fear extinction that we reviewed above. These hypoactivations were significantly more common in PTSD than in the other two anxiety disorders.

Converging evidence comes from structural imaging studies, which have reported decreased gray-matter volumes in patients with PTSD in both dorsal and ventral mPFC (Yamasue *et al.* 2003, Karl *et al.* 2006, Kasai *et al.* 2008). One particularly well-controlled study assessed anterior cingulate volumes in identical twin pairs with similar combat trauma exposure but with only one twin diagnosed with PTSD (Kasai *et al.* 2008). Decreased ACC volumes were associated specifically with the presence of PTSD symptoms.

Of the three disorders, PTSD is considered to be most severe, and it has the most diverse symptomatology. In addition to symptoms of hyperarousal and hypervigilance to trauma-related cues, and avoidance of trauma reminders, all of which may be consistent with a model of anxiety based on inappropriately exuberant fear conditioning, PTSD also presents with a range of symptoms reflecting generalized emotional dysregulation. The latter include emotional numbing, generalization of anxiety reactions to stimuli not closely related with the trauma, intrusive thoughts and memories, rumination, affective instability (e.g., anger outbursts), anhedonia, and a sense of negative foreboding (American Psychiatric Association 2000).

In light of the previous discussion of emotional processing and implicit regulation by the limbic–medial prefrontal circuit, we proposed that the robust hypoactivation in the mPFC in PTSD reflects a deficit in implicit context-based emotion regulation occurring in the absence of deliberate attempts at emotional control (Etkin & Wager 2007). This neural abnormality would therefore be reflected clinically in symptoms of emotion dysregulation and anxiety generalization, rather than being specifically a deficit of fear extinction (Etkin & Wager 2007). Moreover, in the context of the previous discussion of the affective appraisal system, patients with PTSD appear to have dysfunction in both the dorsal affect monitoring/generation and ventral regulation components.

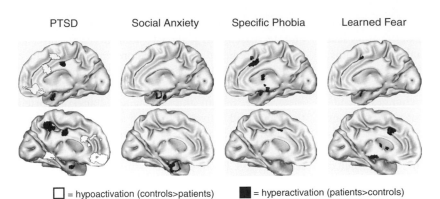

PTSD   Social Anxiety   Specific Phobia   Learned Fear

☐ = hypoactivation (controls>patients)   ■ = hyperactivation (patients>controls)

Figure 17.4. Medial brain surface renderings showing clusters in which significant hyperactivation or hypoactivation was found in patients with PTSD, social anxiety disorder, and specific phobia relative to comparison subjects, and in healthy subjects undergoing fear conditioning. Notable are PTSD-specific hypoactivations in the dorsal and ventral portions of the medial prefrontal cortex. Adapted from Etkin and Wager (2007).

17.7 Generalization of anxiety beyond disorder-related material: PTSD and specific phobia

As discussed above, functional neuroimaging studies of anxiety have employed both disorder-specific and generally negative stimuli. These experiments help determine the extent to which specific types of anxiety manifest through abnormal responses to any negatively valenced stimulus, or whether a response is only elicited to disorder-specific stimuli. For example, different facial expressions can trigger limbic system activation in healthy subjects and can thus be used as a probe of emotional processing in disorders where abnormal social signaling is not a central feature. Patients with PTSD displayed the characteristic pattern of medial prefrontal hypoactivity when viewing fearful compared to neutral or happy faces (Shin *et al.* 2005, Williams *et al.* 2006), counting emotionally negative compared to neutral words (Shin *et al.* 2001), recalling anxious or sad autobiographical events using script-guided imagery (Lanius *et al.* 2003), or viewing pictures of aversive compared to neutral visual scenes (Phan *et al.* 2006). Viewing fearful-expression faces also resulted in amygdalar hyperactivity in PTSD (Shin *et al.* 2005). Patients with specific phobia, meanwhile, showed amygdalar responses to emotional faces similar to those of controls (Wright *et al.* 2003). These data suggest that dysregulation within the limbic–medial prefrontal circuit during the processing of non-disorder-specific negative stimuli may be characteristic of states of generalized emotional dysregulation, such as seen in PTSD, and does not merely reflect the presence of anxiety per se.

It is now also clear, based on a number of imaging studies in healthy subjects, that understanding disorder-related alterations in amygdalar functioning requires separate analyses of emotional processing within and outside of awareness. Several recent studies have shown that elevated generalized anxiety (e.g., trait anxiety) in non-psychiatric populations is associated with exaggerated amygdalar activation, most sensitively detected when emotional stimuli are processed outside of awareness or under the presence of limited attentional resources (Bishop *et al.* 2004, Etkin *et al.* 2004). In PTSD, fearful faces can activate the amygdala even when processed outside of awareness (Rauch *et al.* 2000, Bryant *et al.* 2008a). While similar manipulations of attention or awareness have not been reported in other anxiety disorders, this type of approach will be useful to probe the level at which vigilance or hypersensitivity to threat is already evident in each anxiety disorder.

17.8 Treatment studies

Compared to depression, relatively few neuroimaging-coupled intervention studies have been reported for each anxiety disorder. Of these, most are difficult to interpret because of an absence of important experimental controls. Nonetheless, there are several suggestive studies that open the way to increasingly better designed and more sophisticated approaches. In one such study, Furmark and colleagues (2002) examined patients with SAD treated with either citalopram or cognitive–behavioral therapy (CBT), measuring brain activity in response to having to give a prepared speech in the scanner while in the presence of others, a potent symptom provocation paradigm (Tillfors *et al.* 2001). Improvement in symptoms with treatment was accompanied by decreased activity in the amygdala and the medial temporal lobe. No such changes were seen in wait-list control subjects. Comparing treatment groups with a control group of wait-list patients who received no treatment allowed the authors to rule out changes related only to subject rescanning or simply to the passage of time. Decreases in the activity of the amygdala were seen in both the CBT and the citalopram groups, supporting an important role for this region in the symptoms of SAD. The two treatment groups, however, differed with respect to neural changes outside the amygdala, though interpretation of these findings is hampered by the very small sample sizes (six subjects per group). Interestingly, the degree to which amygdala activity decreased as a result of therapy predicted patients' reduction in symptoms one year later. Along similar lines, though using resting brain metabolic imaging, Baxter and colleagues (1992) noted normalization of caudate hyperactivity in OCD after treatment with either fluoxetine or CBT (nine subjects per group).

Finally, Straube and colleagues (2006) examined subjects with spider phobia and compared the effects of symptom provocation in a group randomized to receive brief, intensive CBT (two four- to five-hour sessions) to a wait-list control group. At baseline, spider phobics hyperactivated the insula and dorsal ACC in response to video clips of spiders. After treatment, the CBT group no longer showed these abnormalities, but they persisted in the wait-list control group. Together, these studies demonstrate that the neural abnormalities associated with symptomatology in anxiety disorders (e.g., amygdala and insula hyperactivation) are corrected after successful clinical interventions. However, much remains unclear, including a more thorough understanding of which neural abnormalities persist after treatment, whether they reflect trait or vulnerability markers, and by what neurobiological mechanisms treatment-related change comes about. It is likely that an understanding of the circuits mediating emotional reactivity and regulation, as outlined above, will be useful in this respect as well. It is interesting in this regard that another study of CBT for spider phobia noted an increase in ventromedial prefrontal activation during symptom provocation after therapy but not in a wait-list control group (Schienle et al. 2007).

Another important aspect of understanding the mechanisms of treatments for anxiety is an appreciation of which subjects are most likely to respond to treatment, whether they respond differentially to various treatments, and why. To this end, two studies have reported results of correlations of pretreatment brain activation during emotional processing with treatment outcome in two anxiety disorders. Whalen and colleagues (2008) reported that increased rostral ACC and decreased amygdala activation to fearful faces at baseline predicted a better response to venlafaxine, a serotonin–norepinephrine reuptake inhibitor commonly used as an antidepressant, in patients with GAD. Meanwhile, Bryant and colleagues (2008b) reported that increased activation in both the rostral ACC and amygdala in response to unconsciously presented fearful faces at baseline was predictive of a favorable response to CBT in patients with PTSD. While these results are preliminary and have not yet been replicated, they raise several interesting possibilities. First, the same brain region (e.g., amygdala) may differentially predict treatment outcome, depending on either the diagnosis or the treatment strategy. Second, a common brain region (e.g., rostral ACC) may be broadly predictive of the likelihood of a patient responding to any treatment. Indeed, treatment-outcome prediction studies in depression have consistently and similarly implicated the rostral ACC across different treatments and imaging modalities (reviewed in Etkin et al. 2005). Even more intriguing, these data suggest that individual differences in the aspects of implicit emotion regulation mediated by the medial PFC may be the ultimate predictor of treatment response across varied treatments and disorders.

17.9 Conclusion

In this chapter, we have outlined limbic–prefrontal neural circuits involved in the reactivity to and regulation of negative emotional stimuli. We focus on a core circuit for negative affective reactivity identified in animal and human studies of fear conditioning. Activity in these regions appears to be modulated by two large-scale, distributed systems. One, the *executive working memory system*, is a set of cortical networks that comprise a system for goal-directed, flexible control over attention and memory. The other, the *affective appraisal system*, is a set of paralimbic cortical and subcortical regions involved in emotion generation and regulation, self-related cognition, long-term memory retrieval, and context-based modulation of conditioned fear.

While it is clear that certain domains have been well studied and that the literature now provides a basis for specific neuroanatomical hypotheses for future experiments, it is also readily apparent that a great deal more work on anxiety disorders and treatment interventions is needed to map basic findings onto clinical conditions. The systems reviewed in this chapter provide a basis for testable outcome measures for therapeutic interventions and provide some guiding principles for establishing the neural circuitry that underlies both vulnerability and resilience to several types of anxiety disorders. This research is in its early stages, and it ultimately may lead to the identification of endophenotypes for genetic vulnerability and other intermediate phenotypes that can be used to both classify disorders and understand individual variability in treatment responses.

Acknowledgments

We would like to thank Lisa Feldman Barrett for her collaborative efforts on the emotion meta-analyses, and for helpful discussions on multilevel analysis and the meta-analytic framework. Software implementing the meta-analyses depicted in this chapter is available from www.columbia.edu/cu/psychology/tor. The work presented here was supported in part by grants NSF 0631637 and R01MH076136 (T.D.W.).

References

American Psychiatric Association (2000). *Diagnostic and Statistical Manual of Mental Disorders*, 4th edn, text revision (DSM-IV-TR). Washington, DC: American Psychiatric Association.

Bandler, R., & Shipley, M. T. (1994). Columnar organization in the midbrain periaqueductal gray: modules for emotional expression? *Trends in Neuroscience*, **17**, 379–389.

Baxter, L. R., Schwartz, J. M., Bergman, K. S., *et al.* (1992). Caudate glucose metabolic rate changes with both drug and behavior therapy for obsessive–compulsive disorder. *Archives of General Psychiatry*, **49**, 681–689.

Behbehani, M. M. (1995). Functional characteristics of the midbrain periaqueductal gray. *Progress in Neurobiology*, **46**, 575–605.

Bishop, S. J., Duncan, J., & Lawrence, A. D. (2004). State anxiety modulation of the amygdala response to unattended threat-related stimuli. *Journal of Neuroscience*, **24**, 10364–10368.

Botvinick, M., Nystrom, L. E., Fissell, K., Carter, C. S., & Cohen, J. D. (1999). Conflict monitoring versus selection-for-action in anterior cingulate cortex. *Nature*, **402**, 179–181.

Bryant, R. A., Kemp, A. H., Felmingham, K. L., *et al.* (2008a). Enhanced amygdala and medial prefrontal activation during nonconscious processing of fear in posttraumatic stress disorder: an fMRI study. *Human Brain Mapping*, **29**, 517–523.

Bryant, R. A., Felmingham, K., Kemp, A., *et al.* (2008b). Amygdala and ventral anterior cingulate activation predicts treatment response to cognitive behaviour therapy for post-traumatic stress disorder. *Psychology and Medicine*, **38**, 555–561.

Buchel, C., & Dolan, R. J. (2000). Classical fear conditioning in functional neuroimaging. *Current Opinions in Neurobiology*, **10**, 219–223.

Buckner, R. L., & Carroll, D. C. (2007). Self-projection and the brain. *Trends in Cognitive Sciences*, **11**, 49–57.

Corcoran, K. A., Desmond, T. J., Frey, K. A., & Maren, S. (2005). Hippocampal inactivation disrupts the acquisition and contextual encoding of fear extinction. *Journal of Neuroscience*, **25**, 8978–8987.

Courtney, S. M., Ungerleider, L. G., Keil, K., & Haxby, J. V. (1997). Transient and sustained activity in a distributed neural system for human working memory. *Nature*, **386**, 608–611.

Critchley, H. D., Wiens, S., Rotshtein, P., Ohman, A., & Dolan, R. J. (2004). Neural systems supporting interoceptive awareness. *Nature Neuroscience*, **7**, 189–195.

Delgado, M. R., Nearing, K. I., Ledoux, J. E., & Phelps, E. A. (2008). Neural circuitry underlying the regulation of conditioned fear and its relation to extinction. *Neuron*, **59**, 829–838.

D'Esposito, M., Postle, B. R., & Rypma, B. (2000). Prefrontal cortical contributions to working memory: evidence from event-related fMRI studies. *Experimental Brain Research*, **133**, 3–11.

Egner, T., & Hirsch, J. (2005a). Cognitive control mechanisms resolve conflict through cortical amplification of task-relevant information. *Nature Neuroscience*, **8**, 1784–1790.

Egner, T., & Hirsch, J. (2005b). The neural correlates and functional integration of cognitive control in a Stroop task. *Neuroimage*, **24**, 539–547.

Egner, T., Etkin, A., Gale, S., & Hirsch, J. (2008). Dissociable neural systems resolve conflict from emotional versus nonemotional distracters. *Cerebral Cortex*, **18**, 1475–1484.

Eisenberg, M., Kobilo, T., Berman, D. E., & Dudai, Y. (2003). Stability of retrieved memory: inverse correlation with trace dominance. *Science*, **301**, 1102–1104.

Etkin, A., & Wager, T. D. (2007). Functional neuroimaging of anxiety: a meta-analysis of emotional processing in PTSD, social anxiety disorder, and specific phobia. *American Journal of Psychiatry*, **164**, 1476–1488.

Etkin, A., Klemenhagen, K. C., Dudman, J. T., *et al.* (2004). Individual differences in trait anxiety predict the response of the basolateral amygdala to unconsciously processed fearful faces. *Neuron*, **44**, 1043–1055.

Etkin, A., Pittenger, C., Polan, H. J., & Kandel, E. R. (2005). Toward a neurobiology of psychotherapy: basic science and clinical applications. *Journal of Neuropsychiatry and Clinical Neuroscience*, **17**, 145–158.

Etkin, A., Egner, T., Peraza, D. M., Kandel, E. R., & Hirsch, J. (2006). Resolving emotional conflict: a role for the rostral anterior cingulate cortex in modulating activity in the amygdala. *Neuron*, **51**, 871–882.

Furmark, T., Tillfors, M., Marteinsdottir, I., *et al.* (2002). Common changes in cerebral blood flow in patients with social phobia treated with citalopram or cognitive–behavioral therapy. *Archives of General Psychiatry*, **59**, 425–433.

Gabbott, P. L., Warner, T. A., Jays, P. R., Salway, P., & Busby, S. J. (2005). Prefrontal cortex in the rat: projections to subcortical autonomic, motor, and limbic centers. *Journal of Computational Neurology*, **492**, 145–177.

Gratton, G., Coles, M. G., & Donchin, E. (1992). Optimizing the use of information: strategic control of activation of responses. *Journal of Experimental Psychology: General*, **121**, 480–506.

Gross, J. J. (1998). The emerging field of emotion regulation: an integrative review. *Review of General Psychology*, **2**, 271–299.

Gusnard, D. A., & Raichle, M. E. (2001). Searching for a baseline: functional imaging and the resting human brain. *Nature Reviews Neuroscience*, **2**, 685–694.

Kalisch, R., Korenfeld, E., Stephan, K. E., *et al.* (2006). Context-dependent human extinction memory is mediated by a ventromedial prefrontal and hippocampal network. *Journal of Neuroscience*, **26**, 9503–9511.

Karl, A., Schaefer, M., Malta, L. S., *et al.* (2006). A meta-analysis of structural brain abnormalities in PTSD. *Neuroscience and Biobehavioral Review*, **30**, 1004–1031.

Kasai, K., Yamasue, H., Gilbertson, M. W., *et al.* (2008). Evidence for acquired pregenual anterior cingulate gray matter loss from a twin study of combat-related posttraumatic stress disorder. *Biological Psychiatry*, **63**, 550–556.

Kerns, J. G., Cohen, J. D., MacDonald, A. W., *et al.* (2004). Anterior cingulate conflict monitoring and adjustments in control. *Science*, **303**, 1023–1026.

Kim, J. J., Rison, R. A., & Fanselow, M. S. (1993). Effects of amygdala, hippocampus, and periaqueductal gray lesions on short-and long-term contextual fear. *Behavioral Neuroscience*, **107**, 1093–1098.

Kober, H., Barrett, L. F., Joseph, J., *et al.* (2008). Functional grouping and cortical-subcortical interactions in emotion: A meta-analysis of neuroimaging studies. *Neuroimage*, **42**, 998–1031.

Kringelbach, M. L., & Rolls, E. T. (2004). The functional neuroanatomy of the human orbitofrontal cortex: evidence from neuroimaging and neuropsychology. *Progress in Neurobiology*, **72**, 341–372.

LaBar, K. S., Gatenby, J. C., Gore, J. C., LeDoux, J. E., & Phelps, E. A. (1998). Human amygdala activation during conditioned fear acquisition and extinction: a mixed-trial fMRI study. *Neuron*, **20**, 937–945.

Lanius, R. A., Williamson, P. C., Hopper, J., *et al.* (2003). Recall of emotional states in posttraumatic stress disorder: an fMRI investigation. *Biological Psychiatry*, **53**, 204–210.

Maren, S., Aharonov, G., & Fanselow, M. S. (1997). Neurotoxic lesions of the dorsal hippocampus and Pavlovian fear conditioning in rats. *Behavioral Brain Research*, **88**, 261–274.

Milad, M. R., & Quirk, G. J. (2002). Neurons in medial prefrontal cortex signal memory for fear extinction. *Nature*, **420**, 70–74.

Milad, M. R., Vidal-Gonzalez, I., & Quirk, G. J. (2004). Electrical stimulation of medial prefrontal cortex reduces conditioned fear in a temporally specific manner. *Behavioral Neuroscience*, **118**, 389–394.

Milad, M. R., Wright, C. I., Orr, S. P., *et al.* (2007). Recall of fear extinction in humans activates the ventromedial prefrontal cortex and hippocampus in concert. *Biological Psychiatry*, **62**, 446–454.

Nee, D. E., Wager, T. D., & Jonides, J. (2007). Interference resolution: Insights from a meta-analysis of neuroimaging tasks. *Cognitive, Affective, and Behavioral Neuroscience*, **7**, 1–17.

Northoff, G., Heinzel, A., de Greck, M., *et al.* (2006). Self-referential processing in our brain: a meta-analysis of imaging studies on the self. *Neuroimage*, **31**, 440–457.

Ochsner, K. N., & Gross, J. J. (2005). The cognitive control of emotion. *Trends in Cognitive Sciences*, **9**, 242–249.

Ochsner, K. N., & Gross, J. J. (2008). Cognitive emotion regulation: Insights from social cognitive and affective neuroscience. *Current Directions in Psychological Science*, **17**, 153–158.

Paxinos, G. (2003). *The Human Nervous System*, 2nd edn. San Diego, CA: Academic Press.

Phan, K. L., Wager, T., Taylor, S. F., & Liberzon, I. (2002). Functional neuroanatomy of emotion: a meta-analysis of emotion activation studies in PET and fMRI. *Neuroimage*, **16**, 331–348.

Phan, K. L., Britton, J. C., Taylor, S. F., Fig, L. M., & Liberzon, I. (2006). Corticolimbic blood flow during nontraumatic emotional processing in posttraumatic stress disorder. *Archives of General Psychiatry*, **63**, 184–192.

Phelps, E. A., Delgado, M. R., Nearing, K. I., & LeDoux, J. E. (2004). Extinction learning in humans: role of the amygdala and vmPFC. *Neuron*, **43**, 897–905.

Quirk, G. J., Russo, G. K., Barron, J. L., & Lebron, K. (2000). The role of ventromedial prefrontal cortex in the recovery of extinguished fear. *Journal of Neuroscience*, **20**, 62256231.

Raichle, M. E., MacLeod, A. M., Snyder, A. Z., *et al.* (2001). A default mode of brain function. *Proceedings of the National Academy of Sciences of the USA*, **98**, 676–682.

Rauch, S. L., Whalen, P. J., Shin, L. M., *et al.* (2000). Exaggerated amygdala response to masked facial stimuli in posttraumatic stress disorder: a functional MRI study. *Biological Psychiatry*, **47**, 769–776.

Schienle, A., Schafer, A., Hermann, A., Rohrmann, S., & Vaitl, D. (2007). Symptom provocation and reduction in patients suffering from spider phobia: an fMRI study on exposure therapy. *European Archives of Psychiatry and Clinical Neuroscience*, **257**, 486–493.

Shin, L. M., Whalen, P. J., Pitman, R. K., *et al.* (2001). An fMRI study of anterior cingulate function in posttraumatic stress disorder. *Biological Psychiatry*, **50**, 932–942.

Shin, L. M., Wright, C. I., Cannistraro, P. A., *et al.* (2005). A functional magnetic resonance imaging study of amygdala and medial prefrontal cortex responses to overtly presented fearful faces in posttraumatic stress disorder. *Archives of General Psychiatry*, **62**, 273–281.

Simmons, A., Stein, M. B., Matthews, S. C., Feinstein, J. S., & Paulus, M. P. (2006). Affective ambiguity for a group recruits ventromedial prefrontal cortex. *Neuroimage*, **29**, 655–661.

Straube, T., Glauer, M., Dilger, S., Mentzel, H. J., & Miltner, W. H. (2006). Effects of cognitive–behavioral therapy on brain activation in specific phobia. *Neuroimage*, **29**, 125–135.

Tillfors, M., Furmark, T., Marteinsdottir, I., *et al.* (2001). Cerebral blood flow in subjects with social phobia during stressful speaking tasks: a PET study. *American Journal of Psychiatry*, **158**, 1220–1226.

Vertes, R. P. (2004). Differential projections of the infralimbic and prelimbic cortex in the rat. *Synapse*, **51**, 32–58.

Wager, T. D., & Smith, E. E. (2003). Neuroimaging studies of working memory: a metaanalysis. *Cognitive, Affective, and Behavioral Neuroscience*, **3**, 255–274.

Wager, T. D., Barrett, L. F., Bliss-Moreau, E., *et al.* (2008a). The neuroimaging of emotion. In M. Lewis, J. M.

Haviland-Jones, & L. F. Barrett, eds., *Handbook of Emotions*, 3rd edn. New York, NY: Guilford Press.

Wager, T. D., Hughes, B., Davidson, M., Lindquist, M. L., & Ochsner, K. N. (2008b). Prefrontal–subcortical pathways mediating successful emotion regulation. *Neuron*, **59**, 1037–1050.

Whalen, P. J., Kagan, J., Cook, R. G., *et al.* (2004). Human amygdala responsivity to masked fearful eye whites. *Science*, **306**, 2061.

Whalen, P. J., Johnstone, T., Somerville, L. H., *et al.* (2008). A functional magnetic resonance imaging predictor of treatment response to venlafaxine in generalized anxiety disorder. *Biological Psychiatry*, **63**, 858–863.

Williams, L. M., Kemp, A. H., Felmingham, K., *et al.* (2006). Trauma modulates amygdala and medial prefrontal responses to consciously attended fear. *Neuroimage*, **29**, 347–357.

Wright, C. I., Martis, B., McMullin, K., Shin, L. M., & Rauch, S. L. (2003). Amygdala and insular responses to emotionally valenced human faces in small animal specific phobia. *Biological Psychiatry*, **54**, 1067–1076.

Yamasue, H., Kasai, K., Iwanami, A., *et al.* (2003). Voxel-based analysis of MRI reveals anterior cingulate gray-matter volume reduction in posttraumatic stress disorder due to terrorism. *Proceedings of the National Academy of Sciences of the USA*, **100**, 9039–9043.

Chapter 18

Cognitive–behavioral treatment of anxiety disorders: model and current issues

James P. Hambrick, Jonathan S. Comer, Anne Marie Albano

18.1 Origins of cognitive–behavioral therapy for anxiety disorders

In 1920, John B. Watson and Rosalie Raynor published the Little Albert experiments, showing that fear can be acquired in humans through associative learning – that is, the pairing of neutral objects with aversive stimuli. In 1924, Mary Cover Jones, then at Teachers' College at Columbia University, demonstrated that fears can also be *removed* through the very same principles of association, establishing the central groundwork for the field of behavior therapy and the evidence-based psychological treatment of anxiety disorders.

Throughout the 1950s, the popularity of behavioral treatment methods grew rapidly, due in large part to Joseph Wolpe's pioneering work in South Africa on "systematic desensitization." This process helped patients overcome phobias by teaching them relaxation skills and then training them to call upon these skills while they are simultaneously confronting increasingly feared material. In the United States, Ogden Lindsley successfully demonstrated the efficacy of Skinnerian concepts of contingent reward and consequence in changing maladaptive behavior patterns in patients with serious mental illness. Among inpatients with schizophrenia, appropriate self-care and related behaviors were promoted by making desired situations or objects (e.g., free time, access to the canteen) directly contingent upon the performance of desired actions (e.g., bathing, brushing teeth). At the same time, Hans Eysenck's writings in England alleged the futility of psychoanalytic and "eclectic" treatment methods (O'Donohue & Krasner 1995). Eysenck (1952) captured a growing dissatisfaction in the middle of the twentieth century regarding psychoanalytic methods, noting that the research to date appeared to suggest an inverse correlation between recovery and psychotherapy – the more psychotherapy, the smaller the recovery rate. Behavioral methods offered a time-limited and goal-directed alternative to the lengthy – and potentially expensive – psychoanalytic methods that were starting to fall out of academic favor.

In the 1960s and 1970s, the seminal works of Beck (e.g., 1967) and Ellis (1962) ushered in a "cognitive revolution," offering another problem-focused alternative to psychoanalytic methods. They placed primary focus on the here and now and on patient attitudes, attributions, interpretations, and beliefs (i.e., patients' inner dialogues) as the most productive targets of clinical intervention. Although early behavioral traditions were unconcerned with patients' mental processes, and early cognitive traditions de-emphasized the role of the environment in shaping behavior, by the early 1980s, clinicians and researchers alike had recognized the tremendous benefits of integrating these two action-oriented therapeutic traditions (Mahoney 1974, Meichenbaum 1977, Kendall & Hollon 1979). Thus, cognitive–behavioral therapy (CBT) was born, merging learning theory's focus on the environmental contingencies of behavior with a critical focus on inner cognitive processes, i.e., the dysfunctional thinking patterns that serve to trigger and maintain patients' emotional and behavioral problems.

Since the early work of Mary Cover Jones, behavioral therapy for anxiety disorders has steadily evolved across generations of clinicians, theoreticians, and researchers. Its extensive research base, drawn from animal models, laboratory studies, and rigorously conducted randomized controlled trials, documents the efficacy of behavioral and cognitive–behavioral approaches for the treatment of anxiety disorders (Barlow 2002). This evolution of behavioral and cognitive treatment methods – from a single case study in the 1920s (Jones 1924) to its position now at the

Anxiety Disorders: Theory, Research, and Clinical Perspectives, ed. Helen Blair Simpson, Yuval Neria, Roberto Lewis-Fernández, Franklin Schneier. Published by Cambridge University Press. © Cambridge University Press 2010.

beginning of the twenty-first century as the psychological treatment of choice for anxiety and related disorders (Roth & Fonagy 2004) – has unfolded across a series of bold scientific movements and spirited paradigm shifts. The present chapter will briefly review the overarching model and standard components of cognitive and behavioral practice and highlight a number of critical issues and academic debates that now face the discipline.

18.2 How anxiety becomes a disorder: the cognitive–behavioral model of anxiety disorders

From the CBT perspective, an individual's vulnerability to experiencing anxiety at a clinical level is considered multidetermined, a combination of biological, psychological, and environmental factors coupled with life experiences (Albano et al. 2003). Genetic predisposition, activation of the neural circuits involved in anxiety and fear, and temperament may predispose an individual to react more readily with anxiety or fear under certain circumstances. Early environmental experiences, particularly parental rearing style (i.e., over-protective and over-controlling), may influence a child's emerging psychology in ways that reinforce self-perceptions of helplessness and incompetence (Chorpita & Barlow 1998).

This emerging cognitive set, coupled with experiences in the wider world (e.g., perceived negative experiences with separation, with peers, or at school), reinforce the negative affectivity and autonomic arousal accompanying anxiety. Escape and avoidance behavior following a period of increased anxiety results in two-factor avoidance conditioning (Mowrer 1947). Initially, classically conditioned, distressing anxiety states accompany a triggering event (e.g., being called on in class induces shaking, stomach distress, blushing). Once the child learns that partial avoidance (e.g., escape by giving a quick answer) or total avoidance (e.g., stay home from school) results in dissipation of the anxiety, then operant conditioning occurs whereby the escape/avoidance is reinforced. Over time, this pattern of arousal and escape/avoidance becomes a fixed pattern in response to anxiety-provoking stimuli. Reinforcement of the various anxious responses by the environment (e.g., coddling by over-protective parents, escape from teasing of peers, engagement of family members in obsessive–compulsive ritual) serves to perpetuate the anxious cycle.

Hence, from the cognitive–behavioral perspective, anxiety is a state of negative affect and dysregulated emotion characterized by a negative feedback cycle of thoughts, feelings, and behaviors. Individuals with anxiety disorders hold certain negative beliefs about themselves and the world, characterized by catastrophic thinking (e.g., "this is the worst thing that can happen") while overestimating the probability of negative events (e.g., "I know I will fail to manage this"). These types of automatic, negative thoughts may stem from more cohesive cognitive schemas, which tend to be thematic (e.g., "I am incapable" or "the world is a dangerous place") and stored in memories that may be readily available (e.g., verbally accessible memories) or non-conscious (e.g., situationally accessible memories) (Brewin et al. 1996). The somatic component incorporates the physiologic aspects of anxiety and fear, experienced by the individual in symptoms such as blushing, concentration disturbance, muscle aches, sweating, shaking, tachycardia, and parasthesias. Behaviorally, anxious individuals tend to avoid the situation or endure it with distress. In either case, the individual does not experience the actual situation in its totality, leaving the perceived situation open to wide misinterpretation of what happened or would have happened (if the person did not escape/avoid). These three components of anxiety (cognitive, affective/somatic, behavioral) together intensify the anxiety experience. Avoidance and escape behavior result in immediate relief from anxiety (and the feared situation), a negative reinforcement paradigm that furthers avoidance behavior and maintenance of anxiety.

18.3 The role of anxious apprehension

A core cognitive and affective experience inherent in the aforementioned CBT model of anxiety is "anxious apprehension" (Barlow 1988, 2002), which is a "future-oriented mood state in which one becomes ready or prepared to attempt to cope with upcoming negative events" (Brown et al. 2001, p. 158). Anxiety disorders are varied in their focus; hence, the feared negative consequences for each disorder are unique. Individuals with social anxiety disorder fear humiliation and rejection; those with panic disorder may fear heart attacks, stroke, or death, and so on.

Basic to anxious apprehension is a sense of being unable to predict the occurrence of negative outcomes (unpredictability) and not having the skills/strategies/abilities needed to prevent a negative outcome (uncontrollability). In response to a perceived threat (whether

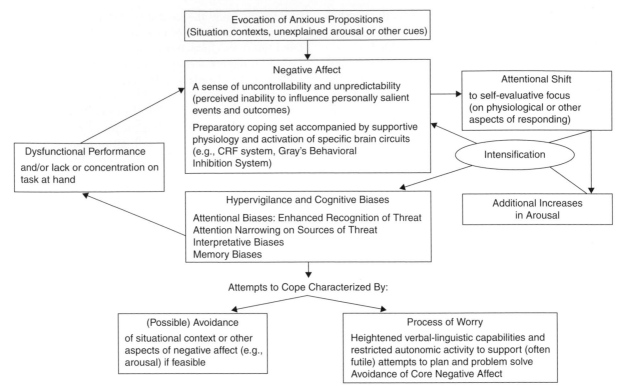

Figure 18.1. The process of anxious apprehension. Reproduced with permission from Barlow (2002).

real or misinterpreted), increases in the experience of unpredictability and uncontrollability are accompanied by heightened physiological arousal. This in turn results in activation of certain brain structures and functions that serve to prepare the individual to deal with danger. If the threat is perceived as possible at some time in the future, hypervigilance results in a somatic state of readiness to take action, stemming from activation of brain circuits associated with Gray's behavioral inhibition system (Gray & McNaughton 1996). This state of future-oriented focus, whereby an individual is ever-ready to deal with upcoming negative events, is commonly referred to as "anxiety" rather than the more specific term "anxious apprehension" (Barlow 2002). As noted by Barlow (2002, p. 64), an individual in this state is thinking, "That terrible event could happen again, and I might not be able to deal with it, but I've got to be ready to try." If, however, the threat is perceived as imminent, such as in the experience of chest pain in panic disorder, engagement of the amygdala results in an immediate activation of specific neural circuits, associated physiological responses characteristic of the "fight or flight" response, and associated experience of fear or panic (Pine *et al.* 2008). Over time, anxiety and fear can render an individual

more vulnerable to misinterpreting cues in the internal (body, mind) or external environment, setting the stage for pathological anxiety states (e.g., generalized anxiety disorder, social anxiety disorder) or the development of fear of fear (panic disorder). The process of anxious apprehension is illustrated in Figure 18.1.

Contact with, or anticipation of exposure to, a fear-provoking stimulus (e.g., an upcoming meeting with superiors, lightheadedness, heights) is the triggering event for an anxiety reaction. Closely associated with the hypervigilance and physiological correlates of anxiety ("negative affect") are additional cognitive, affective, and behavioral components. Anxiety results in a shift of attention toward the self, which increases arousal and negative affect in a self-sustaining feedback loop (Figure 18.1). This attentional shift furthers the individual's hypervigilance for negative outcomes, perceived inadequacies, or inability to manage the situation. Concurrently, behavior may be disrupted as the individual experiences either real or perceived performance deficits in managing the situation and attempts to cope with the situation by escape, avoidance, or non-productive, pathological worry. As noted by Borkovec, pathological worry is associated with increased cognitive activity characterized by low levels of imagery and non-productive problem-solving (Borkovec & Inz 1990, Borkovec 1994). In addition, unproductive worry results in restriction of autonomic activity (suppression of more intense, distressing somatic sensations) and avoidance of more threatening imagery, setting up a cycle of negative reinforcement for the worry (Borkovec 1994).

18.4 Extending the CBT model to emotion (dys)regulation

Recent cognitive–behavioral conceptualizations build upon anxious apprehension and focus on the experience of emotion dysregulation. In the case of generalized anxiety disorder (GAD), for example, Mennin and colleagues offer a theory of worry and emotion regulation whereby the experience and expression of emotion becomes serially dysregulated at multiple levels (Mennin 2004, Mennin *et al.* 2002, 2005). This dysregulation includes heightened emotional arousal; difficulty understanding what emotion is being experienced and/or what triggered that emotion; fear of physiological arousal associated with emotional experience; and maladaptive responses to that experience, such as misinterpretation of one's emotional experience or attempts to over-control that experience through suppression, blunting, or avoidance of emotions. An important component of this theory is the temporally serial nature of the dysregulation: the deficits in emotion regulation begin at the inception of the emotion and cascade down through each subsequent level of the emotional experience as the individual attempts to cope with or modulate the disabling emotional arousal. Worry about, or avoidance of, emotionally evocative circumstances emerges as a primary strategy for regulating emotional experience. In worrying, the person decreases the intensity of the experience (through verbal abstraction) but also fails to extract information from their affective experience that is needed for effective problem solving.

Consider the following vignette, based on an actual therapy session with an individual with GAD:

My boyfriend and I were at home on the couch, watching a romantic movie. I found myself getting really caught up in it, thinking about how amazing the relationship was between the main characters. I was so caught up in it, I didn't notice at first that my boyfriend had fallen asleep. When I noticed that he was asleep, I got so upset. I started worrying that maybe we weren't meant to be together – that we didn't feel the kind of passion they did in the movies. And then I started thinking how wrong that was – I really love him, and I know movies aren't real. So that started getting me wondering if I was ever going to be happy with someone. And then I got upset with myself for not being happy with what I already had. I decided not to say anything to him. He woke up and then we decided to go to bed. On the way to bed, I stepped on a dirty sock, and I just started tearing into him about what a mess his apartment is. I'm so bad – I can't believe I lost it over a little thing like that.

This kind of worry pattern is fairly typical in cases of GAD. According to the emotion dysregulation theory of GAD, the woman's emotional experience (either the positive experience of the romantic memory or the negative experience of upset triggered by the sleeping boyfriend) triggers worry as a way of coping with emotions that she may not even fully understand or be able to identify, except that she feels threatened by the lack of rapport or shared emotion with her boyfriend. Instead of waking him up or attempting to identify and modulate the emotion, she worries in an attempt to problem-solve around what to do with the feelings – is she overreacting, or is the relationship beyond repair? Her worries, intended only to figure out how to manage the feelings, instead increase her appraisals of risk and the problems associated with the relationship. As she becomes less certain of what to do, her anxiety increases, and she becomes more avoidant (e.g., unwilling to discuss her feelings with her boyfriend). However, lacking a sense of closure on the problem (because her worry chain is also suppressing positive emotion cues), she continues to obsess on the problem and worry. Finally, in stepping on the sock, she finds an issue that will permit her to express some aspect of that upset, venting about what she perceives to be a controllable issue, his messiness, and removing the urgency around confrontation of the more substantial problem of lack of intimacy. Any conversation she has at this point, however, will fail to confront the original trigger for the experience, which has already been pushed from awareness.

The emotion dysregulation model predicts that avoidance of emotion through worry may lead to the unattended emotions becoming more intense over time, resulting in higher levels of worry and a constant state of preparedness (anxious apprehension) to hold emotions at bay. At one level, worry acts to suppress emotional arousal and reduce anxiety. Under ideal conditions, this suppression is adaptive, because it permits us to pause and reflect on subsequent action, without each particular solution generating new emotional challenges. It also permits us to avoid being so overwhelmed with emotional arousal that we act impulsively and perhaps disastrously. Simultaneously, the negative affect associated with worry keeps us focused on the task and generating possible solutions. However, if worry becomes a primary source of emotion regulation, problems may result. The suppressive effect of worry is a blunt instrument: it prevents us from detecting not only the negative affect and anxiety associated with a solution, but also the positive affect that lets us know that a solution has been achieved.

In direct tests of this model, individuals with clinical and self-reported GAD reported greater intensity of emotional experience than controls or persons with social anxiety (Mennin *et al.* 2005, Turk *et al.* 2005). In keeping with the expected effect of emotional avoidance, they also reported greater difficulty identifying, describing, and accepting their emotional experience (whether positive or negative), as well as deficits in their ability to soothe themselves when they became distressed. Participants with GAD also reported greater fear of emotional experiences, whether positive or negative. A composite of these variables successfully predicted a diagnosis of GAD after controlling for worry, anxiety, and depression.

These findings regarding the link between GAD and emotion dysregulation also parallel other predictions about relationships between higher intensity of emotional experience, lowered clarity, anxiety about emotional experience, and adaptive problem solving. Individuals with GAD have been found to have lower baseline physiological arousal, which parallels findings about individuals found to be high in affect intensity (Larsen & Diener 1987, Davis *et al.* 2002). Gohm and Clore (2002) found that clarity about one's emotions is associated with beneficial coping styles; conversely, lowered clarity about emotions is associated with being more uncertain and having greater difficulty developing a plan of action. Individuals who are both high in affect intensity and low in emotional clarity appear to be more motivated to attenuate their mood state and are more influenced by mood than individuals who have a clearer understanding of their emotions or experience their emotions less intensely (Gohm 2003). The preconscious bias toward emotional material, regardless of positive or negative valence, supports the notion of felt anxiety around emotional experiences (Mogg *et al.* 1993).

18.5 General principles of CBT for anxiety disorders

Treatment from the CBT perspective is multifaceted and geared towards addressing each of the three components of anxiety (cognitive, affective/somatic, behavioral) through specific, empirically derived techniques. These techniques include psychoeducation, self-monitoring, relaxation, cognitive restructuring, and exposures; they are described in more detail in Table 18.1.

The cornerstone of cognitive–behavioral therapy is assessment (Barrios & Hartmann 1984). That is, case conceptualization and treatment planning is developed and guided by the systematic and ongoing assessment of treatment targets (symptoms, areas of functioning) and progress towards goals. Collaborative empiricism is the process by which the patient and therapist work together, first to uncover maladaptive patterns of functioning that sustain difficulties and then to change these behavioral patterns into coping-focused, adaptive functioning (Beck 1967). This collaboration underlies and fosters the therapeutic alliance in CBT: the therapist uses didactic teaching methods, models and guides participation in facing one's fears, and coaches and encourages the patient to realistically evaluate his or her responses to anxiety-provoking situations through Socratic methods as the treatment progresses. CBT is effective in the treatment of anxiety disorders across a wide age range and in various formats (individual, group, family, couples) (Barlow 2001, Kendall 2005).

Other chapters in this volume describe in detail CBT treatments for distinct anxiety disorders in adult and pediatric populations. Here, we discuss theoretical issues common to all CBT treatments, focusing on matters of measurement, the active components of CBT, the goals of exposure-based tasks, the pacing of treatment, and contributors to outcome that are not specific to the CBT model.

18.5.1 Matters of measurement

A key element that has historically distinguished CBT from other therapeutic approaches is the explicit and regular emphasis on monitoring. CBT is goal-directed, explicitly focusing on measurable change. Treatment begins with a structured baseline evaluation, typically including a diagnostic interview and a functional assessment of symptoms and their contexts, and progress is monitored throughout to inform a continually evolving, evidence-based case conceptualization and treatment plan.

Table 18.1. Basic components of cognitive–behavioral therapy for anxiety disorders

Components of treatment	Therapeutic target and goals
Self-monitoring Daily diary of thoughts, feelings, and behavior SUDS (subjective units of distress) ratings Exposure hierarchy Self-exposure ratings	**Targets**: Identify triggers and contexts eliciting anxious self-talk and misinformation; somatic reactions; avoidance and escape behavior; coping and proactive behavior **Goals**: Education of the patient in uncovering his or her patterns of arousal, avoidance, and factors maintaining the anxiety response; record treatment progress and allow for functional analysis and evaluation of barriers to treatment gains
Psychoeducation	**Targets**: Provide corrective information concerning the nature of anxiety, fear, and threat; origins of anxiety; and role of avoidance behavior in maintaining anxiety; present the CBT model and orient patient to therapy; establish rationale for self-monitoring and ongoing assessment of goals **Goals**: Establish therapeutic alliance and collaborative empiricism; present corrective misinformation and misinterpretation for later cognitive restructuring; develop realistic expectations for therapy
Somatic management techniques Breathing retraining Progressive muscle relaxation training Applied relaxation Meditation	**Targets**: Use of soothing techniques to reduce physiological arousal from increased autonomic nervous system activity **Goals**: Increase ability to detect sources of arousal early (e.g., increased muscle tension) and apply relaxation or slowed breathing to engender a sense of control or mastery
Cognitive restructuring	**Targets**: Automatic thoughts and core schema; change negative, self-defeating internal dialogue to more realistic, coping-focused self-talk **Goals**: Identify automatic thoughts and treat these as hypotheses; develop means to dispute automatic thoughts with realistic evidence and information based on exposures; develop a rational, internal dialogue
Exposure Imaginal In vivo Interoceptive (internal sensations) Virtual	**Targets**: Avoidance and escape behavior **Goals**: Provide experience confronting and interacting with feared situations/stimuli/sensations; allow for the experience of habituation to anxiety in feared situations; gather evidence to refute automatic thoughts; gather experience coping in and with feared stimuli
Specific skills training modules (varies according to diagnosis, age, and patient individual needs) Time management Social skills Problem solving skills Affect regulation skills	**Targets**: Individually identified skill deficits such as social interaction skill, managing problems or multitasking, and management of extreme affective states **Goals**: Develop cognitive and social-emotional skills that may be deficient or absent. Such skill deficits may impede the progress of therapy or render an individual at risk for relapse or attenuated response
Relapse prevention strategies	**Target**: Consolidate and maintain treatment gains **Goals**: Transfer of responsibility to patient for ongoing self-management of anxiety; develop plans for using treatment strategies to manage life changes and challenges that may naturally increase anxiety; reinforce perceptions of control and predictability of anxiety and mastery of anxious responding

No single measure should serve as the sole indicator of a patient's treatment-related gains. Rather, a variety of methods, measures, data sources, and sampling domains should be used to monitor progress and to assess therapy outcomes. Outcomes are more compelling when documented by independent evaluators than when based solely on therapist opinion or on patient self-reports. A multi-informant strategy is preferred, in which perspectives are collected from across multiple reporters (e.g., patient, family members, peers, other adults) in different contexts. This is particularly critical for the assessment of youth. Features of cognitive development may compromise youth self-reports, and children may offer what they believe to be desired responses rather than valid self-reports. At the same time, because anxiety symptoms are partially internal phenomena, some symptoms may be less apparent to parents and teachers, and some observable symptoms may occur in situations outside the home or school.

An inherent liability of multi-informant assessment is that discrepancies among informants are to be expected (Comer & Kendall 2004). Research shows only low to moderate concordance rates among informants in the assessment of anxiety disorders and related symptoms (Choudhury *et al.* 2003, Achenbach *et al.* 2005, De Los Reyes & Kazdin 2005). How best to integrate discrepant reports? Common practice is to employ the "or rule" at the diagnostic level, in which a disorder is considered present if any one of the informants' reports meets criteria for the disorder in question (Albano & Silverman 1996). Employing the "or rule" increases the likelihood that all clinical cases are documented. Given the poor agreement shown across informants (Achenbach *et al.* 2005), the "or rule" seems more practical than the more conservative "and rule," in which a disorder is considered present only if the reports of all informants meet criteria for a given disorder. Reporter discrepancies also highlight the critical importance of incorporating direct behavioral observations and performance-based measures into the assessment of patients.

Practitioners, particularly those working with children, may do well to consider employing the "or rule" at *symptom* level (rather than simply at the diagnostic level), whereby a symptom would be considered present if any of the informants endorse the symptom. Employing the "or rule" at the symptom level may allow for the identification of clinical cases for which no informant's report independently meets criteria for a diagnosis. Such cases may be equal in severity to cases in which at least one informant's report yields a full diagnosis (Comer & Kendall 2004).

Assessing *multiple domains* of functioning provides a comprehensive evaluation of treatment, but treatment rarely produces uniform effects across the domains assessed. Suppose treatment *A*, relative to a control condition, improves depressed clients' level of depression but not their overall psychological well-being. In a randomized controlled trial (RCT) designed to evaluate improved level of depression and psychological well-being, should treatment *A* be deemed efficacious when only one of two measures demonstrated gains? De Los Reyes and Kazdin (2006) propose the Range of Possible Changes model, which calls for a multidimensional conceptualization of intervention change. In this spirit, we recommend that researchers conducting RCTs be explicit about the domains of functioning expected to change and the relative magnitude of expected changes. We also caution consumers of the treatment-outcome literature against simplistic dichotomous appraisals of treatments as efficacious or not.

The central focus of CBT on measurement, symptom monitoring, and observable outcomes has fostered a great deal of research evaluation. However, as an increasingly large body of empirical work documents considerable treatment-related changes associated with cognitive–behavioral treatments, we must question the scope of our traditional measurements and the extent to which they sufficiently tap the relevant domains of functioning in the lives of our patients. Rigorously derived symptom scales may demonstrate solid psychometric properties – including excellent reliability and validity – but may nonetheless shed little light on real-world referents (Kazdin 2006), such as quality of life, marital satisfaction, or job performance. Rarely do patients present for treatment with sole complaints of isolated symptoms devoid of tangible consequences and correlates. As a field, in our remarkable search for statistically significant changes in symptoms of diagnostic constructs, we may be overlooking other, equally important domains of everyday life that carry functional meanings for our patients and are intricately intertwined with treatment satisfaction.

18.5.2 What works? Active components of CBT

As shown in Table 18.1, there are five basic components of any cognitive–behavioral treatment for anxiety:

Psychoeducation teaches the person about his or her disorder, the rationale of cognitive–behavioral therapy, and the course of treatment.

Self-monitoring involves helping the person rate and chart his or her anxiety and mood symptoms over the course of time for the purposes of gathering data about fluctuations across time, charting progress through treatment, and also helping the person identify triggers for the anxiety.

Relaxation training teaches the patient to regulate levels of autonomic arousal through techniques like diaphragmatic breathing or progressive muscle relaxation. In addition to helping regulate autonomic arousal, relaxation training facilitates recognition of somatic triggers of anxious responding.

Cognitive restructuring is a technique through which the patient learns to identify maladaptive thoughts (thoughts that produce or maintain anxiety) and to identify logical errors in those thoughts. Through identification of logical errors, the patient is helped to challenge those thoughts and to come to a more realistic understanding of him- or herself in relation to the world.

Behavioral exposure is the systematic confrontation of feared situations, either through thought (imaginal exposures) or through actually engaging in the feared situation (in-vivo exposures).

There is an unquestionably strong body of evidence supporting CBT's efficacy in treating anxiety disorders. What is less clear is how each component of treatment contributes to (or detracts from) the overall treatment outcome. Unfortunately, because of the complexity and resource demand of studies examining treatment components (dismantling strategies, component analyses), we have relatively little information about how the key components contribute to treatment outcome. Research into the individual contribution of the various components is important because it can suggest ways to make the treatment more efficient (e.g., through streamlining of components that prove to be less critical) or more effective (e.g., by allowing a treatment to play to its strengths, or by offering patients a clearer guide to how treatment works).

A partial picture can be offered by examining meta-analyses of treatment outcomes that compare the relative outcomes of CBT, behavioral exposure, cognitive therapy, and relaxation. In their review of the numerous meta-analyses examining the relative impact of these approaches on treatment outcome, Deacon and Abramowitz (2004) found a mixed picture. In general, the results of the meta-analyses appeared to suggest that combined CBT approaches and specific exposure-based approaches are comparably efficacious in the treatment of anxiety disorders, particularly social anxiety disorder (SAD) and obsessive–compulsive disorder (OCD). In fact, the review authors conclude that the preponderance of evidence clearly makes the case for exposure as the active ingredient in treatment protocols for these anxiety disorders. Meanwhile, cognitive therapy alone, focused primarily on changing the beliefs and attributions of the patient, demonstrated relatively less efficacy.

At the same time, Deacon and Abramowitz suggested a number of factors that make it difficult to fully rule out the impact of cognitive restructuring on successful treatment outcomes. For instance, all meta-analyses run the risk of distorting results by combining a wide range of studies with an often disparate set of methodological approaches. In this review, meta-analyses were further compromised by the fact that there were relatively few studies of the impact of cognitive therapy alone, and even in the studies that purported to focus primarily on cognitive therapy, treatment

descriptions suggested that there was often a behavioral component (and often a cognitive component for the studies described as strictly behavioral therapy). This highlights the fact that CBT, cognitive therapy, and behavior therapy as terms often imply a definitional homogeneity that does not always exist in the literature or in practice.

This kind of variation can also help explain why other investigators have reached somewhat different conclusions. In their randomized controlled trial of cognitive therapy versus exposure versus applied relaxation in the treatment of SAD, Clark and colleagues (2006) found that although they had trouble isolating the active components of CBT, the inclusion of a cognitive component was necessary. Although this was only one controlled trial, it is noteworthy because the components are somewhat better controlled than they were in many of the studies in the meta-analyses. The anomalous and difficult-to-interpret patterns of results, even when synthesized, underscore the need for further research into how the various components contribute to the overall efficacy of CBT.

18.5.3 Goal of exposure: how does it work?

Traditionally, the goal of exposure has been the reduction of fear through habituation or extinction of the fear response (Eelen & Vervliet 2006). This model assumes that fear reduction during an exposure trial is consistent with learning, and that repeated exposure trials consolidate the learning process and form new, coping-focused memories of confronting anxiety-provoking stimuli in the absence of heightened levels of anxiety or fear.

However, theorists have called this traditional perspective into question. Consistent with contemporary emotion regulation theories, Craske and colleagues (2008) recently suggested that fear tolerance may be more critical than reduction of fear. That is, instead of targeting a decrease in subjective units of distress (SUDS) during exposure, the key to fear extinction may be the ability to stay in a feared situation and manage one's behavioral reactions through the process of facilitating inhibitory learning – developing competing, non-threat associations while engaging with the feared stimulus (e.g., Bouton 1993, 2007, Myers & Davis 2007). Thus, the original association of the feared stimulus and anxiety response may remain, but through the process of exposure an individual may also learn that he or she can hold a second association to the feared stimulus, one that represents control and mastery in the situation. While the role of exposure in the treatment of anxiety disorders is not questioned, Craske and colleagues suggest that efforts to foster distress tolerance may prove more durable over time and across contexts for the patient with anxiety.

18.5.4 All at once, or a little bit at a time: how should exposures be timed?

Looking at more specific elements of treatment can help us improve its efficiency and thereby contribute to the improved efficacy of CBT. In the case of behavioral exposures, for example, one question that has been raised is the relative impact of intensive exposure-based treatment (e.g., flooding the patient over the course of several hours, or meeting several times a week) versus distributed practice (e.g., the more traditional, once-a-week model).

More intensive approaches may streamline the course of treatment and help patients get better faster. Intensive treatments may also facilitate access for patients who have to travel to seek treatment and who cannot spend 10, 12, 14, or 20 weeks working on their anxiety disorder (Storch *et al.* 2008). On the other hand, distributed practice may offer improved opportunities to generalize gains, by engaging with anxiety across multiple contexts over time. Furthermore, distributed practice may be more appropriate if the patient is younger or more disabled by his or her anxiety; it can enhance the chance that the patient gains sufficient mastery at each level of the process and prevent confrontation with a situation that may be too challenging for the patient to maintain. Premature exposure to feared objects or situations that are high on a patient's fear hierarchy can lead to feelings of demoralization or, in worst-case scenarios, a treatment breach.

Work with spider-fearful and speech-phobic patients has suggested that conducting a number of exposures in the same day increases short-term gains but fails to have a long-term impact on fears (Rowe & Craske 1998, Tsao & Craske 2000). Intensive treatment has yielded comparable results in OCD, with evidence for comparable or somewhat improved immediate outcomes (Abramowitz *et al.* 2003, Storch *et al.* 2008). However, the study by Abramowitz and colleagues (2003) also found evidence for increased relapse among patients in the intensive treatment group. A pilot study of an eight-day intensive treatment for panic patients found positive outcomes at both conclusion of treatment and at follow-up (assessed at variable times); however, due to the open nature of the trial and the open nature of the follow-up, these conclusions are somewhat tentative (Bitran *et al.* 2008). Results like these lend some support to traditional treatment models emphasizing distributed practice sessions, but also highlight the potential promise and risks of intensive treatment in working with patients.

18.5.5 Beyond the model: other contributors to outcome

Another advantage of examining the specific contributions of the various elements of CBT is that such studies can raise awareness of components that receive less attention but that are also important in contributing to treatment outcome. For example, one variable that typically receives less attention in CBT is the working alliance between the therapist and the patient. Treatment manuals and books place a great deal of emphasis on the role of the therapist in CBT as "coach" or "teacher," but research studies have put relatively little emphasis on examining whether the relationship between therapist and patient exerts any effect on treatment outcome.

The few studies that have looked at this issue have consistently found a small-to-moderate but significant effect (Horvath & Symonds 1991, Martin *et al.* 2000). These studies are notable because they point out the significance of the therapeutic alliance. However, they also point out significant gaps in the literature. Although working alliance is frequently found to be a significant contributor to treatment outcome, it is infrequently assessed in treatment-outcome studies. Further, the clinical trials that have reported working alliance may not be representative.

Another area of potential bias comes from the measures themselves. Many of the measures used to examine working alliance are generic, meant to refer to a variety of treatment approaches. The role of the therapist in CBT, however, is thought to be quite different from the role of the therapist in other treatment approaches. CBT therapists are taught to engage the patient directly, use didactic strategies, question beliefs, model targeted behavior, guide the patient in vivo and in imagination to approach and interact with feared situations, and be flexible and creative in moving the therapeutic process forward. It is unknown whether measures or rating systems that place more specific emphasis on the role definitions valued by CBT might find different results, making working alliance more or less important. Finally, considering that the role of the therapeutic alliance has not been sufficiently studied in the treatment of anxiety, at present we cannot look at key relationship issues between the various treatment components and therapeutic alliance (for a rare exception, see Kendall *et al.* 2009). For example, are patients more willing to engage in exposures or relinquish maladaptive beliefs if they trust the therapist?

18.6 Conclusions

Cognitive–behavioral treatments for the anxiety disorders are steeped in a tradition of learning theory and empiricism, stemming back to the beginning of the twentieth century and standing the test of time in rigorous clinical trials and experimental research. The purpose of the chapter has been to provide an overview of the CBT model of anxiety, to shed light on new conceptualizations of emotion regulation, and to describe how this CBT model of anxiety has led to the evidence-based treatments that we use and study today. While manuals of CBT are necessary for clinical trials, and also have been disseminated into clinical practice, manuals may both help and hinder the community clinician, in that they provide the techniques but not the underlying principles and theory that are considered essential to the practice of CBT. Providing CBT to individuals suffering from anxiety is a complex and continually evolving process. We encourage interested non-CBT trained clinicians to seek educational and supervisory opportunities to become more than merely familiar with this modality – to become experts so that thoughtful, creative, empirically based CBT can be delivered faithfully and with fidelity to patients in need.

References

Abramowitz, J. S., Foa, E. B., & Franklin, M. E. (2003). Exposure and ritual prevention for obsessive–compulsive disorder: effects of intensive versus twice-weekly sessions. *Journal of Consulting and Clinical Psychology*, **71**, 394–398.

Achenbach, T. M., Krukowski, R. A., Dumenci, L., & Ivanova, M. Y. (2005). Assessment of adult psychopathology: meta-analyses and implications of cross-informant correlations. *Psychological Bulletin*, **131**, 361–382.

Albano, A. M., & Silverman, W. K. (1996). *The Anxiety Disorders Interview Schedule for Children for DSM-IV: (Child and Parent Versions): Clinician's Manual*. New York, NY: Oxford University Press.

Albano, A. M., Chorpita, B. F., & Barlow, D. H. (2003). Anxiety disorders. In E.J. Mash & R.A. Barkley, eds., *Child Psychopathology*, 2nd edn. New York, NY: Guilford Press.

Barlow, D. H. (1988). *Anxiety and its Disorders*. New York, NY: Guilford Press.

Barlow, D. H., ed. (2001). *Clinical Handbook of Psychological Disorders*, 3rd edn. New York, NY: Guilford Press.

Barlow, D. H. (2002). *Anxiety and its Disorders*, 2nd edn. New York, NY: Guilford Press.

Barrios, B. A., & Hartmann, D. (1984). Fears and anxieties. In E. J. Mash & L. G. Terdal, eds., *Behavioral Assessment of Childhood Disorders*. New York, NY: Guilford Press.

Beck, A. T. (1967). *Depression: causes and treatment*. Philadelphia, PA: University of Pennsylvania Press.

Bitran, S., Morissette, S. B., Spiegel, D. A., & Barlow, D. H. (2008). A pilot study of sensation-focused intensive treatment for panic disorder with moderate to severe agoraphobia: preliminary outcome and benchmarking data. *Behavior Modification*, **32**, 196–214.

Borkovec, T. D. (1994). The nature, functions, and origins of worry. In G. Davey & F. Tallis, eds., *Worrying: Perspectives on Theory, Assessment, and Treatment*. New York, NY: Wiley.

Borkovec, T. D., & Inz, J. (1990). The nature of worry in generalized anxiety disorder: a preponderance of thought activity. *Behaviour Research and Therapy*, **28**, 153–158.

Bouton, M. E. (1993). Context, time and memory retrieval in the interference paradigms of Pavlovian learning. *Psychological Bulletin*, **114**, 90–99.

Bouton, M. E. (2007). *Learning and Behaviour: a Contemporary Synthesis*. Sunderland, MA: Sinauer Associates.

Brewin, C. R., Dalgleish, T., & Joseph, S. (1996). A dual representation theory of posttraumatic stress disorder. *Psychological Review*, **103**, 670–686.

Brown, T. A., O'Leary, T., & Barlow, D. H. (2001). Generalized anxiety disorder. In D.H. Barlow, ed., *Clinical Handbook of Psychological Disorders*, 3rd edn. New York, NY: Guilford Press.

Chorpita, B. F., & Barlow, D. H. (1998). The development of anxiety: the role of control in the early environment. *Psychological Bulletin*, **124**, 3–21.

Choudhury, M. S., Pimentel, S. S., & Kendall, P. C. (2003). Childhood anxiety disorders: parent–child (dis) agreement using a structured interview for the DSM-IV. *Journal of the American Academy of Child and Adolescent Psychiatry*, **42**, 957–964.

Clark, D. M., Ehlers, A., Hackman, A., *et al.* (2006). Cognitive therapy versus exposure and applied relaxation in social phobia: a randomized controlled trial. *Journal of Consulting and Clinical Psychology*, **75**, 568–578.

Comer, J. S., & Kendall, P. C. (2004). A symptom-level examination of parent–child agreement in the diagnosis of anxious youths. *Journal of the American Academy of Child and Adolescent Psychiatry*, **43**, 878–886.

Craske, M. G., Kircanski, K., Zelikowsky, M., *et al.* (2008). Optimizing inhibitory learning during exposure therapy. *Behaviour Research and Therapy*, **46**, 5–27.

Davis, M., Montgomery, I., & Wilson, G. (2002). Worry and heart rate variables: autonomic rigidity under challenge. *Journal of Anxiety Disorders*, **16**, 639–659.

Deacon, B. J., & Abramowitz, J. S. (2004). Cognitive and behavioral treatments for anxiety disorders: a review of meta-analytic findings. *Journal of Clinical Psychology*, **60**, 429–441.

De Los Reyes, A., & Kazdin, A. E. (2005). Informant discrepancies in the assessment of childhood psychopathology: a critical review, theoretical framework, and recommendations for further study. *Psychological Bulletin*, **131**, 483–509.

De Los Reyes, A., & Kazdin, A. E. (2006). Conceptualizing changes in behavior in intervention research: the range of possible changes model. *Psychological Review*, **113**, 554–583.

Eelen, P., & Vervliet, B. (2006). Fear conditioning and clinical implications: what can we learn from the past? In M. G. Craske, D. Hermans, & D. Vansteenwegen, eds., *Fear and Learning*. Washington, DC, American Psychological Association, pp. 17–35.

Ellis, A. (1962). *Reason and Emotion in Psychotherapy*. Secaucus, NJ: Citadel.

Eysenck, H. J. (1952). The effects of psychotherapy: an evaluation. *Journal of Consulting Psychology*, **16**, 319–324.

Gohm, C. L. (2003). Mood regulation and emotional intelligence: individual differences. *Journal of Personality and Social Psychology*, **84**, 594–607.

Gohm, C. L., & Clore, G. L. (2002). Four latent traits of emotional experience and their involvement in well-being, coping, and attributional state. *Cognition and Emotion*, **16**, 495–518.

Gray, J. A., & McNaughton, N. (1996). The neuropsychology of anxiety: reprise. In D. A. Hope, ed., *Perspectives on Anxiety, Panic and Fear*. Lincoln, NE: University of Nebraska Press.

Horvath, A. O., & Symonds, B. S. (1991). Relation between working alliance and outcome in psychotherapy: a meta-analysis. *Journal of Counseling Psychology*, **38**, 139–149.

Jones, M. C. (1924). A laboratory study of fear: the case of Peter. *Pedagogical Seminary*, **31**, 308–315.

Kazdin, A. E. (2006). Arbitrary metrics: implications for identifying evidence-based treatments. *American Psychologist*, **61**, 42–49.

Kendall, P. C., ed. (2005). *Child and Adolescent Therapy: Cognitive Behavioral Procedures*, 3rd edn. New York, NY: Guilford Press.

Kendall, P. C., & Hollon, S. D., eds. (1979). *Cognitive–behavioral Interventions: theory, research, and procedures*. New York, NY: Academic Press.

Kendall, P. C., Comer, J. S., Marker, C. D., *et al.* (2009). In-session exposure tasks and therapeutic alliance across the treatment of childhood anxiety disorders. *Journal of Consulting and Clinical Psychology*, **77**, 517–525.

Larsen, R. J., & Diener, E. (1987). Affect intensity as an individual difference characteristic: a review. *Journal of Research in Personality*, **21**, 1–39.

Mahoney, M. J. (1974). *Cognition and Behavior Modification*. Cambridge, MA: Ballinger.

Martin, D. J., Garske, J. P., & Davis, M. K. (2000). Relation of the therapeutic alliance with outcome and other variables: a meta-analytic review. *Journal of Consulting and Clinical Psychology*, **68**, 438–450.

Meichenbaum, D. (1977). *Cognitive–Behavior Modification: an Integrative Approach*. New York, NY: Plenum.

Mennin, D. S. (2004). Emotion regulation therapy for generalized anxiety disorder. *Clinical Psychology and Psychotherapy*, **11**, 17–29.

Mennin, D. S., Heimberg, R. G., Turk, C. L., & Fresco, D. M. (2002). Applying an emotion regulation framework to integrative approaches to generalized anxiety disorder. *Clinical Psychology: Science and Practice*, **9**, 85–90.

Mennin, D. S., Heimberg, R. G., Turk, C. L., & Fresco, D. M. (2005). Preliminary evidence for an emotion dysregulation model of generalized anxiety disorder. *Behaviour Research and Therapy*, **43**, 1281–1310.

Mogg, K., Bradley, B., Williams, R., & Mathews A. (1993). Subliminal processing of emotional information in anxiety and depression. *Journal of Abnormal Psychology*, **102**, 304–311.

Mowrer, O. H. (1947). On the dual nature of learning: A reinterpretation of "conditioning" and "problem solving". *Harvard Educational Review*, **17**, 102–148.

Myers, K. M., & Davis, M. (2007). Mechanisms of fear extinction. *Molecular Psychiatry*, **12**, 120–150.

O'Donohue, W., & Krasner, L. (1995). *Theories of Behavior Therapy: Exploring Behavior Change*. Washington, DC: American Psychological Association Press.

Pine, D. S., Helfinstein, S. M., Bar-Haim, Y., Nelson, E., & Fox, N. A. (2008). Challenges in developing novel treatments for childhood disorders: lessons from research on anxiety. *Neuropsychopharmacology Reviews*, 1–16.

Roth, A., & Fonagy, P. (2004). *What Works for Whom? A Critical Review of Psychotherapy Research*, 2nd edn. New York, NY: Guilford Press.

Rowe, M. K., & Craske, M. G. (1998). Effects of an expanding-spaced vs. massed exposure on fear reduction and return of fear. *Behaviour Research and Therapy*, **36**, 701–717.

Storch, E. A., Merlo, L. J., Lehmkuhl, H., *et al.* (2008). Cognitive–behavioral therapy for obsessive–compulsive disorder: a non-randomized comparison of intensive and weekly approaches. *Journal of Anxiety Disorders*, **22**, 1146–1158.

Tsao, J. C. I., & Craske, M. G. (2000). Timing of treatment and return of fear: effects of massed, uniform-, and expanding-spaced exposure schedules. *Behavior Therapy*, **31**, 479–497.

Turk, C. L., Heimberg, R.G., Luterek, J.A., Mennin, D.S., & Fresco, D.M. (2005). Delineating emotion regulation deficits in generalized anxiety disorder: a comparison with social anxiety disorder. *Cognitive Therapy and Research*, **29**, 89–106.

Watson, J., & Raynor, R. (1920). Conditioned emotional reactions. *Journal of Genetic Psychology*, **37**, 394–419.

Chapter 19

The stressor criterion A in posttraumatic stress disorder: issues, evidence, and implications

Bruce P. Dohrenwend

19.1 Introduction

There has been a tendency in the more recent revisions of the *Diagnostic and Statistical Manual* (DSM) of the American Psychiatric Association (APA) and in studies of posttraumatic stress disorder (PTSD) to expand somewhat haphazardly the DSM-III formulation of Criterion A traumatic events. This formulation has evolved from events that are "outside the range of usual human experience" and that "would evoke symptoms in almost everyone" (APA 1980, p. 236), to a much wider range and variety of stressful events that many of us experience at one time or another, such as learning about the unexpected death of a loved one (APA 1994). The purpose of this chapter is to set forth how the field might develop a more rigorous Criterion A definition.

19.2 Background

During World War II, a view developed that psychological symptoms related to combat experiences were normal responses to abnormal situations and were transient unless treated in ways that increased secondary gain (e.g., Wessely 2005). A separate diagnostic category was created for these situationally specific phenomena, and combat-related psychopathology was included in *gross stress reaction* under *transient situational personality disturbance* in DSM-I (APA 1952). Phenomena to be included in this category were described as follows:

> The symptoms are the immediate means used by the individual in his struggle to adjust to an overwhelming situation. In the presence of good adaptive capacity, recession of symptoms generally occurs when the situational stress diminishes. Persistent failure to resolve will indicate a more severe underlying disturbance (APA 1952, p. 40).

In DSM-II (APA 1968) this formulation was carried over under the somewhat different heading of *transient situational disorders* in the section on *adjustment*

reaction of adult life. The diagnosis of posttraumatic stress disorder (PTSD) was introduced with DSM-III (APA 1980) in the context of social and political controversy following the Vietnam War (e.g., Friedman *et al.* 2007a). Unlike the gross stress reactions and transient situational disorders of DSM-I and DSM-II, and also unlike most other diagnoses in DSM-III, DSM-III-R (APA 1987), and DSM-IV (APA 1994), which tend to leave open the question of etiology, DSM-III explicitly required an antecedent traumatic event for a diagnosis of PTSD. In its Criterion A for the diagnosis of PTSD, the adjective "traumatic" is applied to stressors "outside the range of usual human experience" that would "evoke significant symptoms of distress in almost everyone" (APA 1980, p. 236). As will be discussed later, Criterion A is broadened in DSM-IV, but the emphasis on its primacy in the diagnosis is maintained. The primacy of Criterion A stressors is spelled out in DSM-IV as follows:

> *The severity, duration, and proximity of an individual's exposure to the traumatic event are the most important factors affecting the likelihood of developing this disorder.* There is some evidence that social supports, family history, childhood experiences, personality variables, and preexisting mental disorders may influence the development of Posttraumatic Stress Disorder. *This disorder can develop in individuals without any predisposing conditions, particularly if the stressor is especially extreme* (APA 1994, pp. 426–427, italics added).

19.3 Criterion A issues

This formulation implies that traumatic stressors are primary, and not only in the sense of being more important than vulnerability factors. They also are primary because they are both necessary and sufficient (at least when extreme) for the development of the syndrome of PTSD that lasts well beyond the

Anxiety Disorders: Theory, Research, and Clinical Perspectives, ed. Helen Blair Simpson, Yuval Neria, Roberto Lewis-Fernández, Franklin Schneier. Published by Cambridge University Press. © Cambridge University Press 2010.

precipitating stressful situation. As described by Friedman (2005), PTSD symptom responses to traumatic stressors involve "profound and sometimes irreversible changes produced by overwhelming stress. These [changes] include fundamental alterations in perception, cognition, behavior, emotional reactivity, brain function, personal identity, world view, and spiritual beliefs." This assumption about the primacy of the stressor is a main focus of questions about the validity of the PTSD diagnosis as currently formulated. There are strong voices among skeptics who argue that vulnerability factors are more important (e.g., Breslau & Davis 1987, Yehuda & McFarlane 1995). As in DSM-III, the subsequent DSM-III-R and DSM-IV require the presence of traumatic stressors. DSM-III-R provides more examples than DSM-III but defines traumatic stressor similarly as events that are markedly distressing and "outside the range of usual human experience" – especially events that threaten the life or physical integrity of the individual or someone close to him or her; the definition also includes witnessing death or serious injury to others (APA 1987, p. 250).

The definition of traumatic stressors was broadened in DSM-IV. Unlike the previous DSM-III and DSM-III-R, DSM-IV did not require that the stressor be outside the range of usual human experience. Instead, it included events such as learning about the sudden or unexpected death for any reason of a close relative or friend and learning about traumatic events experienced by a close relative or friend. Thus, the broadened definition includes events that indirectly warn the individual of his or her own mortality in addition to events that threaten the individual's life directly. This may dilute, but does not completely obscure, the central focus on fear-inducing life threat in the definition of "traumatic" and the challenging possibility of conceiving and investigating PTSD as a fear circuitry disorder (e.g., Friedman et al. 2007b).

DSM-IV also added, as Criterion A2, a subjective component in the form of self-report that the stressor induced an immediate response of fear, helplessness, or horror. This addition, like the broadening of the previous criterion, now called Criterion A1, has been a source of controversy that I will not go into in great detail here because I think it has a reasonable resolution. Some investigators have pointed out, for example, that such reports may indicate vulnerable predispositions or recall bias and should be considered as separate from the assessment of Criterion A (e.g., Breslau & Kessler 2001). For the same reason, I think

that the subjective A2 criterion should be eliminated as an exposure criterion. Rather, these subjective reactions might be included – perhaps with the addition of other emotions such as sadness, guilt, and anger – under a category of acute subjective reactions, with appropriate cautions about recall issues if contemporary observation is not possible.

None of these diagnostic manuals fully operationalizes Criterion A, nor could the manuals have done so on the basis of existing evidence. As a result, there is considerable argument as to how broad or narrow the definition for Criterion A should be. Advocates for narrow definitions are focused on objectively life-threatening events (e.g., McNally 2003, Weathers & Keane 2007), and advocates for very broad definitions are focused on expanding the range of qualifying events beyond the central focus on objective life threat or other threats to the physical integrity of the individual (e.g., Maier 2007, Rubin et al. 2008).

19.4 State of the evidence

What is reasonably meant by "primacy" of the stressor? The strongest claim to primacy would be for stressors that are necessary and sufficient to elicit the syndrome of PTSD symptoms and signs. Less strong would be stressors that are necessary but not in themselves sufficient to elicit the syndrome or stressors that although not necessary are paramount in a set of risk factors that are sufficient (e.g., stressors that are more strongly related to the syndrome than relevant personal vulnerability factors). Further, there should be evidence that the stressors play the above parts for both onset and course of the syndrome. Additionally, it would be compelling if the above stressors were part of a dose/response continuum in which their importance in comparison with other risk factors (e.g., vulnerability factors) increases with their severity.

19.4.1 Are criterion A exposures necessary for the development of the PTSD symptom syndrome?

Mardi Horowitz (1978) formulated the first two elements of what is now the triad of intrusive/re-experiencing, avoidance/numbing, and arousal symptoms that form the PTSD syndrome. He believed that these types of symptoms were "general response tendencies to stressful events" that "appear after a variety of stress events differing in quantity and quality" (Horowitz 1986, p. 85 ff). Consistent with his view that these symptoms indicate "fairly universal stress response tendencies" and "are not unique to post-traumatic stress disorders" (Horowitz 1986, p. 32), he titled his monograph *Stress Response Syndromes* rather than *Posttraumatic Stress Disorder*.

There have been at least a dozen much more recent studies that, like Horowitz (1978, 1986), have found associations between non-Criterion A stressors, such as divorce and loss of a job, and PTSD symptoms or syndrome. These studies are diverse in the types of samples studied, the procedures for assessing stressors, and the measurement of PTSD symptoms and the PTSD symptom syndrome.

19.4.1.1 Two studies that focus on college students

Two studies draw on college students and are explicitly designed to compare Criterion A events with non-Criterion A events in relation to the PTSD symptom syndrome (Gold *et al.* 2005, Long *et al.* 2008). These studies used checklists of events and checklists of PTSD symptoms (Foa *et al.* 1997). Both studies reported higher rates of "probable PTSD" (Gold *et al.* 2005, Long *et al.* 2008) or greater PTSD symptom severity (Long *et al.* 2008) for the group reporting events that were not consistent with Criterion A (e.g., breakup with a girlfriend or boyfriend) compared to the group who reported Criterion A events.

19.4.1.2 Five studies of samples from general populations

One study of the general population found that loss of farm animals to foot-and-mouth disease was associated with elevated scores on the Impact of Events Scale (IES) (Olff *et al.* 2005). Another study, using a large general population sample, investigated the relatively few non-Criterion A stressful events that were reported in response to the PTSD gatekeeper question in the Diagnostic Interview Schedule (DIS) (Robins *et al.* 1981). This question asked whether the respondents "had experienced an event that frightened them so much that they had one or more of the [PTSD] symptoms listed" (Helzer *et al.* 1987). The investigators found that "discovering a spouse's affair, being poisoned, and having a miscarriage," which were not included by the investigators as Criterion A events, were cited as causes of the PTSD symptom syndrome as measured by the DIS (Helzer *et al.* 1987).

The procedures in the three other studies of general population samples involved administration of checklists of supposedly "traumatic" events that also included an "other" category (Mol *et al.* 2005) or an additional list of events not usually considered "traumatic" (Solomon & Canino 1990, Van Hooff *et al.* 2009). Respondents in two of the studies nominated a "worst" event that was probed in relation to PTSD symptoms measured by either a checklist (Mol *et al.* 2005, Van Hooff *et al.* 2009) or by the Composite International Diagnostic Interview (Van Hooff *et al.* 2009). All three studies found that higher rates of PTSD were associated with non-Criterion A events.

Solomon and Canino (1990) used a PTSD module in the DIS and focused on samples of persons who were exposed to natural disasters. The investigators examined the extent to which the disaster exposure per se predicted PTSD symptoms as compared with other post-disaster stressors (including non-Criterion A events). It seems possible that the non-Criterion A stressors such as "job loss," "money difficulties," and "forced to take someone into household" were the sequelae of more severe disaster exposure and, hence, more strongly correlated with PTSD symptoms than they would have been without the connection to the disaster. It is also possible that this outcome was a "last straw" phenomenon following prior "kindling" (Seidler & Wagner 2006) from the disaster exposure. These results suggest that it is very important to look at linkages between life-threatening and subsequent stressful events of other types over the life course in relation to PTSD symptom outcomes.

19.4.1.3 Five studies focusing solely ($n = 4$) or mainly ($n = 1$) on psychiatric patients

Three studies looked at PTSD in samples of patients with primary diagnoses other than PTSD: 103 respondents in pharmacologic treatment for major depression (Bodkin *et al.* 2007), 45 respondents with social anxiety disorder (Erwin *et al.* 2006), and 53 psychiatric inpatients with a variety of psychiatric diagnoses other than PTSD (Hovens & van der Ploeg 1993). A fourth study investigated patients mainly with disorders other than PTSD, especially depression (Spitzer *et al.* 2000).

Bodkin and colleagues (2007) used the Structured Clinical Interview for DSM-IV (SCID) (First *et al.* 1996) and included subjects who reported only non-Criterion A1 events as well as subjects who provided Criterion A events in response to the event history section of SCID. These investigators found that 78% in the Criterion A1 group and 78% in the other stressful event group met the PTSD symptom syndrome criteria.

Erwin and colleagues (2006) used open-ended questions and checklists to elicit each patient's most distressing socially stressful event (e.g., being ridiculed by a parent) as well as each patient's most distressing Criterion A1 event. The self-report Posttraumatic Diagnostic Scale–revised, based on Foa *et al.* (1997) but administered in an interview with the above section on events, was used for DSM-IV diagnoses. Slightly over a third of patients met PTSD symptom syndrome criteria in relation to their most distressing socially stressful event. Moreover, elevations on the avoidance and arousal symptoms among those who reported no Criterion A1 events (*n* = 16) were similar to the remainder (*n* = 29), who reported Criterion A1 events as well as socially stressful events.

The third study of patients (Hovens & van der Ploeg 1993) asked an open-ended question to assess exposure to stressful events: "Did you ever experience an extremely stressful situation like a holdup, hostage taking, a near fatal accident, war experiences, rape, incestuous or physical abuse? If yes, please describe the situation concisely." The investigators found that 28 of the 53 inpatients described events that met the DSM-III-R criteria for Criterion A; another 12 patients described major negative life events that the investigators judged were not Criterion A stressors. On two PTSD symptom checklists (Keane *et al.* 1984, 1988), the Criterion A stressor patients reported more symptoms than the other stressor patients, who in turn did not differ significantly from patients who reported no "trauma" of either kind. However, the mean scores on the two PTSD symptom scales were high in all three groups. For example, the cut-off for probable PTSD on the Mississippi scale is listed as equal to or greater than 107; the mean for patients meeting Criterion A was 126.47, for those with other stressful events it was 105.8, and for those with neither it was 96.91.

The fourth study, by Spitzer and colleagues (2000), used an adaptation of the Composite International Diagnostic Interview (CIDI) (World Health Organization 1990) to assess PTSD symptoms in the last 12 months in a series of inpatients mainly with depressive, obsessive, and phobic disorders. The opening question on stressors listed a wide variety of experiences that were classified into "high-magnitude" and "low-magnitude" events in much the same way as in the study by Hovens and van der Ploeg (1993). At least one distressing event of either type was reported by 48 of the patients. Among those who nominated "high-magnitude" stressors, 55% met the full symptom syndrome criteria; in the patients who nominated a "low-magnitude" stressor, 57.1% met the full symptom syndrome criteria.

Finally, a fifth study conducted by Kilpatrick and colleagues (1998) as part of the field trials for DSM-IV included mainly patients (*n* = 400) but also a sample from the general population (*n* = 128). The participants were patients seeking mental health treatment at various service settings after exposure to potentially traumatic events. All respondents answered questions from two checklists: one focusing on Criterion A events over the lifetime of the respondent and the other on stressful events in the past year other than those thought to meet Criterion A. The respondents selected a "worst" event from either or both lists. A combination of an early PTSD module from the DIS (Robins *et al.* 1981) and the PTSD section of the Structured Clinical Interview for DSM-III-R (SCID) (Spitzer *et al.* 1987) were used to arrive at PTSD diagnoses. Only a minority of the respondents (*n* = 66) reported experiencing non-Criterion A events but not Criterion A events. Of these respondents, 12.1% received diagnoses of PTSD, that is, they met symptom criteria for the disorder following a non-Criterion A event in the past year.

19.4.1.4 In summary

These studies used a variety of measures of exposure (e.g., Sarason *et al.* 1978, Foa *et al.* 1997, Goodman *et al.* 1998), diverse measures of PTSD and the PTSD symptom syndrome (e.g., Horowitz *et al.* 1979, Robins *et al.* 1981, Spitzer *et al.* 1987, Foa *et al.* 1997, World Health Organization 1997), and samples drawn from such different populations as college students, communities, and patients seeking or receiving treatment. Despite these contrasts in methods and populations, all of the studies suggest that various types of stressors defined by investigators as non-Criterion A are associated with PTSD symptoms or the PTSD symptom syndrome: sudden death of a loved one (Mol *et al.* 2005, Spitzer *et al.* 2000, Long *et al.* 2008); death of a family member or close friend due to illness (Kilpatrick *et al.* 1998, Gold *et al.* 2005); serious physical illness in self (Mol *et al.* 2005) or in self or family member (Kilpatrick *et al.* 1998, Spitzer *et al.* 2000); own divorce (Kilpatrick *et al.* 1998, Spitzer *et al.* 2000, Van Hoof *et al.* 2009); unfaithfulness of spouse (Helzer *et al.* 1987); parental divorce/separation (Gold *et al.* 2005, Mol *et al.* 2005, Van Hoof *et al.* 2009); loss of a job (Kilpatrick *et al.* 1998, Spitzer *et al.* 2000); job stressors (Van Hoof *et al.* 2009); breakup with a girlfriend or boyfriend (Long *et al.* 2008); romantic relationship problems (Gold *et al.* 2005); burglary without confrontation with the burglar (Mol *et al.* 2005); socially stressful events such as being ridiculed by a parent (Erwin *et al.* 2006); and various worries about looks, children, and siblings (Bodkin *et al.* 2007).

These results suggest that Criterion A exposures are not necessary conditions for the development of the PTSD syndrome, as DSM-III, DSM-III-R, and DSM-IV assume. Thus, the findings raise fundamental questions about the diagnosis of PTSD.

19.4.2 Is the diagnosis of "adjustment disorder" a way out of the dilemma?

Weathers and Keane (2007) point out that PTSD symptom syndromes following non-Criterion A events should, according to DSM-IV, be classified as adjustment reactions. This seems arbitrary unless, as Weathers and Keane believe, what is involved is "PTSD-like symptoms" rather than "true" PTSD. They explain, "The fact that some individuals with low-magnitude stressors endorse symptoms of PTSD does not mean they have the disorder … we would conjecture that a syndrome of PTSD-like symptoms precipitated by a low-magnitude stressor is a different clinical entity than PTSD" (Weathers & Keane 2007). There is some support in the literature for this conjecture. Erwin and colleagues (2006) found that the PTSD symptoms reported on the Posttraumatic Diagnostic Scale (PDS) (Foa *et al.* 1997) in response to non-Criterion A socially stressful events were modest in severity compared to symptoms reported in Foa and colleagues' research in response to DSM-III-R Criterion A stressors. Breslau and Kessler (2001) cite research showing that PTSD symptom syndromes in response to the indirectly experienced events that were explicitly added to Criterion A in DSM-IV, such as "learning about an injury to a close relative or friend, or a sudden death of a close relative or friend," had much shorter durations (a median 12.1 months) than syndromes in response to Criterion A events that directly targeted the respondent (a median of 48.1 months). However, Suvak and colleagues (2008) found that both the PTSD Checklist (PCL) (Weathers *et al.* 1993) and the revised IES (Weiss & Marmar 1997) produced similar factor structures in samples of respondents who were indirectly exposed and in respondents who were directly exposed to the September 11th terrorist attacks on the World Trade Center in 2001. These matters need further investigation. Meanwhile, it seems evident that a clear distinction cannot be made as to which present Criterion A and non-Criterion A stressors are necessary to distinguish between the diagnoses of PTSD and adjustment disorder.

19.4.3 The question of sufficiency

Several large-scale epidemiological studies (e.g., Breslau *et al.* 1991, Kessler *et al.* 1995) have included "traumatic events," such as the 12-item checklist from the National Comorbidity Survey (Kessler *et al.* 1995). The studies have found that majorities of respondents reported experiencing one or more of the checklist events during their lifetimes, but only small minorities of these respondents met the study criteria for PTSD (Breslau 2002). On the basis of such results, it has become almost axiomatic for many investigators to conclude that most people exposed to traumatic events do not develop PTSD (e.g., Yehuda & McFarlane 1995, Breslau 2002, Friedman *et al.* 2007a). This interpretation is consistent with the proposition that vulnerability factors may be more important than exposure to traumatic events in the development of PTSD.

There are, however, two interrelated problems with this conclusion on the basis of this kind of evidence. The first is that there is likely to be tremendous variability in the severity of actual events reported in response to the broad checklist categories (Dohrenwend 2006). Consider as an example of this problem of intracategory variability how different the actual experiences could be for individuals replying positively to the first three items on the checklist of Kessler and colleagues (1995). On the one hand, positive responses to "You had direct combat experiences during a war" could be given by veterans who received occasional mortar fire in a relatively safe base camp, as well as by veterans who participated in fire fights, saw comrades killed and wounded, and were wounded themselves, on the other. Positive responses to "You were involved in a life-threatening accident" could be based on being either in a fender bender in which no one was hurt or in a collision involving death and injuries. Positive responses to "You were involved in a fire, flood, or natural disaster" could be given by respondents who were evacuated safely prior to a minor impact on their homes as well as by respondents who were injured, lost loved ones, and had their homes destroyed. Equivalent scores based on responses to such checklist items tend to mask very disparate actual experiences.

The second problem with the conclusion that vulnerability factors are more important is that there are consistent findings of dose/response relationships between severity of exposure and rates of PTSD (e.g., Dohrenwend *et al.* 2006) that are obscured by checklist measures. These dose/response relationships, if of sufficient magnitude, may be consistent with the proposition that the stressor is primary in the development of PTSD. One would expect to find the clearest evidence for the primacy of the stressor in the results of PTSD research on very severe exposure to life-threatening events in hazardous situations, such as in natural disasters and war. It is likely that both the frequency and duration of exposure to stressors in such situations (e.g., Rahe 1988, Rona *et al.* 2007), as well as the kinds of stressors involved, are important in the development of PTSD.

Consider one of the best examples of this research, a study of 56 American men who had been prisoners of the Japanese during World War II compared with 262 prisoners of the Germans who received less harsh treatment (Engdahl *et al.* 1997). The men were systematically sampled from lists of former prisoners of war (POWs) known to be residing in Minnesota, Wisconsin, or North Dakota. They were given diagnostic examinations by experienced clinicians using the Structured Clinical Interview for DSM-III-R (SCID) (Spitzer *et al.* 1987). About 45–50 years after their release, former POWs of the Japanese were found to have a lifetime PTSD prevalence rate of 84% and a current rate of 59%, compared with rates of 44% and 19% for the POWs of the Germans.

These results suggest that long-lasting stressors that are life-threatening are primary in the onset of PTSD, and probably in the persistence or episodic recurrence of PTSD over long periods of time after exposure. However, exposures in such situations are complex. We lack detailed knowledge of what particular combinations of exposures in hazardous situations approach being sufficient for the development of PTSD in previously normal persons. Nor is it clear what types and durations of exposures in hazardous situations lead to a more or less adverse course of the disorder once it develops. Further, we lack information as to whether the events in hazardous situations have counterparts in more usual situations that would help explain why symptoms of PTSD and the PTSD symptom syndrome have been found to be associated with non-Criterion A events in more usual situations of everyday life.

19.5 Toward resolution of criterion A issues

To gain such knowledge, we will need systematic research on the situations in which Criterion A and other stressful events occur, and on the general and

specific characteristics of the diverse-seeming events in such situations.

19.5.1 The situations in which stressful events occur

Stressful events occur along a continuum of situations in which people live their lives. These situations can range from hazardous situations with persistent threat to regular life activities, such as those involved in domestic relationships, education, work, and play. At the hazardous end of the continuum are not only communities in the midst of prolonged natural disaster and racial/ethnic violence, but also family situations characterized by long-standing domestic violence. Next along the continuum might be situations of prolonged poverty, which increase the likelihood that the individual will experience acute events such as eviction from housing and becoming homeless. While situations at the safe and prosperous end of the continuum pose less threat to life, physical integrity, and basic needs for food and shelter, these situations are hardly free of life-threatening events, such as serious physical illnesses and injuries; severe losses, such as deaths of loved ones; and events, such as divorce and loss of job, that threaten important personal goals. There are similarities as well as differences between major negative events in hazardous situations and major negative events in the relatively safe situations.

19.5.2 Major negative events in hazardous situations

Major negative events in hazardous situations have the following general characteristics:

(1) Their *valence* is negative (e.g., they represent loss rather than gain).

(2) The *source* of most of the major negative events is external. The circumstances leading up to them are beyond the control of the individual and uninfluenced by her/his actions, as, for example, being caught in an ambush in a war zone. In the past, I have called these events with external sources "fateful" (e.g., Dohrenwend 1979). For *source*, the crucial distinction is between externally generated events and self-generated events, a distinction that is often a matter of degree. Genetic factors are more likely to influence the onset of the self-generated events (Kendler & Baker 2007).

(3) Onset is often *unpredictable* to the person experiencing the event, as in the ambush above.

221

(4) Some of the events are life-threatening and, hence, most *central* to the needs and goals of the individual.

(5) Some of the events are likely to *exhaust* the individual physically (e.g., being under prolonged enemy attack or, for POWs, being in a long forced march).

(6) The events are large in objective *magnitude*; that is, they are highly likely to bring about great negative changes in the usual activities of the individual (e.g., major casualties in his unit resulting from the ambush). I have postulated that when these negative changes are beyond the individual's ability to control, they are the proximal causes of the onset of disorder (Dohrenwend 1998, 2000).

19.5.3 Major negative events in more usual situations

Examples of major negative events in more usual and less hazardous situations are experiencing the death of a loved one, losing a job, and being a victim of child abuse or rape. Some of the characteristics that define major negative events in hazardous situations occur to some degree in most of these major negative events in more usual situations, though rarely are all of them present. Still, some of the major negative events in more usual circumstances do have most of these characteristics. For example, child abuse and neglect have many of the characteristics of events in hazardous situations and strike at the most vulnerable stages of human development; in the context of prolonged domestic violence, abuse and neglect could be considered an ongoing hazardous situation. Some rape events are not only negative, but also externally generated, unpredictable, and life-threatening. Life-threatening physical illnesses and injuries can have much in common with events in hazardous situations (which can, of course, include life-threatening injuries).

The similarities and contrasts between the above examples and events in hazardous situations are relatively clear-cut. Assessing the points of similarity and contrast between major negative events in hazardous situations and major events in more usual situations of individuals in the general population becomes more complicated when we consider events such as marital separation or divorce, the full variety of events involving job loss (e.g., being fired for cause, as well as becoming unemployed because of a plant shutdown), or some types of physical illness or injury that may not

occur independently of the actions of the individual. The origins of these types of event may as often be in the "stress-generative" behavior of the individual (Hammen 1991) as in the environmental conditions to which the individual is exposed. Still more frequently, a complex mixture of the person's behavior and factors in her/his external environment brings about such events. Moreover, the duration of negative changes in usual activities that follow the event may depend more on the coping ability of the person (e.g., choosing a good divorce lawyer, using a successful strategy of job search following job loss) than on external factors in the wider environment (e.g., soldiers getting reinforcements when outnumbered in a firefight, allied forces liberating concentration-camp survivors).

19.6 Implications

What to include in and exclude from the definition of Criterion A stressors in the next formulation of PTSD should depend on a great deal of systematic research with all types of situations and related negative events. Such research should utilize rigorous diagnoses by experienced clinicians rather than the symptom screening scales currently so widely used, and it should use record-based measures together with labor-intensive narrative/rating measures of exposure rather than self-report checklists of Criterion A and other stressful events that suffer from the problem of intracategory variability (Dohrenwend 2006). This tall order is unlikely to be filled in time for the publication of DSM-5.

In the absence of much of what we would like to have as evidence, I believe that the decision about what to include in Criterion A1 should depend on how strongly we want to adhere to the assumption that the stressors are more important in the development of PTSD than personal vulnerability factors. Full adherence would require Criterion A inclusion on the basis of how nearly we think the externally generated stressors approach being sufficient for the development of the PTSD symptom syndrome. On the basis of existing evidence, priority would be given to stressors with the following general characteristics: negative valence, unpredictability, external source, high centrality involving life threat or threat to physical integrity, large magnitude of uncontrollable negative changes, and strong tendency to exhaust the exposed individual physically. Such events occur with greatest frequency and duration in hazardous situations – such as combat during wartime and prolonged human-made and natural disasters. Such hazardous situations/events are rare in most general populations. Moreover, we know that PTSD symptoms and the PTSD symptom syndrome are associated with quite different events in more usual situations. However, these more common events in more usual situations are unlikely to be sufficient causes of the PTSD symptom syndrome and may not even be more important than some of the vulnerability factors.

Alternatively, if we set aside the primacy assumption about the paramount importance of the exposure, we could do one or more of the following as a basis for creating additional subtypes of PTSD to consider along with, and in comparison to, the prototypical externally generated, life-threatening Criterion A events in hazardous situations above:

(1) Establish subtypes based on the source of the events (externally generated versus self-generated). This would allow inclusion in one of these subtypes of events such as being involved in a life-threatening automobile accident that resulted from the individual's attempting to drive while intoxicated.

(2) Relax the life threat or threat to physical integrity requirement of the prototype. This would let us move down the centrality hierarchy from life threat and threat to physical integrity to events that start with threat to basic needs or threat to social goals. As a result, we could create a subtype that includes mortgage foreclosure, loss of a job, and other types of currently non-Criterion A major negative events that some recent studies have found to be related to the symptom syndrome of PTSD.

(3) Create a subtype consisting of exposure to major negative events that happened to others close to the respondents.

(4) Add a subtype for direct witnessing of serious negative events to others.

(5) Add another subtype consisting of indirect witnessing of life-threatening events, such as repeated television viewing of the World Trade Center attacks, which was found to be strongly associated with symptoms of PTSD (Schlenger *et al.* 2002).

Creation of such subtypes would, of course, complicate the relatively clear-cut starting point of Criterion A in PTSD as described in DSM-III, where stressors were "outside the range of usual human experience" and capable of evoking "significant symptoms of distress in almost everyone." Even in the broadened definitions of DSM-III-R and DSM-IV, there is a continuing central focus on life threat and a central assumption that Criterion A exposure is primary in this disorder. However, the addition of subtypes of exposure to the prototype of Criterion A – externally generated, life-threatening, usually in hazardous situations – would stimulate the kinds of research and clinical observation needed to test basic assumptions about the primacy of the stressor and to systematically specify what ultimately should and should not be included in a definition of Criterion A as part of a diagnosis of something that could reasonably be called "posttraumatic."

Their heuristic value would make the creation of subtypes of exposure and related PTSD symptoms much preferable to consigning arbitrarily to adjustment disorder whatever exposure is associated with the requisite PTSD symptoms but is not included in a haphazardly constructed and rapidly growing list of inclusion criteria for Criterion A. It is possible, for example, that the different subtypes of exposure would be more or less likely to be followed by the PTSD symptom syndrome and be characterized by differences in any or all of the following: biological correlates: profiles of intrusive, avoidance, and arousal symptoms; types and severity of impairment of functioning; types of comorbid disorders; differences in family history of psychiatric disorders, and types of treatment and treatment outcomes. Construction of PTSD syndrome/exposure subtypes and investigation of their correlates could help answer basic questions such as the following:

(1) Should PTSD be classified as a stress-induced fear circuitry disorder? This question could be investigated, because some of the subtypes do not feature stressors that are mainly fear-inducing.

(2) What are the similarities and differences between the PTSD syndrome associated with prototype Criterion A stressors and the PTSD-like syndromes associated with the various other subtypes of situation/event exposures?

(3) What does the present PTSD syndrome have in common with and how does it differ from the syndromes of other disorders in which environmental stressors that do not involve fear-inducing life threat or threat to physical integrity play a strong role?

(4) Which stressors and situations are necessary and which are sufficient for the development of the PTSD symptom syndrome?

(5) Is the PTSD symptom syndrome as currently defined better described as a general stress-response syndrome than as a specific response to "traumatic" stressors?

(6) What are the implications of answers to the above questions for the diagnosis of posttraumatic stress disorder?

Acknowledgments

This work was supported in part by NIMH grant R01-MH059627 and grants from the Spunk Fund, Inc.

References

American Psychiatric Association (1952). *Diagnostic and Statistical Manual of Mental Disorders* (DSM-I). Washington, DC: American Psychiatric Association.

American Psychiatric Association (1968). *Diagnostic and Statistical Manual of Mental Disorders*, 2nd edn (DSM-II). Washington, DC: American Psychiatric Association.

American Psychiatric Association (1980). *Diagnostic and Statistical Manual of Mental Disorders*, 3rd edn (DSM-III). Washington, DC: American Psychiatric Association.

American Psychiatric Association (1987). *Diagnostic and Statistical Manual of Mental Disorders*, 3rd edn., revised (DSM-III-R). Washington, DC: American Psychiatric Association.

American Psychiatric Association (1994). *Diagnostic and Statistical Manual of Mental Disorders*, 4th edn (DSM-IV). Washington, DC: American Psychiatric Association.

Bodkin, J. A., Pope, H. G., Detke, M. J., & Hudson, J. I. (2007). Is PTSD caused by traumatic stress? *Journal of Anxiety Disorders*, **21**, 176–182.

Breslau, N. (2002). Epidemiologic studies of trauma, posttraumatic stress disorder, and psychiatric disorders. *Canadian Journal of Psychiatry*, **47**, 923–929.

Breslau, N., & Davis, G. C., (1987). Posttraumatic stress disorder: The stressor criterion. *Journal of Nervous and Mental Disease*, **175**, 255–264.

Breslau, N., & Kessler, R. C. (2001). The stressor criterion in DSM-IV posttraumatic stress disorder: An empirical investigation. *Biological Psychiatry*, **50**, 699–704.

Breslau, N., Davis, G. C., Andreski, P., & Peterson, E. (1991). Traumatic events and posttraumatic stress disorder in an urban population of young adults. *Archives of General Psychiatry*, **48**, 216–222.

Dohrenwend, B. P. (1979). Stressful life events and psychopathology: some issues of theory and method. In J. F. Barrett, R. M. Rose, & G. L. Klerman, eds., *Stress and Mental Disorder*. New York, NY: Raven Press.

Dohrenwend, B. P. (1998). Theoretical integration. In B. P. Dohrenwend, ed., *Adversity, Stress and Psychopathology*. New York, NY: Oxford University Press.

Dohrenwend, B. P. (2000). The role of adversity and stress in psychopathology: some evidence and its implications for theory and research. *Journal of Health and Social Behavior*, **41**, 1–19.

Dohrenwend, B. P. (2006). Inventorying stressful life events as risk factors for psychopathology: toward resolution of the problem of intracategory variability. *Psychological Bulletin*, **132**, 477–495.

Dohrenwend, B.P., Turner, J.B., Turse, N.A., *et al.* (2006). The psychological risks of Vietnam for U.S. veterans: a revisit with new data and methods. *Science*, **313**, 979–982.

Engdahl, B. Dikel, M. A, Eberly, R., & Blank, A. (1997). Posttraumatic stress disorder in a community group of former prisoners of war: a normative response to severe stress. *American Journal of Psychiatry*, **154**, 1576–1581.

Erwin, B. A., Heimberg, R. G., Marx, B. P., Franklin, M. E. (2006). Traumatic and socially stressful life events among persons with social anxiety disorder. *Journal of Anxiety Disorders*, **20**, 896–914.

First, M. B., Spitzer, R. L., Gibbon, M., & Williams, J. B. W. (1996). *Structured Clinical Interview for DSM-IV Axis I Disorders*. New York, NY: New York State Psychiatric Institute.

Foa, E. B., Cashman, L., Jaycox, L., & Perry, K. (1997). The validation of a self-report measure of posttraumatic stress disorder: the Posttraumatic Diagnostic Scale. *Psychological Assessment*, **9**, 445–451.

Friedman, M. J. (2005). Veterans' mental health in the wake of war. *New England Journal of Medicine*, **352**, 1287–1290.

Friedman, M. J., Resick, P. A., & Keane, T. M. (2007a). PTSD twenty-five years of progress and challenges. In M. J. Friedman, T. M. Keane, & P. A. Resick, eds., *Handbook of PTSD: Science and Practice*. New York, NY: Guilford Press.

Friedman, M. J., Resick, P. A., & Keane, T. M. (2007b). Key questions and an agenda for future research. In M. J. Friedman, T. M. Keane, & P. A. Resick, eds., *Handbook of PTSD: Science and Practice*. New York, NY: Guilford Press.

Gold, S. D., Marx, B. P., Soler-Baillo, J. M., & Loan, D. M. (2005). Is life stress more traumatic than traumatic stress? *Journal of Anxiety Disorders*, **19**, 687–698.

Goodman, L. A., Corcoran, C., Turner, K., Yuan, N., & Green, B. (1998). Assessing traumatic event exposure: general issues and preliminary findings for the Stressful Life Events Screening Questionnaire. *Journal of Traumatic Stress*, **11**, 521–542.

Hammen, C. (1991). Generation of stress in the course of unipolar depression. *Journal of Abnormal Psychology*, **100**, 555–561.

Helzer, J. E., Robins, L. N., & McEvoy, L. (1987). Post-traumatic stress disorder in the general populaton: findings of the Epidemiologic Catchment Area Survey. *New England Journal of Medicine*, **417**, 1630–1634.

Horowitz, M. J. (1978). *Stress Response Syndromes*. Northvale, NJ: Jason Aronson.

Horowitz, M. J. (1986). *Stress Response Syndromes*, 2nd edn. Northvale, NJ: Jason Aronson.

Horowitz, M. J., Winer, N., & Alvarez, W. (1979). Impact of Event Scale: a measure of subjective stress. *Psychosomatic Medicine*, **41**, 209–218.

Hovens, J. E., & van der Ploeg, H. M. (1993). Post-traumatic stress disorder in Dutch psychiatric inpatients. *Journal of Traumatic Stress*, **6**, 91–101.

Keane, T. M., Malloy, P. F., & Fairbank, J. A. (1984). Empirical development of an MMPI subscale for the assessment of combat-related posttraumatic stress disorder. *Journal of Clinical and Consulting Psychology*, **52**, 888–891.

Keane, T. M., Caddel, J. M., & Taylor, K. L. (1988). Mississippi scale for combat-related posttraumatic stress disorder: three studies in reliability and validity. *Journal of Clinical and Consulting Psychology*, **56**, 85–90.

Kendler, K. S., & Baker, J. H. (2007). Genetic influences on measures of the environment. *Psychological Medicine*, **37**, 615–626.

Kessler, R. C., Sonnega, A., Bromet, E., & Nelson, C. B. (1995). Posttraumatic stress disorder in the National Comorbidity Survey. *Archives of General Psychiatry*, **52**, 1048–60.

Kilpatrick, D. G., Resnick, H. S., Freedy, J. R., *et al.* (1998). Posttraumatic stress disorder field trial: evaluation of the PTSD construct. Criteria A through E. In T. Widiger, A. J. Frances, H. A. Pincus, *et al.*, eds., *DSM Sourcebook, Volume 4*. Washington, DC: American Psychiatric Association.

Long, M. E., Elhai, J. D., Schweinle, A., *et al.* (2008). Differences in posttraumatic stress disorder diagnostic rates and symptom severity between Criterion A1 and non-Criterion A1 stressors. *Journal of Anxiety Disorders*, **22**, 1255–1263.

Maier, T. (2007). Weathers' and Keane's "The Criterion A problem revisited: controversies and challenges in defining and measuring psychological trauma". *Journal of Traumatic Stress*, **20**, 915–916.

Maslow, A. H. (1954). *Motivation and Personality*. New York, NY: Harper.

McNally, R. J. (2003). Progress and controversy in the study of posttraumatic stress disorder. *Annual Review of Psychology*, **54**, 229–252.

Mol, S. S. L., Arntz, A., Metsemakers, J. F. M., *et al.* (2005). Symptoms of post-traumatic stress disorder after non-traumatic events: evidence from an open population study. *British Journal of Psychiatry*, **186**, 494–499.

Olff, M., Koeter, M. W. J., Van Haaften, E. H., Kersten, P. H., & Gersons, B. P. R. (2005). Impact of foot and mouth disease crisis on post-traumatic stress symptoms in farmers. *British Journal of Psychiatry*, **186**, 165–166.

Rahe, R. H. (1988). Acute versus chronic reactions to combat. *Military Medicine*, **153**, 365–372.

Robins, L. N., Helzer, J. E., Croughan, J., & Ratcliff, K. S. (1981). The Diagnostic Interview Schedule: Its history, characteristics, and validity. *Archives of General Psychiatry*, **38**, 318–389.

Rona, R. J., Fear, N. T., Hull, L., Greenberg, N., *et al.* (2007). Mental health consequences of overstretch in UK armed forces: first phase of a cohort study. *BMJ*, **335**, 604–609.

Rubin, D. C., Berntsen, D., & Bohni, M. K. (2008). A memory-based model of posttraumatic stress disorder: evaluating basic assumptions underlying the PTSD diagnosis. *Psychological Review*, **115**, 985–1011.

Sarason, I., Johnson, J., & Siegel, J. (1978). Assessing the impact of life changes: development of the life experiences survey. *Journal of Consulting and Clinical Psychology*, **46**, 932–946.

Schlenger, W. E., Caddell, J. M., Ebert, L., *et al.* (2002). Psychological reactions to terrorist attacks: findings from the National Study of Americans' Reactions to September 11. *JAMA*, **288**, 581–588.

Seidler, G. H., & Wagner, F. E. (2006). The stressor criterion in PTSD: notes on the genealogy of a problematic construct. *American Journal of Psychotherapy*, **60**, 261–270.

Solomon, S. D., & Canino, G. J. (1990) Appropriateness of DSM-III-R criteria for posttraumatic stress disorder. *Comprehensive Psychiatry*, **312**, 227–237.

Spitzer, C., Abrahamson G., Reschke K., *et al.* (2000). Posttraumatic stress disorder following high- and low-magnitude stressors in psychotherapeutic inpatients. *Clinical Psychology and Psychotherapy*, **7**, 379–384.

Spitzer, R., Williams, J., & Gibbon, M. (1987). *Structured Clinical Interview for DSM-III-R, Version NP-V*. New York, NY: New York State Psychiatric Institute, Biometrics Research Department.

Suvak, M., Maguen, S., Litz, B. T., Silver, R. C., & Holman, E. A. (2008). Indirect exposure to the September 11 terrorist attacks: Does symptom structure resemble PTSD? *Journal of Traumatic Stress*, **21**, 30–39.

Van Hooff, M., McFarlane, A. C., Baur, J., Abraham, M., & Barnes, D. J. (2009). The stressor criterion-A1 and PTSD: a matter of opinion? *Journal of Anxiety Disorders*, **232**, 77–86.

Weathers, F. W., & Keane, T. M. (2007). The Criterion A problem revisited: controversies and challenges in defining and measuring psychological trauma. *Journal of Traumatic Stress*, **20**, 107–121.

Weathers, F. W., Litz, B. T., Herman, D. S., & Keane, T. M. (1993). The PTSD Checklist (PCL): reliability, validity, and diagnostic utility. Paper presented at the annual meeting of the International Society for Traumatic Stress Studies, San Antonio, Texas.

Weiss, D. S., & Marmar C. R. (1997). The Impact of Event Scale-Revised. In J. P. Wilson & T. M. Keane, eds.,

Assessing Psychological Trauma and PTSD. New York, NY: Guilford Press.

Wessely, S. (2005). Risk, psychiatry and the military. *British Journal of Psychiatry*, **186**, 459–566.

World Health Organization (1990). *Composite International Diagnostic Interview (CIDI)*. Geneva: World Health Organization.

World Health Organization (1997). *Composite International Diagnostic Interview (CIDI)*, Version 2.1. Geneva: World Health Organization.

Yehuda, R., & McFarlane, A. C. (1995). Conflict between current knowledge about posttraumatic stress disorder and its original conceptual basis. *American Journal of Psychiatry*, **152**, 1705–1713.

Chapter 20

Attachment, separation, and anxiety disorders

Elizabeth Sagurton Mulhare, Angela Ghesquiere, M. Katherine Shear

20.1 Introduction

Anxiety is a normal, inborn, adaptive emotion found throughout the animal kingdom. For an organism to function effectively, anxiety should be generated when in a threatening situation. Most animals do not live in isolation, and forming attachment relationships is also a normal, inborn adaptive process that serves, in part, to protect an organism from danger. Across species, the presence of an attachment figure reduces the intensity of anxiety in the face of threat. At the same time, separation from an attachment figure may itself be perceived as a danger and elicit anxiety.

The purpose of this chapter is to describe research pertaining to the association between attachment relationships and vulnerability to anxiety disorders. Anxiety disorders are characterized by the presence of anxiety, often intense, in situations that are not objectively dangerous. In the last decade, investigators have begun to address the role of adult attachment insecurity as a vulnerability factor for DSM-IV anxiety disorders, especially posttraumatic stress disorder (PTSD). Additionally, adult separation anxiety disorder has emerged as a clinically significant condition that requires targeted attention (Fagiolini et al. 1998). In this chapter, we discuss recent research that suggests possible pathways from attachment to anxiety disorders in the areas of emotional regulation, anxiety sensitivity, and cognitive style.

20.2 Defining attachment

The attachment relationship is a specific type of relationship with three defining characteristics. Attachment figures are targets of proximity seeking, serve as a safe haven in times of stress, and serve as a secure base from which the attached person can pursue other life goals. Behaviors of the attachment figure result in different patterns of responses in the attached person, which are then built into his or her attachment systems and tend to persist over time. These individual differences can be broadly characterized as secure or insecure, depending on the degree to which the attachment figure is experienced as predictable, responsive, attuned, and satisfying.

Attachment theory developed from an ethological–evolutionary perspective that identified attachment behaviors as instinctive and necessary for survival and adaptation, with similarities observed between and among animal species and human beings. The bio-behavioral attachment system serves developmental objectives, as well as adult psychophysiological regulatory functions (Hofer 1984, Schore 2000, Schore & Schore 2008). Much of the attachment literature focuses on infants and their caregivers and views attachment as a way of maintaining safety and security during development and into maturity. Attachment theory posits that early interactions between an infant and his or her primary caregivers contribute to the formation of a template for relationship functioning and affect regulation over the life course (Ainsworth 1969, 1991, Bowlby 1969, 1973, 1977, 1980, 1988, Ainsworth et al. 1978, Rciss 1991).

The development and functioning of working models is an integral part of the attachment system (Bowlby 1969, 1973, 1977, 1980, 1988). In early childhood, physical proximity to the caregiver is required to calm anxiety. As a child develops, mental representations, or working models, of the attachment figure are created, and these reduce anxiety in the physical absence of the caregiver. Perception of threat activates the attachment system, leading to proximity-seeking behavior. Secure early attachment experiences are believed to lead to working models that operate efficiently and effectively to resolve anxiety in stress-provoking situations. Conversely, for children with insecure attachment, mental representations of attachment figures are less effective in regulating anxiety derived from perceived

Anxiety Disorders: Theory, Research, and Clinical Perspectives, ed. Helen Blair Simpson, Yuval Neria, Roberto Lewis-Fernández, Franklin Schneier. Published by Cambridge University Press. © Cambridge University Press 2010.

threats, resulting in reduced ability to self-soothe and increased vulnerability to prolonged anxiety states (Bowlby 1973).

Recently, attachment researchers have begun to conceptualize the working model in a way more consistent with what is known about brain functions and with the fact that the quality of relationships often varies over time. Working models are hypothesized to be hierarchical associative memory networks containing exemplars of specific relationships in the form of episodic memories. Models of specific relationships become exemplars of generic relationship schemas. Mikulincer (2007, p. 24) explains:

> everyone possesses models of security attainment, hyperactivation, and deactivation and so can sometimes think about relationships in secure terms and at other times think about them in less secure, more hyperactivating or deactivating terms. Due to differences in relationship histories, dominant working models differ across individuals.

According to Bowlby's theory, working models based on predictable, responsive, attuned, and satisfying interactions between child and caregiver form the basis of a secure generalized attachment style that influences subsequent attachment functioning. However, as Mikulincer's quote illustrates, current attachment research suggests a somewhat more complex and variable model. Studies do support Bowlby's belief that attachment security could change over the life span (Hamilton 2000, Waters *et al.* 2000); it is possible to characterize individual differences in attachment representation, but attachment style is not always stable over time.

20.3 Assessing attachment

Mary Ainsworth (1969, 1991) was the first to systematically measure attachment style. Her Strange Situation evaluation tool classifies early childhood attachment as either secure, insecure–avoidant, insecure–ambivalent, or insecure–disorganized. The Strange Situation consists of a brief evaluation session with a one-year-old child, his or her mother, and a clinician, during which the mother leaves the child alone with the evaluator for a short period and then returns. Bartholomew and Horowitz (1991) measured attachment style using four categories created by intersecting axes of *model of self* and *model of other*, which represent attachment anxiety and attachment avoidance. The *model of self* axis ranges from no fear of rejection or abandonment by others (low anxiety), to intense fear of rejection due to poor self-esteem

and sense of personal unworthiness (high anxiety). The *model of other* axis ranges from trust of other persons (low avoidance), to mistrust and avoidance of others and close interpersonal relationships (high avoidance). According to this framework, securely attached individuals have low anxiety and low avoidance and a positive view of self and others. The other three attachment styles, all considered to be insecure, are dismissive (positive view of self and negative view of others; low anxiety and high avoidance), preoccupied (negative view of self and positive view of others; high anxiety and low avoidance), and fearful (negative view of both self and others; high anxiety and high avoidance).

Several self-report attachment scales have been derived from Bartholemew and Horwitz's (1991) attachment principles. The Relationship Questionnaire (RQ), in which respondents rate the degree to which written descriptions of the four attachment styles describe their own relationship experiences, is commonly used and has high predictive validity. The Experiences in Close Relationships (ECR) scale consists of two 18-item subscales that measure Bartholomew and Horowitz's two underlying components of adult attachment: *view of self* and *view of others* (Watt *et al.* 2005). Other commonly used self-report measures include the Adult Attachment Interview (AAI) (George *et al.* 1985), the Romantic Attachment Scale (Hazan & Shaver 1987), the Adult Attachment Scale (AAS) (Collins & Read 1990), the Revised Adult Attachment Scale (RAAS) (Collins 1996), the Attachment Style Interview (Bifulco *et al.* 2006), and, for adolescents, the Inventory of Parent and Peer Attachment (IPPA) (Armsden & Greenberg 1987).

20.4 Correlates of attachment style

Researchers have studied the relationship between adult attachment style and psychological functioning. Using data from the 1994 National Comorbidity Survey (NCS), Mickelson and colleagues (1997) found that the presence of an adult psychiatric disorder correlated with insecure attachment, both anxious and avoidant, as measured using Hazan and Shaver's (1987) instrument that categorized attachment styles (secure, avoidant, and anxious) on a four-point scale, ranging from not at all like me (score of one) to a lot like me (score of four). The NCS included data from a large representative sample of Americans aged 15–54, with 8098 respondents selected using a stratified random sampling method. About 59% of study subjects were found to have a secure attachment style, 25% an avoidant attachment style, and 11% an anxious attachment style. Respondents classified as secure were more likely to be female, older, married, white, better educated, and better off financially than those classified as insecure. Respondents classified as avoidant were more likely to be male, in the age range 25–44, married or previously married (as opposed to never married), and to be either black or "other" race. Respondents classified as anxious were more likely to be young, previously married, black or Hispanic, less well educated, and less well off financially. In general, anxious attachment style decreased with age.

Mickelson and colleagues (1997) also examined the relationship between adult attachment style and childhood experiences, and found that adverse events in childhood were positively related to insecure attachment in adulthood. Parental divorce/separation, but not other interpersonal loss, was associated with attachment insecurity. Perceptions of maternal and paternal warmth were positively correlated with a secure attachment style and negatively correlated with insecure attachment styles, both avoidant and anxious. Paternal over-protectiveness was related to secure attachment, but maternal over-protectiveness was related to insecure attachment. Secure attachment was associated with high self-esteem, internal locus of control, extroversion, and openness to experience. External locus of control and neuroticism were higher in the avoidant and anxious groups. Overall religiosity was related to secure attachment, while Christian fundamentalism was more related to the anxious attachment style.

Mickelson and colleagues (1997) suggested that attachment insecurity may be most related to adverse events in which adults fail to meet a child's expectations for trust, safety, and reliability (e.g., parental divorce/separation, physical abuse, serious neglect, parents being violent to each other). Childhood exposure to parental psychopathology, such as depression, substance abuse, and personality disorders, may be associated with early internal working models of others as being unsafe and undependable. The connection between attachment and psychopathology suggests that insecure attachment is a predisposing factor for adult psychopathology, including anxiety disorders.

20.5 The role of attachment in emotion regulation

If there is a relationship between attachment security and affect regulation, then attachment insecurity may be a risk factor for anxiety disorders. Beginning with Bowlby, theoretical models included a role for attachment in understanding the effectiveness of emotional regulation (Schore 1996, 2000, 2001, 2002, Schore & Schore 2008). Schore and his colleagues believed that the earliest infant–caregiver relationship is critical to lifelong psychological functioning. These authors argued that communication between infant and caregiver occurs via non-verbal cues and intuitive transmission of affective states described as "intersubjective affective transactions," thought to link pre-verbal, prerational brain structures of both infant and caregiver. According to Schore and Schore (2008), intersubjective affective transactions facilitate postnatal maturation of the infant brain and development of right-brain affective and self-regulatory functions. Fonagy and Target (2005) maintained that a caregiver who perceives, reflects, and modulates an infant's affective states is a key mechanism for the development of self-regulatory capacity, and that this is the primary function of the attachment system.

If Schore and Fonagy are correct, affect regulation that develops in the context of infant attachment relationships may protect against later development of adult mood and anxiety disorders. Conversely, early disturbance in attachment relationships may interfere with optimal development of neurobiological systems that underlie regulation of emotional states, in particular the ability to restore equilibrium following a period of anxious arousal. Right-brain functions hypothesized to be influenced by early attachment are those that play a role in the reception and processing of kinesthetic information received from bodily sensations. Schore and Schore (2008) postulated that attachment experiences during the first and second year of life cause biological changes that affect the development of the corticolimbic system in the prefrontal cortex involved in maintaining emotional regulation. During this period of early life, adverse affective experiences leading to prolonged, unregulated stress can inhibit the optimal development of these corticolimbic circuits, possibly predisposing the individual to psychiatric disorders related to emotional dysregulation. Right-brain functions that are not fully developed could likewise contribute to the heightened sensitivity and maladaptive response to interoceptive cues characteristic of anxiety sensitivity seen in panic and other disorders. While insecure attachment may not be more frequent in panic than in other disorders (Marcaurelle *et al.* 2005, Stewart & Watt 2008), it is possible that anxiety sensitivity may be one pathway to the development of problematic states of adult anxiety.

Since attachment theory postulates that attachment style can be changed, some authors have suggested that the role of attachment in emotional regulation has implications for therapist behavior in the treatment of anxiety and other affective disorders (Sable 2008, Schore & Schore 2008). This point of view emphasizes the soothing and regulatory effect of non-verbal, right-brain to right-brain communication between therapist and patient. These authors suggest that therapists serve functions similar to a secure attachment in providing non-verbal, emotional regulatory functions. Through empathic attunement and response to a patient's non-verbal cues and communications, a secure attachment relationship is created that promotes the development of self-regulatory systems. As the patient internalizes repeated attuned interactions between him- or herself and the therapist, affective self-regulation is fostered. If this idea is valid, it has implications for examining other close relationships in the patient's life. Intervention to improve attachment functioning would be expected to have beneficial effects on anxiety and depression. This is a central principle of interpersonal psychotherapy (Klerman et al. 1984).

Secure attachment may be associated with resilience, and at least one study has shown this to be the case. Neria and colleagues (2001) studied elite Israeli soldiers in real-world stressful situations and found that secure attachment style correlated with high mental health scores and with components of "hardiness," a construct that includes commitment to self-actualization, a sense of control, and positive response to challenges. Avoidant and ambivalent attachment styles were negatively correlated with these "hardiness" components and positively correlated with general psychiatric symptomatology.

20.6 Attachment, cognitive style, and anxiety sensitivity

20.6.1 Anxiety sensitivity and attachment

Much research has identified a correlation between insecure attachment and anxiety sensitivity (Stein et al. 1999, Watt et al. 1998, 2005) and between anxiety sensitivity and anxiety disorders (Taylor et al. 1992, Rector et al. 2007). Anxiety sensitivity refers to the fear that physical and psychological symptoms of anxiety, such as shortness of breath, increased heart rate, trembling, and cognitive confusion will have frightening social,

physical, or psychological consequences. The concept of anxiety sensitivity is derived from Reiss's (1991) expectancy model of fear, panic, and anxiety, which includes components of fear of injury, fear of anxiety, and fear of negative evaluation. Anxiety sensitivity, or "fear of fear," also includes irrational beliefs about the danger posed by anxiety sensations. Anxiety sensitivity can be measured by either the Anxiety Sensitivity Index (ASI) or the Anxiety Sensitivity Index–Revised (ASI-R). The ASI is a 16-item measure composed of lower-order categories of physical concerns, social concerns, and psychological concerns (Watt et al. 2005). The ASI-R is a 36-item self-report measure that assesses the respondent's degree of fear about normal anxiety reactions in the four categories of cardiovascular symptoms, respiratory symptoms, publicly observable anxiety reactions, and cognitive dyscontrol.

Several recent studies have found a positive correlation between insecure attachment and anxiety sensitivity (Watt et al. 1998, 2005, Stein et al. 1999). Weems and colleagues (2002) administered the ASI and the Experiences in Close Relationships (ECR) scale (Bartholomew & Horowitz 1991) to 203 high-school students and 324 university students in southeast Florida (61% Hispanic American, 19% African American, 9% Caucasian, and 3% Asian). Participants with fearful and preoccupied attachment styles were found to have the highest levels of anxiety sensitivity, and more than 75% of participants with elevated ASI scores were classified as fearful or preoccupied. Both fearful and preoccupied attachment styles were associated with a negative view of self. A similar study by Watt and colleagues (2005) examined anxiety sensitivity and attachment styles in all close relationships, not just in romantic relationships. A total of 226 college students completed the ASI, the ECR, the Relationship Questionnaire (RQ), and the State-Trait Anxiety Inventory-Trait Scale (STAI-T). Thirty-nine percent had secure attachment style, with the remainder divided equally across the other three attachment styles. Fearful or preoccupied respondents had higher levels of both anxiety sensitivity and trait anxiety than those with secure or dismissive attachment styles, suggesting that negative self-views, but not negative views of others, are associated with anxiety sensitivity.

20.6.2 Anxiety sensitivity and anxiety disorders

Aggregate scores of 25 or higher on the ASI-R are associated with a high probability of clinically significant anxiety symptoms, while scores of 30 or higher are associated with a likely diagnosis of DSM-IV anxiety disorder, particularly panic disorder, agoraphobia, or PTSD (Weems *et al.* 2002). In the study by Weems and colleagues (2002), a subgroup of 14.3% of the college sample and 15.2% of the high-school sample had ASI scores above 30. This finding is consistent with other research that has found heightened levels of anxiety sensitivity in persons diagnosed with PTSD, generalized anxiety disorder (GAD), obsessive–compulsive disorder, social anxiety disorder (SAD), and panic disorder (Reiss 1991, Taylor *et al.* 1992, Watt *et al.* 2005, Rector *et al.* 2007, Viana & Rabian 2008). Longitudinal studies have found that persons with high anxiety sensitivity are at particularly increased risk for the development of panic disorder (Maller & Reiss 1992, Schmidt *et al.* 1997, 1999).

20.6.3 Cognitive response style as a mediator between attachment and anxiety disorders

According to Reiss's (1991) expectancy model, cognition plays a major role in the development of anxiety. Theorists such as Beck (1985) and Ellis (1962) have long postulated a link between psychopathology and negative, inaccurate thoughts and perceptions, or cognitive errors. A person with a negative cognitive response style tends to interpret interpersonal situations in a negatively distorted manner, creating a propensity to encode selective environmental and interoceptive information as threatening. Negative cognitive response styles are associated with a negative view of self, which is, in turn, associated with high levels of anxiety sensitivity (Bartholomew & Horowitz 1991). Weems and colleagues (2001) also found correlations between cognitive style and anxiety disorders.

Research by Rector and colleagues (2007) examined the relationship between dimensions of anxiety sensitivity and DSM-IV diagnostic categories. The cognitive dimension of the ASI was non-specific and found to be highly correlated with GAD, panic disorder, and major depression. The relationship between panic disorder and cognitive dimensions of anxiety was most prominent in the subgroup of panic disorder patients that presented with worry thoughts of "going crazy" or "losing control." The researchers suggested that distorted perceptions of the uncontrollability and dangerousness of repetitive thought contributed to worry and rumination seen in depression and GAD.

Mikulincer and colleagues (2000) parsed the relationship between cognitive style and anxiety and attachment. In their study of the cognitive accessibility of word groups related to attachment themes, they found higher activation of separation and rejection worry thoughts among persons with insecure versus secure attachment styles. Other investigators have hypothesized that attachment insecurity helps set the stage for cognitive errors associated with a negative cognitive response style, especially in the context of interpersonal experiences. Mikulincer and colleagues outlined a model of how attachment style influences response strategies when a threat is perceived (Mikulincer & Shaver 2003, Mikulincer *et al.* 2003). They suggested that securely attached persons employ strategies that utilize reliable helpful support of others, while anxiously attached persons employ hyperactivating strategies designed to demand more attention from others, and avoidant persons deny the need for others and rely excessively on themselves. These strategies contain cognitive, behavioral, and affective components, and when used regularly in stressful situations they can shape self-image. Dysfunctional cognitive patterns may mediate the development of heightened anxiety sensitivity in persons with insecure attachment styles. In addition to being determined by genetic factors, anxiety sensitivity is likely maintained by negative cognitive patterns that are established and reinforced through repeated unattuned attachment experiences.

Research by Scher and Stein (2003) further supports the role of cognition as mediator between attachment and anxiety pathology. Scher and Stein examined recollected parental attachment experiences and hypothesized that threatening parental behaviors would be associated with anxiety disorders, rejecting behaviors with depressive disorders, and overall negative parental behaviors with anxiety sensitivity. Here, 249 college students completed the ASI, measures to assess current anxiety (the Beck Anxiety Inventory) and depression (the Beck Depression Inventory and the Depression Symptoms Index), and measures that assessed perception of hostile or rejecting parental behaviors (Adult Parental Acceptance–Rejection Questionnaire and Parent Threat Inventory). Results showed that parental behaviors that were recalled to be threatening, hostile, or rejecting showed a small but statistically significant association with anxiety sensitivity. Threatening parental behaviors were associated with fear of publicly observable anxiety symptoms, while hostile and rejecting parental behaviors were related to fears of losing control over one's thoughts. Results of this cross-sectional study raised the possibility that anxiety sensitivity may mediate the relationship between threatening parental behavior in childhood and later development of anxiety-disorder symptomatology, while fear of losing control of one's thoughts may mediate the relationship between hostile and rejecting parental behavior and future depressive symptoms. Parental threatening behaviors were found to have a stronger correlation with anxiety sensitivity than hostile and rejecting behaviors, consistent with the proposition that having unavailable parenting may bias cognitive schemas toward a view of attachment figures as unpredictable and unreliable.

20.7 Attachment relationships and anxiety disorders

20.7.1 Separation anxiety disorder

Separation anxiety disorder (SepAD) is the anxiety disorder most directly linked to attachment relationships. This condition has received most attention as a childhood diagnosis. However, adult separation anxiety disorder has also been identified (Manicavasagar & Silove 1997, Manicavasagar et al. 2000, Cyranowski et al. 2002), and the DSM-5 workgroup is considering whether to include this in the new diagnostic manual. While distress upon separation from an attachment figure is developmentally normal, children with separation anxiety disorder experience anxiety beyond the normal developmental period.

Childhood separation anxiety disorder (C-SepAD) is the most common childhood anxiety disorder. The estimated prevalence of C-SepAD in the general population is 4%, and it is about twice as frequent in females (Shear et al. 2006). C-SepAD has a high spontaneous recovery rate, although children are at some increased risk for the development of other anxiety disorders (Cantwell & Baker 1989, Last et al. 1996, Silove et al. 1996, Aschenbrand et al. 2003). In addition, children with persistent C-SepAD may have an increased risk of developing a depressive disorder (Foley et al. 2004). However, the most common adult anxiety disorder resulting from C-SepAD is adult separation anxiety disorder (A-SepAD) (Shear et al. 2006).

The causes of C-SepAD remain unknown, but, as is the case with anxiety sensitivity, the disorder may develop out of both biological and environmental factors. Animal research indicates that separation distress is a biologically hardwired response, primarily activating the anterior cingulate, when animals are separated from a primary attachment figure (Panksepp 2005). Likewise, Bowlby (1969, 1973) considered separation anxiety as an adaptive, biologically based response that helps keep a vulnerable child close to its caregiver; however, separation anxiety disorder occurs when this response is excessive in frequency, intensity, and duration. Cronk and colleagues utilized twin research to show a significant heritable aspect of C-SepAD (Cronk et al. 2004). In another study, 63% of children diagnosed with juvenile separation anxiety disorder had at least one parent with C-SepAD (Manicavasagar et al. 2001).

Some authors have argued that C-SepAD be conceived as an insecure attachment relationship, with the specific C-SepAD symptoms only an outward manifestation of a deeper orientation (Ollendick et al. 1993). While the argument makes conceptual sense, it is difficult to test, and the existing literature does not clearly discern the cause-and-effect relationship of caregiving and C-SepAD. Though insecure attachment may lead to C-SepAD, it is also possible that a child with C-SepAD may, through his or her behavior, elicit frustration and other negative affects in the parent, thus affecting the relationship. If so, it may be incorrect to attribute the separation anxiety to disturbance in caregiving. While there are few longitudinal data pertaining to the association between attachment style and separation anxiety, a few existing studies do show insecure attachment preceding C-SepAD. Warren and colleagues (1997) found a correlation between the insecure attachment styles of one-year-olds identified using Ainsworth's Strange Situation and later separation anxiety disorder. Similarly, Dallaire and Weinraub (2005) found that children identified at 18 months via the Strange Situation as insecurely attached reported significantly more separation anxiety at age six than did securely attached children.

Although the DSM-IV-TR affirms that adults aged 18 and older can have separation anxiety disorder, few clinicians screen for this condition, and there is a paucity of research on A-SepAD. Manicavasagar and colleagues (1997) discovered a distinct cluster of symptoms, similar to those of child separation anxiety, in a community sample. Symptoms of A-SepAD are similar to those of C-SepAD, though the object of attachment differs. A parent is the most common object for children, whereas partners or children are more often the attachment figure in A-SepAD. Maternal separation anxiety involves excessive anxiety in mothers when separated from their infant children, and it can occur in early childhood or in response to adolescent distancing behavior (Hock et al. 1989, 2001). Moreover, while the criteria for C-SepAD highlight somatic symptoms of anxiety such as stomach aches, physical complaints are reported less frequently in adults (Manicavasagar & Silove 1997). Cyranowski and colleagues (2002) developed a Structured Clinical Interview for Separation Anxiety Symptoms (SCI-SAS) and tested it on a mixed sample of adult psychiatric outpatients and non-psychiatric control subjects. They confirmed a unique group of separation anxiety symptoms prevalent in adults. Wijeratne and Manicavasagar (2003) also identified A-SepAD among a small elderly sample.

Community prevalence of A-SepAD was evaluated in the National Comorbidity Study replication using the SCI-SAS (Shear et al. 2006). Results showed a lifetime prevalence of 6.1%, a rate higher than that found for C-SepAD. Similar to other studies, in about a third of those with childhood-onset SepAD the disorder persisted into adulthood. Among those with A-SepAD, the majority (78%) had onset in adulthood, most commonly in young adulthood. There was a high rate of comorbidity with other anxiety disorders, mood disorders, and substance use disorders. Neither childhood nor adult SepAD was specifically associated with adult panic disorder. Further, there was evidence that A-SepAD was associated with functional impairment even among those who did not have comorbid Axis I conditions.

Not surprisingly, there is also evidence for a relationship between A-SepAD and attachment style. Kobak and Sceery (1988) found that college students who reported secure attachment relationships with their parents adjusted better to college life than those with insecure attachment relationships. Securely attached students reported less separation anxiety, less distress, greater social competence, and a better ability to cope with negative feelings. Armstrong and Roth (1989) discovered high rates of both separation distress and anxious attachment in a population of depressed college students with eating disorders. Hock and colleagues (2001) found that separation anxiety in parents of adolescents was associated with attachment with their children. Mothers with greater separation anxiety reported less comfort with closeness ($B = -0.11$) and less comfort depending on others ($B = -0.23$), while fathers with greater separation anxiety were also less comfortable depending on others ($B = -0.14$) and had more anxiety about relationship rejection and abandonment ($B = 0.18$).

The subjective distress, impact on relationships, and possible disruption of family functioning all point to the importance of understanding and treating all forms of separation anxiety disorder. We found no published treatment studies of A-SepAD, but cognitive–behavioral treatments that focus on graded exposure to the separation experience have been studied in C-SepAD (Weems & Carrion 2003). Here, a hierarchy of feared events is created in collaboration with the child, and graded exposure is conducted. During the exposure process, anxiety responses are gradually extinguished and coping skills increased. Usually, a behavioral contract is written specifying that the child will receive a particular reward, such as a favorite food or a toy, upon completion of a particular exposure. Teachers and school counselors may be enrolled to assist in the process by providing rewards for school attendance. Cognitive–behavioral therapy (CBT) has been found to be an effective treatment for C-SepAD (Kendall 1994, Silverman et al. 1999, Masi et al. 2001).

Studies also suggest that medications can treat C-SepAD. Studies by Birmaher and colleagues (2003) and by the Research Unit on Pediatric Psychopharmacology (2001) found selective serotonin reuptake inhibitors (SSRIs) to be efficacious for C-SepAD. A recent study compared CBT, sertraline, and the combination for children with C-SepAD. Combination treatment was superior to either CBT or sertraline alone. Medication results did not differ from those of CBT (Walkup et al. 2008).

Weems and Carrion have developed an intervention based on the attachment perspective, and proposed that this might be used to enhance adherence to CBT treatments for C-SepAD (Weems & Carrion 2003). Therapists explain to parents and their anxious children that children form a bond with their parents. If this bond is disrupted, children feel insecure and react in certain ways to ensure that their parents stay close. The goal of CBT is therefore to teach the child ways to feel safe and secure even when the parent is not there. In a case report, Weems and Carrion (2003) reported that a child treated in this manner showed a 50% decrease in C-SepAD symptoms at the end of treatment, with continued gains at a six-month follow-up assessment.

20.7.2 Attachment style and posttraumatic stress disorder

Researchers have studied attachment style among people with PTSD. Dieperink and colleagues (2001) administered the RQ and the PTSD Checklist Military Version (PCL-M) for DSM-IV (Blanchard *et al.* 1996) to 107 former prisoner-of-war (POW) veterans. Those with insecure attachment styles scored significantly higher on measures of PTSD than did those with secure style. Insecure attachment was a stronger predictor of PTSD symptom intensity than was severity of the traumas experienced. O'Connor and Elklit (2008) administered the RAAS to 328 Danish students and simultaneously measured PTSD using the Trauma Symptom Checklist (TSC) (Briere & Runtz 1989). They found a strong association between insecure attachment style and number of PTSD symptoms.

Declercq and Palmans (2006) studied 544 Dutch adults who were either employees of a security company or volunteers with the Belgian Red Cross. These investigators measured adult attachment using the RQ and PTSD using the Zelf Inventarisatie Lijst (ZIL), a 22-item Dutch self-report questionnaire. Results showed a strong relationship between PTSD and both the insecure–fearful avoidant and insecure–preoccupied types. Solomon and colleagues (1998) interviewed 164 Israeli ex-POWs and 184 matched controls, who completed a battery of questionnaires 18 years after the 1973 Yom Kippur War. Subjects were interviewed about their subjective experience of captivity, current mental health status, and characteristic attachment style. Attachment styles were assessed via a questionnaire that was a modified version of Hazan and Shaver's (1987) description of how people typically feel in close relationships. Veterans with both avoidant and ambivalent attachment styles reported significantly more PTSD symptoms, more intense war-related intrusions and avoidance behaviors, and more difficulties in functioning than did secure veterans. Taken together, these data suggest that insecure attachment may be a risk factor for the development of PTSD.

20.7.3 Attachment style and other anxiety disorders

Data on attachment and other anxiety disorders, while sparse, do support a link between insecure attachment and a broad range of anxiety disorders. The study by Mickelson and colleagues (1997), using data from the NCS, showed a positive relationship between avoidant and anxious attachment styles and panic disorder, agoraphobia, SAD, simple phobia, and GAD. The magnitude of the correlation did not differ significantly for avoidant versus anxious attachment styles, with the exception of GAD, where the positive correlation with avoidant attachment style was much greater than the positive correlation with anxious attachment style. Viana and Rabian (2008) found that both the "mother alienation" and "peer alienation" components of the Inventory of Parent and Peer Attachment (IPPA) were significantly positively related to scores on the Penn State Worry Questionnaire (PSWQ); the authors concluded that insecure attachment increased the likelihood of worry and GAD symptoms. As noted previously, other research has established strong links between attachment and anxiety sensitivity, and between anxiety sensitivity and anxiety disorders. More research is needed, however, to elucidate specific relationships between attachment and other DSM-IV anxiety disorders.

20.8 Conclusions

Attachment theory posits that humans are predisposed to seek and maintain attachment relationships throughout the life span. Attachment figures provide a safe haven in times of stress and a secure base from which children and adults learn and explore the world, develop autonomy, and enjoy satisfying affiliative relationships. Attachment security has wide-ranging effects on psychological functioning, and insecure attachment may comprise a risk factor for certain childhood and adult anxiety disorders. Attachment relationships are thought to be incorporated into mental functioning in a way that influences overall sense of safety and well-being. Attachment security is dependent upon experiences with caregivers who are available and responsive. If such persons are not available, the internalized attachment representation is insecure, and there may be excessive anxiety about the availability of the attachment figure and/or attachment avoidance. Insecure attachment styles, stemming from early childhood and/or experiences later in life, may lead to expectations of others as undependable and result in chronic feelings of anxiety or difficulty regulating emotional responsiveness to stress. Insecure attachment correlates with anxiety sensitivity, which is elevated in most anxiety disorders. The experience of insecure attachment may also lead to cognitive errors about the objective threat of anxiety symptoms. These maladaptive cognitive biases may mediate a relationship between early attachment experiences and childhood or adult anxiety disorders.

Empirical support for the relationship between attachment and anxiety disorders is still limited, and longitudinal studies are needed to determine causality. Psychoanalytic theories regarding the role of the attachment system in the development of brain capacity to regulate emotions also need to be tested in longitudinal studies of brain functioning. It remains unclear to what extent insecure attachment and anxiety sensitivity are causal factors for anxiety disorders, as opposed to co-occurring, or even resulting, conditions. There is, for instance, a strong correlation between SAD and anxious insecure attachment, but research has not yet established insecure attachment as a causal factor for SAD. For SAD, as with other anxiety disorders, a bidirectional, reciprocal relationship seems likely as a maintaining factor regardless of the underlying precipitating factor.

A greater understanding of the causes of anxiety disorders can inform the development of efficacious treatments for these debilitating conditions. Attachment-theory principles can be integrated into psychotherapeutic approaches, such as CBT. Identifying a client's attachment style can also enhance the clinician's ability to form a therapeutic alliance and help guide the foci of treatment.

References

Ainsworth, M. (1969). Object relations, dependency and attachment: a theoretical review of the infant–mother relationship. *Child Development*, **40**, 969–1025.

Ainsworth, M. (1991). An ethological approach to personality development. *American Psychologist*, **46**, 333–341.

Ainsworth, M., Blehar, M. C., Waters, E., & Wall, S. (1978). *Patterns of Attachment: a Psychological Study of the Strange Situation*. Hillsdale, NJ: Lawrence Erlbaum.

Armsden, G. C., & Greenberg, M. T. (1987). The inventory of parent and peer attachment: Individual differences and their relationship to psychological well-being in adolescence. *Journal of Youth and Adolescence*, **16**, 427–454.

Armstrong, S., & Roth, D. (1989). Attachment and separation difficulties in eating disorders: A preliminary investigation. *International Journal of Eating Disorders*, **8**, 141–155.

Aschenbrand, S. G., Kendall, P. C., Webb, A., Safford, S. M., & Flannery-Schroeder, E. (2003). Is childhood separation anxiety disorder a predictor of adult panic disorder and agoraphobia? A seven-year longitudinal study. *Journal of the American Academy of Child and Adolescent Psychiatry*, **42**, 1478–1485.

Bartholomew, K., & Horowitz, L. M. (1991). Attachment styles among young adults: a test of a four-category model. *Journal of Personality and Social Psychology*, **61**, 226–244.

Beck, A. T. (1985). *Cognitive Therapy and the Emotional Disorders*. New York, NY: International Universities Press.

Bifulco, A., Kwon, J., Jacobs, C., *et al.* (2006). Adult attachment styles as mediator between childhood neglect/abuse and adult depression and anxiety. *Social Psychiatry and Psychiatric Epidemiology*, **41**, 796–805.

Birmaher, B., Axelson, D. A., Monk, K., *et al.* (2003). Fluoxetine for the treatment of childhood anxiety disorders. *Journal of the American Academy of Child and Adolescent Psychiatry*, **42**, 415–423.

Blanchard, E. B., Jones-Alexander, J., Buckley, T. C., & Forneris, C. A. (1996). Psychometric properties of the PTSD Checklist (PCL). *Behavior Research and Therapy*, **34**, 669–673.

Bowlby, J. (1969). *Attachment and Loss, Vol. 1: Attachment*. New York, NY: Basic Books.

Bowlby, J. (1973). *Attachment and Loss, Vol. 2: Separation: Anxiety and Anger*. New York, NY: Basic Books.

Bowlby, J. (1977). The making and breaking of affectional bonds. *British Journal of Psychiatry*, **130**, 201–210.

Bowlby, J. (1980). *Attachment and Loss. Vol. 3: Loss, Sadness and Depression*. New York, NY: Basic Books.

Bowlby, J. (1988). *A Secure Base*. New York, NY: Basic Books.

Briere, J., & Runtz, M. G. (1989). The Trauma Symptom Checklist (TSC-33): early data on a new scale. *Journal of Interpersonal Violence*, **4**, 151–163.

Cantwell, D. P., & Baker, L. (1989). Stability and natural history of DSM-III childhood diagnoses. *Journal of the American Academy of Child and Adolescent Psychiatry*, **28**, 691–700.

Collins, N. L. (1996). Working models of attachment: Implications for explanation, emotion, and behavior. *Journal of Personality and Social Psychology*, **71**, 810–832.

Collins, N. L., & Read, S. J. (1990). Adult attachment, working models, and relationship quality in dating couples. *Journal of Personality and Social Psychology*, **58**, 644–663.

Cronk, N. J., Slutske, W. S., Madden, P. A., Bucholz, K. K., & Heath, A. C. (2004). Risk for separation anxiety disorder among girls: paternal absence, socioeconomic disadvantage, and genetic vulnerability. *Journal of Abnormal Psychology*, **113**, 237–247.

Cyranowski, J. M., Shear, M. K., Rucci, P., *et al.* (2002). Adult separation anxiety: psychometric properties of a new structured clinical interview. *Journal of Psychiatric Research*, **36**, 77–86.

Dallaire, D. H., & Weinraub, M. (2005). Predicting children's separation anxiety at age 6: the contributions of infant–mother attachment security, maternal sensitivity, and maternal separation anxiety. *Attachment and Human Development*, 7, 393–408.

Declercq, F., & Palmans, V. (2006). Two subjective factors as moderators between critical incidents and the occurrence of post traumatic stress disorders: adult attachment and perception of social support. *Psychology and Psychotherapy*, 79, 323–337.

Dieperink, M., Leskela, J., Thuras, P., & Engdahl, B. (2001). Attachment style classification and posttraumatic stress disorder in former prisoners of war. *American Journal of Orthopsychiatry*, 71, 374–378.

Ellis, A. (1962). *Reason and Emotion in Psychotherapy*. Secaucus, NJ: Citadel Press.

Fagiolini A., Shear, M. K., Cassano, G. B., & Frank E. (1998). Is lifetime separation anxiety a manifestation of panic spectrum? *CNS Spectrums*, 3, 63–72.

Foley, D. L., Pickles, A., Maes, H. M., Silberg, J. L., & Eaves, L. J. (2004). Course and short-term outcomes of separation anxiety disorder in a community sample of twins. *Journal of the American Academy of Child and Adolescent Psychiatry*, 43, 1107–1114.

Fonagy, P, & Target, M. (2005). Bridging the transmission gap: an end to an important mystery of attachment research? *Attachment and Human Development*, 7, 333–343.

George, C., Kaplan, N., & Main, M. (1985). *The Berkeley Adult Attachment Interview*. Berkeley, CA: University of California.

Hamilton, C. E. (2000). Continuity and discontinuity of attachment from infancy through adolescence. *Child Development*, 71, 690–694.

Hazan, C., & Shaver, P. (1987). Romantic love conceptualized as an attachment process. *Journal of Personality and Social Psychology*, 52, 511–524.

Hock, E., McBride, S, & Gnezda, M. (1989). Maternal separation anxiety: mother–infant separation from the maternal perspective. *Child Development*, 60, 79–802.

Hock, E., Eberly, M., Bartle-Haring, S., Ellwanger, P., & Widaman, K. F. (2001). Separation anxiety in parents of adolescents: theoretical significance and scale development. *Child Development*, 72, 284–298.

Hofer, M. (1984). Relationships as regulators: a psychobiologic perspective on bereavement. *Psychosomatic Medicine*, 46, 183–197.

Kendall, P. C. (1994). Treating anxiety disorders in children: results of a randomized clinical trial. *Journal of Consulting and Clinical Psychology*, 62, 100–110.

Klerman, G., Weissman, M., Rounseville, B., & Chevron, E. S. (1984). *Interpersonal Psychotherapy for Depression*. New York, NY: Basic Books.

Kobak, R. R., & Sceery, A. (1988). Attachment in late adolescence: working models, affect regulation, and representations of self and others. *Child Development*, 59, 135–146.

Last, C. G., Perrin, S., Hersen, M., & Kazdin, A. E. (1996). A prospective study of childhood anxiety disorders. *Journal of the American Academy of Child and Adolescent Psychiatry*, 35, 1502–1510.

Maller, R G, & Reiss, S. (1992). Anxiety sensitivity in 1984 and panic attacks in 1987. *Journal of Anxiety Disorders*, 6, 241–247.

Manicavasagar, V., & Silove, D. (1997). Is there an adult form of separation anxiety disorder? A brief clinical report. *Australian and New Zealand Journal of Psychiatry*, 31, 299–303.

Manicavasagar, V., Silove, D., & Curtis, J. (1997). Separation anxiety in adulthood: a phenomenological investigation. *Comprehensive Psychiatry*, 38, 274–282.

Manicavasagar, V., Silove, D., Curtis, J., & Wagner, R. (2000). Continuities of separation anxiety from early life into adulthood. *Journal of Anxiety Disorders*, 14, 1–18.

Manicavasagar, V., Silove, D., Rapee, R., Waters, F., & Momartin, S. (2001). Parent–child concordance for separation anxiety: a clinical study. *Journal of Affective Disorders*, 65, 81–84.

Marcaurelle, R., Belanger, C., Marchand, A., Katerelos, T. E., & Mainguy, N. (2005). Marital predictors of symptom severity in panic disorder with agoraphobia. *Journal of Anxiety Disorders*, 19, 211–232.

Masi, G., Mucci, M., & Millepiedi, S. (2001). Separation anxiety disorder in children and adolescents: Epidemiology, diagnosis and management. *CNS Drugs*, 15, 93–104.

Mickelson, K. D., Kessler, R. C., & Shaver, P. (1997). Adult attachment in a nationally representative sample. *Journal of Personality and Social Psychology*, 73, 1092–1106.

Mikulincer, M., & Shaver, P. R. (2007). *Attachment in Adulthood: Structure, Dynamics, and Change*. New York, NY: Guilford Press.

Mikulincer, M., & Shaver, P. (2003). The attachment behavioral system in adulthood: activation, psychodynamics, and interpersonal processes. In M. P. Zanna, ed., *Advances in Experimental Social Psychology, Vol. 35*. New York, NY: Academic Press, pp. 53–152.

Mikulincer, M., Birnbaum, G., Woddis, D., & Nachmias, O. (2000). Stress and accessibility of proximity-related thoughts: exploring the normative and intraindividual components of attachment theory. *Journal of Personality and Social Psychology*, 78, 509–523.

Mikulincer, M., Shaver, P., & Pereg, D. (2003). Attachment theory and affect regulation: The dynamics, development, and cognitive consequences of attachment-related strategies. *Motivation and Emotion*, 27, 77–102.

Neria, Y., Guttman-Steinmetz, S., Koenen, K., *et al.* (2001). Do attachment and hardiness relate to each other and to mental health in real life stress? *Journal of Social and Personal Relationships*, **18**, 844–858.

O'Connor, M., & Elklit, A. (2008). Attachment styles, traumatic events, and PTSD: a cross-sectional investigation of adult attachment and trauma. *Attachment and Human Development*, **10**, 59–71.

Ollendick, T. H., Lease, C., & Cooper, C. (1993). Separation anxiety in young adults: a preliminary examination. *Journal of Anxiety Disorders*, **7**, 293–305.

Panksepp, J. (2005). Why does separation distress hurt? Comment on MacDonald and Leary (2005). *Psychological Bulletin*, **131**, 224–230; author reply 237–240.

Rector, N. A., Szacun-Shimizu, K., & Leybman, M. (2007). Anxiety sensitivity within the anxiety disorders: disorder-specific sensitivities and depression comorbidity. *Behaviour Research and Therapy*, **45**, 197–1975.

Reiss, S. (1991). Expectancy model of fear, anxiety, and panic. *Clinical Psychology Review*, **11**, 141–153.

Research Unit on Pediatric Psychopharmacology Anxiety Study Group (2001). Fluvoxamine for the treatment of anxiety disorders in children and adolescents. *New England Journal of Medicine*, **344**, 1279–1285.

Sable, P. (2008). What is adult attachment? *Clinical Social Work Journal*, **36**, 21–30.

Scher, C. D., & Stein, M. B. (2003). Developmental antecedents of anxiety sensitivity. *Anxiety Disorders*, **17**, 253–269.

Schmidt, N. B., Lerew, D. R., & Jackson, R. J. (1997). The role of anxiety sensitivity in the pathogenesis of panic: prospective evaluation of spontaneous panic attacks during acute stress. *Journal of Abnormal Psychology*, **106**, 355–364.

Schmidt, N. B., Lerew, D. R., & Jackson, R. J. (1999). Prospective evaluation of anxiety sensitivity in the pathogenesis of panic: replication and extension. *Journal of Abnormal Psychology*, **108**, 532–537.

Schore, A. N. (1996). The experience-dependent maturation of a regulatory system in the orbital prefrontal cortex and the origin of developmental psychopathology. *Development and Psychopathology*, **8**, 59–87.

Schore, A. N. (2000). Attachment and the regulation of the right brain. *Attachment and Human Development*, **2**, 23–47.

Schore, A. N. (2001). The effects of a secure attachment relationship on right brain development, affect regulation, and infant mental health. *Infant Mental Health Journal*, **22**, 7–66.

Schore, A. N. (2002). Advances in neuropsychoanalysis, attachment theory, and trauma research: implications for self psychology. *Psychoanalytic Inquiry*, **22**, 433–484.

Schore, J., & Schore, A. (2008). Modern attachment theory: the central role of affect regulation in development and treatment. *Clinical Social Work Journal*, **36**, 9–20.

Shear, K., Jin, R., Ruscio, A. M., Walters, E. E., & Kessler, R. C. (2006). Prevalence and correlates of estimated DSM-IV child and adult separation anxiety disorder in the National Comorbidity Survey Replication. *American Journal of Psychiatry*, **163**, 1074–1083.

Silove, D., Manicavasagar, V., Curtis, J., & Blaszczynski, A. (1996). Is early separation anxiety a risk factor for adult panic disorder? A critical review. *Comprehensive Psychiatry*, **37**, 167–179.

Silverman, W. K., Kurtines, W. M., Ginsburg, G. S., *et al.* (1999). Treating anxiety disorders in children with group cognitive–behaviorial therapy: a randomized clinical trial. *Journal of Consulting and Clinical Psychology*, **67**, 995–1003.

Solomon, Z., Ginzburg, K., Mikulincer, M., Neria, Y., & Ohry, A. (1998). Coping with war captivity: the role of attachment style. *European Journal of Personality*, **12**, 271–285.

Stein, M. B., Jang, K. L., & Livesley, W. J. (1999). Heritability of anxiety sensitivity: a twin study. *American Journal of Psychiatry*, **156**, 246–251.

Stewart, S. H., & Watt, M. C. (2008). Introduction to the special issue on interoceptive exposure in the treatment of anxiety and related disorders: novel applications and mechanisms of action. *Journal of Cognitive Psychotherapy*, **22**, 291–302.

Taylor, S., Koch, W. J., & McNally, R. J. (1992). How does anxiety sensitivity vary across the anxiety disorders? *Journal of Anxiety Disorders*, **6**, 249–259.

Viana, A. G., & Rabian, B. (2008). Perceived attachment: relations to anxiety sensitivity, worry, and GAD symptoms. *Behaviour Research and Therapy*, **46**, 737–747.

Walkup, J. T., Albano, A. M., Piacentini, J., *et al.* (2008). Cognitive behavioral therapy, sertraline, or a combination in childhood anxiety. *New England Journal of Medicine*, **359**, 2753–2766.

Warren, S. L., Huston, L., Egeland, B., & Sroufe, L. A. (1997). Child and adolescent anxiety disorders and early attachment. *Journal of the American Academy of Child and Adolescent Psychiatry*, **36**, 637–644.

Waters, E., Weinfield, N. S., & Hamilton, C. E. (2000). The stability of attachment security from infancy to adolescence and early adulthood: general discussion. *Child Development*, **71**, 703–706.

Watt, M. C., Stewart, S. H., & Cox, B. J. (1998). A retrospective study of the learning history origins of anxiety sensitivity. *Behaviour Research and Therapy*, **36**, 505–525.

Watt, M. C., McWilliams, L. A., & Campbell, A. G. (2005). Relations between anxiety sensitivity and attachment style dimensions. *Journal of Psychopathology and Behavioral Assessment*, **27**, 191–200.

Weems, C., & Carrion, V. (2003). The treatment of separation anxiety disorder employing attachment theory and cognitive behavior therapy techniques. *Clinical Case Studies*, **2**, 188–198.

Weems, C., Berman, S., Silverman, W., & Saavedra, L. (2001). Cognitive errors in youth with anxiety disorders: the linkages between negative cognitive errors and anxious symptoms. *Cognitive Therapy and Research*, **25**, 559–575.

Weems, C., Berman, S., Silverman, W., & Rodriquez, E. (2002). The relation between anxiety sensitivity and attachment style in adolescence and early adulthood. *Journal of Psychopathology and Behavioral Assessment*, **24**, 159–168.

Wijeratne, C., & Manicavasagar, V. (2003). Separation anxiety in the elderly. *Journal of Anxiety Disorders*, **17**, 695–702.

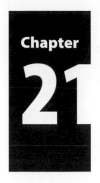

Non-human primate models in understanding anxiety

Navin A. Natarajan, Ranjeeb Shrestha, Jeremy D. Coplan

21.1 Why non-human primates?

Non-human primates share a great deal of phylogenic proximity to humans and exhibit similar behavioral and physiological responses to anxiety-producing situations (Barros & Tomaz 2002). Both species experience an extended postnatal period of development that is characterized by social and cognitive adaptations from infancy to full maturation (Nelson & Winslow 2009). Non-human primates have significant biological and behavioral markers that correspond to human developmental milestones, allowing researchers to make cross-species interpretations (Kalin & Shelton 2003). Furthermore, humans and non-human primates share genetic make-up and essentially the same serotonin transporter gene along with its functional polymorphism. These similarities facilitate understanding of complex gene-by-environment interactions (Suomi 2006).

21.2 Significance of the mother–infant dyad

Infant monkeys exhibit a sequence of developmental milestones similar to humans. At the age of two months, they explore their physical and social surroundings using their mother as a base from which to venture out while remaining near physical contact (Suomi 2006). By three months of age, the rhesus brain is developmentally similar to a human brain of one year (Kalin 2004). The infant is able to learn appropriate adaptive defensive responses to specific types of threat, such as remaining still or freezing when confronted by a human intruder (Kalin *et al.* 1991). Their ability to regulate defensive behavior has been correlated with the maturation of the hypothalamic–pituitary–adrenal (HPA) axis, as studied through autoradiography (Kalin 2004).

The hypothalamus regulates levels of the steroid hormone cortisol from the adrenal gland (Herman *et al.* 2003) through the release of corticotropin-releasing hormone (CRH). Dysregulation of the HPA axis has been associated with multiple human somatic and psychiatric illnesses, including depression and anxiety (Sanchez 2006). Studies in rodents have shown that postnatal maternal care is required for proper maturation of HPA response to stress (Meaney & Szyf 2005). Based on clinical and biological research in human samples, the proper maturation and regulation of the HPA axis is considered integral to mental well-being.

21.3 Parental separation models

Relatively few naturalistic animal studies have attempted to inform understanding of the development of anxiety disorders. At the National Institutes of Health Animal Center in Maryland, Stephen Suomi and colleagues observed that 20% of rhesus macaques growing up in naturalistic settings consistently respond to stressful situations with unusually anxious and fearful behavior. In these fearful infant monkeys, the investigators saw a delay in the age of onset for explorative behavior, reluctance to engage with peers, and increased time spent with the mother. This constellation of behaviors was associated with prolonged HPA activation leading to elevation of both salivary and plasma cortisol (Suomi 2006). When temporarily separated from their mothers, these highly reactive monkeys exhibited far greater behavioral distress and HPA activation in comparison to non-fearful controls. As juveniles, these monkeys continued to express increased lethargy, eating and sleeping difficulties, social withdrawal, holding a fetal position for hours, and other behavioral symptoms when faced with stress (Suomi 1997). When researchers looked at biological correlates, they discovered prolonged HPA axis activation, rapid noradrenergic turnover, greater selective immunosuppression, and elevated sympathetic arousal (Suomi 1997).

Anxiety Disorders: Theory, Research, and Clinical Perspectives, ed. Helen Blair Simpson, Yuval Neria, Roberto Lewis-Fernández, Franklin Schneier. Published by Cambridge University Press. © Cambridge University Press 2010.

To systematically investigate such naturalistic findings, multiple methods have been implemented to experimentally modify early mother–infant experiences in a controlled setting. Harry Harlow in the 1960s published his work with infant rhesus macaques separated from their mothers at the time of birth and placed in complete isolation. With complete deprivation from all contact, these infant monkeys displayed bizarre behavioral abnormalities and significant emotional and social deficits that were persistent (Suomi 1997). Later studies have implemented a modified separation paradigm to create a rhesus monkey model that could be better translated into human experience. The infant was removed from its mother at time of birth and hand-reared for a month. It was then placed with same-aged peers until the age of six months, after which it was introduced to the larger community to interact with both peer-reared and mother-reared infants. In observing attachment styles, peer-reared infants were noted to have strong social attachment with their peers, as did mother-reared infants. Peer-reared subjects were also found to be similar in physical and motor development to mother-reared infants and did not exhibit bizarre behavior. However, though they had relatively normal social interactions, the peer-reared infants exhibited anxious behaviors, such as reluctance to explore novel environments and interact with unfamiliar peers. They were also found to occupy the bottom ranks of the dominance hierarchies (Goldberg et al. 1995). In identifying the biological features of peer-reared macaques, Suomi (2006) found many patterns similar to those of spontaneously fearful subjects found in naturalistic settings. Suomi postulated that social experiences of maternal deprivation can have long-lasting biological and behavioral effects of equivalent magnitude to any individual difference related to heritable factors (Suomi 2006).

Maestripieri and colleagues (2006) attempted to understand the impact of impaired mother–infant dyads through the model of maternal abuse. The researchers studied two groups of rhesus monkeys. One group was cross-fostered with non-biological mothers, and a control group was raised by their biological mothers. Twelve of the non-cross-fostered/biologically reared and eight of the cross-fostered infants were rejected by the mothers. Rejection by mothers included limited time and duration of contact and decreased carrying and suckling of the infant. Nurturing mothers were protective of their infants; they restricted them from exploration and cradled, groomed, and initiated

contact with them. The researchers discovered that the infants who were reared with maternal rejection in both cross-fostered and non-cross-fostered groups exhibited behavioral responses such as increased solitary play along with a lower cerebrospinal fluid (CSF) level concentration of the serotonin metabolite 5-hydroxyindoleacetic acid (5-HIAA) (Maestripieri et al. 2006). The CSF 5-HIAA concentration was also found to negatively correlate with scratching, a sign indicating anxiety. They also found no significant fostering effects on the CSF 5-HIAA concentration of the protective parental group. Based on their work, the authors described the significance of a dysfunctional serotonergic system in relation to maternal rejection and the development of anxious behavior.

Looking at alternative ways to examine the behavioral and biological effects of an altered mother–infant relationship, Sanchez and her group (2005) examined the short- and long-term effects of repeated, brief, unpredictable maternal separation in rhesus monkeys between the ages of three and six months. They found that repeated separation produced a higher cortisol response than in non-separated controls, reflecting an initial sensitization of the infant's HPA axis to the separation. This sensitization of the HPA axis persisted into the juvenile age, leading to a flattened diurnal rhythm of cortisol (Sanchez 2006). The latter finding was interesting, as high cortisol response to infant separation correlated with low basal cortisol levels as juveniles. When the infant was returned to its mother following separation, the dyad reunited quickly and remained in close physical contact for an extended duration of time. Sanchez and colleagues (2001) found that intensity of the mother–infant contact at the time of the reunion buffered HPA axis reactivity and predicted better outcome for long-term HPA axis function. Therefore, the quality of maternal contact appeared to buffer the effect of early adverse experience in infant stress response.

21.4 Variable foraging demand model

The variable foraging demand (VFD) model for the study of primate behavior was developed by Rosenblum and Paully in 1984. In contrast to the frank maternal separation studied by Harlow, it provided a more indirect approach, mimicking a real-life situation (Harlow & Suomi 1974). The aims of these VFD studies were to follow how maternal stress resulted in disturbed mother–infant attachment pattern and further resulted in psychopathology in offspring. The effect of stress on the infant in the VFD model was indirect and was intended to be communicated via disruption of mothering following her stress response to unpredictable foraging conditions. Over the years, the basic premise of the model has remained the same but it has become more biologically focused than earlier research, which focused mainly on behavior.

Rosenblum and Paully (1984, 1987) developed three different experimental rearing conditions for the bonnet macaque monkeys. Cohorts of infant monkeys and their breastfeeding mothers were assigned randomly to three different foraging conditions for either a 12- or a 16-week period. In the first rearing condition, which was designated low foraging demand (LFD), the mothers of the infant monkeys were exposed to conditions where food was easily available. In the second condition, high foraging demand (HFD), food was difficult to find: it had to be dug out of clean wood-chip bedding that hid the less-abundant food located within "mobile foraging carts." In the third condition, which was called variable foraging demand (VFD), the availability of food switched between LFD and HFD every two weeks. Sufficient food was always available throughout the period of the experiments, and food deprivation was not a factor. Weekly weight measures and daily health checks were performed to ensure normal growth and health in all infants and their mothers. Interestingly, there was no difference in the behavioral and biological findings in monkeys raised in HFD and LFD. However, there was a significant difference in the behavioral and biological manifestations of being raised under the VFD condition when compared to LFD/HFD. Researchers hypothesized that VFD stress was transmitted to the offspring via disruption of maternal attachment and normative affective reciprocity.

The VFD-reared monkeys, as compared to the LFD-reared monkeys, showed a range of behavior abnormalities at successive stages of maturation. During infancy, in dyadic assessment shortly after the rearing experience, VFD rearing adversely affected the subject's ability to separate from mother to explore a novel physical environment. VFD-reared infants manifested timidity, social subordinance, and increased separation despair (Rosenblum & Paully 1984, 1987). These features have commonality with symptoms of human anxiety disorders. When VFD-reared monkeys were tested in late adolescence with a social challenge paradigm, they exhibited diminished capacity for affiliative social engagement relative to LFD monkeys, possibly akin to social anxiety disorder in humans (Rosenblum et al. 2001).

In addition, in unperturbed home-cage behavioral observations, in comparison to LFD-reared subjects, VFD juvenile subjects exhibited reduced social engagement, increased affective withdrawal, and social timidity. Taken together, these observations demonstrated a persistently abnormal behavioral profile analogous to certain aspects of anxiety and depression seen in humans.

Coplan and colleagues explored the neurobiological sequelae of exposure to this adverse rearing environment. They looked into abnormalities of serotonergic and noradrenergic systems, both of which have been implicated in mood and anxiety disorders. VFD-reared subjects were found to exhibit abnormal behavioral responsivity to yohimbine, a noradrenergic probe, and m-chlorophenylpiperazine (mCPP), a serotonin agonist (Coplan et al. 1992, Rosenblum et al. 1994). VFD-reared subjects were hyper-responsive to the anxiogenic effects of yohimbine and hypo-responsive to the behavioral effects of mCPP. When compared with controls, VFD-reared monkeys exhibited elevated concentrations of cisternal CSF somatostatin, as well as serotonin and dopamine metabolites (Coplan et al. 1998). This diffuse excitatory influence could be mediated by the ubiquitous excitatory amino acid glutamate along with its regulatory activity of the neuropeptide CRH, which acts as the intermediate vehicle of excitation (Mathew et al. 2001).

CRH, as mentioned above, is a neuropeptide which coordinates the body's behavioral, neuroendocrine, and neuroimmunologic response to stress, and it has been implicated in the pathophysiology of mood and anxiety disorders (Nemeroff & Vale 2005). Juvenile VFD-reared subjects exhibited persistently elevated concentrations of CSF CRH with concomitant HPA axis suppression in comparison to both LFD- and HFD-reared subjects (Coplan et al. 1996). Growth hormone (GH) is a pituitary hormone that has been associated with positive trophic state (Cirulli et al. 2009). In anxiety and mood disorders, GH secretion has been found to be reduced when challenged with the alpha-2-agonist clonidine (Coplan et al. 2000). Interestingly, the serial CSF CRH concentrations in VFD-reared subjects inversely predicted the GH response to clonidine challenge. This finding suggests that persistent activation of the central CRH system in VFD monkeys is associated with an antitrophic state. In addition, this supports the hypothesis that central CRH elevation may contribute to the blunted GH response to clonidine, as observed in humans with mood and anxiety disorders.

Glutamate is a ubiquitous amino acid with a diffuse excitatory influence in the brain. The VFD model has also been used to assess if glutamate is integral in activation of noradrenergic and central CRH systems in the bonnet macaque (Coplan *et al.* 2001). Researchers tested whether administration of LY354740, a metabotropic presynaptic receptor agonist of glutamate, blocked acute yohimbine-induced cortisol increases by down-modulating the HPA axis. Intravenous LY354740 attenuated the acute cortisol and 3-methoxy-4-hydroxyphenylglycol (a monoamine metabolite) responses. Daily oral administration of this drug led to reduction in cortisol several weeks into treatment. However, no rearing-group difference was noted in this experiment. Despite the group similarity, this study supports the notion that glutamate excess could underlie norepinephrine excess and limbic HPA axis activation, perhaps even compromising the neurotrophic state (Coplan *et al.* 2001).

Transforming growth factor beta 1 (TGF-β1) is a potent anti-inflammatory cytokine that inhibits T-cell activation (Sternberg 1997). TGF-β1 was examined in VFD-reared subjects due to its regulatory action on HPA axis through adrenocortical steroidogenesis and blockade of acetylcholine-induced release of CRH in the amygdala and hippocampus (Smith *et al.* 2001). Furthermore, these cytokines act as immunoregulatory mediators and are stimulated by glucocorticoids, which suggests a potential mechanism of stress-induced glucocorticoid-mediated immunosuppression (AyanlarBatuman *et al.* 1991). Serum TGF-β1 and plasma cortisol were found to be elevated in juvenile VFD-reared primates, relative to age-matched, normally reared controls, after exposure to moderate stress (Smith *et al.* 2002). Further studies using gene microarray methods on monocytes indicate that VFD-reared macaques are characterized by an imbalance in inflammatory homeostasis, as evidenced by a shift in global gene expression to a proinflammatory state in response to stress and a marked decrease in gene expression of TGF-β1.

Significant work has been done on the effect of stress and HPA axis activity on hippocampal neurogenesis (Mirescu & Gould 2006). In primate studies, hippocampal neurogenesis has been found to decrease in response to stress (Gould *et al.* 1998). This relationship has led researchers to look at neurotrophic factors, such

as brain-derived neurotrophic factor (BDNF), which are critical regulators in the formation and plasticity of neuronal networks (Onen Sertoz *et al.* 2008). Recent findings have shown decreased BDNF concentration in Alzheimer's dementia, type 2 diabetes, and depression (Krabbe *et al.* 2007). Using the VFD-reared sample, Kaufman and colleagues (2007) found that peripubertal VFD juveniles exhibited weight gain with elevated BMI and insulin resistance during euglycemic-clamp studies. These findings reflect the potential involvement of decreased BDNF level as a pathogenic factor leading to a cluster of these conditions.

The use of neuroimaging has led to increased understanding of the neurobiological and neuroanatomical effects of adverse rearing. An elegant study by Mathew and colleagues (2003) using magnetic resonance spectroscopic imaging (MRSI) of the brains of VFD-reared primates showed marked changes in neuronal viability in regions that have been found to have metabolic irregularities in human affective and anxiety disorders. They assessed the impact of VFD-rearing on neurotrophic state through measurement of cerebral metabolites and markers reflecting neuronal density and integrity. Based on prior studies, *N*-acetylaspartate (NAA) was used as a marker of neuronal density and functioning, and choline-containing compounds (Cho) for cell membrane integrity. These compounds were placed in a ratio with the neurometabolite creatine (Cr), which is the standard denominator for MRSI ratio analysis. Glutamate-glutamine-gamma-aminobutyric acid (Glx), which is a spectral signal representing mainly glutamate (Prost *et al.* 1997), was also assessed to identify the correlation of heightened glutamatergic neurotransmission with decreased neuronal viability. Regions of interest were the medial temporal lobes and the anterior cingulate cortex (De Bellis *et al.* 2000, Schuff *et al.* 2001). The study showed that NAA was significantly decreased while Glx was significantly increased in the anterior cingulate cortex. Glx/Cr ratio was negatively correlated with NAA/Cr, suggesting that higher glutamatergic states may exert an antineurotrophic effect within the anterior cingulate cortex. The mean Cho/Cr ratio was found to be elevated in the hippocampus of VFD-reared subjects. In another study by Coplan and colleagues involving volumetric magnetic resonance imaging (MRI) analysis, VFD-reared subjects were shown to have decreased hippocampal volume with a higher right/left ratio when compared to LFD subjects.

Diffusion tensor imaging is another tool used to understand brain pathology, and white matter in particular. In intact myelinated fibers, water molecules drift along the internal membranes of the fiber rather than the thick wall of lipids and proteins. In pathological and deteriorative states, the integrity of the myelin sheath becomes compromised, leading to non-bidirectional diffusion of water molecules. Therefore, the reduction in the diffusion anisotropy (fractional anisotropy, FA) is indicative of white-matter deterioration. Greenberg and colleagues (2008) looked at the differences in the fractional anisotropy of VFD versus non-VFD subjects. Their region of interest was the anterior limb of the internal capsule, which is a site for deep brain stimulation in refractory depression and obsessive–compulsive disorder. They found a decrement in fractional anisotropy in both the right and left anterior limbs of the internal capsule in the VFD-reared sample. This finding provides further evidence for multiple structural and functional abnormalities of cortical regions due to the aneurotrophic effect of early adverse rearing.

The functional polymorphism of the serotonin transporter gene has been implicated in the development of anxiety and depression disorders (Holmes *et al.* 2003). This polymorphism alters transcription of the serotonin transporter gene, which in turn regulates serotonin function in the brain by terminating its action in the synapse via reuptake. The variant site is commonly known as *5-HTTLPR* (serotonin-transporter-linked polymorphic region) with two common functional alleles, the short (s) allele and the long (l) allele. The s allele encodes an attenuated promoter segment and is associated with reduced transcription and functional capacity of the serotonin transporter relative to the l allele (Perlis *et al.* 2003, Perna *et al.* 2005). Serotonin transporter genotyping was available on infant male macaques that underwent the 16-week VFD protocol. During the final LFD/HFD cycle, repeated observations were performed to identify the extent of infant attachment to its mother. The researchers found that infants with the s allele of the *5-HTTLPR* exhibited a significantly greater degree of proximity to mother than their l-allele counterparts. This difference was not noted for the HFD period. These preliminary findings suggest an influence of serotonin transporter genotype on infant behavior within the context of the VFD paradigm.

Additional differences were noted in VFD-reared primates carrying the s allele in comparison to VFD-reared primates carrying the l allele and LFD carrying either the l allele or s allele. When compared with the control primates, the VFD s-allele carriers were found to exhibit elevated CRH (J. D. Coplan *et al.* unpublished). There was also a difference in the cross-sectional area of the corpus callosum, where the s-allele VFD subjects showed much smaller areas than their control-group counterparts (A. P. Jackowski *et al.* unpublished). Amygdalar volume has also been correlated with the serotonin transporter gene (Serretti *et al.* 2006). In a meta-analysis looking at the amygdala volume of mood disorders in human samples, studies have shown conflicting evidence with marked heterogeneity (Hajek *et al.* 2009). In VFD-reared s-allele-carrying primates, in comparison to control subjects, an increased amygdala volume was noted (J. D. Coplan *et al.* unpublished). In addition, a ratio of amygdala/hippocampal volume was found to be elevated in the s-allele-carrying VFD primates in comparison to the control groups. Further research looking into the interaction of genotype and phenotype in response to early life stress can provide greater understanding into the etio-pathogenesis of various disorders.

21.5 Brain lesion model

Researchers have attempted to understand the complex interactions between brain regions in the expression of emotional and cognitive behavior by examining the effect of stress after targeted destruction of specific regions. Functional imaging studies in humans have indicated the involvement of the amygdala and orbitofrontal cortex (OFC) in the adaptive process of emotion and in psychopathology (Drevets 2000, Davidson *et al.* 2002). Within the amygdala, the central nucleus (CeA) has been a region of much interest, as its neurons project to sites involved in mediating stress response, including the hypothalamus, brainstem, and basal forebrain (Price & Amaral 1981). In order to examine the role of the amygdala in mediating anxiety response, Kalin and colleagues (2004) induced excitotoxic lesions of the CeA and observed the behavioral and physiological responses to anxiety-provoking stimuli. Using rhesus macaques, the researchers induced bilateral amygdalar lesion in one group and compared them with a unilateral lesion group. The lesions were specific to damage only the neurons and not the fibers of passage passing through the amygdala. When exposed to snake and human intruder stimuli, the bilateral lesion group displayed significantly less fear-related behavior upon exposure to a snake and less freezing behavior when faced by a human intruder. They also were noted to have decreased CSF concentration of CRH, reflecting a blunted CRH response to the anxiogenic stimuli (Kalin *et al.* 2004).

The OFC has been related to anxious temperament, as it mediates emotional responses to goal-directed behavior (Izquierdo *et al.* 2004, Rolls 2004). In addition, the medial regions of the OFC have been bidirectionally linked to the most dense projections from the amygdala (Amaral & Price 1984). To assess the role of OFC in anxiety, Kalin and colleagues (2007) examined the effect of lesions to the OFC sites that were linked to the amygdala and assessed the behavioral response to snake fear, threat-induced freezing, and CSF concentrations of CRH, reflecting central CRH activity. The findings showed that OFC lesions significantly decreased threat-induced freezing and marginally decreased fear in response to snakes. Furthermore, the lesions did not significantly decrease HPA activity or the CRH concentration. The findings provide researchers with further understanding of the complex relationship between OFC and CeA in mediating acute anxiety response and anxious temperament.

21.6 Stress inoculation and resilience

Resilience may be defined as an individual's capacity to cope with stressful events, unforeseen circumstances, and catastrophe. Thus, resilience may be conceptualized as an anti-stress factor. Stress plays an important role in producing anxiety and depression; by extension, resilience may be protective against anxiety and depression. A primate model of resilience has been developed by a group of researchers at Stanford University. Just like a vaccine that strengthens natural defenses against infections to which a person may be exposed later in life, stress inoculation via exposure to early life stress can enhance resilience. Experiments on rodents, primates, and humans have shown that early stressful events, regardless of their severity, have the capacity to alter emotional, cognitive, and HPA axis function (Suomi 1997, Glaser 2000, Kaufman *et al.* 2000). Extreme stressors may be so overwhelming that they can overcome the individual's ability to cope. Therefore, in order to enhance resilience, a stressor needs to be challenging enough to elicit emotional activation without overwhelming the individual's capacity to cope. The Stanford investigators further hypothesized that a level of stress of this intermediate magnitude could stimulate

cognitive processing and make future coping strategies more efficient (Fergus & Zimmerman 2005).

In a series of experiments, squirrel monkeys were raised in cohorts of three to four mother–infant pairs and randomized to a stress-inoculation group or a no-stress control group at the age of 17 weeks (Parker *et al.* 2004). The infants in the stress-inoculation protocol were separated from their mothers for one hour at a time every week for 10 consecutive weeks. The monkeys were placed individually in a setting containing toys and could see, hear, smell, but not touch other unfamiliar monkeys. This was meant to provide opportunities for emotional activation and cognitive processing without overwhelming the capacity for coping with adversity (Parker *et al.* 2004). At the age of nine months, each monkey was tested along with its mother for 30 minutes on five consecutive days in a novel environment. Interestingly, stress-inoculated monkeys, compared to non-inoculated monkeys, appeared to be less anxious, as evidenced by less clinging behavior, greater object exploration, and better regulation of arousal (Parker *et al.* 2004). In addition, monkeys that had been stress-inoculated were found to have a greater degree of curiosity when tested at two-and-a-half years of age (Parker *et al.* 2007). This is important, because information-seeking and exploration behaviors are keys to maintenance of resilience. Stress-inoculated monkeys were more willing to explore a new environment, were faster to explore it, and spent more time doing so.

Squirrel monkeys that underwent the stress-inoculation protocol also demonstrated lower plasma adrenocorticotropic hormone (ACTH) and cortisol at baseline when tested at 15 months of age (Parker *et al.* 2004). They also exhibited a blunted HPA response when exposed to a novel situation. Interestingly, research by Gunnar and colleagues (1996) has suggested that securely attached children have lower basal cortisol level as compared with children who are not securely attached.

Increase in prefrontal activity has been shown to correspond with a decrease in the activity of the amygdala, one of the key components in the anxiety circuitry (Gorman *et al.* 2000). Furthermore, enhanced prefrontal activation has been shown to be associated with better cognitive control of emotions (Ochsner & Gross 2005, Taylor *et al.* 2006). Patients with anxiety and depressive disorders have been described as having deficits in prefrontal functions (Etkin & Wager 2007). One of the theories that researchers have explored is the mechanism by which stress inoculation can improve prefrontal functioning, leading to decreased in anxiety in later life. Studies have suggested that stress inoculation may have specific effects on cortical development. In a response inhibition test designed to assess prefrontal brain-dependent cognitive–behavioral control, stress-inoculated monkeys performed better than the non-stress-exposed monkeys, suggesting that stress inoculation may lead to enhancement of prefrontal function (Parker *et al.* 2005a). Further support for this finding comes from an earlier MRI study that showed that juvenile monkeys that had undergone stress inoculation went on to develop larger prefrontal cortical volumes with no corresponding impact on hippocampal volumes (Lyons *et al.* 2001, 2002).

One of the questions that researchers attempted to clarify was whether the development of resilience was mediated by maternal behavior or whether it was due to the direct effect of stress on the infant. Maternal-mediated resilience would mean that the resilience in the infant was primarily enhanced by the increased attention provided by the mother after each separation, rather than by the separation per se. To address this possible confounding factor, researchers developed a set of new paradigms examining stress resistance following exposure to brief intermittent infant stress, mother–infant stress, or no stress between postnatal weeks 17 and 27 (Parker *et al.* 2006). The results showed that although the mother–infant stress group received less maternal care, the intermittent infant stress and the no-stress group were the ones to develop stress resistance. Both groups of separated juveniles – those who were separated alone and those who were separated along with their mothers – developed neuroendocrine signs of resilience as manifested by a diminished cortisol response to novel environmental stressors. The findings supported the stress-inoculation hypothesis and rejected the maternal-mediated hypothesis.

The Stanford team also explored the role of oxytocin in the development of resilience (Parker *et al.* 2005b). Social relationships play an important role in how an individual handles stress and may be protective against stress and anxiety. Oxytocin is thought to play a role in the development of social bonds and may foster social relationships that in turn enhance stress responsiveness (Heinrichs *et al.* 2003). Intranasal oxytocin was administered to a cohort of squirrel monkeys while saline-treated monkeys were used as controls. Both groups of monkeys were then exposed to stress. Oxytocin-treated monkeys exhibited lower ACTH concentrations, possibly reflecting its anti-stress effects (Parker *et al.* 2005b).

21.7 Summary

Understanding the complex pathogenesis of an anxiety disorder continues to be an area of intense research. Through the aid of non-human primates, researchers have been able to make significant strides in learning about causative and modifiable factors. Through naturalistic and laboratory studies, researchers were able to identify a specific subgroup of monkeys that exhibited hyper-responsiveness to anxiety-promoting situations. These subjects shared behavioral features as well as biological changes, such as the dysregulation of HPA axis. The significance of maternal–infant attachment has been seen as a significant factor in the development and maturation of biological systems. Impaired attachment through parental deprivation, repeated separation, abuse, and disruption through unpredictable foraging demand leads to significant neurobiological and behavioral sequelae. Of significance, infant monkeys who were adversely reared had persistent neurobiological changes that continued into the juvenile years. Neuroimaging and functional studies have identified certain regions of significance and, together with lesion studies, have provided insight into complex neural circuitry. Findings have also shown the influence of serotonin transporter gene polymorphisms in expression of symptoms when exposed to stress. Non-human primates have also aided in understanding resilience through exploration of stress inoculation and maternal–infant relation.

References

Amaral, D. G., & Price, J. L. (1984). Amygdalo-cortical projections in the monkey (Macaca fascicularis). *Journal of Computational Neurology*, **230**, 465–496.

AyanlarBatuman, O., Ferrero, A. P., Diaz, A., & Jimenez, S. A. (1991). Regulation of transforming growth factor-beta 1 gene expression by glucocorticoids in normal human T lymphocytes. *Journal of Clinical Investigation*, **88**, 1574–1580.

Barros, M., & Tomaz, C. (2002). Non-human primate models for investigating fear and anxiety. *Neuroscience and Biobehavioral Review*, **26**, 187–201.

Cirulli, F., Francia, N., Branchi, I., *et al.* (2009). Changes in plasma levels of BDNF and NGF reveal a gender-selective vulnerability to early adversity in rhesus macaques. *Psychoneuroendocrinology*, **34**, 172–180.

Coplan, J. D., Rosenblum, L. A., Friedman, S., Bassoff, T. B., & Gorman, J. M. (1992). Behavioral effects of oral yohimbine in differentially reared nonhuman primates. *Neuropsychopharmacology*, **6**, 31–37.

Coplan, J. D., Andrews, M. W., Rosenblum, L. A., *et al.* (1996). Persistent elevations of cerebrospinal fluid concentrations of corticotropin-releasing factor in adult nonhuman primates exposed to early-life stressors: implications for the pathophysiology of mood and anxiety disorders. *Proceedings of the National Academy of Sciences of the USA*, **93**, 1619–1623.

Coplan, J. D., Trost, R. C., Owens, M. J., *et al.* (1998). Cerebrospinal fluid concentrations of somatostatin and biogenic amines in grown primates reared by mothers exposed to manipulated foraging conditions. *Archives of General Psychiatry*, **55**, 473–477.

Coplan, J. D., Smith, E. L., Trost, R. C., *et al.* (2000). Growth hormone response to clonidine in adversely reared young adult primates: relationship to serial cerebrospinal fluid corticotropin-releasing factor concentrations. *Psychiatry Research*, **95**, 93–102.

Coplan, J. D., Mathew, S. J., Smith, E. L., *et al.* (2001). Effects of LY354740, a novel glutamatergic metabotropic agonist, on nonhuman primate hypothalamic-pituitary-adrenal axis and noradrenergic function. *CNS Spectrums*, **6**, 607–612, 617.

Davidson, R. J., Lewis, D. A., Alloy, L. B., *et al.* (2002). Neural and behavioral substrates of mood and mood regulation. *Biological Psychiatry*, **52**, 478–502.

De Bellis, M. D., Keshavan, M. S., Spencer, S., & Hall, J. (2000). N-Acetylaspartate concentration in the anterior cingulate of maltreated children and adolescents with PTSD. *American Journal of Psychiatry*, **157**, 1175–1177.

Drevets, W. C. (2000). Functional anatomical abnormalities in limbic and prefrontal cortical structures in major depression. *Progress in Brain Research*, **126**, 413–431.

Etkin, A., & Wager, T. D. (2007). Functional neuroimaging of anxiety: a meta-analysis of emotional processing in PTSD, social anxiety disorder, and specific phobia. *American Journal of Psychiatry*, **164**, 1476–1488.

Fergus, S., & Zimmerman, M. A. (2005). Adolescent resilience: a framework for understanding healthy development in the face of risk. *Annual Review of Public Health*, **26**, 399–419.

Glaser, D. (2000). Child abuse and neglect and the brain: a review. *Journal of Child Psychology and Psychiatry*, **41**, 97–116.

Goldberg, S., Muir, R., & Kerr, J. (1995). *Attachment Theory: Social, Developmental, and Clinical Perspectives*. Hillsdale, NJ: Analytic Press.

Gorman, J. M., Kent, J. M., Sullivan, G. M., & Coplan, J. D. (2000). Neuroanatomical hypothesis of panic disorder, revised. *American Journal of Psychiatry*, **157**, 493–505.

Gould, E., Tanapat, P., McEwen, B. S., Flugge, G., & Fuchs, E. (1998). Proliferation of granule cell precursors in the dentate gyrus of adult monkeys is diminished by stress.

Proceedings of the National Academy of Sciences of the USA, **95**, 3168–3171.

Greenberg, B. D., Askland, K. D., & Carpenter, L. L. (2008). The evolution of deep brain stimulation for neuropsychiatric disorders. *Frontiers in Bioscience*, **13**, 4638–4648.

Gunnar, M. R., Brodersen, L., Nachmias, M., Buss, K., & Rigatuso, J. (1996). Stress reactivity and attachment security. *Developmental Psychobiology*, **29**, 191–204.

Hajek, T., Kopecek, M., Kozeny, J., *et al.* (2009). Amygdala volumes in mood disorders: meta-analysis of magnetic resonance volumetry studies. *Journal of Affective Disorders*, **115**, 395–410.

Harlow, H. F., & Suomi, S. J. (1974). Induced depression in monkeys. *Behavioral Biology*, **12**, 273–296.

Heinrichs, M., Baumgartner, T., Kirschbaum, C., & Ehlert, U. (2003). Social support and oxytocin interact to suppress cortisol and subjective responses to psychosocial stress. *Biological Psychiatry*, **54**, 1389–1398.

Herman, J. P., Figueiredo, H., Mueller, N. K., *et al.* (2003). Central mechanisms of stress integration: hierarchical circuitry controlling hypothalamo–pituitary–adrenocortical responsiveness. *Frontiers in Neuroendocrinology*, **24**, 151–180.

Holmes, A., Murphy, D. L., & Crawley, J. N. (2003). Abnormal behavioral phenotypes of serotonin transporter knockout mice: parallels with human anxiety and depression. *Biological Psychiatry*, **54**, 953–959.

Izquierdo, A., Suda, R. K., & Murray, E. A. (2004). Bilateral orbital prefrontal cortex lesions in rhesus monkeys disrupt choices guided by both reward value and reward contingency. *Journal of Neuroscience*, **24**, 7540–7548.

Kalin, N. H. (2004). Studying non-human primates: a gateway to understanding anxiety disorders. *Psychopharmacological Bulletin*, **38** (Suppl. 1), 8–13.

Kalin, N. H., & Shelton, S. E. (2003). Nonhuman primate models to study anxiety, emotion regulation, and psychopathology. *Annals of the New York Academy of Sciences*, **1008**, 189–200.

Kalin, N. H., Shelton, S. E., & Takahashi, L. K. (1991). Defensive behaviors in infant rhesus monkeys: ontogeny and context-dependent selective expression. *Child Development*, **62**, 1175–1183.

Kalin, N. H., Shelton, S. E., & Davidson, R. J. (2004). The role of the central nucleus of the amygdala in mediating fear and anxiety in the primate. *Journal of Neuroscience*, **24**, 5506–5515.

Kalin, N. H., Shelton, S. E., & Davidson, R. J. (2007). Role of the primate orbitofrontal cortex in mediating anxious temperament. *Biological Psychiatry*, **62**, 1134–1139.

Kaufman, J., Plotsky, P. M., Nemeroff, C. B., & Charney, D. S. (2000). Effects of early adverse experiences on brain structure and function: clinical implications. *Biological Psychiatry*, **48**, 778–790.

Kaufman, D., Banerji, M. A., Shorman, I., *et al.* (2007). Early-life stress and the development of obesity and insulin resistance in juvenile bonnet macaques. *Diabetes*, **56**, 1382–1386.

Krabbe, K. S., Nielsen, A. R., Krogh-Madsen, R., *et al.* (2007). Brain-derived neurotrophic factor (BDNF) and type 2 diabetes. *Diabetologia*, **50**, 431–438.

Lyons, D. M., Yang, C., Sawyer-Glover, A. M., Moseley, M. E., & Schatzberg, A. F. (2001). Early life stress and inherited variation in monkey hippocampal volumes. *Archives of General Psychiatry*, **58**, 1145–1151.

Lyons, D. M., Afarian, H., Schatzberg, A. F., Sawyer-Glover, A., & Moseley, M. E. (2002). Experience-dependent asymmetric variation in primate prefrontal morphology. *Behavioral Brain Research*, **136**, 51–59.

Maestripieri, D., McCormack, K., Lindell, S. G., Higley, J. D., & Sanchez, M. M. (2006). Influence of parenting style on the offspring's behaviour and CSF monoamine metabolite levels in crossfostered and noncrossfostered female rhesus macaques. *Behavioral Brain Research*, **175**, 90–95.

Mathew, S. J., Coplan, J. D., Schoepp, D. D., *et al.* (2001). Glutamate-hypothalamic-pituitary-adrenal axis interactions: implications for mood and anxiety disorders. *CNS Spectrums*, **6**, 555–556, 561–554.

Mathew, S. J., Shungu, D. C., Mao, X., *et al.* (2003). A magnetic resonance spectroscopic imaging study of adult nonhuman primates exposed to early-life stressors. *Biological Psychiatry*, **54**, 727–735.

Meaney, M. J., & Szyf, M. (2005). Maternal care as a model for experience-dependent chromatin plasticity? *Trends in Neuroscience*, **28**, 456–463.

Mirescu, C., & Gould, E. (2006). Stress and adult neurogenesis. *Hippocampus*, **16**, 233–238.

Nelson, E. E., & Winslow, J. T. (2009). Non-human primates: model animals for developmental psychopathology. *Neuropsychopharmacology*, **34**, 90–105.

Nemeroff, C. B., & Vale, W. W. (2005). The neurobiology of depression: inroads to treatment and new drug discovery. *Journal of Clinical Psychiatry*, **66** (Suppl. 7), 5–13.

Ochsner, K. N., & Gross, J. J. (2005). The cognitive control of emotion. *Trends in Cognitive Science*, **9**, 242–249.

Onen Sertoz, O., Tolga Binbay, I., Koylu, E., *et al.* (2008). The role of BDNF and HPA axis in the neurobiology of burnout syndrome. *Progress in Neuropsychopharmacology and Biological Psychiatry*, **32**, 1459–1465.

Parker, K. J., Buckmaster, C. L., Schatzberg, A. F., & Lyons, D. M. (2004). Prospective investigation of stress inoculation in young monkeys. *Archives of General Psychiatry*, **61**, 933–941.

Parker, K. J., Buckmaster, C. L., Justus, K. R., Schatzberg, A. F., & Lyons, D. M. (2005a). Mild early life stress enhances prefrontal-dependent response inhibition in monkeys. *Biological Psychiatry*, **57**, 848–855.

Parker, K. J., Buckmaster, C. L., Schatzberg, A. F., & Lyons, D. M. (2005b). Intranasal oxytocin administration attenuates the ACTH stress response in monkeys. *Psychoneuroendocrinology*, **30**, 924–929.

Parker, K. J., Buckmaster, C. L., Sundlass, K., Schatzberg, A. F., & Lyons, D. M. (2006). Maternal mediation, stress inoculation, and the development of neuroendocrine stress resistance in primates. *Proceedings of the National Academy of Sciences of the USA*, **103**, 3000–3005.

Parker, K. J., Rainwater, K. L., Buckmaster, C. L., *et al.* (2007). Early life stress and novelty seeking behavior in adolescent monkeys. *Psychoneuroendocrinology*, **32**, 785–792.

Perlis, R. H., Mischoulon, D., Smoller, J. W., *et al.* (2003). Serotonin transporter polymorphisms and adverse effects with fluoxetine treatment. *Biological Psychiatry*, **54**, 879–883.

Perna, G., Favaron, E., Di Bella, D., Bussi, R., & Bellodi, L. (2005). Antipanic efficacy of paroxetine and polymorphism within the promoter of the serotonin transporter gene. *Neuropsychopharmacology*, **30**, 2230–2235.

Price, J. L., & Amaral, D. G. (1981). An autoradiographic study of the projections of the central nucleus of the monkey amygdala. *Journal of Neuroscience*, **1**, 1242–1259.

Prost, R. W., Mark, L., Mewissen, M., & Li, S. J. (1997). Detection of glutamate/glutamine resonances by 1H magnetic resonance spectroscopy at 0.5 tesla. *Magnetic Resonance in Medicine*, **37**, 615–618.

Rolls, E. T. (2004). The functions of the orbitofrontal cortex. *Brain and Cognition*, **55**, 11–29.

Rosenblum, L. A., & Paully, G. S. (1984). The effects of varying environmental demands on maternal and infant behavior. *Child Development*, **55**, 305–314.

Rosenblum, L. A., & Paully, G. S. (1987). Primate models of separation-induced depression. *Psychiatric Clinics of North America*, **10**, 437–447.

Rosenblum, L. A., Coplan, J. D., Friedman, S., *et al.* (1994). Adverse early experiences affect noradrenergic and serotonergic functioning in adult primates. *Biological Psychiatry*, **35**, 221–227.

Rosenblum, L. A., Forger, C., Noland, S., Trost, R. C., & Coplan, J. D. (2001). Response of adolescent bonnet macaques to an acute fear stimulus as a function of early rearing conditions. *Developmental Psychobiology*, **39**, 40–45.

Sanchez, M. M. (2006). The impact of early adverse care on HPA axis development: nonhuman primate models. *Hormones and Behavior*, **50**(4), 623–631.

Sanchez, M. M., Ladd, C. O., & Plotsky, P. M. (2001). Early adverse experience as a developmental risk factor for later psychopathology: evidence from rodent and primate models. *Developmental Psychopathology*, **13**, 419–449.

Sanchez, M. M., Noble, P. M., Lyon, C. K., *et al.* (2005). Alterations in diurnal cortisol rhythm and acoustic startle response in nonhuman primates with adverse rearing. *Biological Psychiatry*, **57**, 373–381.

Schuff, N., Neylan, T. C., Lenoci, M. A., *et al.* (2001). Decreased hippocampal N-acetylaspartate in the absence of atrophy in posttraumatic stress disorder. *Biological Psychiatry*, **50**, 952–959.

Serretti, A., Calati, R., Mandelli, L., & De Ronchi, D. (2006). Serotonin transporter gene variants and behavior: a comprehensive review. *Current Drug Targets*, 7, 1659–1669.

Smith, E. L., Batuman, O. A., Coplan, J. D., & Rosenblum, L. A. (2001). Stress, peer affiliation, and transforming growth factor-β1 in differentially reared primates. *CNS Spectrums*, **6**, 573–578.

Smith, E. L., Batuman, O. A., Trost, R. C., Coplan, J. D., & Rosenblum, L. A. (2002). Transforming growth factor-beta 1 and cortisol in differentially reared primates. *Brain Behavioral Immunology*, **16**, 140–149.

Sternberg, E. M. (1997). Neural–immune interactions in health and disease. *Journal of Clinical Investigation*, **100**, 2641–2647.

Suomi, S. J. (1997). Early determinants of behaviour: evidence from primate studies. *British Medical Bulletin*, **53**, 170–184.

Suomi, S. J. (2006). Risk, resilience, and gene × environment interactions in rhesus monkeys. *Annals of the New York Academy of Sciences*, **1094**, 52–62.

Taylor, S. E., Eisenberger, N. I., Saxbe, D., Lehman, B. J., & Lieberman, M. D. (2006). Neural responses to emotional stimuli are associated with childhood family stress. *Biological Psychiatry*, **60**, 296–301.

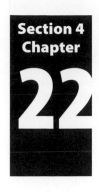

Evidence-based treatment for patients with obsessive–compulsive disorder: questions and controversies

Carolyn I. Rodriguez, Helen Blair Simpson

22.1 Introduction

Obsessive–compulsive disorder (OCD) is a debilitating mental illness characterized by intrusive thoughts (obsessions) and compelling repetitive behaviors (compulsions) (Murray & Lopez 1996). The lifetime prevalence rate is about 2% in the general population (Kessler *et al.* 2005, Ruscio *et al.* 2010). There are two evidence-based monotherapies for patients with OCD: pharmacotherapy with serotonin reuptake inhibitors (SRIs, which consist of clomipramine and the selective serotonin reuptake inhibitors, SSRIs) and cognitive–behavioral therapy (CBT), consisting of exposure and response prevention (typically referred to as ERP or EX/RP in the literature).

The American Psychiatric Association (APA) practice guidelines for treatment of adults with OCD (Koran *et al.* 2007) recommend offering CBT (ERP) monotherapy to every OCD patient when available, and that it be the first treatment used with patients with milder OCD. SSRI monotherapy or combined SSRI and CBT (ERP) treatment is recommended for adults with more severe OCD (Koran *et al.* 2007).

Despite these general guidelines, for the average clinician many questions and controversies regarding optimal treatment for adults with OCD still remain. In this chapter, we examine the available evidence regarding choosing a treatment modality, efficacy within modality classes, special groups (patients with primary hoarding symptoms or with obsessions without overt rituals), and augmentation strategies. We also review the latest advances in treatment.

22.2 Pharmacotherapy questions and controversies

22.2.1 Which is the most efficacious treatment, SRI monotherapy, CBT (ERP) monotherapy, or combination therapy?

CBT (ERP) and SRI monotherapy (including clomipramine and SSRIs) have each been shown in multiple randomized controlled trials to be efficacious for adults with OCD. However, which treatment is most effective or whether the combination of ERP and SRI is superior to either treatment alone has been examined in only a handful of randomized controlled trials (Marks *et al.* 1980, 1988, Cottraux *et al.* 1990, Hohagen *et al.* 1998, van Balkom *et al.* 1998, Foa *et al.* 2005).

In two separate studies, Marks and colleagues (1980, 1988) assessed the effectiveness of combined therapy by comparing oral clomipramine (CMI) or pill placebo (PBO) to psychotherapy of exposure in vivo (ERP) or a control therapy (relaxation therapy in the 1980 study and self-controlled exposures in the 1988 study). Both studies showed a slight additive effect of CMI and ERP; however, complex study designs and small samples make conclusions tentative. Cottraux and colleagues (1990) randomized 60 OCD patients to fluvoxamine plus ERP (FLV+ERP), fluvoxamine plus anti-exposure instructions (FLV+AE), or placebo (PBO+ERP) for 24 weeks but found no significant differences between these groups for OCD measures, perhaps due to inadequate statistical power or the suboptimal (i.e., weekly) delivery of ERP. Hohagen and colleagues (1998) randomized 58 OCD patients to either FLV+ERP or PBO+ERP. Both groups improved significantly and comparably on compulsions, but the combination FLV+ERP group improved significantly more on obsessions and comorbid depression. The ERP included elements other than exposure (e.g., cognitive restructuring), and therapist adherence to the treatment manual was not formally assessed. Van Balkom and colleagues (1998) randomized 117 OCD patients to FLV+ERP, ERP, cognitive therapy (CT), FLV+CT, or wait-list control (WL), and found that ERP alone was as efficacious as FLV+ERP. The authors concluded that for patients without comorbid depression and with overt compulsions, ERP monotherapy was preferred to combination treatment; however, limitations include suboptimal pharmacotherapy and ERP delivery and the possibility that some treatment groups contained treatment-refractory patients. Foa and colleagues (2005) randomized 122 OCD patients to intensive ERP, CMI, CMI+ERP, or PBO, and found that combined CMI+ERP treatment was significantly more effective than CMI monotherapy but was not more effective than ERP alone. Importantly, this study excluded patients with significant symptoms of depression, and the ERP was delivered intensively.

Certain conclusions can be drawn from these studies. First, both SRIs and ERP are effective monotherapies treatments for OCD. Second, how SRIs or ERP are delivered can affect their efficacy as monotherapy as well as how effective they are in combination (Simpson & Liebowitz 2005). Third, although combination treatment is not required by all patients with OCD (Franklin 2005), the available data suggest that in particular populations combination therapy can be superior to monotherapy in some OCD patients. In particular, in OCD patients with comorbid depression or with prominent obsessions, combination therapy has been shown to be superior to ERP monotherapy (Hohagen et al. 1998). In OCD patients without comorbid depression, combination therapy has also been shown to be superior to SRI monotherapy (Foa et al. 2005).

In sum, the APA practice guidelines recommend that SRIs and CBT (ERP) be the first-line treatments for OCD. Combination treatment is recommended in OCD patients to treat a comorbid and SRI-responsive disorder (e.g., depression), to augment a partial response to either SRI or CBT monotherapy, and to decrease relapse when SRI is discontinued (Koran et al. 2007).

22.2.2 What is known about time to SRI response?

SRIs (including clomipramine and SSRIs, e.g., fluoxetine, fluvoxamine, sertraline, paroxetine, citalopram) have been shown to be more effective than pill placebo for OCD in multisite randomized controlled trials (Koran et al. 2007). Although all of the aforementioned SRIs function by blocking the serotonin reuptake inhibitor, clomipramine additionally blocks the norepinephrine reuptake inhibitor. Roughly 40–60% of OCD patients who complete an adequate trial of an SRI will have, on average, a 20–40% reduction in their OCD symptoms (Greist et al. 1995, Pigott & Seay 1999). Several meta-analyses have shown that of the SRIs, clomipramine has the greatest efficacy (Jenike et al. 1990, Ackerman & Greenland 2002, Eddy et al. 2004); however, since the CMI studies were conducted earlier than the SSRI studies, the CMI studies may have included more treatment-naive patients. In head-to-head comparator studies, clomipramine was not found to be superior to fluoxetine, fluvoxamine, or paroxetine (Pigott et al. 1990, Freeman et al. 1994, Koran et al. 1996, Lopez-Ibor et al. 1996, Zohar & Judge 1996, Mundo et al. 2000).

Given that head-to-head comparisons show similar efficacy, and SSRIs have fewer side effects than clomipramine, the APA recommends that SSRIs be used as a first-line agent, and that a second SSRI should be tried before clomipramine. The decision of which SSRI to try first, given that they all have similar efficacy, will depend on the patient's prior treatment response and side-effect profile, and on the potential for drug interactions.

22.2.3 What is known about time to response for SRI?

Expert consensus guidelines have determined what defines an adequate SRI trial for OCD. An adequate SRI trial requires an adequate dose (e.g., clomipramine [$\geq$ 225 mg/day], fluoxetine [$\geq$ 60 mg/day], paroxetine [$\geq$ 60 mg/day], sertraline [$\geq$ 200 mg/day], fluvoxamine [$\geq$ 250 mg/day], citalopram [$\geq$ 60 mg/day], escitalopram [$\geq$ 30 mg/day], or paroxetine CR [$\geq$ 75 mg/day]) for a minimum of 8–12 weeks, with at least six weeks of the maximum dose comfortably tolerated (Koran et al. 2007). These guidelines are informed by the fact that randomized controlled trials of SRIs for OCD do not show significant difference between placebo and active medication before six weeks.

It is unclear why the response time with SRI for OCD patients takes longer than for depression. El Mansari and Blier (2006) have proposed that SRIs decrease

OCD symptoms by increasing synaptic serotonin in the orbitofrontal cortex. In order for SRIs to increase serotonin, the autoreceptors that initially work against this increase must first be desensitized. Animal studies indicate that terminal autoreceptor desensitization of the orbitofrontal cortex requires eight weeks, whereas in other parts of the brain this process only takes three weeks (El Mansari & Blier 2006).

22.2.4 Are serotonin–norepinephrine reuptake inhibitors (SNRIs) other than clomipramine effective in OCD?

Venlafaxine has been tested in several randomized studies, but the findings from these studies conflict. Yaryura-Tobias and Neziroglu (1996) randomized 30 OCD patients to venlafaxine and placebo and found no significant difference; limitations included small sample size, suboptimal dose (225 mg/day) and short duration of the trial (eight weeks). Two other 12-week trials compared venlafaxine (225–300 mg/day) to paroxetine (Denys et al. 2003) or clomipramine (Albert et al. 2002) and found venlafaxine to be equal in efficacy in each case; however, there was no placebo group in either study. Denys and colleagues (2004a) compared paroxetine non-responders switched to venlafaxine (19% responded) versus venlafaxine non-responders switched to paroxetine (56% responded), and found paroxetine to be more efficacious than venlafaxine in patients with poor response to the other medication. The latter study suggests that venlafaxine is less effective for OCD, at least in paroxetine non-responders.

The only published study of duloxetine in OCD is a case series of four patients with OCD who had either a partial or no response to an SRI; three patients responded after being switched to duloxetine up to 120 mg/day (Dell'osso et al. 2008). Larger controlled studies of duloxetine are needed.

In sum, there is conflicting evidence regarding the use of venlafaxine in OCD and little evidence supporting the use of duloxetine. However, in clinical practice, venlafaxine is often tried in OCD patients who have not responded to several SSRIs and cannot tolerate clomipramine.

22.2.5 What are psychopharmacological augmentation strategies for partial response to SRIs?

If a patient has had a partial response to an SRI (i.e., failed to respond to a maximal dose of a SRI for at least 12 weeks), then the clinician should consider two strategies: psychopharmacological augmentation with antipsychotics psychological augmentation with CBT (ERP). Here, we review psychopharmacological augmentation strategies.

Several randomized controlled trials have shown antipsychotics (i.e., haloperidol, risperidone, quetiapine, and olazapine) to be effective for augmenting SRIs (McDougle et al. 1994, 2000, Bystritsky et al. 2004, Denys et al. 2004b). There are also negative findings from trials of quetiapine (Carey et al. 2005) and olanzapine (Shapira et al. 2004), but these may have been due to study limitations. A case report of a patient with an incomplete response to combined CBT and setraline who showed good response to aripiprizole suggests aripiprizole may be a good augmentation strategy (Storch et al. 2008). However, a randomized controlled study will be necessary to make a more definitive conclusion. According to a systematic review of antipsychotic augmentation that combined nine double-blind, randomized controlled clinical trials, roughly one-third of OCD patients will be helped by antipsychotic augmentation (Bloch et al. 2006). Of the antipsychotics, haloperidol and risperidone had the strongest evidence (Bloch et al. 2006).

Many questions remain regarding the use of antipsychotic augmentation for OCD. Although it is known that low antipsychotic doses appear effective (e.g., < 3 mg for risperidone or the equivalent), and the time to response is about two to four weeks, there is no evidence for which antipsychotic is most effective, their long-term efficacy, or the risk of relapse upon discontinuation. A retrospective study showed high relapse rates upon antipsychotic discontinuation in a 15-patient sample (Maina et al. 2003).

Many other medications have been tested to see if they can augment the effects of SRIs in OCD; these include lithium, buspirone, clonazepam, L-triiodothyronine, pindolol, and desipramine. Although some of these agents appeared promising in open trials, none showed clear efficacy for OCD in small placebo-controlled trials (Koran et al. 2007). The current list of promising medications include SSRI augmentation with clomipramine (Szegedi et al. 1996), glutamate-modulating agents like riluzole (Coric et al. 2005) and N-acetylcysteine (Lafleur et al. 2006), the anticonvulsant topiramate (Van Ameringen et al. 2006), and morphine sulfate (Koran et al. 2005a). These compounds require further study in randomized controlled trials.

22.2.6 What are the options for a patient with no response to an SRI trial?

As outlined previously, APA guidelines suggest that patients should receive two SSRI trials before switching to clomipramine, because of estimates that up to 50% of patients may benefit from SSRI switching. However, the effectiveness of switching diminishes as the number of failed adequate trials increases (Koran et al. 2007). If, despite several SRI trials (including clomipramine), a patient still has no response, options include adding an antipsychotic, switching to venlafaxine or duloxetine (as discussed previously), or switching to other classes of pharmacological agents. These other classes include mirtazapine (an agent with complex actions on both serotonergic and noradrenergic receptors), based on a small double-blind discontinuation study (Koran et al. 2005b); tramadol (an opioid that also works on the noradrenergic and serotonergic systems), based on an open-label study (Shapira et al. 1997); and stimulants (and specifically D-amphetamine), based on several small studies (Insel et al. 1983, Joffe & Swinson 1987, Joffe et al. 1991). If medication options have been exhausted, and patients have also failed an adequate course of CBT, transcranial magnetic stimulation, deep brain stimulation, and ablative neurosurgery may be considered, per APA guidelines (Koran et al. 2007).

22.2.7 What are the latest pharmacological treatments?

Many OCD patients, though not all, will respond to an adequate trial of an SRI (clomipramine and SSRIs); however, in those who do respond, SRIs rarely produce complete remission of symptoms. As a result, there is a need for new pharmacological treatments. Available data suggest that OCD may be caused in part by an excess of glutamate in the orbitofrontal/basal-ganglia brain circuits (Graybiel & Rauch 2000, Pittenger et al. 2006). Glutamate is the most common excitatory neurotransmitter in the nervous system and functions via N-methyl-D-aspartate (NMDA), alpha-amino-3-hydroxy-5-methyl-4-isonazole propionic acid (AMPA), kainate subtypes, and G-protein-coupled receptors. Several medications that modulate glutamate have recently been show in either case reports or small open-label trials to improve OCD symptoms. These agents usually have been used to augment SRI response and not as monotherapy. In particular, there has been a positive open-label retrospective case series of topiramate,

which blocks AMPA/kainite receptors (Van Ameringen et al. 2006). Open-label trials of glutamate modulating agents such as N-acetylcysteine and riluzole (Riluteck) suggest that these agents can augment SRI response in people with OCD (Coric et al. 2005, Lafleur et al. 2006, Pittenger et al. 2008). Placebo-controlled randomized studies of both N-acetylcysteine and riluzole are currently under way and will yield more definitive results on the usefulness of glutamate modulators in OCD.

22.3 Psychotherapy questions and controversies

22.3.1 What is cognitive–behavioral therapy (CBT) for OCD?

Other than pharmacotherapy with a serotonin reuptake inhibitor, cognitive–behavioral therapy (CBT) is the only other first-line treatment for adults (Koran et al. 2007). In general, CBT can focus on either behavioral techniques, such as exposure and response prevention (ERP), or cognitive techniques (CT). Of these two, ERP-based CBT has the best evidentiary support for OCD. ERP-based CBT consists of patients voluntarily exposing themselves to feared objects or ideas (real or imagined) while refraining from performing their compulsive, ritualized response. The theory is that as the patient is exposed to the fearful stimulus, this response will habituate, and the patient will experience less anxiety over time.

22.3.2 How effective is ERP for OCD?

ERP therapy has been shown to be superior when compared to other treatments and control conditions in randomized controlled trials, including pill placebo (Foa et al. 2005), anxiety management therapy (Lindsay et al. 1997), self-guided relaxation therapy (Greist et al. 2002), therapist-guided progressive muscle relaxation (Fals-Stewart et al. 1993), and wait-list control (van Balkom et al. 1998). Randomized studies have also shown group ERP to be better than progressive muscle relaxation (Fals-Stewart et al. 1993) and wait-list control (Cordioli et al. 2003). In clinical trials of ERP, about 60% of those who enter treatment will respond with up to 55% symptom reduction (Foa et al. 2005).

Several factors are thought to affect ERP outcome, including the number and intensity of sessions (Abramowitz et al. 2002, Foa et al. 2005, Sorensen et al. 2005), adherence to ERP procedures (Greist & Baer 2002), the presence of certain comorbid conditions (e.g., severe depression, comorbid posttraumatic stress disorder) (Foa *et al.* 1983), and the degree of insight (Foa *et al.* 1999). Whether addressing any of these factors before or during ERP treatment can lead to better outcome needs further study.

Few studies have examined the long-term outcome of ERP. A review of 16 studies describing long-term outcome of adult OCD patients after ERP treatment suggested that 76% maintained their response (Foa & Kozak 1996); however, the studies reviewed were typically naturalistic follow-up, and they used varying definitions of how gains are maintained. Simpson and colleagues (2004) examined the relapse rate after ERP discontinuation with evaluators blind to original treatment assignment; 12 weeks after discontinuation, the relapse rate was significantly lower (12% vs. 45%), and the time to relapse was significantly longer for patients who responded to ERP (with or without concomitant CMI) than for patients who responded to CMI alone. Data suggest that relapse prevention techniques maintain the gains of ERP therapy (Hiss *et al.* 1994).

In sum, ERP is an effective monotherapy for OCD. However, not all patients will respond to treatment or maintain their gains. How to optimize ERP outcome is an active area of research.

22.3.3 Is cognitive therapy (CT) effective for OCD?

Cognitive therapy (CT), another form of cognitive–behavioral therapy, has also been used in OCD. In CT, patient and therapist work together to identify distorted patterns of thinking that lead to emotional reactions and then challenge and alter their ways of thinking in order to change their emotional response.

Several randomized trials have compared ERP to CT for OCD. Emmelkamp and colleagues randomized OCD patients (*n* = 18 in the 1988 study and *n* = 21 in 1991) to a form of CT called rational emotive therapy, consisting of analyzing irrational thoughts, or to self-controlled ERP (Emmelkamp *et al.* 1988, Emmelkamp & Beens 1991). They found no significant differences in outcomes in either study; however, the sample sizes were very small. Van Oppen and colleagues (1995) randomized 71 OCD patients to self-controlled ERP or CT with behavioral experiments for 16 weeks; both treatments were similarly effective. Using some of the same patients, van Balkom and colleagues (1998) randomized 117 OCD patients to self-controlled ERP, CT with behavioral experiments, fluvoxamine + ERP, fluvoxamine + CT, or wait-list control for 16 weeks;

again, all active treatments were similarly effective. However, self-controlled exposure is not the optimal way of delivering ERP. Cottraux and colleagues (2001) found no significant difference in outcome between 65 patients randomized to therapist-guided ERP (two-hour sessions delivered twice per week for four weeks, followed by 40-minute booster sessions delivered biweekly for 12 weeks) or CT that included behavioral experiments (20 one-hour sessions delivered over 16 weeks), but the study had limited power to detect differences. Whittal and colleagues (2005) randomized 59 OCD patients to individual ERP (which permitted habituation during exposure but not cognitive restructuring) or CT (which included behavioral experiments) and found both to be equally effective; however, when delivered in group format, ERP was superior (McLean *et al.* 2001).

These studies are difficult to interpret for many reasons, including the fact that standard ERP (Kozack & Foa 1997) includes informal cognitive techniques (e.g., relapse prevention, cognitive restructuring during exposures), and standard CT includes behavioral experiments that can resemble exposures. Thus, separating these treatments is procedurally difficult. Yet only some of these studies monitored therapist adherence to the treatment procedures, and none included a placebo group other than a wait-list control.

Taken together, the data suggest that CT that includes behavioral experiments is similar in efficacy to ERP when it is not optimally delivered (e.g., 45-minute weekly sessions, self-guided exposure, exposures that focus only on habituation). A more recent open trial suggested that CT in the absence of behavioral experiments can help some OCD patients (Wilhelm *et al.* 2005). However, there are no large placebo-controlled studies demonstrating that CT (with or without behavioral exposures) is as effective as standard ERP (Kozack & Foa 1997). As a result, ERP remains the first-line psychotherapy for OCD.

22.3.4 Are there ways to enhance ERP to improve patient outcome?

As discussed previously, ERP is an effective treatment. However, the therapy requires a substantial time commitment on the part of the patient, is labor-intensive, and requires full adherence to treatment procedures for full effects. Patients have to be willing to tolerate high levels of anxiety during the exposure procedures. In addition, certain types of OCD patient (e.g., those with compulsive hoarding or without overt compulsions) are thought to have a poorer response to standard ERP procedures (Saxena 2008). To address these issues, several research groups have attempted to enhance ERP outcome by improving adherence using motivational interviewing, increasing the rate of extinction learning with D-cycloserine, developing adaptations for specific OCD subtypes, and devising different ways of delivering ERP to increase accessibility to the therapy.

Increasing patient adherence can improve the outcome of ERP, and there are several ways to approach this. One way is to address any ambivalence the patient may have about change or ERP itself. Motivational interviewing (MI), originally developed to treat alcoholics, is a goal-oriented therapeutic technique for enhancing intrinsic motivation to change by exploring and resolving ambivalence (Miller & Rollnick 2002, Miller *et al.* 2006). In a small controlled trial, Matlby and Tolin (2005) found that a multimodal intervention that included MI procedures provided prior to ERP increased acceptance of ERP treatment. However, this intervention as a prelude to ERP appeared insufficient to prevent subsequent dropout (Maltby & Tolin 2005). Preliminary data from Simpson and colleagues (2008) suggest that MI can be integrated into standard ERP introductory sessions and exposure sessions as needed; the researchers are currently testing the hypothesis that MI+ERP leads to better adherence and outcome when compared to ERP in an ongoing randomized controlled trial. Other interventions, such as a schema-based CBT to target domains proposed to be relevant to OCD (e.g. perfectionism, inflated responsibility, vulnerability, response to unpredictability, change), also have been developed and are being tested to see if they can increase the patient's capacity to engage in ERP (Sookman & Pinard 1999, 2007).

Another way to improve ERP outcome is to enhance what patients learn during sessions. With the goal of enhancing extinction learning during ERP sessions, researchers have sought to potentiate the effects of the NMDA receptors, which have long been implicated in learning and memory. D-Cycloserine (DCS), a partial agonist of the glycine site at the NMDA glutamatergic receptor, stimulates the glycine site, which is required (along with glutamate) for full activation of the NMDA receptor. Known to facilitate fear extinction in animal models, DCS has been shown to improve response to exposure treatment in acrophobics (Ressler *et al.* 2004) and in social-phobics (Hofmann *et al.* 2006). Two OCD studies have found that DCS led to faster time to response and less dropout (Kushner *et al.* 2007,

Wilhelm *et al.* 2008), but another study found that DCS had no such effects (Storch *et al.* 2007). The discrepancy may be due to the fact that in the latter study, the DCS was given hours before the session and at higher doses. At higher doses, DCS blocks full activation of the glycine site, acting as a full glycine antagonist. Shim and colleagues (2008) have proposed that with full glycine agonists, such as glycine and D-serine, a greater effect may be achieved. Other medications that might also facilitate extinction learning and thereby enhance CBT outcome are being investigated (Davis *et al.* 2006, Ressler & Mayberg 2007).

Another approach to improving outcome in OCD patients is to tailor ERP for certain subtypes of OCD patients that have been considered "resistant to treatment." For example, an intervention for compulsive hoarding has been developed (Tolin *et al.* 2007). In this method, patients received 26 individual sessions (with frequent home visits) of ERP with cognitive restructuring. The cognitive restructuring component is specifically focused to address problems with motivation and organizing, acquiring, and removing clutter by targeting three key issues in hoarding: information processing deficits, such as difficulty categorizing their own possessions, maladaptive beliefs about and emotional attachment to possessions, and emotional distress and avoidance (Saxena 2008, Tolin *et al.* 2007).

Freeston and colleagues (1997) developed a tailored CBT approach to patients with obsessions as the primary concern. Their intervention was standard ERP with cognitive restructuring targeted to four dysfunctional patterns of thinking: the overimportance of thoughts and magical thinking, exaggerated responsibility for negative consequences, perfectionistic expectations, and inflated estimates of probability of severe consequences associated with feared stimulus. Compared with wait-list patients, patients receiving therapy improved significantly on measures of severity of obsessions, current functioning, self-report obsessive–compulsive symptoms, and anxiety. Although both of the above studies are limited by lack of adequate control groups (no control group in Tolin *et al.* and only wait-list control in Freeston *et al.*), they are important steps in improving outcome by designing "tailored" approaches to specific subtypes of OCD.

Whether ERP can be delivered in different formats and thereby enhance outcome or improve access is also under study. For example, ERP delivered in a group format has been shown to be effective in several studies (Fals-Stewart *et al.* 1993, Himle *et al.* 2001). However, the relative efficacy of group versus individual ERP is not clear. Also, several web- and computer-based ERP therapies, including CT-STEPS (comprehensive therapy steps; Jazz Pharmaceuticals) and BT-STEPS (behavior therapy steps), have also been developed (Greist *et al.* 2002, Baer *et al.* 2007). Greist and colleagues conducted a randomized controlled trial of 218 OCD patients who were assigned to ERP therapy, guided either by computer (BT-STEPS) or by therapist, or to systematic relaxation (control). The authors found computer-guided ERP therapy to be significantly better than the control relaxation therapy; however, clinician-guided ERP therapy was found to be significantly better than computer-guided ERP (Greist *et al.* 2002).

In sum, many promising avenues of research are being explored relative to making ERP more accessible and more efficacious for different types of patients with OCD.

22.3.5 What other psychotherapies are available?

To date, the only form of psychotherapy shown to be effective in controlled trials is CBT. However, other therapies are being investigated. For example, several small studies have investigated acceptance and commitment therapy (ACT) in the treatment of OCD. ACT differs from traditional CT in that rather than challenging and altering their ways of thinking in order to change their emotional response, ACT teaches patients to "just notice," accept, and embrace their intrusive and unwanted thoughts, feelings, and images. Twohig and colleagues (2006) evaluated the effectiveness of an eight-session ACT for OCD in a non-concurrent, multiple-baseline, across-participants design, which showed that the intervention produced clinically significant reductions in compulsions by the end of treatment for all participants, with results maintained at three-month follow-up. However, limitations include the small sample size and complex design (Twohig *et al.* 2006). Moreover, some researchers have questioned whether the active ingredients in ACT might not be similar to ERP (Tolin 2008). In addition, mindfulness meditation is also being investigated as a way for patients to learn to notice their thoughts and emotions without trying to escape, avoid, or change them. The goal of this approach is to help people lead satisfying lives without expending emotional energy on actively changing the content of their thoughts (Bishop 2002, Baer 2004, Patel *et al.* 2007). There is no evidence that psychodynamic psychotherapy or psychoanalysis reduce OCD symptoms, but it may be helpful to address personal and interpersonal conflicts preventing patients from seeking treatment or treatment adherence (Koran *et al.* 2007).

22.4 Summary

OCD is a severe and debilitating illness. Whether patients are treated with SRI medication or CBT therapy, there are several common issues and limitations across treatments. First, the format of delivery matters: how often treatment is delivered in therapy and the dosage and duration of medication are important to achieving the optimal symptoms reduction. In addition to optimization of current treatments, future research should also be directed towards developing novel types of medications, such as pharmacotherapies targeting the dopamine and glutamate systems. Second, a common theme in our current treatment portfolio is that there is evidence that certain types of OCD patient (e.g., those with compulsive hoarding) may have a poorer response to standard treatment. Understanding and further defining subtypes of OCD will not only improve the chances of finding underlying genetic and neurobiological mechanisms, but also will allow for better treatments. Exciting avenues for future work include personalized medicine, in which patients with specific, definable clinical characteristics could be prescribed tailored medication based on their predicted treatment response. A third common theme is that we know little about how our treatments work at the level of the nervous system. Although brain imaging studies have linked hyperactivation of certain brain circuits in OCD, much more research needs to be done to elucidate the etiology and pathophysiology of OCD. New horizons for research include development of clinical correlates, or endophenotypes, of OCD symptoms in order to understand the underlying mechanism of disease. Translational approaches, such as developing mouse models of OCD and neuroimaging of the serotonin, dopamine, and glutamate neurotransmitter systems, will help us to understand better how neural substrates are linked to OCD and how our treatments affect these neural systems and reduce OCD symptoms.

References

Abramowitz, J. S., Franklin, M. E., Zoellner, L. A., & DiBernardo, C. L. (2002). Treatment compliance and outcome in obsessive–compulsive disorder. *Behavior Modification*, **26**, 447–463.

Ackerman, D. L., & Greenland, S. (2002). Multivariate meta-analysis of controlled drug studies for obsessive–compulsive disorder. *Journal of Clinical Psychopharmacology*, **22**, 309–317.

Albert, U., Aguglia, E., Maina, G., & Bogetto, F. (2002). Venlafaxine versus clomipramine in the treatment of obsessive–compulsive disorder: a preliminary single-blind, 12-week, controlled study. *Journal of Clinical Psychiatry*, **63**, 1004–1009.

Baer, L., Greist, J., & Marks, I. M. (2007). Computer-aided cognitive behaviour therapy. *Psychotherapy and Psychosomatics*, **76**, 193–195.

Baer, R. (2004). Mindfulness training as a clinical intervention: a conceptual and empirical review. *Clinical Psychology: Science and Practice*, **10**, 125–143.

Bishop, S. R. (2002). What do we really know about mindfulness-based stress reduction? *Psychosomatic Medicine*, **64**, 71–84.

Bloch, M. H., Landeros-Weisenberger, A., Kelmendi, B., *et al.* (2006). A systematic review: antipsychotic augmentation with treatment refractory obsessive–compulsive disorder. *Molecular Psychiatry*, **11**, 622–632.

Bystritsky, A., Ackerman, D. L., Rosen, R. M., *et al.* (2004). Augmentation of serotonin reuptake inhibitors in refractory obsessive–compulsive disorder using adjunctive olanzapine: a placebo-controlled trial. *Journal of Clinical Psychiatry*, **65**, 565–568.

Carey, P. D., Vythilingum, B., Seedat, S., Muller, J. E., Van Ameringen, M., & Stein, D. J. (2005). Quetiapine augmentation of SRIs in treatment refractory obsessive–compulsive disorder: a double-blind, randomised, placebo-controlled study [ISRCTN83050762]. *BMC Psychiatry*, **5**, 5.

Cordioli, A. V., Basso de Sousa, M., & Bochi, D. B. (2003). Intravenous clomipramine in severe and refractory obsessive–compulsive disorder. *Journal of Clinical Psychopharmacology*, **23**, 665–666.

Coric, V., Taskiran, S., Pittenger, C., Wasylink, S., *et al.* (2005). Riluzole augmentation in treatment-resistant obsessive–compulsive disorder: an open-label trial. *Biological Psychiatry*, **58**, 424–428.

Cottraux, J., Mollard, E., Bouvard, M., *et al.* (1990). A controlled study of fluvoxamine and exposure in obsessive–compulsive disorder. *International Clinical Psychopharmacology*, **5**, 17–30.

Cottraux, J., Note, I., Yao, S. N., *et al.* (2001). A randomized controlled trial of cognitive therapy in obsessive–compulsive disorder. *Psychotherapy and Psychosomatics*, **70**, 288–297.

Davis, M., Myers, K. M., Chhatwal, J., & Ressler, K. J. (2006). Pharmacological treatments that facilitate extinction of fear: relevance to psychotherapy. *NeuroRx*, **3**, 82–96.

Dell'osso, B., Mundo, E., Marazziti, D., & Altamura, A. C. (2008). Switching from serotonin reuptake inhibitors to duloxetine in patients with resistant obsessive compulsive disorder: a case series. *Journal of Psychopharmacology*, **22**, 210–213.

Denys, D., van der Wee, N., van Megen, H. J., & Westenberg, H. G. (2003). A double blind comparison of venlafaxine and paroxetine in obsessive–compulsive disorder. *Journal of Clinical Psychopharmacology*, **23**, 568–575.

Denys, D., van Megen, H. J., van der Wee, N., & Westenberg, H. G. (2004a). A double-blind switch study of paroxetine and venlafaxine in obsessive–compulsive disorder. *Journal of Clinical Psychiatry*, **65**, 37–43.

Denys, D., de Geus, F., van Megen, H. J., & Westenberg, H. G. (2004b). A double-blind, randomized, placebo-controlled trial of quetiapine addition in patients with obsessive–compulsive disorder refractory to serotonin reuptake inhibitors. *Journal of Clinical Psychiatry*, **65**, 1040–1048.

Eddy, K. T., Dutra, L., Bradley, R., & Westen, D. (2004). A multidimensional meta-analysis of psychotherapy and pharmacotherapy for obsessive–compulsive disorder. *Clinical Psychology Review*, **24**, 1011–1030.

El Mansari, M., & Blier, P. (2006). Mechanisms of action of current and potential pharmacotherapies of obsessive–compulsive disorder. *Progress in Neuropsychopharmacology and Biological Psychiatry*, **30**, 362–373.

Emmelkamp, P. M., & Beens, H. (1991). Cognitive therapy with obsessive–compulsive disorder: a comparative evaluation. *Behaviour Research and Therapy*, **29**, 293–300.

Emmelkamp, P. M., Visser, S., & Hoekstra, R. J. (1988). Cognitive therapy vs exposure in vivo in the treatment of obsessive–compulsives. *Cognitive Therapy and Research*, **12**, 103–114.

Fals-Stewart, W., Marks, A. P., & Schafer, J. (1993). A comparison of behavioral group therapy and individual behavior therapy in treating obsessive–compulsive disorder. *Journal of Nervous and Mental Disease*, **181**, 189–193.

Foa, E. B., & Kozak, M. J. (1996). Psychological treatment for obsessive–compulsive disorder. In M. R. Mavissakalian & R. F. Prien, eds., *Long-Term Treatments of Anxiety Disorders*. Washington, DC: American Psychiatric Press.

Foa, E. B., Grayson, J. B., Steketee, G. S., *et al.* (1983). Success and failure in the behavioral treatment of obsessive–compulsives. *Journal of Consulting and Clinical Psychology*, **51**, 287–297.

Foa, E. B., Dancu, C. V., Hembree, E. A., *et al.* (1999). A comparison of exposure therapy, stress inoculation training, and their combination for reducing posttraumatic stress disorder in female assault victims. *Journal of Consulting and Clinical Psychology*, **67**, 194–200.

Foa, E. B., Liebowitz, M. R., Kozak, M. J., *et al.* (2005). Randomized, placebo-controlled trial of exposure and ritual prevention, clomipramine, and their combination in the treatment of obsessive–compulsive disorder. *American Journal of Psychiatry*, **162**, 151–161.

Franklin, M. E. (2005). Combining serotonergic medication with cognitive–behavior therapy: is it necessary for all OCD patients? In J. S. Abramowitz and A. C. Houts, eds.,

Concepts and Controversies in Obsessive–Compulsive Disorder. New York, NY: Springer, pp. 377–389.

Freeman, C. P., Trimble, M. R., Deakin, J. F., Stokes, T. M., & Ashford, J. J. (1994). Fluvoxamine versus clomipramine in the treatment of obsessive compulsive disorder: a multicenter, randomized, double-blind, parallel group comparison. *Journal of Clinical Psychiatry*, **55**, 301–305.

Freeston, M. H., Ladouceur, R., Gagnon, F., *et al.* (1997). Cognitive–behavioral treatment of obsessive thoughts: a controlled study. *Journal of Consulting and Clinical Psychology*, **65**, 405–413.

Graybiel, A. M., & Rauch, S. L. (2000). Toward a neurobiology of obsessive–compulsive disorder. *Neuron*, **28**, 343–347.

Greist, J. H., & Baer, L. (2002). Psychotherapy for obsessive–compulsive disorder. In D. J. Stein & E. Hollander, eds., *Textbook of Anxiety Disorders*. Washington, DC: American Psychiatric Publishing.

Greist, J. H., Jefferson, J. W., Kobak, K. A., Katzelnick, D. J., & Serlin, R. C. (1995). Efficacy and tolerability of serotonin transport inhibitors in obsessive–compulsive disorder: a meta-analysis. *Archives of General Psychiatry*, **52**, 53–60.

Greist, J. H., Marks, I. M., Baer, L., *et al.* (2002). Behavior therapy for obsessive–compulsive disorder guided by a computer or by a clinician compared with relaxation as a control. *Journal of Clinical Psychiatry*, **63**, 138–145.

Himle, J. A., Rassi, S., Haghighatgou, H., *et al.* (2001). Group behavioral therapy of obsessive–compulsive disorder: seven vs. twelve-week outcomes. *Depression and Anxiety*, **13**, 161–165.

Hiss, H., Foa, E. B., & Kozak, M. J. (1994). Relapse prevention program for treatment of obsessive–compulsive disorder. *Journal of Consulting and Clinical Psychology*, **62**, 801–808.

Hofmann, S. G., Meuret, A. E., Smits, J. A., *et al.* (2006). Augmentation of exposure therapy with d-cycloserine for social anxiety disorder. *Archives of General Psychiatry*, **63**, 298–304.

Hohagen, F., Winkelmann, G., Rasche-Raeuchle, H., *et al.* (1998). Combination of behaviour therapy with fluvoxamine in comparison with behaviour therapy and placebo: results of a multicentre study. *British Journal of Psychiatry*, **173** (Suppl. 35), 71–78.

Insel, T. R., Hamilton, J. A., Guttmacher, L. B., & Murphy, D. L. (1983). D-amphetamine in obsessive–compulsive disorder. *Psychopharmacology (Berlin)*, **80**, 231–235.

Jenike, M. A., Baer, L., & Greist, J. H. (1990). Clomipramine versus fluoxetine in obsessive–compulsive disorder: a retrospective comparison of side effects and efficacy. *Journal of Clinical Psychopharmacology*, **10**, 122–124.

Joffe, R. T., & Swinson, R. P. (1987). Methylphenidate in primary obsessive–compulsive disorder. *Journal of Clinical Psychopharmacology*, **7**, 420–422.

Joffe, R. T., Swinson, R. P., & Levitt, A. J. (1991). Acute psychostimulant challenge in primary obsessive–compulsive disorder. *Journal of Clinical Psychopharmacology*, **11**, 237–241.

Kessler, R. C., Berglund, P., Demler, O., *et al.* (2005). Lifetime prevalence and age-of-onset distributions of DSM-IV disorders in the National Comorbidity Survey Replication. *Archives of General Psychiatry*, **62**, 593–602.

Koran, L. M., McElroy, S. L., Davidson, J. R., *et al.* (1996). Fluvoxamine versus clomipramine for obsessive–compulsive disorder: a double-blind comparison. *Journal of Clinical Psychopharmacology*, **16**, 121–129.

Koran, L. M., Aboujaoude, E., Bullock, K. D., *et al.* (2005a). Double-blind treatment with oral morphine in treatment-resistant obsessive–compulsive disorder. *Journal of Clinical Psychiatry*, **66**, 353–359.

Koran, L. M., Gamel, N. N., Choung, H. W., Smith, E. H., & Aboujaoude, E. N. (2005b). Mirtazapine for obsessive–compulsive disorder: an open trial followed by double-blind discontinuation. *Journal of Clinical Psychiatry*, **66**, 515–520.

Koran, L. M., Hanna, G. L., Hollander, E., Nestadt, G., & Simpson, H. B. (2007). Practice guideline for the treatment of patients with obsessive–compulsive disorder. *American Journal of Psychiatry*, **164** (7 Suppl.), 5–53.

Kozack, M. J., & Foa, E. B. (1997). *Mastery of Obsessive–Compulsive Disorder: a Cognitive Behavioral Approach. Therapist Guide*. Oxford: Oxford University Press.

Kushner, M. G., Kim, S. W., Donahue, C., *et al.* (2007). D-cycloserine augmented exposure therapy for obsessive–compulsive disorder. *Biological Psychiatry*, **62**, 835–838.

Lafleur, D. L., Pittenger, C., Kelmendi, B., *et al.* (2006). N-acetylcysteine augmentation in serotonin reuptake inhibitor refractory obsessive–compulsive disorder. *Psychopharmacology (Berlin)*, **184**, 254–256.

Lindsay, M., Crino, R., & Andrews, G. (1997). Controlled trial of exposure and response prevention in obsessive–compulsive disorder. *British Journal of Psychiatry*, **171**, 135–139.

Lopez-Ibor, J. J., Saiz, J., Cottraux, J., *et al.* (1996). Double-blind comparison of fluoxetine versus clomipramine in the treatment of obsessive compulsive disorder. *European Neuropsychopharmacology*, **6**, 111–118.

Maina, G., Albert, U., Ziero, S., & Bogetto, F. (2003). Antipsychotic augmentation for treatment resistant obsessive–compulsive disorder: what if antipsychotic is discontinued? *International Clinical Psychopharmacology*, **18**, 23–28.

Maltby, N., & Tolin, D. F. (2005). A brief motivational intervention for treatment-refusing OCD patients. *Cognitive Behavior Therapy*, **34**, 176–184.

Marks, I. M., Stern, R. S., Mawson, D., Cobb, J., & McDonald, R. (1980). Clomipramine and exposure for obsessive–compulsive rituals: i. *British Journal of Psychiatry*, **136**, 1–25.

Marks, I. M., Lelliott, P., Basoglu, M., *et al.* (1988). Clomipramine, self-exposure and therapist-aided exposure for obsessive–compulsive rituals. *British Journal of Psychiatry*, **152**, 522–534.

McDougle, C. J., Goodman, W. K., Leckman, J. F., *et al.* (1994). Haloperidol addition in fluvoxamine-refractory obsessive–compulsive disorder: a double-blind, placebo-controlled study in patients with and without tics. *Archives of General Psychiatry*, **51**, 302–308.

McDougle, C. J., Epperson, C. N., Pelton, G. H., Wasylink, S., & Price, L. H. (2000). A double-blind, placebo-controlled study of risperidone addition in serotonin reuptake inhibitor-refractory obsessive–compulsive disorder. *Archives of General Psychiatry*, **57**, 794–801.

McLean, P. D., Whittal, M. L., Thordarson, D. S., *et al.* (2001). Cognitive versus behavior therapy in the group treatment of obsessive–compulsive disorder. *Journal of Consulting & Clinical Psychology*, **69**, 205–214.

Miller, W. R., & Rollnick, S. (2002). *Motivational Interviewing: Preparing People for Change*, 2nd edn. New York, NY: Guilford Press.

Miller, W. R., Sorensen, J. L., Selzer, J. A., & Brigham, G. S. (2006). Disseminating evidence-based practices in substance abuse treatment: a review with suggestions. *Journal of Substance Abuse and Treatment*, **31**, 25–39.

Mundo, E., Maina, G., & Uslenghi, C. (2000). Multicentre, double-blind, comparison of fluvoxamine and clomipramine in the treatment of obsessive–compulsive disorder. *International Clinical Psychopharmacology*, **15**, 69–76.

Murray, C. J. L., & Lopez, A. D. (1996). *The Global Burden of Disease: a Comprehensive Assessment of Mortality and Disability from Diseases, Injuries, and Risk Factors in 1990 and Projected to 2020*. Cambridge, MA: Harvard University Press.

Patel, S., Carmody, J., & Simpson, H. B. (2007). Adapting mindfulness-based stress reduction for the treatment of obsessive–compulsive disorder: a case report. *Cognitive and Behavioral Practice*, **14**, 375–380.

Pigott, T. A., & Seay, S. M. (1999). A review of the efficacy of selective serotonin reuptake inhibitors in obsessive–compulsive disorder. *Journal of Clinical Psychiatry*, **60**, 101–106.

Pigott, T. A., Pato, M. T., Bernstein, S. E., *et al.* (1990). Controlled comparisons of clomipramine and fluoxetine in the treatment of obsessive–compulsive disorder. Behavioral and biological results. *Archives of General Psychiatry*, **47**, 926–932.

Pittenger, C., Krystal, J. H., & Coric, V. (2006). Glutamate-modulating drugs as novel pharmacotherapeutic agents in the treatment of obsessive–compulsive disorder. *NeuroRx*, **3**, 69–81.

Pittenger, C., Kelmendi, B., Wasylink, S., Bloch, M. H., & Coric, V. (2008). Riluzole augmentation in treatment-refractory obsessive–compulsive disorder: a series of 13 cases, with long-term follow-up. *Journal of Clinical Psychopharmacology*, **28**, 363–367.

Ressler, K. J., & Mayberg, H. S. (2007). Targeting abnormal neural circuits in mood and anxiety disorders: from the laboratory to the clinic. *Nature Neuroscience*, **10**, 1116–1124.

Ressler, K. J., Rothbaum, B. O., Tannenbaum, L., *et al.* (2004). Cognitive enhancers as adjuncts to psychotherapy: use of d-cycloserine in phobic individuals to facilitate extinction of fear. *Archives of General Psychiatry*, **61**, 1136–1144.

Ruscio, A. M., Stein, D. J., Chiu, W. T., & Kessler, R. C. (2010). The epidemiology of obsessive–compulsive disorder in the National Comorbidity Survey Replication. *Molecular Psychiatry*, **15**, 53–63.

Saxena, S. (2008). Recent advances in compulsive hoarding. *Current Psychiatry Reports*, **10**, 297–303.

Shapira, N. A., Keck, P. E., Goldsmith, T. D., *et al.* (1997). Open-label pilot study of tramadol hydrochloride in treatment-refractory obsessive–compulsive disorder. *Depression and Anxiety*, **6**, 170–173.

Shapira, N. A., Ward, H. E., Mandoki, M., *et al.* (2004). A double-blind, placebo-controlled trial of olanzapine addition in fluoxetine-refractory obsessive–compulsive disorder. *Biological Psychiatry*, **55**, 553–555.

Shim, S. S., Hammonds, M. D., & Vrabel, M. M. (2008). D-cycloserine augmentation for behavioral therapy. *American Journal of Psychiatry*, **165**, 1050.

Simpson, H. B., & Liebowitz, M.R. (2005). Combining pharmacotherapy and cognitive-beharvioral therapy in the treatment of OCD. In J. S. Abramowitz & A. C. Houts, eds., *Concepts and Controversies in Obsessive–Compulsive Disorder*. New York, NY: Springer.

Simpson, H. B., Liebowitz, M. R., Foa, E. B., *et al.* (2004). Post-treatment effects of exposure therapy and clomipramine in obsessive–compulsive disorder. *Depression and Anxiety*, **19**, 225–233.

Simpson, H. B., Zuckoff, A., Page, J. R., Franklin, M. E., & Foa, E. B. (2008). Adding motivational interviewing to exposure and ritual prevention for obsessive–compulsive disorder: an open pilot trial. *Cognitive Behavior Therapy*, **37**, 38–49.

Sookman, D., & Pinard, G. (1999). Integrative cognitive therapy for obsessive compulsive disorder which focuses on multiple schemas. *Cognitive and Behavioral Practice*, **6**, 351–361.

Sookman, D., & Pinard, G. (2007). Specialized cognitive behavior therapy for resistant obsessive–compulsive disorder: elaboration of a schema-based model. In D. J. Stein, ed., *Cognitive Schemas and Core Beliefs in Psychological Problems: a Scientist–Practitioner Guide*. New York, NY: American Psychological Association.

Sorensen, C., Drummond, M., Kanavos, P., & McGuire, A. (2005). *National Institute for Health and Clinical Excellence (NICE) Clinical Guidelines of Obsessive Compulsive Disorder*. London: NICE.

Storch, E. A., Merlo, L. J., Bengtson, M., *et al.* (2007). D-cycloserine does not enhance exposure-response prevention therapy in obsessive–compulsive disorder. *International Clinical Psychopharmacology*, **22**, 230–237.

Storch, E. A., Lehmkuhl, H., Geffken, G. R., Touchton, A., & Murphy, T. K. (2008). Aripiprazole augmentation of incomplete treatment response in an adolescent male with obsessive–compulsive disorder. *Depression and Anxiety*, **25**, 172–174.

Szegedi, A., Wetzel, H., Leal, M., Hartter, S., & Hiemke, C. (1996). Combination treatment with clomipramine and fluvoxamine: drug monitoring, safety, and tolerability data. *Journal of Clinical Psychiatry*, **57**, 257–264.

Tolin, D. F. (2008). Alphabet Soup: ERP, CT, and ACT for OCD. *Cognitive Behavioral Practice*, **9**, 1–9.

Tolin, D. F., Frost, R. O., & Steketee, G. (2007). An open trial of cognitive–behavioral therapy for compulsive hoarding. *Behavior Research and Therapy*, **45**, 1461–1470.

Twohig, M. P., Hayes, S. C., & Masuda, A. (2006). Increasing willingness to experience obsessions: acceptance and commitment therapy as a treatment for obsessive–compulsive disorder. *Behavior Therapy*, **37**, 3–13.

Van Ameringen, M., Mancini, C., Patterson, B., & Bennett, M. (2006). Topiramate augmentation in treatment-resistant obsessive–compulsive disorder: a retrospective, open-label case series. *Depression and Anxiety*, **23**, 1–5.

van Balkom, A. J., de Haan, E., van Oppen, P., *et al.* (1998). Cognitive and behavioral therapies alone versus in combination with fluvoxamine in the treatment of obsessive compulsive disorder. *Journal of Nervous and Mental Disease*, **186**, 492–499.

van Oppen, P., de Haan, E., van Balkom, A. J., *et al.* (1995). Cognitive therapy and exposure in vivo in the treatment of obsessive compulsive disorder. *Behaviour Research and Therapy*, **33**, 379–390.

Whittal, M., Thordarson, D., & McLean, P. (2005). Treatment of obsessive–compulsive disorder: cognitive behavior therapy vs. exposure and response prevention. *Behaviour Research and Therapy*, **43**, 1559–1576.

Wilhelm, S., Steketee, G., Reilly-Harrington, N. A., *et al.* (2005). Effectiveness of cognitive therapy for obsessive–compulsive disorder: an open trial. *Journal of Cognitive Psychotherapy*, **19**, 173–179.

Wilhelm, S., Buhlmann, U., Tolin, D. F., *et al.* (2008). Augmentation of behavior therapy with d-cycloserine for obsessive–compulsive disorder. *American Journal of Psychiatry*, **165**, 335–341; quiz 409.

Yaryura-Tobias, J. A., & Neziroglu, F. A. (1996). Venlafaxine in obsessive–compulsive disorder. *Archives of General Psychiatry*, **53**, 653–654.

Zohar, J., & Judge, R. (1996). Paroxetine versus clomipramine in the treatment of obsessive–compulsive disorder. OCD Paroxetine Study Investigators. *British Journal of Psychiatry*, **169**, 468–474.

Chapter 23

Treatment of social anxiety disorder

Franklin Schneier, Kristin Pontoski, Richard G. Heimberg

23.1 Introduction

Over the past three decades, a dramatic expansion of research on social anxiety disorder (SAD), also known as social phobia, has yielded an emerging consensus on first-line evidence-based pharmacotherapy and psychotherapy (Ballenger *et al.* 1998, Ipser *et al.* 2008, Powers *et al.* 2008). Selective serotonin reuptake inhibitors (SSRIs) and the serotonin–norepinephrine reuptake inhibitor (SNRI) venlafaxine (Effexor XR) each help a majority of patients with SAD, as demonstrated in short-term randomized controlled trials of 8–12 weeks. Cognitive–behavioral therapy (CBT) in several forms, administered over 12–24 weeks, yields roughly similar response rates in controlled trials. Gains have been shown to be well maintained during continuation therapy with medication for up to a year (e.g., Stein *et al.* 2003) and at follow-up assessments after a course of CBT for up to five years (e.g., Heimberg *et al.* 1993).

Beyond this consensus, however, many aspects of the treatment of SAD remain poorly understood. Little is known about predictors of response to specific treatments. Relapse after treatment discontinuation appears more common after pharmacotherapy, but individualized predictors of which patients are vulnerable to relapse are lacking. Although SAD tends to be highly chronic, few treatment studies have followed patients for more than a year, and although SAD usually occurs with comorbid disorders, few studies have examined the impact of comorbidity on treatment outcome. SAD typically has an age of onset in the mid-teens; however, most clinical trials have excluded adolescents. Many patients do not respond fully to SSRI/SNRI medication or CBT, but alternative medications and psychosocial treatments are much less well studied. Although pharmacotherapy and CBT treatments are each usually partially effective, and they employ quite different approaches, efforts to demonstrate additive or synergistic effects of combined treatment have so far yielded inconclusive results.

This chapter will review evidence from randomized controlled trials for the efficacy of medication and psychotherapy treatments of SAD, highlight important clinical issues in the treatment of SAD, and discuss the unresolved issue of how best to combine medication and CBT approaches.

23.2 Cognitive–behavioral therapy (CBT) and other psychosocial treatments

Individuals with SAD fear that they will do or say something to elicit negative evaluation or that they will appear excessively anxious to others (American Psychiatric Association 2000). Rapee and Heimberg (1997) suggest that the perception of an evaluative audience leads the individual with SAD to focus on a negatively distorted mental representation of how he or she appears to others. The person becomes hypervigilant to internal and external negative cues associated with this representation, and this initiates a cycle of increasing anxiety in the anticipation of negative outcomes. Clark and Wells (1995) present a similar conceptualization, and also suggest that avoidance behavior contributes to the maintenance of anxiety in social situations over time. Both models recommend providing experiences that allow the patient to re-evaluate his or her cognitive construction of the self and others. Therefore, exposure, cognitive restructuring, and their combination have been the most commonly examined approaches to modifying patients' schemas and reducing symptoms of social anxiety.

Anxiety Disorders: Theory, Research, and Clinical Perspectives, ed. Helen Blair Simpson, Yuval Neria, Roberto Lewis-Fernández, Franklin Schneier. Published by Cambridge University Press. © Cambridge University Press 2010.

23.2.1 Exposure and cognitive strategies

Exposure therapy is designed to encourage socially anxious patients to approach their feared social situations via imagery or direct confrontation, thus allowing habituation and disconfirmation of maladaptive beliefs to occur. Exposure has been recognized as an essential component of most successful treatments for anxiety (Chambless & Ollendick 2001), and it has most often been combined with cognitive techniques in the treatment of SAD. A growing body of research supports the efficacy of treatments incorporating both cognitive techniques and exposure (Magee *et al.* 2009). Historically, additional behavioral strategies such as applied relaxation (see Öst 1987 for a review) and social skills training (see Franklin *et al.* 1999 for a review) have also been utilized, but their efficacy is less well established, and they will not be discussed further here.

23.2.2 Heimberg's cognitive–behavioral group therapy

A diverse literature investigating the efficacy of cognitive–behavioral group therapy (CBGT) (Heimberg & Becker 2002) has accumulated over the past two decades. CBGT typically consists of 12 weekly 2.5-hour group sessions that provide psychoeducation, foster rapport and group cohesion, and teach cognitive restructuring concepts to integrate with exposure. Through this process, patients learn to recognize, examine, and challenge their negative and inaccurate thoughts while participating in role plays of feared social situations in the group. Treatment ultimately focuses on exploring core beliefs that underlie and maintain each patient's social concerns, and on adopting achievable and objective goals in social situations. Patients also engage in exposures between sessions and practice applying cognitive restructuring skills to situations in the real world.

A series of investigations contributed to the development of this treatment protocol and the establishment of its efficacy. CBGT was first compared to a psychosocial control condition, educational-supportive group therapy (ES). Significantly more CBGT patients were classified as responders, and they were more likely to have maintained gains at a six-month follow-up (Heimberg *et al.* 1990) and at another follow-up five years later (Heimberg *et al.* 1993). CBGT was recently compared to a meditation-based stress reduction program (MBSR) (Koszycki *et al.* 2007). Both CGBT and MBSR demonstrated clinically meaningful changes on measures of social anxiety, depression, and quality of life. However, patients receiving CBGT demonstrated greater reductions in self-reported and clinician-rated social anxiety. Response and remission rates were also superior for CBGT. Other studies have compared CBGT to pharmacotherapy for SAD, and these are discussed below.

Heimberg and colleagues have adapted CBGT to an individual format (Hope *et al.* 2000, 2006). This workbook-driven individual CBT involves 16 one-hour weekly sessions, conducted over 16–20 weeks, and it comprises the same components as CBGT – psychoeducation, cognitive restructuring, and in-session and in-vivo exposure. Ledley and colleagues (2009) demonstrated that this individualized CBT provided superior outcomes to a wait-list control and produced effect sizes similar to the group package.

23.2.3 Clark's individual CBT

Clark's treatment protocol, based on the Clark and Wells (1995) model, consists of 12–16 weekly individual sessions focused on the identification of thoughts, images, attentional strategies, and safety behaviors (behaviors that maintain social anxiety symptoms by fostering avoidance and preventing new learning). Several techniques are employed based on this personalized model, including role plays of feared situations with and without the use of safety behaviors, external shifting of attention, the use of video feedback, or other behavioral experiments.

Clark's protocol has demonstrated efficacy in randomized controlled trials. It was recently compared to exposure plus applied relaxation (but without cognitive restructuring, EXP+AR) and a wait list (Clark *et al.* 2006). Both active treatments were superior to wait list on most measures, and CBT was superior to EXP+AR on measures of social anxiety. These gains were maintained at one-year follow-up, and patients receiving CBT were twice as likely as those receiving EXP+AR to be characterized as treatment responders.

In summary, both Heimberg's and Clark's CBT treatments are efficacious first-line interventions that articulate the need for socially anxious individuals to re-evaluate their negative self-construction using exposure and cognitive restructuring techniques. No studies to date have directly compared the efficacy of the two treatments.

23.2.4 Group versus individual CBT

Some efforts have been made to compare the efficacy of delivering CBT for SAD in group (CBGT) versus individual CBT formats. Lucas and Telch (1993) found that both CBGT and individual CBT were similarly efficacious and superior to ES. Stangier and colleagues (2003) compared Clark's CBT to a group treatment based on the Clark and Wells model. Although both groups improved, those receiving individual CBT showed significantly larger gains on social anxiety measures. Mortberg and colleagues (2007) compared Clark's CBT to an intensive short-term variant of group therapy and treatment with an SSRI. All therapies showed some efficacy, and individual CBT was superior to the other groups. However, these results are difficult to interpret because the group therapy was delivered in an intensive three-week timeframe instead of in weekly sessions over four months. Meta-analyses of the larger literature, described below, failed to show any differences between group and individual formats. Individual therapy's potential advantages, such as greater acceptability to patients, ease of scheduling, and increased attention to an individual's unique issues, contrast with group therapy's potential benefits of group support and ease of conducting group role plays within sessions. The choice of modality may ultimately be a matter of preference or the feasibility of conducting group therapy within particular clinical settings, given the lack of strong support for differences in efficacy.

23.2.5 Meta-analytic findings

Over the past decade, several meta-analytic reviews of studies of cognitive–behavioral techniques have demonstrated that CBT – most notably all treatments that include exposure techniques with or without cognitive restructuring – are superior to control conditions and roughly equivalent to treatment with an SSRI. Individual and group CBT treatments fare equally well (Feske & Chambless 1995, Taylor 1996, Gould et al. 1997, Fedoroff & Taylor 2001, Hofmann & Smits 2008, Powers et al. 2008).

23.2.6 Effects of comorbidity on treatment outcome

Several studies have found comorbid mood disorders to be related to greater severity of social anxiety (e.g., Erwin et al. 2002) and poorer treatment outcome (e.g., Ledley et al. 2005). However, the slope of change in the severity of social anxiety does not appear to differ for patients with a principal diagnosis of SAD with and without depression (Erwin et al. 2002). Furthermore, in another study, reductions in depressive symptoms

followed reductions in social anxiety symptoms, but changes in social anxiety did not follow changes in depression (Moscovitch et al. 2005).

SAD also tends to co-occur frequently with alcohol use disorders, and individuals with SAD often report the use of alcohol to reduce their anxiety in stressful situations (Buckner et al. 2006), but most studies of CBT for SAD have excluded persons actively abusing alcohol. Augmenting CBT with motivational enhancement therapy (Miller et al. 1992) could help motivate individuals with comorbid social anxiety and alcohol use disorders to start and continue in therapy and thus increase the efficacy of CBT for SAD. A recent clinical case study (Buckner et al. 2008) supports the efficacy of this combination of techniques and makes a case for a future randomized controlled trial. Future research should investigate other comorbid disorders, including Axis II disorders.

23.2.7 Other psychological treatments for SAD

CBT is by far the most extensively researched psychosocial treatment for SAD. However, in clinical practice, other approaches are often utilized. Although a full discussion of these practical techniques is beyond the scope of this chapter, there is a small literature on the efficacy of these approaches, including – but not limited to – supportive–expressive therapy (Leichsenring et al. 2007), interpersonal psychotherapy (Borge et al. 2008, Lipsitz et al. 2008), acceptance and commitment therapy (Ossman et al. 2006, Dalrymple & Herbert 2007), and MBSR (Koszycki et al. 2007). Future research should examine the efficacy of these techniques compared to or in combination with CBT.

23.3 Medication treatments for social anxiety disorder

23.3.1 Serotonergic medications

Findings from more than 30 randomized placebo-controlled trials of six different SSRIs and the SNRI venlafaxine support the efficacy of these medications for SAD. Recent meta-analyses confirm that SSRIs and venlafaxine yield increased response rates and greater magnitude of improvement compared to placebo (Blanco et al. 2003, Ipser et al. 2008). Four medications are approved by the US Food and Drug Administration (FDA) for social anxiety disorder: paroxetine (Paxil, Paxil CR), sertraline (Zoloft), venlafaxine (Effexor

XR), and fluvoxamine (Luvox CR). There is no consistent evidence for superiority of any SSRI or SNRI medication, although support may be weakest for fluoxetine (Prozac), with only one positive study (Davidson *et al.* 2004) and two studies failing to demonstrate efficacy (Kobak *et al.* 2002, Clark *et al.* 2003) in SAD. Fluoxetine and venlafaxine ER have been shown in randomized controlled trials to be effective for the treatment of SAD in children aged 6–17 (Birmaher *et al.* 2003, Wagner *et al.* 2004, March *et al.* 2007).

Among other serotonergic (but non-SSRI) antidepressants, mirtazapine (Remeron) appeared effective for women with SAD in one controlled trial (Muehlbacher *et al.* 2005), but nefazodone (Serzone) was not superior to placebo in a single trial in adults (Van Ameringen *et al.* 2007). The serotonergic anxiolytic buspirone (Buspar) has not appeared effective for SAD in two low-dose trials (Clark & Agras 1991, van Vliet *et al.* 1997).

23.3.2 Generalizability of clinic trials

In considering the generalizability of this research, it is useful to recognize that most patients in these studies have had a principal diagnosis of the generalized type of SAD, without current major depression, recent substance abuse, or lifetime psychosis. Most trials have been of 8–12 weeks' duration, with dose gradually escalated to a prototypical antidepressant dose over several weeks of treatment and then adjusted as clinically indicated. Response has often been assessed by the Liebowitz Social Anxiety Scale (Liebowitz 1987), a clinician-administered instrument that assesses fear and avoidance of 24 social or performance situations, and by the Clinical Global Impression Change Scale, on which persons who are much improved or very much improved are typically considered responders. In most of the large multicenter SSRI/SNRI trials, 40–60% of participants have been treatment responders at endpoint, and about half of these responders have been rated very much improved (i.e., virtually symptom-free). Placebo response rates tend to run 20–30 percentage points lower than SSRI/SNRI response rates. These medications are generally well tolerated by persons with SAD, with common adverse effects including nausea, insomnia, fatigue, sexual dysfunction, or weight gain.

With respect to time course, improvement in some studies has been shown to continue beyond the first eight weeks (Stein *et al.* 2002a). Three studies have randomized responders in an acute 12–20-week trial of SSRIs/SNRIs to either continuation of active treatment or switch to placebo (Walker *et al.* 2000, Stein *et al.* 2002b, Montgomery *et al.* 2005). They demonstrate that response is well maintained during six months of continuation treatment, with relapse rates under 25% – significantly lower than the relapse rates of 36–50% in persons switched to placebo.

23.3.3 Benzodiazepines

Benzodiazepines also are widely used for SAD as monotherapy or in conjunction with SSRI/SNRI medication (Vasile *et al.* 2005), but they have been much less studied. The best evidence for efficacy exists for clonazepam (Klonopin), which appeared highly efficacious in one randomized controlled trial (Davidson *et al.* 1993) and several open trials. Dose is gradually titrated upward to a typical range of 2–4 mg/day in standing divided doses. Alprazolam (Xanax) appeared more modestly efficacious in one trial (Gelernter *et al.* 1991). An advantage of benzodiazepines is their rapid onset of action, which allows them to also be used on an as-needed basis. Disadvantages include lack of efficacy for comorbid depressive symptoms and potential adverse effects of sedation, incoordination, falls, and potential for abuse. Slow taper of benzodiazepines prior to their discontinuation, commonly over a period of weeks to months, is usually required to minimize the risk of withdrawal symptoms and rebound anxiety (Connor *et al.* 1998). Because the adverse-effect profile of benzodiazepines is largely complementary to that of SSRIs, combined treatment may be well tolerated, and one controlled study found a trend for an advantage in efficacy for combined clonazepam and SSRI treatment over SSRI treatment alone (Seedat & Stein 2004).

23.3.4 Other medications

Medications from several other classes have demonstrated efficacy for SAD. The calcium channel alpha-2-delta ligands gabapentin (Neurontin) and pregabalin (Lyrica) have each appeared effective for SAD in single trials (Pande *et al.* 1999, 2004). The antipsychotics olanzapine and quetiapine have also appeared promising in very small controlled trials (Barnett *et al.* 2002, Vaishnavi *et al.* 2007) and need further study.

Monoamine oxidase inhibitors (MAOIs) were among the first medications to be studied in SAD. Earlier they had been shown efficacious for the atypical form of depression, which shares with SAD the feature of prominent interpersonal sensitivity. Phenelzine (Nardil) has appeared highly effective for SAD in several controlled trials (e.g., Liebowitz *et al.* 1992), but it is now generally reserved for treatment-refractory cases, because of the risk of hypertensive reactions and the attendant need for dietary restrictions. The reversible MAOI moclobemide is safer and has been marketed for SAD outside of the United States, but several controlled trials suggest that its efficacy in SAD is less than that of the SSRIs (Blanco *et al.* 2003)

Beta-adrenergic blockers given on a daily schedule have appeared ineffective for generalized SAD in two controlled trials (Liebowitz *et al.* 1992, Turner *et al.* 1994), but they remain widely used on an as-needed basis for non-generalized SAD or performance anxiety. While there are no controlled trials of beta-blockers for diagnosed non-generalized SAD, their efficacy is supported by studies of anxious performers (Liebowitz *et al.* 1985). The beta-blocker propranolol (Inderal) is typically given in a 20 mg dose about an hour before an anticipated performance.

23.3.5 Medication treatment with comorbid conditions

A few studies have addressed medication treatment of SAD that presents with common comorbid conditions. In patients with SAD and comorbid depression, depressive symptoms have been observed to respond more rapidly than SAD symptoms to SSRI treatment (Schneier *et al.* 2003). Persons with SAD and pathological sweating (hyperhidrosis) were shown to benefit from augmentation of SSRI treatment with botulinum toxin treatment for sweating (Connor *et al.* 2006). Among patients with SAD and comorbid alcohol use disorders, the SSRI paroxetine remains efficacious for SAD but does not effectively treat the alcohol use disorder (Book *et al.* 2007).

23.4 CBT and pharmacotherapy compared and combined

23.4.1 Evidence from clinical trials

A natural progression in the study of SAD treatment has been to examine the relative efficacy of CBT and pharmacotherapy and then combine the most efficacious psychological and pharmacological treatments to see if they offer an additive effect. Several early studies compared CBT and pharmacotherapies, but these trials were either uncontrolled (e.g., Otto *et al.* 2000), compared CBT to medications that were not themselves superior to placebo (e.g., Clark & Agras 1991,

Turner *et al.* 1994), or modified the CBT procedure such that its efficacy may have been reduced (Gelernter *et al.* 1991).

Heimberg and colleagues (1998) completed a two-site study in which 133 patients were randomized to CBGT, the MAOI phenelzine, educational support, or pill placebo. After 12 weeks of treatment, CBGT and phenelzine produced similar proportions of treatment responders (75% and 77%, respectively), and both active treatments had higher proportions of responders than the placebo or educational-support conditions (41% and 35%, respectively). However, phenelzine patients were significantly more improved than CBGT patients on some dimensional measures of social anxiety, such as the Liebowitz Social Anxiety Scale. After the 12-week acute treatment phase, patients responding to CBGT or phenelzine received maintenance treatment for six months, which was followed by a six-month follow-up (Liebowitz *et al.* 1999). Over the course of maintenance and follow-up, patients with generalized SAD treated with CBGT were significantly less likely to relapse than were patients treated with phenelzine (0% vs. 50%). Thus, phenelzine may provide somewhat more immediate relief, but CBGT may provide greater protection against relapse.

Clark and colleagues (2003) compared Clark's CBT to fluoxetine plus self-exposure (FLU+SE) and placebo plus self-exposure (PBO+SE). After 16 weeks, there were significant improvements from all three treatments, but CBT was superior to both medication and placebo at mid-treatment, post-treatment, and 12-month follow-up.

A variant of CBGT, comprehensive cognitive–behavioral group therapy (CCBT) was recently compared to fluoxetine (FLU), placebo (PBO), and their combinations (CCBT+FLU and CCBT+PBO) in a large, multisite sample of individuals with generalized SAD (Davidson *et al.* 2004). CCBT includes exposure and cognitive restructuring and an additional emphasis on social skills training. After 14 weeks of treatment, all active treatments were superior to placebo, with no differences among them. Combined treatment did not confer additional efficacy over the monotherapies.

To investigate the efficacy of combining CBT with phenelzine, Blanco and colleagues (2010) completed a multisite randomized controlled trial comparing the efficacy of CBGT, phenelzine, combined CBGT–phenelzine, and placebo in 128 patients with SAD. The combined treatment outperformed placebo on all measures, fared better than phenelzine on some measures of social anxiety, and always did better than CBGT alone. However, the monotherapies in this study were notable in that they resulted in much less satisfying outcomes than the same treatments in the study by Heimberg and colleagues (1998). Thus, whereas this study suggests the greater efficacy of combined treatment, the performance of the monotherapies in previous studies suggests caution in making this interpretation.

Blomhoff and colleagues (2001) investigated the efficacy of the SSRI sertraline, exposure therapy, and their combination compared to placebo in 387 general medical practice patients with SAD. Patients were randomized to one of four groups and received sertraline or placebo for 24 weeks; those in the exposure groups received eight 15–20-minute sessions of exposure therapy during the first 12 weeks of medication or placebo treatment. These sessions consisted of identification of feared social situations, discussion of gradual exposure to those situations, and utilization of an exposure homework diary. Both sertraline groups were significantly improved after 24 weeks compared to placebo patients. There was a trend for the combination group to demonstrate added benefit beyond the efficacy of sertraline alone. However, at one-year follow-up, patients in the sertraline-only and combined sertraline–exposure groups demonstrated greater deterioration than the exposure-only group (Haug et al. 2003).

In summary, CBT – delivered on a weekly basis over a period of 12–16 weeks and containing exposure and cognitive-restructuring components – and pharmacotherapy with SSRIs fare well as first-line treatments for SAD. The combination of these techniques sometimes fares better than either therapy alone, but the use of such combined therapies is not necessarily recommended as a first-line treatment in clinical practice. Foa and colleagues (2002) reviewed combined treatment for anxiety disorders and concluded that, across the anxiety disorders, combining treatments does not enhance outcome. Given this judgment, it is worthwhile to examine the assumptions that have led the field to its interest in combined treatments. We study combined treatment because we hypothesize that it would be superior to the monotherapies of which it is composed, but is there reasonable justification for this hypothesis? It rests on an assumption that two treatments are better than one, but this is only one of a number of possible results of combining treatments, and it truly makes sense only if we can demonstrate that the two monotherapies have different mechanisms of action or target different symptoms. It is not clear that this is the case, mostly because research on mechanisms of action, especially comparing multiple treatments, is extremely rare. One example of such a study was conducted by Furmark and colleagues (2002). Patients with SAD were treated with either the SSRI citalopram or CBGT or assigned to a wait list. Treated patients improved more than wait-list patients, but there was no difference between citalopram and CBGT. Positron emission tomography studies conducted before and after treatment showed that response to treatment was associated with decreases in regional cerebral blood flow in several sites in the amygdala, hippocampus, and neighboring cortical areas, but type of treatment did not influence these changes.

23.4.2 Hypotheses and study design for combined treatment

In the absence of compelling evidence that there is benefit to combined treatments, we need to examine other hypotheses. For instance, it is possible that combined treatment might add nothing to each monotherapy precisely because combining the monotherapies represents duplication of effort (i.e., they work in the same way or the same places). Alternatively, one treatment may detract from the efficacy of the other treatment. Certain medications (especially those that have acute sedating effects) might inhibit the ability of the patient to generate sufficient anxiety to fully engage in the exposure process (Foa & Kozak 1986). It is also possible that a patient who believes that the medication is the more important treatment may put less effort into learning CBT skills or conducting homework assignments for in-vivo exposure, thereby impeding his or her own chances for a successful treatment outcome. Yet another twist on this hypothesis is that the explanations that a patient makes to himself or herself about improvements experienced in combined CBT–medication treatment might have an impact on the maintenance of gains after medication discontinuation. Although this hypothesis has not been examined in SAD, in a study of panic disorder with agoraphobia (Basoglu et al. 1994) patients receiving combined alprazolam and exposure treatment who attributed their treatment success to the medication were more likely to relapse than were patients who attributed success to their own efforts. Clearly, combination treatments are not as straightforward as 1 + 1 = 2!

Additionally, it is questionable whether combined treatments have been combined in the most efficacious manner in randomized controlled trials. All the studies reviewed above started both treatments at the same time and discontinued them at the same time. However, one might consider augmentation, starting with one treatment (perhaps an SSRI as the first-line medication treatment and one that is easily available) and augmenting with the other if there is not sufficient response to the initial treatment. In one study, Joorman and colleagues (2005) found that individuals with SAD and comorbid depression receiving CBT for social anxiety improved on measures of social anxiety but not on measures of depression following treatment, suggesting that such individuals could benefit from an augmentation treatment that targets depressive symptoms (but see Erwin *et al.* 2002).

In a more general sense, however, augmentation is a good strategy for several reasons. First, combined treatments use more resources, and it is unclear that the greater resource expenditure is justified. Second, patients who show a very positive response to the first treatment have shown that they do not need the second treatment, and those who do not respond to the first treatment might well receive a different monotherapy without a combination approach, an option that is foreclosed by simultaneous administration of two or more treatments. Third, augmentation allows a patient to adjust to one treatment before having to incorporate the demands of the second treatment. Preliminary results from a study from our collaborating clinics appear to demonstrate that augmenting paroxetine among partial responders to a 12-week open trial with 16 weeks of CBT (while paroxetine is continued) results in higher rates of response and remission than continued paroxetine alone. However, augmentation strategies are in their infancy in the treatment of SAD, and more research is required.

23.4.3 Studies of D-cycloserine as CBT enhancer

Recent studies of D-cycloserine (DCS) and CBT for SAD and other anxiety disorders have generated excitement for a new paradigm in combining medication and CBT treatments. Unlike the medications that have been shown to be effective as monotherapies before being studied in tandem with CBT, DCS does not appear to be efficacious as an independent treatment for anxiety. Originally marketed as an antituberculosis drug, it had more recently been found to be a partial agonist at the N-methyl-D-aspartate

(NMDA) receptor, which is involved in conditioned learning. Animal studies have shown that the process of extinction of conditioned fear, the same process believed crucial to the mechanism of exposure therapy in humans, is facilitated by DCS administered just before the extinction trial.

After an initial human trial suggested that DCS enhanced CBT for the treatment of height phobia, two published studies have found that DCS can also enhance the effects of a brief CBT treatment of SAD. Hofmann and colleagues (2006) treated 27 SAD patients with significant public speaking anxiety with five CBT sessions. After the introductory session, participants engaged in four weekly sessions involving exposure to increasingly challenging public speaking assignments with videotaped feedback of performances. One hour prior to each session, participants received a single dose of DCS 50 mg or placebo. Blind conditions were maintained, as patients were unable to distinguish DCS from placebo. After the fifth session, patients who had received DCS showed significantly greater improvement on self-report measures than those who had received placebo, and this superior response was maintained one month after treatment had ended.

Guastella and colleagues (2008) replicated these findings in a sample of 56 patients with SAD, following a protocol that adhered closely to that of the earlier study. After the fifth session, patients who had received DCS showed significantly greater improvement on three of four self-report measures, and this effect was maintained at one-month follow-up. Further analysis showed that patients assigned to DCS, but not patients assigned placebo, exhibited a significant relationship between improvement in self-appraisals of speech performance after each exposure session and lower post-treatment severity of social anxiety. This is consistent with the theoretical prediction that DCS facilitates the generalization of learning that occurs within each exposure/extinction session.

These findings support the principle of a new approach using cognition-enhancing medications to augment CBT treatments. However, important questions about the clinical utility of this approach remain to be answered, such as whether DCS's enhancement of brief, attenuated CBT will also extend to enhancement of compliance and magnitude of improvement with a full course of CBT. Parameters of optimal dosage and timing of each element of the combined treatment need more study. While DCS's availability as a marketed drug made it a logical first choice for this paradigm, its success may open the door for study of a new generation of medications that supplement CBT through cognitive enhancement.

23.5 Conclusions

In summary, the SSRIs and the SNRI venlafaxine have been established as first-line medication treatments for SAD, and CBT, as studied in several formats, is well established as the preferred psychosocial treatment. Medication and CBT treatments appear to be of roughly comparable efficacy, although medications may work more rapidly while CBT has more lasting effects after treatment is discontinued. Alternative medications that have appeared efficacious in controlled trials include benzodiazepines, mirtazapine, gabapentin, and pregabalin. Beta-blockers are commonly used in the treatment of performance anxiety in non-generalized SAD.

More research is needed on treatment of patients with inadequate response to first-line treatments. The results of several studies combining CBT and medication treatments have been inconsistent, but they suggest that some patients benefit from combined treatment more than either monotherapy. In the absence of reliable predictors of which patients will need combined treatment, it is probably most cost-effective to reserve it for non-responders to a monotherapy. Two controlled studies of the cognitive enhancer DCS combined with CBT suggest promise for this new approach to combined treatment. Further studies of augmentation strategies in combining medication and psychosocial treatments, and greater attention to methods for treatment of patients with comorbid disorders, are sorely needed.

References

American Psychiatric Association (2000). *Diagnostic and Statistical Manual of Mental Disorders*, 4th edn, text revision (DSM-IV-TR). Washington, DC: American Psychiatric Association.

Ballenger, J. C., Davidson, J. R., Lecrubier, Y., *et al.* (1998). Consensus statement on social anxiety disorder from the International Consensus Group on Depression and Anxiety. *Journal of Clinical Psychiatry*, **59** (Suppl. 17), 54–60.

Barnett, S. D., Kramer, M. L., Casat, C. D., Connor, K. M., & Davidson, J. R. (2002). Efficacy of olanzapine in social anxiety disorder: a pilot study. *Journal of Psychopharmacology*, **16**, 365–368.

Basoglu, M., Marks, I. M., Kilic, C., Brewin, C. R., & Swinson, R. P. (1994). Alprazolam and exposure for panic disorder with agoraphobia: attribution of improvement to medication predicts subsequent relapse. *British Journal of Psychiatry*, **164**, 652–659.

Birmaher, B., Axelson, D. A., Monk, K., *et al.* (2003). Fluoxetine for the treatment of childhood anxiety disorders. *Journal of the American Academy of Child and Adolescent Psychiatry*, **42**, 415–423.

Blanco, C., Schneier, F. R., Schmidt, A., *et al.* (2003). Pharmacological treatment of social anxiety disorder: a meta-analysis. *Depression and Anxiety*, **18**, 29–40.

Blanco, C., Heimberg, R. G., Schneier, F. R., *et al.* (2010). A placebo-controlled trial of phenelzine, cognitive behavioral group therapy and their combination for social anxiety disorder. *Archives of General Psychiatry*, **67**, 286–295.

Blomhoff, S., Haug, T. T., Hellstrøm, K., *et al.* (2001). Randomized controlled general practice trial of setraline, exposure therapy, and combined treatment in generalized social phobia. *British Journal of Psychiatry*, **179**, 23–30.

Book, S. W., Thomas, S. E., Randall, P. W., & Randall, C. L. (2007). Paroxetine reduces social anxiety in individuals with a co-occurring alcohol use disorder. *Journal of Anxiety Disorders*, **22**, 310–318.

Borge, F. M., Hoffart, A., Sexton, H., *et al.* (2008). Residential cognitive therapy versus residential interpersonal therapy for social phobia: a randomized clinical trial. *Journal of Anxiety Disorders*, **22**, 991–1010.

Buckner, J. D., Eggleston, A. M., & Schmidt. N. B. (2006). Social anxiety and problematic alcohol consumption: the mediating role of drinking motives and situations. *Behavior Therapy*, **37**, 381–391.

Buckner, J. D., Ledley, D. R., Heimberg, R. G., & Schmidt, N. B. (2008). Treating comorbid social anxiety and alcohol use disorders: combining motivation enhancement therapy with cognitive–behavioral therapy. *Clinical Case Studies*, 7, 208–223.

Chambless, D. L., & Ollendick, T. H. (2001). Empirically supported psychological interventions: Controversies and evidence. *Annual Review of Psychology*, **52**, 685–716.

Clark, D. B., & Agras, S. (1991). The assessment and treatment of performance anxiety in musicians. *American Journal of Psychiatry*, **148**, 598–605.

Clark, D. M., & Wells, A. (1995). A cognitive model of social phobia. In R. G. Heimberg, M. R. Liebowitz, D. A. Hope, & F. R. Schneier, eds., *Social Phobia: Diagnosis, Assessment, and Treatment*. New York, NY: Guilford Press.

Clark, D. M., Ehlers, A., McManus, F., *et al.* (2003). Cognitive therapy versus fluoxetine in generalized social phobia: a randomized placebo-controlled trial. *Journal of Consulting and Clinical Psychology*, **71**, 1058–1067.

Clark, D. M., Ehlers, A., Hackman, A., *et al.* (2006). Cognitive therapy versus exposure plus applied relaxation in social phobia: a randomized controlled trial. *Journal of Consulting and Clinical Psychology*, **74**, 568–578.

Connor, K. M., Davidson, J. R. T., Potts, N. L. S., *et al.* (1998). Discontinuation of clonazepam in the treatment of social phobia. *Journal of Clinical Psychopharmacology*, **18**, 373–378.

Connor, K. M., Cook, J. L., & Davidson, J. R. (2006). Botulinum toxin treatment of social anxiety disorder with hyperhidrosis: A placebo-controlled double-blind trial. *Journal of Clinical Psychiatry*, **67**, 30–36.

Dalrymple, K. L., & Herbert, J. D. (2007). Acceptance and commitment therapy for generalized social anxiety disorder. *Behavior Modification*, **31**, 543–568.

Davidson, J. R., Potts, N. L., Richichi, E., *et al.* (1993). Treatment of social phobia with clonazepam and placebo. *Journal of Clinical Psychopharmacology*, **13**, 423–428.

Davidson, J. R., Foa, E. B., Huppert, J. D., *et al.* (2004). Fluoxetine, comprehensive cognitive behavioral therapy, and placebo in generalized social phobia. *Archives of General Psychiatry*, **61**, 1005–1013.

Erwin, B. A., Heimberg, R. G., Juster, H., & Mindlin, M. (2002). Comorbid anxiety and mood disorders among persons with social anxiety disorder. *Behaviour Research and Therapy*, **40**, 19–35.

Fedoroff, I. C., & Taylor, S. (2001). Psychological and pharmacological treatments for social anxiety disorder: a meta-analysis. *Journal of Clinical Psychopharmacology*, **21**, 311–324.

Feske, U., & Chambless, D. L. (1995). Cognitive behavioral versus exposure only treatment for social phobia: A meta-analysis. *Behavior Therapy*, **26**, 695–720.

Foa, E. B., & Kozak, M. J. (1986). Emotional processing of fear: exposure to corrective information. *Psychological Bulletin*, **99**, 20–35.

Foa, E. B., Franklin, M. E., & Moser, J. (2002). Context in the clinic: how well do cognitive–behavioral therapies and medications work in combination? *Biological Psychiatry*, **52**, 987–997.

Franklin, M. E., Jaycox, L. H., & Foa, E. B. (1999). Social skills training. In M. Hersen & A. S. Bellack, eds., *Handbook of Comparative Interventions for Adult Disorders*, 2nd edn. Hoboken, NJ: Wiley.

Furmark, T., Tillfors, M., Marteinsdottir, I., *et al.* (2002). Common changes in cerebral blood flow in patients with social phobia treated with citalopram or cognitive–behavioral therapy. *Archives of General Psychiatry*, **59**, 425–433.

Gelernter, C. S., Uhde, T. W., Cimbolic, P., *et al.* (1991). Cognitive–behavioral and pharmacological treatments of social phobia: a controlled study. *Archives of General Psychiatry*, **48**, 938–945.

Gould, R. A., Buckminster, S., Pollack, M. H., Otto, M., & Yap, L (1997). Cognitive behavioral and pharmacological

treatment for social phobia: a meta-analysis. *Clinical Psychology: Science and Practice*, **4**, 291–306.

Guastella, A. J., Richardson, R., Lovibond, P. F., *et al.* (2008). A randomized controlled trial of d-cycloserine enhancement of exposure therapy for social anxiety disorder. *Biological Psychiatry*, **63**, 544–549.

Haug, T. T., Blomhoff, S., Hellstrøm, K., *et al.* (2003). Exposure therapy and sertraline in social phobia: 1-year follow-up of a randomised controlled trial. *British Journal of Psychiatry*, **182**, 312–318.

Heimberg, R. G., & Becker, R. E. (2002). *Cognitive–Behavioral Group Therapy for Social phobia: Basic Mechanisms and Clinical Strategies*. New York, NY: Guilford Press.

Heimberg, R. G., Dodge, C. S., Hope, D. A., *et al.* (1990). Cognitive–behavioral group treatment of social phobia: comparison to a credible placebo control. *Cognitive Therapy and Research*, **14**, 1–23.

Heimberg, R. G., Salzman, D. G., Holt, C. S., & Blendell, K. A. (1993). Cognitive–behavioral group treatment for social phobia: Effectiveness at five-year follow-up. *Cognitive Therapy and Research*, **17**, 325–339.

Heimberg, R. G., Liebowitz, M. R., Hope, D. A., *et al.* (1998). Cognitive–behavioral group therapy versus phenelzine in social phobia: 12 week outcome. *Archives of General Psychiatry*, **55**, 1133–1141.

Hofmann, S. G., & Smits, J. A. J. (2008). Cognitive–behavioral therapy for adult anxiety disorders: a meta-analysis of randomized placebo-controlled trials. *Journal of Clinical Psychiatry*, **69**, 621–632.

Hofmann, S. G., Meuret, A. E., Smits, J. A. J., *et al.* (2006). Augmentation of exposure therapy with d-cycloserine for social anxiety disorder. *Archives of General Psychiatry*, **63**, 298–304.

Hope, D. A., Heimberg, R. G., Juster, H., & Turk, C. L. (2000). *Managing social anxiety: a Cognitive–Behavioral Therapy Approach (Client Workbook)*. New York, NY: Oxford University Press.

Hope, D. A., Heimberg, R. G., & Turk, C. L. (2006). *Managing Social Anxiety: a Cognitive–Behavioral Therapy Approach (Therapist Guide)*. New York, NY: Oxford University Press.

Ipser, J. C., Kariuki, C. M., & Stein, D. J. (2008). Pharmacotherapy for social anxiety disorder: a systematic review. *Expert Reviews in Neurotherapeutics*, **8**, 235–257.

Joormann, J., Kosfelder, J., & Schulte, D. (2005). The impact of comorbidity of depression on the course of anxiety treatments. *Cognitive Therapy and Research*, **29**, 561–591.

Kobak, K. A., Griest, J. H., Jefferson, J. W., & Katzelnick, D. J. (2002). Fluoxetine in social phobia: a double-blind placebo controlled pilot study. *Journal of Clinical Psychopharmacology*, **22**, 257–262.

Koszycki, D., Benger, M., Shlik, J., & Bradwejn, J. (2007). Randomized trial of a meditation-based stress reduction program and cognitive behavior therapy in generalized social anxiety disorder. *Behaviour Research and Therapy*, **45**, 2518–2526.

Ledley, D. R., Huppert, J. D., Foa, E. B., *et al.* (2005). Impact of depressive symptoms on the treatment of generalized social anxiety disorder. *Depression and Anxiety*, **22**, 161–167.

Ledley, D. R., Heimberg, R. G., Hope, D. A., *et al.* (2009). Efficacy of a manualized and workbook-driven individual treatment for social anxiety disorder. *Behavior Therapy*, **40**, 414–424.

Leichsenring, F., Beutel, M., & Leibing, E. (2007). Psychodynamic psychotherapy for social phobia: A treatment based on supportive-expressive therapy. *Bulletin of the Menninger Clinic*, **71**, 56–83.

Liebowitz, M. R. (1987). Social phobia. *Modern Problems in Pharmacopsychiatry*, **22**, 141–173.

Liebowitz, M. R., Gorman, J. M., Fyer, A. J., & Klein, D. F. (1985). Social phobia: review of a neglected anxiety disorder. *Archives of General Psychiatry*, **42**, 729–736.

Liebowitz, M. R., Schneier, F., Campeas, R., *et al.* (1992). Phenelzine vs atenolol in social phobia. A placebo-controlled comparison. *Archives of General Psychiatry*, **49**, 290–300.

Liebowitz, M. R., Heimberg, R. G., Schneier, F. R., *et al.* (1999). Cognitive–behavioral group therapy versus phenelzine in social phobia: Long-term outcome. *Depression and Anxiety*, **10**, 89–98.

Lipsitz, J. D., Gur, M., Vermes, D., *et al.* (2008). A randomized trial of interpersonal therapy versus supportive therapy for social anxiety disorder. *Depression and Anxiety*, **25**, 542–553.

Lucas, R. A., & Telch, M. J. (1993). Group versus individual treatment of social phobia. Paper presented at the annual meeting of the Association for Advancement of Behavior Therapy, Atlanta, GA, November 1993.

Magee, L., Erwin, B. A., & Heimberg, R. G. (2009). Psychological treatment of social anxiety disorder and specific phobia. In M. M. Antony & M. B. Stein, eds., *Oxford Handbook of Anxiety and Related Disorders*. New York, NY: Oxford University Press.

March, J. S., Entusah, A.R., Rynn, M., Albano, A. M., & Tourian, K. A. (2007). A randomized controlled trial of venlafaxine ER versus placebo in pediatric social anxiety disorder. *Biological Psychiatry*, **62**, 1149–1154.

Miller, W. R., Zweben, A., DiClemente, C. C., & Rychtarik, R. G. (1992). *Motivational Enhancement Therapy Manual: a Clinical Research Guide for Therapists Treating Individuals with Alcohol Abuse and Dependence*. Rockville, MD: National Institute on Alcohol Abuse and Alcoholism.

Montgomery, S. A., Nil, R., Dürr-Pal, N., Loft, H., & Boulenger, J.P. (2005). A 24-week randomized, double-blind, placebo-controlled study of escitalopram for the prevention of generalized social anxiety disorder. *Journal of Clinical Psychiatry*, **66**, 1270–1278.

Mörtberg, E., Clark, D. M., Sundin, Ö., & Wistedt, A. A. (2007). Intensive group cognitive treatment and individual cognitive therapy vs. treatment as usual in social phobia: a randomized controlled trial. *Acta Psychiatrica Scandinavica*, **115**, 142–154.

Moscovitch, D. A., Hofmann, S. G., Suvak, M. K., & In-Albon, T. (2005). Mediation of changes in anxiety and depression during treatment of social phobia. *Journal of Consulting and Clinical Psychology*, **73**, 945–952.

Muehlbacher, M., Nickel, M. K., Nickel, C., *et al.* (2005). Mirtazapine treatment of social phobia in women: A randomized, double-blind, placebo-controlled study. *Journal of Clinical Psychopharmacology*, **25**, 580–583.

Ossman, W. A., Wilson, K. G., Storaasli, R. D., & McNeill, J. W. (2006). A preliminary investigation of the use of acceptance and commitment therapy in a group treatment for social phobia. *International Journal of Psychology and Psychological Therapy*, **6**, 397–416.

Öst, L.-G. (1987). Applied relaxation: description of a coping technique and review of controlled studies. *Behaviour Research and Therapy*, **25**, 397–409.

Otto, M. W., Pollack, M. H., Gould, R. A., *et al.* (2000). A comparison of the efficacy of clonazepam and cognitive–behavioral group therapy for the treatment of social phobia. *Journal of Anxiety Disorders*, **14**, 345–358.

Pande, A. C., Davidson, J. R., Jefferson, J. W., *et al.* (1999). Treatment of social phobia with gabapentin: a placebo-controlled study. *Journal of Clinical Psychopharmacology*, **19**, 341–348.

Pande, A. C., Feltner, D. E., Jefferson, J. W., *et al.* (2004). Efficacy of the novel anxiolytic pregabalin in social anxiety disorder: a placebo-controlled, multicenter study. *Journal of Clinical Psychopharmacology*, **24**, 141–149.

Powers, M. B., Sigmarsson, S. R., & Emmelkamp, P. M. G. (2008). A meta-analytic review of psychological treatments for social anxiety disorder. *International Journal of Cognitive Therapy*, **1**, 94–113.

Rapee, R. M & Heimberg, R. G. (1997). A cognitive–behavioral model of anxiety in social phobia. *Behavior Research and Therapy*, **35**, 741–756.

Schneier, F. R., Blanco, C., Campeas, R., *et al.*(2003). Citalopram treatment of social anxiety disorder and comorbid major depression. *Depression and Anxiety*, **17**, 191–196.

Seedat, S., & Stein, M. B. (2004). Double-blind, placebo-controlled assessment of combined clonazepam with paroxetine compared with paroxetine monotherapy for generalized social anxiety disorder. *Journal of Clinical Psychiatry*, **65**, 244–248.

Stangier, U., Heidenreich, T., Peitz, M., Lauterbach, W., & Clark, D. M. (2003). Cognitive therapy for social phobia: Individual versus group treatment. *Behaviour Research and Therapy*, **41**, 991–1007.

Stein, D. J., Stein, M. B., Pitts, C. D., Kumar, R., & Hunter, B. (2002a). Predictors of response to pharmacotherapy in social anxiety disorder: an analysis of 3 placebo-controlled paroxetine trials. *Journal of Clinical Psychiatry*, **63**, 152–155.

Stein, D. J., Versiani M., Hair, T., & Kumar, R. (2002b). Efficacy of paroxetine for relapse prevention in social anxiety disorder. *Archives of General Psychiatry*, **59**, 1111–1118.

Stein, D. J., Westenberg, H. G., Yang, H., Li, D., & Barbato, L. M. (2003). Fluvoxamine CR in the long-term treatment of social anxiety disorder: the 12- to 24-week extension phase of a multicentre, randomized, placebo-controlled trial. *International Journal of Neuropsychopharmacology*, **6**, 317–23.

Taylor, S. (1996). Meta-analysis of cognitive–behavioral treatments for social phobia. *Journal of Behavior Therapy and Experimental Psychiatry*, **27**, 1–9.

Turner, S. M., Beidel, D. C., & Jacob, R. G. (1994). Social phobia: a comparison of behavior therapy to atenolol. *Journal of Consulting and Clinical Psychology*, **62**, 350–358.

Vaishnavi, S., Alamy, S., Zhang, W., Connor, K. M., & Davidson, J. R. (2007). Quetiapine as monotherapy for social anxiety disorder: a placebo-controlled study. *Progress in Neuropsychopharmacology and Biological Psychiatry*, **31**, 1464–1469.

Van Ameringen, M., Mancini, C., Oakman, J., *et al.* (2007). Nefazodone in the treatment of generalized social phobia: a randomized, placebo-controlled trial. *Journal of Clinical Psychiatry*, **68**, 288–295.

van Vliet, I. M., den Boer, J. A., Westenberg, H. G. M., & Pian, K. L. (1997). Clinical effects of buspirone in social phobia: a double-blind placebo-controlled study. *Journal of Clinical Psychiatry*, **58**, 164–168.

Vasile, R. G., Bruce, S. E., Goisman, R. M., Pagano, M., & Keller, M. B. (2005). Results of a naturalistic longitudinal study of benzodiazepine and SSRI use in the treatment of generalized anxiety disorder and social phobia. *Depression and Anxiety*, **22**, 59–67.

Wagner, K. D., Berard, R., Stein, M. B., *et al.* (2004). A multicenter, randomized, double-blind, placebo-controlled trial of paroxetine in children and adolescents with social anxiety disorder. *Archives of General Psychiatry*, **61**, 1153–1162.

Walker, J. R., Van Ameringen, M. A., Swinson, R., *et al.* (2000). Prevention of relapse in generalized social phobia: Results of a 24-week study in responders to 20 weeks of sertraline treatment. *Journal of Consulting and Clinical Psychology*, **33**, 448–457.

Chapter 24

Treatment of posttraumatic stress disorder

Gregory M. Sullivan, Eun Jung Suh, Yuval Neria

24.1 Introduction

Posttraumatic stress disorder (PTSD) is a common psychiatric disorder (Kessler *et al.* 1995) that is also among the most functionally impairing (Brunello *et al.* 2001, Druss *et al.* 2008). Among the first to recognize PTSD as a discrete clinical entity were physicians treating combat veterans of World War I, World War II, and the Korean War. PTSD was first officially characterized as a distinct psychiatric disorder in 1980 (American Psychiatric Association 1980). More recently, it has became evident that an array of traumatic exposures beyond combat can result in PTSD, including childhood abuse, abuse in interpersonal relationships, physical assaults, rape, life-threatening accidents, and disasters. As per the current DSM-IV-TR (American Psychiatric Association 2000), the index traumatic exposure must have involved actual or threatened death or serious injury (Criterion A1) to self or another person (i.e., "witnessing"). Also requisite is that the emotional response to the trauma involves intense fear, helplessness, or horror (Criterion A2).

The constellation of PTSD symptoms includes greater than one month of (1) *re-experiencing* the event (Criterion B), which can take the form of trauma-related intrusive images, recollections, flashbacks, or nightmares; (2) *avoidance* of stimuli associated with the event and *emotional numbing* symptoms (Criterion C); and (3) *increased arousal* symptoms (Criterion D), manifesting as poor concentration, irritability, sleep disturbance, hypervigilence, and/or enhanced startle. Dissociation, somatization, and disturbances of affect regulation have also been recognized as common phenomena in a substantial portion of those with non-combat-related traumas, particularly childhood physical and sexual abuse (van der Kolk *et al.* 1996, Oquendo *et al.* 2005, Carballo *et al.* 2008). Comorbidity levels are strikingly high in PTSD, particularly for mood and substance use disorders (Neria & Bromet 2000), and elevated rates of suicidal ideation and suicide attempts are reported in PTSD (Neria *et al.* 2000, 2006, Oquendo *et al.* 2003, 2005, Sareen *et al.* 2005).

Diagnosis of PTSD is established through a comprehensive clinical interview by a licensed mental-health professional. Commonly employed psychometric assessment scales for PTSD include the PTSD module of the Structured Clinical Interview for DSM-IV (SCID) (First *et al.* 1994), the Composite International Diagnostic Interview (CIDI) (Andrews & Peters 1998), and what has become the gold standard in clinical trials, the Clinician-Administered PTSD Scale (CAPS) (Blake *et al.* 1990, 1995). The interview version of the PTSD Symptom Scale (PSS-I) is a similarly reliable and valid alternative to the CAPS, with significantly reduced administration time (Foa & Tolin 2000). Self-report scales such as the patient version of the PSS (PSS-SR) (Foa *et al.* 1993), the Impact of Events Scale (IES) (Horowitz *et al.* 1979), and the PTSD Checklist (PCL) (Blanchard *et al.* 1996) are also important screening tools for PTSD. Clinical trials also often include an assessment of global improvement, such as in the Clinical Global Impression scale (National Institute of Mental Health 1970).

This chapter reviews evidence-based pharmacotherapeutic and psychotherapeutic treatments for PTSD and highlights some of the ongoing controversies regarding them. We review the pharmacological literature, mainly placebo-controlled randomized clinical trials (RCTs) that targeted global symptom reduction in PTSD. One section looks at some clinical trials that have targeted one particular symptom cluster or individual symptoms associated with PTSD, such as sleep disturbance and nightmares, and the chapter also looks at efforts made to prevent PTSD in recently traumatized individuals. We also address the results of psychotherapy trials in PTSD.

Anxiety Disorders: Theory, Research, and Clinical Perspectives, ed. Helen Blair Simpson, Yuval Neria, Roberto Lewis-Fernández, Franklin Schneier. Published by Cambridge University Press. © Cambridge University Press 2010.

24.2 Neurobiological findings in PTSD and approaches to treatment

24.2.1 Salient neurobiological findings

To date, there are no validated biomarkers for PTSD that can aid in diagnosis, treatment selection, or monitoring of clinical progress. Notable biological findings in PTSD include (1) derangements in the two main branches of the stress response system, the noradrenergic/sympathetic central nervous systems and the hypothalamic–pituitary–adrenal axis (Southwick *et al.* 1994); (2) increased cerebrospinal fluid concentrations of corticotropin-releasing hormone (CRH) (Bremner *et al.* 1997, Baker *et al.* 1999); (3) lower volume of the hippocampus (Bremner *et al.* 1995, Gilbertson *et al.* 2002, Smith 2005); (4) functional differences in activation of the fear-system brain regions, such as hyperactivation of the amygdala and hypoactivation of the prefrontal cortex (Pissiota *et al.* 2002, Vermetten & Bremner 2002, Shin *et al.* 2004); (5) sleep disturbances (Breslau *et al.* 2004); (6) measures of hyperarousal in response to stimuli and of delayed habituation to loud noises (Orr *et al.* 2003); (7) impaired conditioned fear extinction (Milad *et al.* 2006, 2008).

Such findings have firmly grounded the psychopathology of PTSD in neurobiological dysfunctions, thereby suggesting routes for pharmacotherapeutic intervention (Yehuda & LeDoux 2007). Importantly, findings of impaired conditioned fear extinction in PTSD have added support to the psychotherapeutic technique known as exposure, in which trauma-associated stimuli and memories are introduced in safe contexts for the purpose of extinguishing conditioned fear reactions (Rothbaum & Davis 2003).

24.2.2 Impact of basic science studies of emotional learning on PTSD treatments

Preclinical neuroscience studies of emotional learning and memory have suggested that pharmacotherapies may prevent the development of PTSD (Pitman *et al.* 2002, Stein *et al.* 2007). Along a similar vein, efforts are being made in particular anxiety disorders, including PTSD, to enhance the learning and memory processes believed to be central to the efficacy of specific psychotherapies, such as cognitive–behavioral therapy (CBT). These investigations promise to speed up response to CBT and other prolonged exposure-based therapies (Norberg *et al.* 2008).

24.3 Treatment selection in PTSD

24.3.1 First-line treatment for PTSD: serotonin-reuptake inhibitor monotherapy, psychotherapy, or combination of pharmaco- and psychotherapy?

Agents that enhance serotonergic neurotransmission, such as the selective serotonin reuptake inhibitors (SSRIs), appear to attenuate several of the prominent symptoms of PTSD (see section 24.4.1). However, the RCTs published to date have, at best, demonstrated limited efficacy (Institute of Medicine 2008, Sullivan & Neria 2009) with relatively small effect sizes (Cohen's *d* statistic < 0.5), even from the more methodologically sound pharmacotherapy RCTs (National Institute for Clinical Excellence 2005). Yet the overall conclusion of a recent meta-analysis conducted by the Cochrane Collaboration was that medication treatments are superior to placebo in reducing the severity of PTSD symptom clusters, as well as comorbid depression and disability (Stein *et al.* 2006).

24.4 Pharmacotherapy questions and controversies

Several different classes of psychotropic medications have been tested in PTSD patients over the past several decades. In this section we review results from a number of RCTs and discuss several RCTs aimed at particular symptoms associated with PTSD, such as sleep disturbance, hyperarousal, and co-occurring psychotic symptoms. Additionally, we briefly review efforts at prevention of PTSD in individuals recently exposed to significant traumas.

24.4.1 Which SSRI is most effective for PTSD?

The efficacy of SSRIs has been tested in RCTs for PTSD in a variety of trauma exposure types, including combat, physical and sexual abuse, assault, accident, and witnessing exposures in others (van der Kolk *et al.* 1994, 2007, Brady *et al.* 2000, Hertzberg *et al.* 2000, Davidson *et al.* 2001a, Marshall *et al.* 2001, 2007, Tucker *et al.* 2001, Martenyi *et al.* 2002a, Zohar *et al.* 2002, Friedman *et al.* 2007). In large RCTs, the SSRIs sertraline ($n = 208$) and paroxetine ($n = 551$) were more effective in the treatment of PTSD than placebo, and both are now approved by the US Food and Drug Administration (FDA) for PTSD. It is notable that only paroxetine had demonstrated superiority over placebo in all three PTSD symptom clusters (i.e., re-experiencing, numbing/avoidance, and hyperarousal) (Marshall *et al.* 2001).

Several of the larger RCTs demonstrating therapeutic effects of SSRIs have been conducted in mostly civilian samples (Brady *et al.* 2000, Davidson *et al.* 2001a, Tucker *et al.* 2001, Martenyi *et al.* 2002a), making extrapolation to combat veteran samples difficult. In two of the larger RCTs of mostly veterans with chronic PTSD, SSRIs were not more effective than placebo (Zohar *et al.* 2002, Friedman *et al.* 2007), suggesting that this population may be less responsive to SSRIs than non-veteran populations. Little is known about response rates to SSRIs in veterans with PTSD from recent exposure. Also, not all studies in civilians have demonstrated efficacy of SSRI pharmacotherapy (van der Kolk *et al.* 2007).

Despite the efficacy of the SSRIs, the overall effect sizes in PTSD medication trials, with rare exceptions, have not been greater than 0.5, prompting the United Kingdom's National Institute for Clinical Excellence to recommend that medication treatments not be used as routine first-line treatments in preference to a trial of a trauma-focused psychological therapy (National Institute for Clinical Excellence 2005). However, while it is certainly true that effect sizes have generally been small, the choice of 0.5 as a lower limit of clinical effectiveness is somewhat arbitrary as there is no direct translation of the effect size statistic to clinical efficacy (Stein *et al.* 2006). Therefore, it is our belief that *both* (1) a combination of psychotherapy and pharmacotherapy *and* (2) psychotherapy-alone should be considered first-line approaches, while pharmacotherapy-alone is only recommended in the circumstance when proven efficacious psychotherapies are not available.

24.4.2 Optimal treatment length with SSRIs to avoid relapse

There is a paucity of data on optimal treatment length when using SSRIs for PTSD, although several maintenance studies provide some guidance. Continuation of an SSRI for six months after a 12-week acute phase is reported to prevent relapse at a significantly higher rate than placebo (Martenyi *et al.* 2002b, Martenyi & Soldatenkova 2006). Other work has indicated that continuing an SSRI for 6–8 months after an initial 6–9 months of treatment is also significantly more likely to

prevent relapse than placebo (Davidson *et al.* 2001b, 2005). Thus, the limited available data suggest a treatment course with an SSRI of at least nine months, but extended treatment of one year or more also confers continued protection from relapse. Additionally, the typical pharmacological trial length of 12 weeks or less is inadequate to observe improvement in a subset of patients with more severe PTSD symptoms; 54% of acute phase non-responders converted to responder status during a 24-week, open-label continuation phase (Londborg *et al.* 2001). Therefore, even in absence of observable treatment response to an SSRI, continuation of a treatment trial for more than 12 weeks appears warranted in this subgroup.

24.4.3 SNRIs

To date, there have been only two large published trials in PTSD using the dual-action serotonin–norepinephrine reuptake inhibitor (SNRI) venlafaxine extended-release (ER), involving 329 and 538 patients, respectively (Davidson *et al.* 2006a, 2006b). Between the two studies, venlafaxine ER has been shown to be superior to placebo on all three PTSD symptom clusters. As with studies on SSRIs in PTSD, the effect sizes were small, in the range of 0.3. Also, both studies had notably high dropout rates of over 30%.

24.4.4 Tricyclic antidepressants and monamine oxidase inhibitors

RCTs of the tricyclic antidepressants (TCAs) and the irreversible monoamine oxidase inhibitors (MAOIs) were mostly conducted in the 1980s, when psychiatric pharmacological trials were in relative infancy. Thus the methodological shortcomings were great, and most also suffered from inadequate sample sizes (Shestatzky *et al.* 1988, Reist *et al.* 1989, Davidson *et al.* 1990, Kosten *et al.* 1991). Although these studies indicate that TCAs and irreversible MAOIs may have efficacy in PTSD, the evidence is quite limited. Larger, more methodologically sound RCTs are clearly needed to definitely demonstrate efficacy. Given the generally higher risks of adverse events from these agents (and the dietary restrictions necessary for the safe use of the irreversible MAOIs), they cannot currently be recommended as first-line treatments for PTSD. The reversible MAOI brofaromine has undergone two large multicenter RCTs (Katz *et al.* 1994, Baker *et al.* 1995). In both, brofaromine failed to demonstrate significant effects for the primary outcome measure of overall PTSD symptoms.

24.4.5 Other second-generation antidepressants

Although alternatives to SSRIs and mixed SNRIs in PTSD are needed, few data support the use of other antidepressants. An RCT of bupropion sustained-release (SR) in a sample of PTSD with diverse types of traumatic exposure ("mixed trauma") failed to be distinct from placebo (Becker *et al.* 2007). Mirtazapine, an alpha-2-adrenergic antagonist, produced mixed results in a small study with limited power. Overall, mirtazapine was not superior to placebo, although the authors emphasized a better response rate for mirtazapine among eight-week completers (11 of 14 in the mirtazapine group vs.one of six in the placebo group) on the SCID global measure employed. A 12-week RCT of nefazodone, which is both an SRI and a 5-HT_{2A} receptor antagonist, demonstrated greater reduction in CAPS total score and hyperarousal subscale score compared with placebo (Davis *et al.* 2004); however, post-marketing association between nefazodone and hepatotoxicity makes adoption of first-line use of nefazodone in PTSD unlikely (Stewart 2002).

24.4.6 Benzodiazepines

Benzodiazepines are commonly prescribed for their anti-anxiety and hypnotic properties, but little empirical research has been conducted with benzodiazepines among patients with PTSD. A recent systematic review of controlled trials in anxiety disorders, including PTSD, noted that there has been a major change in prescribing patterns from benzodiazepines to newer antidepressants despite the absence of comparative data (Berney *et al.* 2008). Remarkably, only one small RCT in PTSD was identified by the authors. The study involved 10 subjects in a five-week cross-over design of alprazolam in a mixed trauma population with PTSD (Braun *et al.* 1990) and failed to show an effect on PTSD-specific symptoms. A naturalistic treatment study of 370 veterans with PTSD looked at benzodiazepine prescription patterns, one-year outcome after discharge, and healthcare utilization, and also considered presence or absence of comorbid substance abuse (Kosten *et al.* 2000). The rate of benzodiazepine prescriptions among substance-abusing participants was about half that of non-substance-abusers. Benzodiazepine treatment was not associated with adverse effects on one-year outcome, although among substance abusers there was less improvement of violent behaviors and substance use in the benzodiazepine subgroup. Benzodiazepine use was associated with lower outpatient healthcare utilization.

The paucity of RCT data for benzodiazepines in PTSD prevents firm conclusions about their role in PTSD treatment. At this point, judicious use of benzodiazepines in PTSD should involve careful consideration of comorbid substance use disorders and risk of dependence. Systematic, methodologically sound large trials of benzodiazepines in PTSD are clearly needed.

24.4.7 Anticonvulsants

The limited existing data assessing anticonvulsants in PTSD, such as lamotrigine (Hertzberg *et al.* 1999), topiramate (Tucker *et al.* 2007), tiagabine (Davidson *et al.* 2007), and divalproex (Davis *et al.* 2008), have not been promising, although methodological shortcomings limit the generalizability of the RCTs reported to date. Therefore, existing evidence does not suggest a role for anticonvulsants in the treatment of PTSD at this time. However, further RCTs of particular anticonvulsants may be warranted.

24.4.8 Atypical antipsychotics

Several RCTs of atypical antipsychotics in PTSD have been reported, yet in some the use has been adjunctive to an antidepressant (Stein *et al.* 2002, Rothbaum *et al.* 2008), and in others the reduction in overall PTSD symptomatology has not been the main outcome measure (Hamner *et al.* 2003). Generally, there is only limited evidence supporting use of atypical antipsychotics as monotherapy in PTSD (Butterfield *et al.* 2001), and data on their use as an augmentation strategy to SSRIs are equivocal (Stein *et al.* 2002, Rothbaum *et al.* 2008). Risperidone may be helpful in selected cases in which comorbid psychotic symptoms are present (see section 24.5), and some evidence suggests further study of these agents is warranted for specific PTSD symptom clusters, such as re-experiencing and hyperarousal (Reich *et al.* 2004, Bartzokis *et al.* 2005, Padala *et al.* 2006).

24.4.9 NMDA receptor system

Preclinical evidence implicates the N-methyl-D-aspartate (NMDA) subtype of glutamatergic receptors in fear extinction and reconsolidation. D-Cycloserine (a partial agonist at a glycine regulatory site of the NMDA receptor) was tested in a four-week RCT in civilians with PTSD (Heresco-Levy *et al.* 2002) and showed no differential group-level reductions in CAPS scores. RCTs in progress are investigating whether the effectiveness of CBT (with an exposure component) can be enhanced by combination with D-cycloserine in PTSD. Thus, it is not yet possible to suggest a role for this agent in PTSD treatment.

24.5 PTSD-associated symptoms

In a study evaluating the effect of atypical antipsychotics on comorbid psychotic features in PTSD, a significantly greater decrease in psychotic symptoms was demonstrated with the use of these agents, while the reduction in CAPS total score did not differ between groups (Hamner et al. 2003). Another study in combat veterans focused on the effect of risperidone in a small subsample with notably high hyperarousal (cluster D) symptoms. In a six-week placebo-controlled trial of low-dose (0.5–2 mg/day) risperidone, use of this agent resulted in significantly greater reductions in irritability and intrusive thoughts (Monnelly et al. 2003).

Nightmares and sleep disturbances affect up to 70% of PTSD patients, and this has been attributed in part to noradrenergic system dysfunction (Raskind et al. 2003). Prazosin, an alpha-1-antagonist that attenuates noradrenergic-mediated suppression of REM sleep in preclinical work (Hilakivi & Leppavuori 1984), has been tested in PTSD in several RCTs, assessing impact on nightmares, insomnia, and global clinical status (Raskind et al. 2003, 2007, Taylor et al. 2008). Improvement in all three measures in veterans with chronic PTSD has been reported with prazosin treatment, with minimal adverse events and large effect sizes of around 1.0. Via home sleep monitoring, prazosin-induced reductions in nighttime PTSD symptoms were shown to be accompanied by an increase in total sleep time, REM sleep time, and mean REM period duration. However, prazosin did not have a sedative-like effect on sleep onset latency (Taylor et al. 2008).

24.6 Prevention of PTSD development in recently traumatized individuals

There are currently no pharmacotherapy treatments that can be recommended for the prevention of PTSD development post-trauma, though some studies show promise for this area. Animal models of traumatic stress may have particular relevance for preventing the development of PTSD after trauma exposure. Noradrenergic signaling in the amygdala is critically involved in the modulatory effects of acute stress on formation of traumatic memories (McGaugh et al. 1996). Inhibition of such noradrenergic modulation was the basis for an RCT aimed at preventing the development of PTSD by interfering with memory consolidation, achieved by administering the beta-adrenergic antagonist propranolol within six hours of the trauma (Pitman et al. 2002). Neither CAPS score at one month nor PTSD rate at three months demonstrated superiority over placebo, although exposure to trauma script-driven imagery led to greater physiological responsivity in the placebo group. Another RCT compared propranolol, the anticonvulsant gabapentin, and placebo, beginning within 48 hours of injury at a surgical trauma center (Stein et al. 2007). No significant benefit over placebo was found with respect to PTSD and depressive symptoms at one, four, and eight months post-injury for either medication.

A small, non-randomized trial of benzodiazepines for PTSD prevention in recently traumatized subjects received much attention because the group receiving benzodiazepines ($n = 13$) developed higher rates of PTSD at six months than a matched control group (Gelpin et al. 1996). However, the methodology was insufficient due to lack of randomization or placebo group (the control group was a sample of the same size matched for gender and trauma severity). By contrast, a second prevention trial in recently traumatized subjects involving a one-week RCT of temazepam ($n = 11$ in each group) failed to demonstrate a group effect on rates of PTSD or PTSD symptoms at six-week assessment (Mellman et al. 2002).

Opiates acutely inhibit the noradrenergic system in brain regions believed to be responsible for traumatic memory consolidation. The effect of morphine, administered as an analgesic, on post-trauma emergence of PTSD symptoms was investigated in children hospitalized for acute burns (Saxe et al. 2001). An inverse relationship was identified between change in the Child PTSD Reaction Index score and mean morphine dose per hospital day, suggesting that further investigation of the use of morphine or other opioids in the prevention of PTSD may be warranted.

24.7 Psychotherapy questions and controversies

Substantial empirical evidence has amassed over the past several decades to support the efficacy of psychological treatments of PTSD (Bisson et al. 2007). Among these are prolonged exposure (PE), eye movement desensitization and reprocessing (EMDR), stress inoculation therapy (SIT), trauma management therapy, cognitive therapy, and others (Foa *et al.* 1991, 1999, 2005, Van Etten & Taylor 1998, Devilly & Spence 1999, Taylor *et al.* 2003, Bisson & Andrew 2005, Bradley *et al.* 2005, Bisson *et al.* 2007). In this section, we highlight evidence-based psychological treatments for PTSD and discuss the more important research evaluating these treatments.

24.7.1 Cognitive–behavioral therapies (CBT) for PTSD

CBT for PTSD falls into three general subtypes: exposure-based therapies, anxiety management, and cognitive therapies. In exposure therapies, such as prolonged exposure (PE) therapy (Foa & Rothbaum 1998), trauma-related fearful responding and avoidant behaviors are addressed by progressive desensitization using two components of exposure: (1) imaginal exposure, which involves recounting the trauma in the safety of the therapy sessions, and (2) in-vivo exposure, in which avoided situations are confronted in a hierarchical manner through homework assignments between sessions. These two components aim to elicit emotional processing pathways that extinguish problematic traumatic memories and avoidances. Anxiety management approaches, such as stress inoculation training (SIT) (Meichenbaum 1974), include relaxation training and self-distraction techniques (e.g., thought stopping) that are aimed at improved coping skills and affect regulation. Another approach is cognitive treatment, such as cognitive processing therapy (Resick *et al.* 2002), in which dysfunctional and erroneous cognitions are challenged, with the aim to replace them with more functional and realistic ones.

24.7.2 Effectiveness of cognitive–behavioral approaches

In a pioneering comparative psychotherapy study, Brom and colleagues (1989) randomized individuals ($n = 112$) with PTSD of no greater than five years' duration to one of four groups: desensitization therapy (similar to PE), hypnotherapy, brief dynamic therapy, or wait-list control. No significant differences were found between the three therapies, and all were superior to the control condition. Desensitization therapy had the largest numerical effect: on the Impact of Events Scale it reduced symptoms by 41.4%, compared to 33.7% for hypnotherapy and 29.4% for dynamic therapy.

Foa and colleagues (1991) conducted several clinical trials in female assault victims with PTSD. In the first, rape victims with chronic PTSD were randomly assigned to nine biweekly sessions of PE, SIT, or supportive counseling (SC) or to a wait-list control group (five weeks). The SC treatment emphasized problem-solving in the "here-and-now" and discouraged detailed discussion of the traumatic experience. In the 45 participants who completed the study treatments, 40% of those receiving PE still met PTSD symptom criteria, compared to 50% in SIT, 90% in SC, and 100% in the wait-list group. On immediate post-treatment PTSD severity, SIT was significantly superior to the SC and wait-list conditions, while PE did not significantly differ from each other. At follow-up 14 weeks after treatment termination, there were no significant differences in improvement between the active treatment groups (67% SIT, 56% PE, 33% SC).

Hypothesizing that combination therapy might be more effective, Foa and colleagues (1999) compared the efficacy of nine twice-weekly sessions of PE/SIT to PE and SIT alone, as well as to a wait-list comparison group in 96 female assault victims with PTSD. However, at trial completion there were no differences on PSS-I score between active treatments, and all were superior to a wait-list group. In the intent-to-treat sample, composite endpoint of high end-state functioning was achieved by 52% in PE, 31% in SIT, and 27% in the PE/SIT groups, but in 0% of the wait-list group. At one-year follow-up ($n = 46$), there were no statistically significant differences between active treatments on high end-state functioning (52% PE, 42% SIT, 36% PE/SIT). The effect sizes in the intent-to-treat sample on the PSS-I were higher for PE than for the other groups.

Foa and colleagues (2005) also compared the efficacy of PE alone with a program that combined PE plus cognitive restructuring (PE/CR) in female assault survivors ($n = 171$) with chronic PTSD. In intent-to-treat and completer analyses, both treatments reduced PTSD severity compared with the wait-list condition, but the two psychotherapies did not differ significantly. For the majority of patients, treatment gains were maintained at follow-up out to 12-months.

In a similar study, Marks and colleagues (1998) compared exposure therapy (E) and cognitive restructuring (CR) alone with combination therapy (E/CR) and relaxation training (RT) in adults with PTSD with mixed trauma types. Intent-to-treat analyses were not reported, but data on those completing at least six weeks of treatment were analyzed ($n = 76$). Immediately post-treatment, the E, CR, and E/CR groups all appeared superior to RT.

Tarrier and colleagues (1999) conducted a randomized trial of imaginal exposure (IE) versus cognitive therapy (CT) after a four-week evaluation and monitoring period ($n = 72$). Both treatments resulted in significant improvement compared to baseline. The authors concluded that there were no significant differences in efficacy between PE and CT.

Thus, considering exposure therapies, cognitive therapies, and stress inoculation treatments in PTSD, all appear superior to wait-list control conditions. Further, some evidence suggests that exposure and stress inoculation approaches are better than supportive therapy, and that exposure and cognitive restructuring are superior to relaxation therapy.

24.7.3 Efficacy of eye movement desensitization and reprocessing (EMDR) therapy

Eye movement desensitization and reprocessing (EMDR) involves processing and reappraisal of traumatic memories while performing sets of saccadic eye movements (Shapiro 1989, 1995, 2001). Traumatic images and memories are accessed and evaluated for their aversive qualities, and focus is placed on generation of alternative cognitive appraisals of these images and memories.

Rothbaum and colleagues (Rothbaum *et al.* 2005) compared EMDR with exposure therapy in female rape victims with PTSD and essentially found similar gains between the two treatments, although exposure therapy produced a numerically (but not statistically) higher treatment response rate at six-month follow-up. Similarly, Devilly and Spence (1999) compared EMDR (eight sessions) to exposure-based CBT (Trauma Treatment Protocol [TTP], nine sessions) for individuals with non-combat-related PTSD ($n = 32$), with no significant differences found between treatments on multiple analyses. Yet here too, symptom reduction as measured by the PTSD symptom scale was numerically better for the exposure group, 60% for TTP and 29.8% for EMDR, and treatment gains at three-month follow-up were stable in the former.

Shapiro, who developed the EMDR approach, has argued that EMDR is particularly effective for patients who develop PTSD after single-trauma exposure, producing resolution of the diagnosis in 84–100% of subjects in only three sessions and with no in-vivo exercises (Shapiro 1999). However, there is no evidence of superiority of EMDR over other effective approaches.

A meta-analysis encompassing 34 studies of EMDR in a variety of populations, including 20 studies of PTSD or a trauma memory, concluded that while EMDR is superior to non-exposure therapies and no-treatment control conditions, it is no more effective than other exposure therapies (Davidson & Parker 2001).

24.7.4 Current controversy over optimal psychotherapies for PTSD

Based on numerous randomized clinical trials and meta-analyses, it is clear that several psychological treatments of PTSD are superior to control conditions. However, there is no consensus on the relative efficacy of these treatments. Several experts have concluded that exposure therapy has received more empirical support than other psychotherapies (Foa *et al.* 2004, Robertson *et al.* 2004, Nemeroff *et al.* 2006). However, the Department of Veterans Affairs and the Department of Defense recommend various psychotherapies (CT, ET, SIT, and EMDR) for treatment of PTSD in military and non-military populations (Department of Veteran Affairs 2004). In contrast, the Substance Abuse and Mental Health Services Administration (SAMHSA) has selected PE therapy as a model treatment for dissemination to clinics nationwide (Nemeroff *et al.* 2006). PE has been found to be clear and easy to learn, even for those clinicians without previous experience in CBT (Amsel *et al.* 2005).

Others have argued that there is insufficient evidence to suggest that psychological treatments specifically designed for PTSD are superior to other empirically supported psychotherapies targeting PTSD symptomatology (McFarlane & Yehuda 2000, Lee *et al.* 2006, Benish *et al.* 2008). A meta-analysis by Benish and colleagues (2008) addressed this problem by including only bona fide psychotherapies (treatments that were intended to be therapeutic rather than "control" psychotherapies not expected to be efficacious), avoiding categorization of psychotherapies and utilizing only direct comparison studies. They found no evidence to suggest outcome differences between bona fide psychotherapies (effect sizes were homogenously distributed around zero) for any outcome measure, including PTSD symptoms. They cautioned against recommending one particular treatment over another, as patients may benefit from increased access to the variety of psychotherapies with demonstrated efficacy for PTSD.

Patients with PTSD present to therapy with a variety of motives, symptom clusters, abilities, worldviews, cultural backgrounds, and life experiences, and these factors may determine the more preferable and tolerable individualized treatment. In the absence of differential effectiveness between psychotherapies, Wampold (2001) suggests that congruence between patients' illness explanations and the treatment rationale should be a criterion for choosing an appropriate psychotherapy, as this may result in greater improvement.

24.7.5 Potential future directions for psychotherapies for PTSD

Resick and colleagues (2007) suggest that trauma research would greatly benefit from identifying what types of patients respond to specific treatments and under what circumstances. Substantial evidence has accumulated that cognitive–behavioral approaches significantly decrease symptoms of chronic PTSD and prevent relapse. Nevertheless, as many as 50% of patients in efficacy studies still meet diagnostic criteria for PTSD at the end of treatment and at follow-up assessments (Bradley *et al.* 2005). Certain PTSD symptoms, such as emotional numbing, have been less responsive to existing treatments. More comprehensive studies specifically targeting non-responders and a better understanding of the characteristics of study dropouts may yield modifications in therapy that can increase completion rates and possibly improve outcomes.

Exploration of alternative psychotherapies for PTSD or novel treatment approaches may also lead to improvements. For example, Markowitz and colleagues are currently investigating the relative efficacy of interpersonal psychotherapy (IPT), a brief, manualized psychotherapy that addresses interpersonal issues, and PE for PTSD under controlled conditions (Bleiberg & Markowitz 2005). Unlike CBT treatments for PTSD, IPT does not encourage within-session re-experiencing or out-of-session exposure. Another example is combining treatments for complex trauma and their sequencing in time (Cloitre *et al.* 2002). Here, the initial phase of treatment focuses skills training in emotional regulation and establishing a strong therapeutic alliance, and the second phase includes a modified prolonged exposure approach.

24.8 Summary and conclusions

We reviewed RCTs that examined the efficacy of pharmacotherapy and psychotherapy for PTSD. Many pharmacotherapy studies have been limited by small sample sizes, high dropout rates, and inadequate statistical methodologies applied for missing data. Despite these shortcomings, and especially for civilian populations, two SSRIs – sertraline and paroxetine – have demonstrated reasonable efficacy in the treatment of PTSD as compared to placebo. Findings among veteran populations, however, suggest that SSRIs are not more effective than placebo, especially among service members with long-standing, disabling PTSD. Research on the efficacy of longer trials of SSRIs for veterans with severe PTSD may hold some promise. In addition to SSRIs, research has shown some effectiveness for venlafaxine extended-release (ER) for PTSD and more robust efficacy for prazosin, an alpha-1-antagonist, for veterans with trauma-related nightmares and insomnia.

While pharmacotherapy research in PTSD has yet to provide conclusive results for other classes of medications, psychotherapy research conducted in the last two decades has shown impressive support for a number of psychotherapies, including prolonged exposure (PE), eye movement desensitization and reprocessing (EMDR), stress inoculation therapy (SIT), and trauma management therapy. Some evidence suggests that PE and EMDR are superior to other forms of psychotherapy for PTSD; however, there is, as yet, little evidence for a difference in efficacy between these two treatment types (Bisson *et al.* 2007). On the other hand, high dropout rates and the fact that almost half of the treated populations in most RCTs still meet diagnostic criteria for PTSD at the end of treatment and at follow-up assessments (Bradley *et al.* 2005) should encourage ongoing research. In particular, investigators should focus on how to tailor treatment type (i.e., which psychotherapy and/or pharmacotherapy to be used) to patient-specific clinical scenarios and needs. In addition, more studies should target non-responders. Novel therapies for PTSD are urgently needed (Bleiberg & Markowitz 2005, Litz *et al.* 2007). Treatments for PTSD that target interpersonal functioning, moral injury, post-trauma adaptation, and combinations of treatments (e.g., combination of drugs, drug and psychotherapy, combination of psychotherapies) are also highly needed in order to advance the field and ensure that all PTSD patients receive effective treatments.

References

American Psychiatric Association (1980). *Diagnostic and Statistical Manual of Mental Disorders*, 3rd edn (DSM-III). Washington, DC: American Psychiatric Association.

American Psychiatric Association (2000). *Diagnostic and Statistical Manual of Mental Disorders*, 4th edn, text revision (DSM-IV-TR). Washington, DC: American Psychiatric Association.

Amsel, L. V., Neria, Y., Marshall, R. D., & Suh, E. J. (2005). Training therapists to treat the psychological consequences of terrorism: Disseminating psychotherapy research and researching psychotherapy dissemination. *Journal of Aggression, Maltreatment and Trauma*, **10**, 633–647.

Andrews, G., & Peters, L. (1998). The psychometric properties of the Composite International Diagnostic Interview. *Social Psychiatry and Psychiatric Epidemiology*, **33**, 80–88.

Baker, D. G., Diamond, B. I., Gillette, G., *et al.* (1995). A double-blind, randomized, placebo-controlled, multi-center study of brofaromine in the treatment of post-traumatic stress disorder. *Psychopharmacology (Berlin)*, **122**, 386–389.

Baker, D. G., West, S. A., Nicholson, W. E., *et al.* (1999). Serial CSF corticotropin-releasing hormone levels and adrenocortical activity in combat veterans with posttraumatic stress disorder. *American Journal of Psychiatry*, **156**, 585–588.

Bartzokis, G., Lu, P. H., Turner, J., Mintz, J., & Saunders, C. S. (2005). Adjunctive risperidone in the treatment of chronic combat-related posttraumatic stress disorder. *Biological Psychiatry*, **57**, 474–479.

Becker, M. E., Hertzberg, M. A., Moore, S. D., *et al.* (2007). A placebo-controlled trial of bupropion SR in the treatment of chronic posttraumatic stress disorder. *Journal of Clinical Psychopharmacology*, **27**(2), 193–197.

Benish, S. G., Imel, Z. E., & Wampold, B. E. (2008). The relative efficacy of bona fide psychotherapies for treating post-traumatic stress disorder: a meta-analysis of direct comparisons. *Clinical Psychology Review*, **28**, 746–758.

Berney, P., Halperin, D., Tango, R., Daeniker-Dayer, I., & Schulz, P. (2008). A major change of prescribing pattern in absence of adequate evidence: benzodiazepines versus newer antidepressants in anxiety disorders. *Psychopharmacology Bulletin*, **41** (3), 39–47.

Bisson, J., & Andrew, M. (2005). Psychological treatment of post-traumatic stress disorder (PTSD). *Cochrane Database of Systematic Reviews* (2), CD003388.

Bisson, J. I., Ehlers, A., Matthews, R., *et al.* (2007). Psychological treatments for chronic post-traumatic stress disorder. Systematic review and meta-analysis. *British Journal of Psychiatry*, **190**, 97–104.

Blake, D. D., Weathers, F. W., Nagy, L. M., *et al.* (1990). A clinician rating scale for assessing current and lifetime PTSD: the CAPS-1. *Behavioral Therapy*, **13**, 187–188.

Blake, D. D., Weathers, F. W., Nagy, L. M., *et al.* (1995). The development of a clinician-administered PTSD scale. *Journal of Traumatic Stress*, **8**, 75–90.

Blanchard, E. B., Jones-Alexander, J., Buckley, T. C., & Forneris, C. A. (1996). Psychometric properties of the PTSD Checklist (PCL). *Behaviour Research and Therapy*, **34**, 669–673.

Bleiberg, K. L., & Markowitz, J. C. (2005). A pilot study of interpersonal psychotherapy for posttraumatic stress disorder. *American Journal of Psychiatry*, **162**, 181–183.

Bradley, R., Greene, J., Russ, E., Dutra, L., & Westen, D. (2005). A multidimensional meta-analysis of psychotherapy for PTSD. *American Journal of Psychiatry*, **162**, 214–227.

Brady, K., Pearlstein, T., Asnis, G. M., Baker, D., *et al.* (2000). Efficacy and safety of sertraline treatment of posttraumatic stress disorder: a randomized controlled trial. *JAMA*, **283**, 1837–1844.

Braun, P., Greenberg, D., Dasberg, H., & Lerer, B. (1990). Core symptoms of posttraumatic stress disorder unimproved by alprazolam treatment. *Journal of Clinical Psychiatry*, **51**, 236–238.

Bremner, J. D., Randall, P., Scott, T. M., *et al.* (1995). MRI-based measurement of hippocampal volume in patients with combat-related posttraumatic stress disorder. *American Journal of Psychiatry*, **152**, 973–981.

Bremner, J. D., Licinio, J., Darnell, A., *et al.* (1997). Elevated CSF corticotropin-releasing factor concentrations in posttraumatic stress disorder. *American Journal of Psychiatry*, **154**, 624–629.

Breslau, N., Roth, T., Burduvali, E., *et al.* (2004). Sleep in lifetime posttraumatic stress disorder: a community-based polysomnographic study. *Archives of General Psychiatry*, **61**, 508–516.

Brom, D., Kleber, R. J., & Defares, P. B. (1989). Brief psychotherapy for posttraumatic stress disorders. *Journal of Consulting and Clinical Psychology*, **57**, 607–612.

Brunello, N., Davidson, J. R., Deahl, M., *et al.* (2001). Posttraumatic stress disorder: diagnosis and epidemiology, comorbidity and social consequences, biology and treatment. *Neuropsychobiology*, **43**, 150–162.

Butterfield, M. I., Becker, M. E., Connor, K. M., *et al.* (2001). Olanzapine in the treatment of post-traumatic stress disorder: a pilot study. *International Clinical Psychopharmacology*, **16**, 197–203.

Carballo, J. J., Harkavy-Friedman, J., Burke, A. K., *et al.* (2008). Family history of suicidal behavior and early traumatic experiences: additive effect on suicidality and course of bipolar illness? *Journal of Affective Disorders*, **109**, 57–63.

Cloitre, M., Koenen, K. C., Cohen, L. R., & Han, H. (2002). Skills training in affective and interpersonal regulation followed by exposure: a phase-based treatment for PTSD related to childhood abuse. *Journal of Consulting and Clinical Psychology*, **70**, 1067–1074.

Davidson, J., Kudler, H., Smith, R., *et al.* (1990). Treatment of posttraumatic stress disorder with amitriptyline and placebo. *Archives of General Psychiatry*, **47**, 259–266.

Davidson, J., Rothbaum, B. O., van der Kolk, B. A., Sikes, C. R., & Farfel, G. M. (2001a). Multicenter, double-blind comparison of sertraline and placebo in the treatment of posttraumatic stress disorder. *Archives of General Psychiatry*, **58**, 485–492.

Davidson, J., Pearlstein, T., Londborg, P., *et al.* (2001b). Efficacy of sertraline in preventing relapse of posttraumatic stress disorder: results of a 28-week double-blind, placebo-controlled study. *American Journal of Psychiatry*, **158**, 1974–1981.

Davidson, J., Connor, K. M., Hertzberg, M. A., *et al.* (2005). Maintenance therapy with fluoxetine in posttraumatic stress disorder: a placebo-controlled discontinuation study. *Journal of Clinical Psychopharmacology*, **25**, 166–169.

Davidson, J., Baldwin, D., Stein, D. J., *et al.* (2006a). Treatment of posttraumatic stress disorder with venlafaxine extended release: a 6-month randomized controlled trial. *Archives of General Psychiatry*, **63**, 1158–1165.

Davidson, J., Rothbaum, B. O., Tucker, P., *et al.* (2006b). Venlafaxine extended release in posttraumatic stress disorder: a sertraline- and placebo-controlled study. *Journal of Clinical Psychopharmacology*, **26**, 259–267.

Davidson, J., Brady, K., Mellman, T. A., Stein, M. B., & Pollack, M. H. (2007). The efficacy and tolerability of tiagabine in adult patients with post-traumatic stress disorder. *Journal of Clinical Psychopharmacology*, **27**, 85–88.

Davidson, P. R., & Parker, K. C. (2001). Eye movement desensitization and reprocessing (EMDR): a meta-analysis. *Journal of Consulting and Clinical Psychology*, **69**, 305–316.

Davis, L. L., Jewell, M. E., Ambrose, S., *et al.* (2004). A placebo-controlled study of nefazodone for the treatment of chronic posttraumatic stress disorder: a preliminary study. *Journal of Clinical Psychopharmacology*, **24**, 291–297.

Davis, L. L., Davidson, J. R., Ward, L. C., *et al.* (2008). Divalproex in the treatment of posttraumatic stress disorder: a randomized, double-blind, placebo-controlled trial in a veteran population. *Journal of Clinical Psychopharmacology*, **28**, 84–88.

Devilly, G. J., & Spence, S. H. (1999). The relative efficacy and treatment distress of EMDR and a cognitive–behavior trauma treatment protocol in the amelioration of posttraumatic stress disorder. *Journal of Anxiety Disorders*, **13**, 131–157.

Druss, B. G., Hwang, I., Petukhova, M., *et al.* (2008). Impairment in role functioning in mental and chronic medical disorders in the United States: results from the National Comorbidity Survey Replication. *Molecular Psychiatry*, **14**, 728–737

First, M. B., Spitzer, R. L., Gibbon, M., & Williams, J. B. W. (1994). *Structured Clinical interview for DSM-IV Axis I disorders, Patient Edition. SCID-I/P, Version 2.0.* New York, NY: Biometrics Research, New York State Psychiatric Institute.

Foa, E. B., & Rothbaum, B. O. (1998). *Treating the Trauma of Rape: Cognitive–Behavioral Therapy for PTSD.* New York, NY: Guilford Press.

Foa, E. B., & Tolin, D. F. (2000). Comparison of the PTSD Symptom Scale–Interview Version and the Clinician-Administered PTSD Scale. *Journal of Traumatic Stress*, **13**, 181–191.

Foa, E. B., Rothbaum, B. O., Riggs, D. S., & Murdock, T. B. (1991). Treatment of posttraumatic stress disorder in rape victims: a comparison between cognitive–behavioral procedures and counseling. *Journal of Consulting and Clinical Psychology*, **59**, 715–723.

Foa, E. B., Riggs, D. S., Dancu, C. V., & Rothbaum, B. O. (1993). Reliability and validity of a brief instrument for assessing post-traumatic stress disorder. *Journal of Traumatic Stress*, **6**, 459–473.

Foa, E. B., Dancu, C. V., Hembree, E. A., *et al.* (1999). A comparison of exposure therapy, stress inoculation training, and their combination for reducing posttraumatic stress disorder in female assault victims. *Journal of Consulting and Clinical Psychology*, **67**, 194–200.

Foa, E. B., Keane, T. M., & Friedman, M. J. (2004). *Effective Treatments for PTSD: Practice Guidelines from the International Society for Traumatic Stress Studies.* New York, NY: Guilford Press.

Foa, E. B., Hembree, E. A., Cahill, S. P., *et al.* (2005). Randomized trial of prolonged exposure for posttraumatic stress disorder with and without cognitive restructuring: outcome at academic and community clinics. *Journal of Consulting and Clinical Psychology*, **73**, 953–964.

Friedman, M. J., Marmar, C. R., Baker, D. G., Sikes, C. R., & Farfel, G. M. (2007). Randomized, double-blind comparison of sertraline and placebo for posttraumatic stress disorder in a Department of Veterans Affairs setting. *Journal of Clinical Psychiatry*, **68**, 711–720.

Gelpin, E., Bonne, O., Peri, T., Brandes, D., & Shalev, A. Y. (1996). Treatment of recent trauma survivors with benzodiazepines: a prospective study. *Journal of Clinical Psychiatry*, **57**, 390–394.

Gilbertson, M. W., Shenton, M. E., Ciszewski, A., *et al.* (2002). Smaller hippocampal volume predicts pathologic vulnerability to psychological trauma. *Nature Neuroscience*, **5**, 1242–1247.

Department of Veteran Affairs (2004). *VA/DoD Clinical Practice Guideline for the Management of Post-Traumatic Stress.* Washington, DC: Department of Defense. www.healthquality.va.gov/Post_Traumatic_Stress_Disorder_PTSD.asp (accessed February 2010).

Hamner, M. B., Faldowski, R. A., Ulmer, H. G., *et al.* (2003). Adjunctive risperidone treatment in post-traumatic stress disorder: a preliminary controlled trial of effects on comorbid psychotic symptoms. *International Clinical Psychopharmacology*, **18**, 1–8.

Heresco-Levy, U., Kremer, I., Javitt, D. C., *et al.* (2002). Pilot-controlled trial of d-cycloserine for the treatment of post-traumatic stress disorder. *International Journal of Neuropsychopharmacology*, **5**, 301–307.

Hertzberg, M. A., Butterfield, M. I., Feldman, M. E., *et al.* (1999). A preliminary study of lamotrigine for the treatment of posttraumatic stress disorder. *Biological Psychiatry*, **45**, 1226–1229.

Hertzberg, M. A., Feldman, M. E., Beckham, J. C., Kudler, H. S., & Davidson, J. R. (2000). Lack of efficacy for fluoxetine in PTSD: a placebo controlled trial in combat veterans. *Annals of Clinical Psychiatry*, **12**, 101–105.

Hilakivi, I., & Leppavuori, A. (1984). Effects of methoxamine, and alpha-1 adrenoceptor agonist, and prazosin, an alpha-1 antagonist, on the stages of the sleep-waking cycle in the cat. *Acta Physiologica Scandinavica*, **120**, 363–372.

Horowitz, M., Wilner, N., & Alvarez, W. (1979). Impact of Event Scale: a measure of subjective stress. *Psychosomatic Medicine*, **41**, 209–218.

Institute of Medicine (2008). *Treatment of Posttraumatic Stress Disorder: an Assessment of the Evidence.* Washington, DC: National Academies Press.

Katz, R. J., Lott, M. H., Arbus, P., *et al.* (1994). Pharmacotherapy of post-traumatic stress disorder with a novel psychotropic. *Anxiety*, **1**, 169–174.

Kessler, R. C., Sonnega, A., Bromet, E., Hughes, M., & Nelson, C. B. (1995). Posttraumatic stress disorder in the National Comorbidity Survey. *Archives of General Psychiatry*, **52**, 1048–1060.

Kosten, T. R., Frank, J. B., Dan, E., McDougle, C. J., & Giller, E. L. (1991). Pharmacotherapy for posttraumatic stress disorder using phenelzine or imipramine. *Journal of Nervous and Mental Disease*, **179**, 366–370.

Kosten, T. R., Fontana, A., Sernyak, M. J., & Rosenheck, R. (2000). Benzodiazepine use in posttraumatic stress disorder among veterans with substance abuse. *Journal of Nervous and Mental Disease*, **188**, 454–459.

Lee, C. W., Taylor, G., & Drummond, P. D. (2006). The active ingredient in EMDR: is it traditional exposure or dual focus of attention? *Clinical Psychology and Psychotherapy*, **13**, 97–107.

Litz, B. T., Engel, C. C., Bryant, R. A., & Papa, A. (2007). A randomized, controlled proof-of-concept trial of an Internet-based, therapist-assisted self-management treatment for posttraumatic stress disorder. *American Journal of Psychiatry*, **164**, 1676–1683.

Londborg, P. D., Hegel, M. T., Goldstein, S., *et al.* (2001). Sertraline treatment of posttraumatic stress disorder: results of 24 weeks of open-label continuation treatment. *Journal of Clinical Psychiatry*, **62**, 325–331.

Marks, I., Lovell, K., Noshirvani, H., Livanou, M., & Thrasher, S. (1998). Treatment of posttraumatic stress disorder by exposure and/or cognitive restructuring: a controlled study. *Archives of General Psychiatry*, **55**, 317–325.

Marshall, R. D., Beebe, K. L., Oldham, M., & Zaninelli, R. (2001). Efficacy and safety of paroxetine treatment for chronic PTSD: a fixed-dose, placebo-controlled study. *American Journal of Psychiatry*, **158**, 1982–1988.

Marshall, R. D., Lewis-Fernández, R., Blanco, C., *et al.* (2007). A controlled trial of paroxetine for chronic PTSD, dissociation, and interpersonal problems in mostly minority adults. *Depression and Anxiety*, **24**, 77–84.

Martenyi, F., & Soldatenkova, V. (2006). Fluoxetine in the acute treatment and relapse prevention of combat-related post-traumatic stress disorder: analysis of the veteran group of a placebo-controlled, randomized clinical trial. *European Neuropsychopharmacology*, **16**, 340–349.

Martenyi, F., Brown, E. B., Zhang, H., Prakash, A., & Koke, S. C. (2002a). Fluoxetine versus placebo in posttraumatic stress disorder. *Journal of Clinical Psychiatry*, **63**, 199–206.

Martenyi, F., Brown, E. B., Zhang, H., Koke, S. C., & Prakash, A. (2002b). Fluoxetine v. placebo in prevention of relapse in post-traumatic stress disorder. *British Journal of Psychiatry*, **181**, 315–320.

McFarlane, A. C., & Yehuda, R. (2000). Clinical treatment of posttraumatic stress disorder: conceptual challenges raised by recent research. *Australian and New Zealand Journal of Psychiatry*, **34**, 940–953.

McGaugh, J. L., Cahill, L., & Roozendaal, B. (1996). Involvement of the amygdala in memory storage: interaction with other brain systems. *Proceedings of the National Academy of Sciences of the USA*, **93**, 13508–13514.

Meichenbaum, D. (1974). Self-instructional methods. In F. H. Kanfer & A. P. Goldstein, eds., *Helping People Change*. New York, NY: Pergamon Press, pp. 357–391.

Mellman, T. A., Bustamante, V., David, D., & Fins, A. I. (2002). Hypnotic medication in the aftermath of trauma. *Journal of Clinical Psychiatry*, **63**, 1183–1184.

Milad, M. R., Rauch, S. L., Pitman, R. K., & Quirk, G. J. (2006). Fear extinction in rats: implications for human brain imaging and anxiety disorders. *Biological Psychology*, **73**, 61–71.

Milad, M. R., Orr, S. P., Lasko, N. B., *et al.* (2008). Presence and acquired origin of reduced recall for fear extinction in PTSD: results of a twin study. *Journal of Psychiatric Research*, **42**, 515–520.

Monnelly, E. P., Ciraulo, D. A., Knapp, C., & Keane, T. (2003). Low-dose risperidone as adjunctive therapy for irritable aggression in posttraumatic stress disorder. *Journal of Clinical Psychopharmacology*, **23**, 193–196.

National Institute for Clinical Excellence (2005). *Post-Traumatic Stress Disorder (PTSD): the Management of PTSD in Adults and Children in Primary and Secondary Care*. Clinical Guideline 26. London: NICE. www.nice.org.uk/CG026NICEguideline (accessed February 2010).

National Institute of Mental Health (1970). CGI: Clinical Global Impressions. In W. Guy & R. R. Bonato, eds., *Manual for the ECDEU Assessment Battery*. Chevy Chase, MD: National Institute of Mental Health, Vol. 2, pp. 12-11–12-16.

Nemeroff, C. B., Bremner, J. D., Foa, E. B., *et al.* (2006). Posttraumatic stress disorder: a state-of-the-science review. *Journal of Psychiatric Research*, **40**, 1–21.

281

Neria, Y., & Bromet, E. J. (2000). Comorbidity of PTSD and depression: linked or separate incidence. *Biological Psychiatry*, **48**, 878–880.

Neria, Y., Solomon, Z., Ginzburg, K., *et al.* (2000). Posttraumatic residues of captivity: a follow-up of Israeli ex-prisoners of war. *Journal of Clinical Psychiatry*, **61**, 39–46.

Neria, Y., Gross, R., Olfson, M., *et al.* (2006). Posttraumatic stress disorder in primary care one year after the 9/11 attacks. *General Hospital Psychiatry*, **28**, 213–222.

Norberg, M. M., Krystal, J. H., & Tolin, D. F. (2008). A meta-analysis of d-cycloserine and the facilitation of fear extinction and exposure therapy. *Biological Psychiatry*, **63**, 1118–1126.

Oquendo, M. A., Friend, J. M., Halberstam, B., *et al.* (2003). Association of comorbid posttraumatic stress disorder and major depression with greater risk for suicidal behavior. *American Journal of Psychiatry*, **160**, 580–582.

Oquendo, M., Brent, D. A., Birmaher, B., *et al.* (2005). Posttraumatic stress disorder comorbid with major depression: factors mediating the association with suicidal behavior. *American Journal of Psychiatry*, **162**, 560–566.

Orr, S. P., Metzger, L. J., Lasko, N. B., *et al.* (2003). Physiologic responses to sudden, loud tones in monozygotic twins discordant for combat exposure: association with posttraumatic stress disorder. *Archives of General Psychiatry*, **60**, 283–288.

Padala, P. R., Madison, J., Monnahan, M., *et al.* (2006). Risperidone monotherapy for post-traumatic stress disorder related to sexual assault and domestic abuse in women. *International Clinical Psychopharmacology*, **21**, 275–280.

Pissiota, A., Frans, O., Fernández, M., *et al.* (2002). Neurofunctional correlates of posttraumatic stress disorder: a PET symptom provocation study. *European Archives of Psychiatry and Clinical Neuroscience*, **252**, 68–75.

Pitman, R. K., Sanders, K. M., Zusman, R. M., *et al.* (2002). Pilot study of secondary prevention of posttraumatic stress disorder with propranolol. *Biological Psychiatry*, **51**, 189–192.

Raskind, M. A., Peskind, E. R., Kanter, E. D., *et al.* (2003). Reduction of nightmares and other PTSD symptoms in combat veterans by prazosin: a placebo-controlled study. *American Journal of Psychiatry*, **160**, 371–373.

Raskind, M. A., Peskind, E. R., Hoff, D. J., *et al.* (2007). A parallel group placebo controlled study of prazosin for trauma nightmares and sleep disturbance in combat veterans with post-traumatic stress disorder. *Biological Psychiatry*, **61**, 928–934.

Reich, D. B., Winternitz, S., Hennen, J., Watts, T., & Stanculescu, C. (2004). A preliminary study of risperidone in the treatment of posttraumatic stress disorder related to childhood abuse in women. *Journal of Clinical Psychiatry*, **65**, 1601–1606.

Reist, C., Kauffmann, C. D., Haier, R. J., *et al.* (1989). A controlled trial of desipramine in 18 men with posttraumatic stress disorder. *American Journal of Psychiatry*, **146**, 513–516.

Resick, P. A., Nishith, P., Weaver, T. L., Astin, M. C., & Feuer, C. A. (2002). A comparison of cognitive-processing therapy with prolonged exposure and a waiting condition for the treatment of chronic posttraumatic stress disorder in female rape victims. *Journal of Consulting and Clinical Psychology*, **70**, 867–879.

Resick, P. A., Monson, C. M., & Gutner, C. (2007). Psychosocial treatments for PTSD. In M. J. Friedman, T. M. Keane, & P. A. Resick, eds., *Handbook of PTSD: Science and Practice*. New York, NY: Guilford Press.

Robertson, M., Humphreys, L., & Ray, R. (2004). Psychological treatments for posttraumatic stress disorder: recommendations for the clinician based on a review of the literature. *Journal of Psychiatric Practice*, **10**, 106–118.

Rothbaum, B. O., & Davis, M. (2003). Applying learning principles to the treatment of post-trauma reactions. *Annals of the New York Academy of Sciences*, **1008**, 112–121.

Rothbaum, B. O., Astin, M. C., & Marsteller, F. (2005). Prolonged exposure versus eye movement desensitization and reprocessing (EMDR) for PTSD rape victims. *Journal of Traumatic Stress*, **18**, 607–616.

Rothbaum, B. O., Killeen, T. K., Davidson, J. R., *et al.* (2008). Placebo-controlled trial of risperidone augmentation for selective serotonin reuptake inhibitor-resistant civilian posttraumatic stress disorder. *Journal of Clinical Psychiatry*, **69**, 520–525.

Sareen, J., Houlahan, T., Cox, B. J., & Asmundson, G. J. (2005). Anxiety disorders associated with suicidal ideation and suicide attempts in the National Comorbidity Survey. *Journal of Nervous and Mental Disease*, **193**, 450–454.

Saxe, G., Stoddard, F., Courtney, D., *et al.* (2001). Relationship between acute morphine and the course of PTSD in children with burns. *Journal of the American Academy of Child and Adolescent Psychiatry*, **40**, 915–921.

Shapiro, F. (1989). Eye movement desensitization: a new treatment for post-traumatic stress disorder. *Journal of Behavioral Therapy and Experimental Psychiatry*, **20**, 211–217.

Shapiro, F. (1995). *Eye Movement Desensitization and Reprocessing: Basic Principles, Protocols, and Procedures*. New York, NY: Guilford Press.

Shapiro, F. (1999). Eye movement desensitization and reprocessing (EMDR) and the anxiety disorders: clinical and research implications of an integrated psychotherapy treatment. *Journal of Anxiety Disorders*, **13**, 35–67.

Shapiro, F. (2001). *Eye Movement Desensitization and Reprocessing: Basic Principles, Protocols, and Procedures*, 2nd edn. New York, NY: Guilford Press.

Shestatzky, M., Greenberg, D., & Lerer, B. (1988). A controlled trial of phenelzine in posttraumatic stress disorder. *Psychiatry Research*, **24**, 149–155.

Shin, L. M., Orr, S. P., Carson, M. Λ., et al. (2004). Regional cerebral blood flow in the amygdala and medial prefrontal cortex during traumatic imagery in male and female Vietnam veterans with PTSD. *Archives of General Psychiatry*, **61**, 168–176.

Smith, M. E. (2005). Bilateral hippocampal volume reduction in adults with post-traumatic stress disorder: a meta-analysis of structural MRI studies. *Hippocampus*, **15**, 798–807.

Southwick, S. M., Bremner, D., Krystal, J. H., & Charney, D. S. (1994). Psychobiologic research in post-traumatic stress disorder. *Psychiatric Clinics of North America*, **17**, 251–264.

Stein, D. J., Ipser, J. C., & Seedat, S. (2006). Pharmacotherapy for post traumatic stress disorder (PTSD). *Cochrane Database of Systematic Reviews*, (1), CD002795.

Stein, M. B., Kline, N. A., & Matloff, J. L. (2002). Adjunctive olanzapine for SSRI-resistant combat-related PTSD: a double-blind, placebo-controlled study. *American Journal of Psychiatry*, **159**, 1777–1779.

Stein, M. B., Kerridge, C., Dimsdale, J. E., & Hoyt, D. B. (2007). Pharmacotherapy to prevent PTSD: results from a randomized controlled proof-of-concept trial in physically injured patients. *Journal of Traumatic Stress*, **20**, 923–932.

Stewart, D. E. (2002). Hepatic adverse reactions associated with nefazodone. *Canadian Journal of Psychiatry*, **47**, 375–377.

Sullivan, G. M., & Neria, Y. (2009). Pharmacotherapy in post-traumatic stress disorder: evidence from randomized controlled trials. *Current Opinion in Investigational Drugs*, **10**, 35–45.

Tarrier, N., Pilgrim, H., Sommerfield, C., et al. (1999). A randomized trial of cognitive therapy and imaginal exposure in the treatment of chronic posttraumatic stress disorder. *Journal of Consulting and Clinical Psychology*, **67**, 13–18.

Taylor, F. B., Martin, P., Thompson, C., et al. (2008). Prazosin effects on objective sleep measures and clinical symptoms in civilian trauma posttraumatic stress disorder: a placebo-controlled study. *Biological Psychiatry*, **63**, 629–632.

Taylor, S., Thordarson, D. S., Maxfield, L., et al. (2003). Comparative efficacy, speed, and adverse effects of three PTSD treatments: exposure therapy, EMDR, and relaxation training. *Journal of Consulting and Clinical Psychology*, **71**, 330–338.

Tucker, P., Zaninelli, R., Yehuda, R., et al. (2001). Paroxetine in the treatment of chronic posttraumatic stress disorder: results of a placebo-controlled, flexible-dosage trial. *Journal of Clinical Psychiatry*, **62**, 860–868.

Tucker, P., Trautman, R. P., Wyatt, D. B., et al. (2007). Efficacy and safety of topiramate monotherapy in civilian posttraumatic stress disorder: a randomized, double-blind, placebo-controlled study. *Journal of Clinical Psychiatry*, **68**, 201–206.

van der Kolk, B. A., Dreyfuss, D., Michaels, M., et al. (1994). Fluoxetine in posttraumatic stress disorder. *Journal of Clinical Psychiatry*, **55**, 517–522.

van der Kolk, B. A., Pelcovitz, D., Roth, S., et al. (1996). Dissociation, somatization, and affect dysregulation: the complexity of adaptation of trauma. *American Journal of Psychiatry*, **153** (7 Suppl.), 83–93.

van der Kolk, B. A., Spinazzola, J., Blaustein, M. E., et al. (2007). A randomized clinical trial of eye movement desensitization and reprocessing (EMDR), fluoxetine, and pill placebo in the treatment of posttraumatic stress disorder: treatment effects and long-term maintenance. *Journal of Clinical Psychiatry*, **68**, 37–46.

Van Etten, M. L., & Taylor, S. (1998). Comparative efficacy of treatments for post-traumatic stress disorder: A meta-analysis. *Clinical Psychology and Psychotherapy*, **5**, 126–144.

Vermetten, E., & Bremner, J. D. (2002). Circuits and systems in stress. II. Applications to neurobiology and treatment in posttraumatic stress disorder. *Depression and Anxiety*, **16**, 14–38.

Wampold, B. E. (2001). *The Great Psychotherapy Debate: Models, Methods, and Findings*. Mahwah, NJ: L. Erlbaum Associates.

Yehuda, R., & LeDoux, J. (2007). Response variation following trauma: a translational neuroscience approach to understanding PTSD. *Neuron*, **56**, 19–32.

Zohar, J., Amital, D., Miodownik, C., et al. (2002). Double-blind placebo-controlled pilot study of sertraline in military veterans with posttraumatic stress disorder. *Journal of Clinical Psychopharmacology*, **22**, 190–195.

Chapter 25

Panic disorder and agoraphobia

Smit S. Sinha, Donald F. Klein

25.1 Introduction

Panic disorder (PD) is a common and debilitating anxiety disorder, with lifetime prevalence ranging from 1.3% (with agoraphobia) to 4.7% (without agoraphobia). Women are affected more often than men (Kessler *et al.* 2006). Importantly, many epidemiologic estimates of agoraphobia *without* panic disorder significantly overestimate prevalence, due to the use of criteria that erroneously also capture social and simple phobia (Mannuzza *et al.* 1990, Horwath *et al.* 1993). Since these evaluations are conducted largely by non-clinicians using a checklist, both false positives and false negatives occur. Clinical cross-checks are rare and have their own methodological problems. Therefore, epidemiological findings cannot be accepted at face value and do not clarify the nosology of panic disorder and agoraphobia.

There is a bimodal age of onset of PD, with the first, largest peak in the early twenties and a second, smaller peak around age 30 (Pollack 2002). PD is highly comorbid with other psychiatric and medical disorders (Katon 1996, Candilis *et al.* 1999). Severe PD has been linked to an increased risk of suicide attempts (not completed suicides) and substance abuse problems (Weissman *et al.* 1989, Kessler *et al.* 1998).

Systematic research of PD over the past 40 years has led to enormous advances regarding our understanding of the disorder. This chapter provides an overview of fundamental diagnostic and clinical considerations, discusses specific methodological issues relevant to panic treatment research, and reviews the current status of pharmacotherapy, psychotherapy, and combination treatment. Given the limitations of epidemiological studies and meta-analyses, we focus on findings from randomized controlled trials (RCTs).

25.2 Diagnostic and clinical overview

PD was officially introduced into the psychiatric nomenclature by the DSM-III (American Psychiatric Association 1980), based in part on the seminal observation of imipramine's specific anti-panic effects (Klein 1964). However, panic attacks were well described by Freud in 1895, though misattributed to blocked libidinal discharge, and many earlier descriptions date back to Plato but were confusingly labeled "hysteria."

Klein's "pharmacological dissection" of panic attacks (Klein 1981) reconceptualized panic on the basis of its pattern of therapeutic response to imipramine. Imipramine's efficacy for panic attacks was qualitatively distinct from its effects on severe anxiety or normal fear, thus contrasting with the prevailing continuum model of anxiety. This was a key theoretical advance for anxiety research and also led to the original formulation of generalized anxiety disorder (GAD). Klein's observation allowed him to conceptualize three distinct phenomena: spontaneous panic attacks, anticipatory anxiety, and agoraphobic avoidance.

The core clinical feature of PD is the unexpected panic attack. Panic attacks by definition occur "out of the blue" without *overt* environmental, emotional, or situational triggers. Panic attacks are paroxysmal, discrete events, lasting only a few to several minutes. There is usually a rapid crescendo of intense fear or discomfort associated with intense physical and cognitive symptoms, such as palpitations, shortness of breath, sweating, chest pain, nausea, dizziness, fears of dying, going crazy, or losing control. The criteria for a full panic attack are met if four or more of these symptoms are present, although most clinical attacks far exceed this threshold. Defining duration is subjectively difficult because panic attacks cause great anticipatory

Anxiety Disorders: Theory, Research, and Clinical Perspectives, ed. Helen Blair Simpson, Yuval Neria, Roberto Lewis-Fernández, Franklin Schneier. Published by Cambridge University Press. © Cambridge University Press 2010.

fear and flight to help, which are often considered part of the panic rather than its consequences. However, physiological and, in particular, respiratory measurements indicate that panic attacks last well under 10 minutes. Astute patients can exactly report the timing of panic offset. Patients who insist their panic lasts all day require careful diagnostic evaluation, which regularly finds them to not have PD.

Two important variants of panic attacks are limited symptom (larval) attacks and nocturnal attacks. Limited symptom attacks fall below the four-symptom threshold. Nocturnal panic attacks typically occur in deepening stage 2 sleep (non-REM) and are highly specific for the diagnosis of PD (McNally 1994). It is noteworthy that panics do not occur during nightmares, which is out of keeping with theories attributing panics to unrecognized frightening stimuli. The DSM-IV (American Psychiatric Association 1994) also identifies situationally *bound* panic attacks, which occur regularly in certain situations, and situationally *predisposed* attacks, which are probabilistically linked to specific situations but may not occur.

Panic attacks are extremely frightening experiences that often lead patients to seek out immediate help. The flight to emergency rooms, primary care settings, and cardiac clinics often leads to incorrect treatment strategies and poor outcomes (Fleet *et al.* 2000). Panic attacks are also ubiquitous phenomena that occur in a wide range of psychiatric and medical disorders (lifetime prevalence of 11% in the general population). However, the experience of panic attacks alone does not constitute panic disorder. To meet the diagnosis of PD, patients must experience recurrent, unexpected attacks. Attempts to specify a minimum number of attacks have been arbitrary and not based on data.

As attacks recur, patients develop highly variable degrees of worry about the occurrence or consequences of future attacks, known as anticipatory, chronic, or inter-attack anxiety. Anticipatory anxiety leads some to avoid situations where they fear that upon having a panic, escape would be difficult or embarrassing. This avoidance behavior is known as "agoraphobia," a misnomer because the phenomenon is not simply a fear of open or crowded places. Severe cases render the patient housebound (American Psychiatric Association 1994, Pollack *et al.* 2003). This is not simple conditioning, because patients often become phobic of a situation, such as flying in a plane or sitting in the middle of a crowded theater row, without ever having panicked in that setting. Their mere anticipation

of possibly panicking and having difficulty fleeing to help is sufficient for the development of a set of phobic avoidances.

The diagnosis of PD can be made with or without agoraphobia, but whether agoraphobia occurs without antecedent PD is controversial. Clinically investigated series regularly affirm that PD antecedes or is concurrent with agoraphobia, whereas this is not the case for epidemiologic studies. This discrepancy indicates the importance of differing criterion sets and the experience of the data gatherers (Klein 1973, 1981, Klein & Klein 1989).

25.3 Methodological issues in panic disorder treatment research

Clinical trial research in PD has typically emphasized reduction in frequency of attacks and percentage of patients panic-free as primary outcome measures. This has occurred for several reasons. First, as recurrent panic attacks are the key feature of the illness, changes in panic attack frequency should logically provide the most informative measure of outcome. Moreover, elimination of panic attacks is often the first step in a sequential pattern of response identified in PD: An initial reduction in panic attack frequency and severity is followed by decreased inter-attack anxiety and subsequent reduction in agoraphobic avoidance. However, the latter symptoms may persist well beyond the end of a 6–8-week trial (Klein 1996).

Though frequency of panic attacks is a likely candidate for reliable measurement, the self-report of panic attack frequency is not a reliable measure for status or outcome because it is easily confused with crescendos of anticipatory anxiety, yielding a powerful recall bias (Bandelow *et al.* 1995). Additionally, panic attack frequency has been inconsistently defined across studies. For example, patients who experience attacks with less than four symptoms may be designated as panic-free or, alternatively, as still experiencing limited symptom attacks. Estimates of panic severity have proven far more useful as an outcome measure, regularly showing substantial benefits for severe attacks, with far less benefit for lesser attacks. To some degree this may be an artifact of scaling or misdiagnosis.

Improvement across symptom domains does not usually occur in parallel. Panic attacks can remit while significant agoraphobia persists (Shear *et al.* 2001a). It is essential that in addition to panic attacks, clinical trials measure the other symptom domains of anticipatory anxiety, phobic avoidance, and overall level of functional impairment to adequately describe PD.

To address the complexities of tracking illness progression and evaluating treatment outcome in PD, Shear and colleagues (1997) developed the Panic Disorder Severity Scale (PDSS). Modeled after the Yale–Brown Obsessive Compulsive Scale, the PDSS assesses PD severity and associated features by rating the following seven items: panic frequency, panic distress, anticipatory anxiety, agoraphobic fear/avoidance, interoceptive fear/avoidance, work impairment/distress, and social impairment/distress. It is notable that agoraphobia was included as a component of the PDSS although it is not part of the definition of PD. The authors found that a two-factor solution best fit their data, derived from a study of patients with PD and mild agoraphobia. One factor included panic frequency and distress, and the other comprised the remaining five non-panic-attack items. The item for interoceptive fear (fear of bodily sensations), which is based on cognitive misattribution, had the lowest loading.

A follow-up study by Shear and colleagues (2001b) assessed use of the PDSS to categorically assign the presence/absence of DSM-IV PD in a sample of 104 outpatients with one or more current Axis I mood and/or anxiety disorders (including 54 that met criteria for current PD). They found the optimal cut-off score to identify patients with current PD was eight (with a sensitivity of 83.3% and a specificity of 64%) and concluded that there was "a satisfactory performance of the PDSS." However, these specificity data show a high false-positive rate (36%), and using these estimates in a mixed sample of anxiety disorders containing the optimal proportion of 50% PD would increase the false-positive rate to 44%. In addition, the former item "interoceptive fear/avoidance" was replaced by "panic-related sensation fear/avoidance," which does not seem to refer to the same concept. Scaling seems useful for severity measures within an already diagnosed group, but it may not discriminate diagnoses well. Clearly, more work is necessary in this area.

Several other important methodological limitations in panic research need to be considered when evaluating efficacy in clinical trials. Pharmacological trials often have a very high dropout rate due to PD patients' exquisite sensitivity to side effects. In addition, the placebo response rate in PD is among the highest in psychiatry, exceeding that of major depression (Ninan 1997). Further, psychotherapy efficacy studies have often permitted the concomitant use of medication that may inflate efficacy (Bandelow et al. 2007). The lack of a credible control group has been problematic in a large number of cognitive–behavioral therapy (CBT) studies (Nadiga et al. 2003). To sum up, methodological problems abound, so each report must be critically assessed in the context of related reports.

25.4 Pharmacotherapy

25.4.1 Cyclic antidepressants

Imipramine and clomipramine have been the most extensively studied tricyclic antidepressants (TCAs) for PD. Klein (1964) was the first to demonstrate imipramine's anti-panic efficacy, and numerous controlled studies have since replicated this finding for both short- and long-term treatment (Sheehan et al. 1980, Mavissakalian & Perel 1999). The largest, the Cross-National Collaborative Panic Study (CNCPS) (1992) compared imipramine, alprazolam, and placebo in 1112 patients over eight weeks of treatment. Improvement on imipramine was independent of the presence of affective symptoms. Interestingly, and highly relevant to the false suffocation alarm theory of the pathophysiology of PD (Klein 1993), Briggs and colleagues (1993) found that PD patients with significant respiratory symptoms during panic were more responsive to imipramine than to alprazolam. The converse was true for non-respiratory panickers.

Clomipramine, a strongly serotonergic TCA, is also highly efficacious in treating PD (Lecrubier et al. 1997), but it is limited by poor tolerability. Two studies have suggested superior efficacy of clomipramine compared to imipramine (Modigh et al. 1992, Gentil et al. 1993), though Modigh and colleagues (1992) used a comparatively low dose of imipramine. Meta-analyses of RCTs (Wilkinson et al. 1991, Boyer 1995) have reported moderate effect sizes on multiple outcome measures for both imipramine and clomipramine.

Other TCAs have been much less rigorously studied. Desipramine in a 12-week study was superior to placebo on phobic avoidance and Hamilton Anxiety Scale ratings but not on panic attack ratings (Lydiard et al. 1993). This has not been replicated.

25.4.2 Monoamine oxidase inhibitors (MAOIs)

Systematic study of the irreversible monoamine oxidase inhibitors (MAOIs) has been limited, owing to their drawbacks of dietary restrictions and side-effect profile.

Sheehan and colleagues (1980) randomized 77 patients with endogenous anxiety (panic plus agoraphobia) to receive phenelzine (45 mg), imipramine (150 mg), or placebo; they found comparable efficacy across most outcome measures and an advantage for phenelzine on overall severity, avoidance, and functional impairment. Results for reversible MAOIs (RIMAs) have been quite promising, though these medications are not marketed in the USA. No differences in efficacy were found between brofaromine and fluoxetine in an eight-week trial (van Vliet *et al.* 1996), or between moclobemide and fluoxetine (Tiller *et al.* 1999).

25.4.3 Selective serotonin reuptake inhibitors (SSRIs)

Selective serotonin reuptake inhibitors (SSRIs) have supplanted all other medication classes as the first-line treatment for PD, due to a confluence of two factors. First, SSRIs have a superior side-effect profile compared to older medications, particularly in respect to relative safety in overdose. Klein (2006) has demonstrated that the recent US Food and Drug Administration (FDA) "black box" warning for increased risk of suicide has limited empirical substantiation. SSRIs also have notably less anticholinergic, histaminergic, and cardiovascular effects (Otto *et al.* 2001). Concern has been expressed that long-term SSRI use may interfere with dopamine-fueled incentive motivation, resulting in an apathetic attitude. A pilot trial showed that bromocriptine, a dopaminergic agent that is not considered to be a stimulant, reversed such effects (McGrath *et al.* 1995). Unfortunately, this has not been replicated.

The second factor influencing the dominance of SSRIs as first-line treatment is their demonstrated efficacy in randomized controlled trials. Four SSRIs have been FDA-approved for the treatment of PD: paroxetine, fluvoxamine, fluoxetine, and sertraline. Ballenger and colleagues (1998) found that paroxetine IR (immediate-release) 40 mg/day, but not 10 or 20 mg, was effective in significantly reducing panic attacks within four weeks of treatment. Paroxetine CR (controlled-release) has also been found superior to placebo for reduction in panic attacks and improvement on the Clinical Global Impression Scale (CGI) (Sheehan *et al.* 2005). Superiority to placebo has been found for fluoxetine (Michelson *et al.* 2001), fluvoxamine (Black *et al.* 1993, Sharp *et al.* 1996), and sertraline (Pollack *et al.* 1998, Rapaport *et al.* 2001). Citalopram and escitalopram have also appeared effective in RCTs (Wade *et al.* 1997, Stahl *et al.* 2003).

There has been much interest in determining whether SSRIs are in fact superior in efficacy to the older cyclic antidepressants or other classes, such as serotonin–norepinephrine reuptake inhibitors (SNRIs). Mavissakalian (2003) found that sertraline and imipramine were equally efficacious, and that imipramine yielded a faster rate of improvement. Otto and colleagues (2001) conducted a meta-analysis on the effect sizes of 12 RCTs of SSRIs (fluvoxamine, paroxetine, sertraline, and citalopram) and compared this to results of a large meta-analysis of non-SSRI treatment effect sizes in PD (Gould *et al.* 1995). Mean effect sizes for acute treatment outcome for SSRIs (0.55) were not significantly different from those for antidepressants in general (0.55) or imipramine specifically (0.48). Bakker and colleagues (2002) also found no difference in the short-term efficacy of SSRIs and TCAs in a meta-analysis of 43 studies, but SSRI treatments had a significantly lower dropout rate. In summary, treatment evidence does not demonstrate specific advantages for the SSRIs other than enhanced tolerability and safety.

There exists no convincing evidence that any individual SSRI is superior to the others for the treatment of panic, and studies directly comparing SSRIs have shown few differences (Dannon *et al.* 2007) There is, however, emerging anecdotal evidence of a differential side-effect profile among SSRIs. Paroxetine, for example, has a greater likelihood of causing significant weight gain as well as early extrapyramidal symptoms. When choosing an SSRI, a clinician's primary considerations should be the individual's medication history, and family history of response may be useful as well.

25.4.4 Serotonin–norepinephrine reuptake inhibitors (SNRIs)

The SNRI venlafaxine exerts therapeutic effect through inhibition of both serotonin and norepinephrine reuptake. Both venlafaxine immediate-release (IR) and extended-release (ER) have proven efficacious in treating PD, and the ER form is FDA-approved for PD. Pollack and colleagues (1996) found venlafaxine IR superior to placebo in an eight-week trial. Bradwejn and colleagues (2005) randomized 361 PD patients to venlafaxine ER (75–225 mg/day) or placebo for 10 weeks. The venlafaxine ER group had lower mean panic attack frequency, anticipatory anxiety, and phobic avoidance, as well as a greater proportion of subjects free of limited symptom attacks (but not full symptom attacks). Other trials have confirmed the efficacy of venlafaxine for PD (Pollack *et al.* 1996, Liebowitz *et al.* 2004).

Two important studies have compared an SSRI and SNRI in the treatment of PD. Pollack and colleagues (2007a) randomly assigned 664 PD patients to fixed-dosed venlafaxine ER 75mg or 150 mg/day, paroxetine 40 mg/day, or placebo for 12 weeks. The percentages of patients panic-free were significantly higher in all three treatment groups than in the placebo group and were not significantly different from each other (venlafaxine ER 75mg 54.4%, venlafaxine ER 150 mg 59.7%, paroxetine 60.9%). There were also no differences between the groups on limited symptom attacks or remission rates. Another study compared a higher dose of venlafaxine ER (225 mg/day) to 75 mg/day venlafaxine ER, paroxetine 40 mg, or placebo in 653 patients (Pollack *et al.* 2007b). At endpoint, the venlafaxine 225 mg dose group, but not the 75 mg dose group, had a significantly higher percentage of patients free of full symptom attacks compared with the paroxetine group (70% vs. 58.3%) and significantly lower PDSS total scores. The 225 mg dose of venlafaxine potentiates noradrenergic effects relative to lower dosages, which are primarily serotonergic. Combined noradrenergic and serotonergic activity at the higher dosage of venlafaxine ER may provide stronger anti-panic activity.

25.4.5 Benzodiazepines

Although current American Psychiatric Association guidelines denote the SSRIs as a first-line treatment for PD, benzodiazepines remain widely used. Bruce and colleagues (2003) demonstrated in a sample of 433 panic patients that from 1991 to 2001, benzodiazepines were the most commonly used medications, surpassing SSRIs or TCAs.

Two high-potency benzodiazepines have been approved by the FDA for the treatment of PD: alprazolam and clonazepam. Alprazolam has a shorter half-life, necessitating multiple daily doses and a significant attendant risk of interdose rebound anxiety. By contrast, clonazepam can often be administered on a once-daily dose schedule but can be quite sedative. Some patients find it useful as a single dose at hour of sleep (hs). Alprazolam XR was designed to increase duration of therapeutic effect and improve tolerability by reaching maximum plasma concentrations over 4–12 hours and maintaining a steadier plasma concentration of drug (decreasing the normal peaks and troughs of the IR formulation) (Susman & Klee 2005).

Efficacy of the high-potency benzodiazepine alprazolam has been evaluated in several large RCTs (Ballenger *et al.* 1988, CNCPS 1992). The CNCPS randomly assigned 481 patients to flexible-dose alprazolam (mean dose 5.7 mg/day) or placebo for eight weeks. Alprazolam was superior to placebo on measures of panic attacks, anticipatory anxiety, and phobic avoidance. Other studies suggest the optimal dose of alprazolam to be 2–4 mg/day (Uhlenhuth *et al.* 1999). Studies have shown alprazolam to be uniformly better tolerated than imipramine and to have a quicker onset of therapeutic effect.

Clonazepam has also been shown to be superior to placebo in RCTs. Rosenbaum and colleagues (1997) found that 74% of patients treated with 1 mg clonazepam twice daily were panic-free compared to 56% treated with placebo in a nine-week trial, and they suggested a 1–2 mg dose range as optimal. Tesar and colleagues (1991) found that clonazepam (mean 2.5 mg/day) and alprazolam (mean 5.3 mg/day) were similarly efficacious in reducing panic attacks and improving global function. Lorazepam and diazepam have not been as well studied in PD but have also shown efficacy (Dunner *et al.* 1986, Charney & Woods 1989).

Though many clinicians are concerned about the potential for benzodiazepine abuse and dependence, most PD patients are able to use these drugs responsibly. Initially effective dosage often needs to be increased to maintain benefits, but most PD patients do not persistently develop increasing tolerance to the anti-panic effects of benzodiazepines (Schweizer *et al.* 1993, Soumerai *et al.* 2003). However, withdrawal upon discontinuation may cause clinically significant symptomatology. Sudden insomnia and weakness usefully distinguish withdrawal from recurrent anxiety disorder. Rickels and colleagues (1993) found that after about eight months of treatment with alprazolam (mean dose 5.6 mg) 63% of PD patients experienced significant withdrawal during a four-week taper, and 33% were unable to discontinue medication.

Benzodiazepines co-administered with SSRIs during the first month of treatment have been shown to effectively augment the anti-panic action of SSRIs and increase study retention rates (Goddard *et al.* 2001). PD patients were treated with sertraline, co-administered with either clonazepam 0.5 mg or placebo, during the initial four weeks of treatment, followed by a three-week taper and discontinuation of the clonazepam or placebo. The sertraline/clonazepam group had a higher response rate than the sertraline/placebo group at week one and week three (41% vs. 4%, 63% vs. 32%, respectively).

Pollack and colleagues (2003) randomized 60 patients with PD to 12 weeks of paroxetine plus clonazepam, five weeks of paroxetine plus clonazepam followed by clonazepam taper, or five weeks of paroxetine plus placebo. Patients receiving paroxetine plus clonazepam improved the fastest; however, continued treatment beyond the fifth week did not lead to further improvement. After 12 weeks, all three groups showed equivalent efficacy, suggesting lack of advantage for concurrent benzodiazepines after the first month of acute stabilization.

In summary, high-potency benzodiazepines are highly effective anti-panic drugs. The main indications for their use in panic are: (1) use in cases of severe illness necessitating rapid amelioration of panic (within 1–2 weeks), (2) use during the first few weeks of antidepressant treatment as a prophylaxis against hypersensitivity to the acute anxiogenic effects of antidepressants, (3) use as an adjunct medication for patients partially responsive to antidepressants, and (4) use as a second-line treatment for patients who cannot tolerate antidepressants.

25.5 How long should panic patients be treated with medication?

The optimal duration of pharmacotherapy for PD is not known. Further, PD is a phasic illness (Simon *et al.* 2002), in contrast to disorders such as social anxiety disorder and generalized anxiety disorder. Recrudescence of symptoms can emerge after varying periods of stable remission, either triggered by stressful life events or arising spontaneously, perhaps by as-yet-unknown fluctuations in neurobiological sensitivity (Brown & Barlow 1995). For each of the major classes of anti-panic drugs, researchers have addressed whether maintenance of treatment beyond the acute phase is associated with sustained or enhanced improvement in symptoms, and whether discontinuation is linked to relapse.

Rapaport and colleagues (2001) randomly assigned 183 completers of a year of open-label sertraline for PD to an additional 28 weeks of sertraline or switch to placebo. In the sertraline group, 69% completed the 28 weeks compared to 49.4% in the placebo group, and rate of relapse was significantly lower in the sertraline group (12%) than in the placebo group (24%).

Mavissakalian and Perel (1999) randomly assigned 56 panic patients who were in stable remission after six months of acute-phase treatment with imipramine (2.25 mg/kg/day) to either double-blind maintenance treatment or placebo for one year, finding that maintenance treatment with imipramine had a significant protective effect. Mavissakalian and Perel (2002)

attempted to further clarify optimal duration of imipramine treatment of PD. Fifty-one panic patients in remission after six months of treatment were randomly assigned to discontinue medication either after an additional six months or after a 12- to 30-month range of additional treatment. The two groups, however, did not differ significantly in relapse rates.

Ferguson and colleagues (2007) randomly assigned responders to 12–26 weeks of venlafaxine ER or placebo. The venlafaxine ER group had a 22.5% relapse rate, compared to 50% for placebo, and 76% maintained panic-free status, compared to 55% of the placebo group. All secondary measures indicated significant worsening in the placebo group compared to the venlafaxine group.

The evidence suggests that maintenance therapy is a very important consideration in PD treatment, with continued treatment for at least one year after acute therapy conferring advantages over treatment discontinuation. Current APA practice guidelines recommend continuation of treatment for approximately 12–18 months beyond the acute phase (American Psychiatric Association 2009).

25.6 Psychotherapy

25.6.1 Exposure therapy

Exposure is a behavioral therapy technique that is effective in treating agoraphobia but has not been established as a treatment for panic attacks. Further, the efficacy of exposure for agoraphobia is enhanced in the context of reduced panic attacks. In-vivo situational exposure involves exposing the patient in a graded fashion to increasingly feared situations (e.g., elevators, crowds, etc.). Through repeated exposure exercises, patients habituate to the evoked anxiety, facilitating their ability to again approach previously avoided situations.

Relatively few studies have systematically evaluated exposure-based therapy alone for the treatment of PD. Fava and colleagues (1995) followed up 90 patients who had received 12 sessions of graduated exposure therapy over a six-month period, identifying 87% as panic-free and much improved. There was also evidence of longer-term benefit, as 96% of responders maintained gains over two years. These data have not been replicated.

25.6.2 Cognitive–behavioral therapy

The cognitive model of PD assumes that the genesis of spontaneous panic attacks is an antecedent, catastrophizing cognitive set that misinterprets innocuous bodily sensations as having serious medical consequences (Clark *et al.* 1994). A classic positive-feedback mechanism is postulated whereby misinterpretation leads to increased physiological arousal, leading to further catastrophizing, and spiraling into a full-blown panic attack. However, the empirical basis for antecedent catastrophizing cognitions has not been established for PD (Barlow 2002) and seems unlikely as a necessary feature.

Cognitive–behavioral therapy (CBT) for PD involves four core components (Craske & Barlow 2001). Psychoeducation explains symptoms of PD and how panic attacks originate. Cognitive restructuring identifies maladaptive cognitions and introduces strategies for replacing these with adaptive cognitions. Interoceptive exposure involves exercises to promote habituation to purposely provoked feared physical sensations (palpitations, shortness of breath). Situational or in-vivo exposure involves graded exposure to feared or avoided situations, such as subways, shopping malls, or crowds, and is especially important for agoraphobic avoidance. Breathing retraining and applied relaxation are often added to the core techniques.

The efficacy of CBT has been reported in numerous controlled but flawed studies (Barlow *et al.* 2000). For example, Klosko and colleagues (1990) compared CBT to alprazolam, pill placebo, and wait-list control. Among patients in the CBT condition, 87% achieved panic-free status, compared to 50% for alprazolam, 33% for placebo, and 33% for the wait-list control group. This study is highly problematic because the response rate to alprazolam, an established anti-panic medication, was not significantly different from placebo. Such a flaw actually renders this study unusable by current FDA standards, yet this study is typically cited as evidence for CBT's efficacy. Further, as a result of the claims of CBT efficacy, the American Psychiatric Association practice guidelines (2009) consider CBT a first-line treatment.

A meta-analysis of 43 trials that used a range of cognitive–behavioral interventions (Gould *et al.* 1995) found CBT that included interoceptive exposure had the highest effect sizes (0.88). In a meta-analysis of 124 studies, Mitte (2005) demonstrated that both CBT and behavioral therapy were more effective than placebo in several symptom domains. Other meta-analyses demonstrate comparable efficacy between CBT and pharmacotherapy (Westen & Morrison 2005). Meta-analyses by Chambless and Gillis (1993) and Clum

and colleagues (1993), found the highest effect sizes for cognitive interventions coupled with exposure techniques; however, these meta-analyses are problematic because they include few head-to-head comparisons. Instead, within-study effect sizes are aggregated and compared. This puts a misleading statistical gloss on naturalistic data that can be erroneously considered as if they were the product of experimental controlled contrasts (Klein 2000).

25.6.3 Relaxation therapy

Two major types of relaxation therapy have also been evaluated for PD: progressive relaxation and applied relaxation. Progressive muscle relaxation (PMR) involves training patients to alternate between tensing and relaxing different muscle groups. Applied relaxation (AR) involves applying the above techniques during graduated exposure to progressively fearful situations. Both PMR and AR often include deep diaphragmatic breathing.

Öst (1987) directly compared AR with PMR in 14 PD patients with agoraphobia. After acute treatment, 100% of the AR group was panic-free, compared to 71% of the PMR group, and the gains with AR were better maintained at 19-month follow-up. Öst and colleagues (1993) randomly assigned 45 patients with PD with agoraphobia to receive AR, in-vivo exposure, or cognitive therapy. Comparable efficacy was demonstrated across the three treatment groups, with benefits maintained at one-year follow up.

Four studies that directly compared CBT and relaxation therapy for panic showed superiority for CBT in all panic domains (Barlow *et al.* 1989, Beck *et al.* 1994, Clark *et al.* 1994, Arntz & van den Hout 1996). However, it is possible that comparisons using relaxation as a control are flawed (Klein 1993).

25.7 Direct comparisons of antidepressant pharmacotherapy and psychotherapy

Most head-to-head comparisons of pharmacotherapy and CBT have shown either no differences or superiority of medication during acute treatment. Black and colleagues (1993) randomly assigned 75 moderate-to-severe PD patients to receive eight weeks of fluvoxamine, cognitive therapy, or placebo. Fluvoxamine was superior to cognitive therapy on all measures of frequency, general anxiety, global functioning, and depression, with the exception of panic attack severity. Fluvoxamine produced earlier benefit as well: at week four, 57% of fluvoxamine patients were rated moderately improved or better, compared to 40% with cognitive therapy and 22% with placebo. At week eight, 81% of fluvoxamine subjects were panic-free, compared to 53% for cognitive therapy.

In a 12-week RCT, Bakker and colleagues (1999) assigned 131 panic patients to receive paroxetine, clomipramine, placebo, or cognitive therapy. Paroxetine was shown to be superior to cognitive therapy on all measures with the exception of panic frequency. The poor performance of cognitive therapy may have been because moderate-to-severe agoraphobics comprised 52% of the sample; CBT studies regularly exclude such patients. Overall, this study suggests that medication may be superior to cognitive therapy in the more severely ill patient group typical of clinical practice.

Other studies have detected no significant differences between antidepressant and CBT monotherapies, but these are also flawed (Sharp *et al.* 1996, Barlow *et al.* 2000). A meta-analysis by Mitte (2005) demonstrated that CBT and behavioral therapy were as effective as pharmacotherapy, and all were superior to placebo. Gould and colleagues (1995) found that CBT interventions were the most successful at maintaining long-term treatment gains. However, the analysis by Gould *et al.* failed to include the study by Black and colleagues (1993) (whose findings directly contradict the conclusions of Gould *et al.*), and they included nine studies that did not have a contrast group (Klein 2000). Moreover, Gould and colleagues included only two studies (5%) that directly compared pharmacotherapy with psychotherapy; Clum and colleagues (1993) used only one. These serious flaws limit estimation of the relative efficacies of the two modalities. In any case, these are naturalistic rather than experimental conclusions.

25.8 Combination therapy

25.8.1 Combination of antidepressant pharmacotherapy and psychotherapy

Combination treatment with medication and psychotherapy is often expected to be superior to monotherapy, since it combines two demonstrably successful treatment modalities with putative additive or synergistic effects. However, the literature shows only modest support for this hypothesis.

Barlow and colleagues (2000) randomly assigned 312 panic patients with mild or no agoraphobia to receive imipramine, CBT, placebo, CBT plus imipramine, or CBT plus placebo. Patients were assessed by the PDSS and CGI as the primary outcome measures. Both imipramine alone and CBT alone were significantly better than placebo on the PDSS, and there were no differences in efficacy after three months of treatment. However, response was defined as 40% reduction on the PDSS, which is an arbitrary and comparatively low threshold for improvement that may have obscured important differences between drug therapy and psychotherapy. A secondary analysis of subjects categorized as responders (defined by CGI as much improved and rated as having mild disorder) found that responders to imipramine had significantly lower PDSS scores than responders to CBT in the acute phase. Combination treatment had no advantage over CBT plus placebo in the acute phase; however, in a six-month maintenance phase, those receiving combined treatment had significantly lower PDSS scores than those receiving CBT plus placebo. At six-month follow-up only the CBT groups were more effective at maintaining self-reported responder status.

Van Apeldoorn and colleagues (2008) randomized 150 panic patients with or without agoraphobia to CBT, SSRI, or CBT plus SSRI. No differences were found between monotherapies. Combination treatment was superior to SSRI on three measures in the completer analysis and no measures in the intention-to-treat (ITT) analysis; combination was superior to CBT monotherapy on all measures in the ITT. There were no compelling differences between CBT plus SSRI and SSRI alone.

Sharp and colleagues (1996) compared CBT plus fluvoxamine, CBT, fluvoxamine, CBT plus placebo, and placebo in 190 panic patients for 12 weeks. No superiority for the combination treatment versus monotherapies was demonstrated. Otto and colleagues (2005) have argued that benefits of CBT learned in the context of medication are often not maintained once medication is discontinued, due to a "changed internal context." Overall, there is limited evidence to support the use of a combined antidepressant–psychotherapeutic approach in PD. It is noteworthy that these studies do not emphasize the possibility that psychotherapy may improve patient adherence with taking medication or may induce positive verbal response biases.

25.8.2 Combination of benzodiazepines with psychotherapy

State-dependent learning may be a reason for concern about the combination of benzodiazepines with psychotherapy. Also, benzodiazepines may suppress anxious states needed for exposure tasks to facilitate extinction (Spiegel & Bruce 1997, Otto *et al.* 2002).

Marks and colleagues (1993) randomized 143 PD patients to alprazolam (mean dose 5.8 mg/day) or placebo combined with in-vivo exposure or relaxation therapy. Alprazolam only marginally enhanced treatment during the eight-week acute phase, and there was also statistically significant deterioration during six months of follow-up after drug discontinuation, which the authors suggested may have been due to state-dependent learning. Overall, there is no evidence that combining benzodiazepines with CBT improves short- or long-term outcome; similarly, such a combination is not likely to reduce attrition in CBT trials. There may be limited benefit for severely ill patients with high levels of anxiety and increased severity of panic attacks.

CBT may facilitate discontinuation of benzodiazepines, but it is unclear if this is a specific effect. Otto and colleagues (1993) found that 76% of patients who received CBT during alprazolam and clonazepam taper were able to discontinue drug use, compared to 25% that did not receive CBT. There were no comparisons with alternative psychotherapies or even supportive measures. Similarly, Spiegel and colleagues (1994) found that 50% of patients who had tapered alprazolam (mean dose 2.2 mg/day) without CBT relapsed over six-month follow-up, compared to none in the alprazolam plus CBT group. That there were no relapses at all in the alprazolam–CBT group suggests that mechanisms independent of specific CBT components may have facilitated reported discontinuation.

25.9 Conclusions

This chapter has highlighted several of the advances made in panic disorder treatment research. Recognition of methodological problems inherent to the area has led to the development and dissemination of standardized assessment instruments that may enable more precise investigation. RCTs affirm that panic disorder is a profoundly treatable condition and that pharmacotherapy is the mainstay. No clear differences in efficacy have emerged among the several different medication classes. However, long-term therapy is extremely important to maintain treatment gains. Though psychotherapy, in particular CBT, has been claimed to be an effective treatment modality, the evidence from RCTs is not compelling, and meta-analyses comparing pharmacotherapy with psychotherapy are invalid. In addition, combining modalities has not been shown to enhance outcome.

Rigorous systematic studies are still needed in PD. Studying flawed existing trials can be enormously useful in improving the methodologies for future trials. In addition, novel therapeutic agents, such as glutamate antagonists, should be evaluated in pilot studies. Patients who demonstrate clinical benefit with these agents would form an ideal group for studies addressing theories of PD pathophysiology.

References

American Psychiatric Association (1980). *Diagnostic and Statistical Manual of Mental Disorders*, 3rd edn (DSM-III). Washington, DC: American Psychiatric Association.

American Psychiatric Association (1994). *Diagnostic and Statistical Manual of Mental Disorders*, 4th edn (DSM-IV). Washington, DC: American Psychiatric Association.

American Psychiatric Association (2009). *Practice Guideline for the Treatment of Patients with Panic Disorder*, 2nd edn. Washington, DC: American Psychiatric Association.

Arntz, A., & van den Hout, M. (1996). Psychological treatments of panic disorder without agoraphobia: cognitive therapy versus applied relaxation. *Behavior Research and Therapy*, **40**, 325–341.

Bakker, A., van Dyck, R., Spinhoven, P., & van Balkom, A. J. L. M. (1999). Paroxetine, clomipramine and cognitive therapy in the treatment of panic disorder. *Journal of Clinical Psychiatry*, **60**, 831–838.

Bakker, A., van Balkom, A. J. L. M., & Spinhoven, P. (2002). SSRIs vs. TCAs in the treatment of panic disorder: a meta-analysis. *Acta Psychiatrica Scandinavica*, **106**, 163–167.

Ballenger, J. C., Burrows, G. D., Dupont, R. L., *et al.* (1988). Alprazolam in panic disorder and agoraphobia:results from a multicentre trial. *Archives of General Psychiatry*, **45**, 413–422.

Ballenger, J. C., Wheadon, D. E., Steiner, M., Bushnell, W., & Gergel, I. P. (1998). Double blind, fixed dose, placebo controlled study of paroxetine in the treatment of panic disorder. *American Journal of Psychiatry*, **155**, 36–42.

Bandelow, B., Hajak, G., Holzrichter, S., Kunert, H. J., & Ruther, E. (1995). Assessing the efficacy of treatments for panic disorder and agoraphobia I. Methodological problems. *International Clinical Psychopharmacology*, **10**, 83–93.

Bandelow, B., Seidler-Brandler, U., Becker, A., Wedekind, D., & Ruther, E. (2007). Meta-analysis of randomized controlled comparisons of psychopharmacological and psychological treatments for anxiety disorders. *World Journal of Biological Psychiatry*, **8**, 175–87.

Barlow, D. H. (2002). *Anxiety and its Disorders*, 2nd edn. New York, NY: Guilford Press.

Barlow, D. H., Craske, M. G., & Cerny, J. A. (1989). Behavioral treatment of panic disorder. *Behavior Therapy*, **20**, 261–281.

Barlow, D. H., Gorman, J. M., Shear, M. K., & Woods, S. W. (2000). Cognitive–behavioral therapy, imipramine, or their combination for panic disorder: a randomized controlled trial. *JAMA*, **283**, 2529–2536.

Beck, J. G., Stanley, M. A., Baldwin, L. E., Deagle, E. A., & Averill, P. M. (1994). Comparison of cognitive therapy and relaxation training for panic disorder. *Journal of Consulting and Clinical Psychology*, **62**, 818–826.

Black, D. W., Wesner, R., Bowers, W., & Gabel, J. (1993). A comparison of fluvoxamine, cognitive therapy and placebo in the treatment of panic disorder. *Archives of General Psychiatry*, **50**, 44–40.

Boyer, W. (1995) Serotonin uptake inhibitors are superior to imipramine and alprazolam in alleviating panic attacks: a meta-analysis. *International Clinical Psychopharmacology*, **10**, 45–49.

Bradwejn, J., Emilien, G., & Whitaker, T. (2005) Treatment of panic disorder with venlafaxine XR. *British Journal of Psychiatry*, **187**, 352–359.

Briggs, A. C., Stretch, D. D., & Brandon, S. (1993). Subtyping of panic by symptom profile. *British Journal of Psychiatry*, **163**, 201–209.

Brown, T. A., & Barlow, D. H. (1995). Long term outcome in cognitive behavioral treatment of panic disorder: clinical predictors and alternative strategies for assessment. *Journal of Consulting and Clinical Psychology*, **63**, 754–765.

Bruce, S. E., Vasile, R. G., Goisman, R. M., *et al.* (2003). Are benzodiazepines still the medication of choice for patients with panic disorder with or without agoraphobia? *American Journal of Psychiatry*, **160**, 1432–1438.

Candilis, P. J., Mclean, R. Y., Otto, M. W. (1999). Quality of life in patients with panic disorder. *Journal of Nervous and Mental Disease*, **187**, 429–434.

Chambless, D. L., & Gillis, M. M. (1994). Cognitive therapy of anxiety disorders. *Journal of Consulting and Clinical Psychiatry*, **61**, 248–260.

Charney, D. S., & Woods, S. W. (1989). Benzodiazepine treatment of panic disorder: a comparison of alprazolam and lorazepam. *Journal of Clinical Psychiatry*, **50**, 418–423.

Clark, D. M., Salkovskis, P. M., Hackmann, A., *et al.* (1994). A comparision of cognitive therapy, applied relaxation and imipramine in the treatment of panic disorder. *British Journal of Psychiatry*, **164**, 759–769.

Clum, G. A., Clum, G. A., & Surls R. (1993). A meta-analysis of treatments for panic disorder. *Journal of Consulting and Clinical Psychology*, **61**, 317–326.

Craske, M. G., & Barlow, D. H. (2001). Panic disorder and agoraphobia. In D. H. Barlow, ed., *Clinical Handbook of Psychological Disorders*, 3rd edn. New York, NY: Guilford Press.

Cross-National Collaborative Panic Study (CNCPS) (1992). Second phase investigators, drug treatment of panic disorder: comparative efficacy of alprazolam, imipramine and placebo. *British Journal of Psychiatry*, **160**, 191–202.

Dannon, P. N., Iancu, I., Lowengrub, K., *et al.* (2007). A naturalistic long term comparison study of selective serotonin reuptake inhibitors in the treatment of panic disorder. *Clinical Neuropharmacology*, **30**, 326–334.

Dunner, D. L., Ishiki, D., Avery, D. H., Wilson, L. G., & Hyde, T. S. (1986). Effect of alprazolam and diazepam on anxiety and panic attacks in panic disorder: a controlled study. *Journal of Clinical Psychiatry*, **47**, 458–460.

Fava, G. A., Zielezny, M., & Savron, G. (1995). Long-term effects of behavioral treatment for panic disorder with agoraphobia. *British Journal of Psychiatry*, **166**, 87–92.

Ferguson, J. M., Khan, A., Mangano, R., Entsuah, R., & Izanis, E. (2007). Relapse prevention of panic disorder in adult outpatient responders to treatment with venlafaxine extended release. *Journal of Clinical Psychiatry*, **68**, 58–68.

Fleet, R. P., Martel, J. P., Lavoie, K. L., Dupuis, G., & Beitman, R. D. (2000). Non-fearful panic disorder: a variant of panic in medical patients? *Psychosomatics*, **41**, 311–320.

Gentil, V., Lotufo-Neto, F., Andrade, L., *et al.* (1993). Clomipramine, a better reference drug for panic/agoraphobia. I. Effectiveness comparison with imipramine. *Journal of Psychopharmacology*, **7**, 316–324.

Goddard, A. W., Brouette, T., & Almai, A. (2001) Early coadministration of clonazepam with sertraline for panic disorder. *Archives of General Psychiatry*, **58**, 681–686.

Gould, R. A., Otto, M. W., & Pollack, M. H. (1995). A meta-analysis of treatment outcome for panic disorder. *Clinical Psychology Reviews*, **15**, 819–844.

Horwath, E., Lish, J. D., Johnson, J., Hornig, C. D., & Weissman, M. M. (1993). Agoraphobia without panic: clinical reappraisal of an epidemiologic finding. *American Journal of Psychiatry*, **150**, 1496–1501.

Katon, W. (1996). Panic disorder: relationship to high medical utilization, unexplained physical symptoms, and medical costs. *Journal of Clinical Psychiatry*, **57** (Suppl. 10), 11–18.

Kessler, R., Stang, P. E., Wittchen, H., *et al.* (1998) Lifetime panic-depression comorbidity in the National Comorbidity Survey. *Archives of General Psychiatry*, **55**, 801–808.

Kessler, R. C., Chiu, W. T., Jin, R., *et al.* (2006). The epidemiology of panic attacks, panic disorder, and agoraphobia in the National Comorbidity Survey Replication. *Archives of General Psychiatry*, **63**, 415–424.

Klein, D. F. (1964). Delineation of two drug-responsive anxiety syndromes. *Psychopharmacology (Berlin)*, **5**, 346–354.

Klein, D. F. (1973). Drug therapy as a means of syndromal identification and nosological revision. In J. O. Cole, A. M. Freedman, & A. J. Friedhoff, eds., *Psychopathology and Psychopharmacology*. Baltimore, MD: Johns Hopkins University Press, pp. 143–160.

Klein, D. F. (1981) Anxiety reconceptualized. In D. F. Klein & J. Rabkin, eds., *Anxiety: New Research and Changing Concepts*. New York, NY: Raven Press, pp. 235–263.

Klein, D. F. (1993). False suffocation alarms, spontaneous panics, and related conditions: an integrative hypothesis. *Archives of General Psychiatry*, **50**, 306–317.

Klein, D. F. (1996). Panic disorder and agoraphobia: hypothesis hothouse. *Journal of Clinical Psychiatry*, **57** (Suppl. 6), 21–27.

Klein, D. F. (2000) Flawed metaanalyses comparing psychotherapy with pharmacotherapy. *American Journal of Psychiatry*, **157**, 1204–1211.

Klein, D. F. (2006). The flawed basis for FDA postmarketing safety decisions:the example of antidepressants and children. *Neuropsychopharmacology*, **31**, 689–699.

Klein, D. F., & Klein, H. M. (1989). The substantive effect of variations in panic measurement and agoraphobia definition. *Journal of Anxiety Disorders*, **3**, 45–46.

Klosko, J. S., Barlow, D. H., Tassinari, R., & Cerny, J. A. (1990). A comparison of alprazolam and behavior therapy in the treatment of panic disorder. *Journal of Consulting and Clinical Psychology*, **58**, 77–84.

Lecrubier, Y., Baker, A., Dunbar, G., & Judge, R. (1997). A comparison of paroxetine, clomipramine and placebo in the treatment of panic disorder. Collaborative Paroxetine Panic Study Investigators. *Acta Psychiatrica Scandinavia*, **95**, 145–152.

Liebowitz, M., Asnis, G., Tsanis, E., & Whitaker, T. (2004) A double blind placebo controlled trial of venlafaxine XR in the short term treatment of panic disorder. *European Neuropsychopharmacology*, **14** (Suppl. 3), s305–306.

Lydiard, R. B., Morton, W. A., Emmanuel, N. P., *et al.* (1993). Preliminary report: placebo controlled, double-blind study of the clinical and metabolic effects of desipramine in panic disorder. *Psychopharmacology Bulletin*, **29**, 183–188.

Mannuzza, S., Fyer, A. J., Liebowitz, M. R., & Klein, D. F. (1990). Delineating the boundaries of social phobia: Its relationship to panic disorder and agoraphobia. *Journal of Anxiety Disorders*, **4**, 41–59.

Marks. I. M., Swinson, R. P., Basoglu, M., *et al.* (1993). Alprazolam and exposure alone and combined in panic disorder with agoraphobia. *British Journal of Psychiatry*, **162**, 776–787.

Mavissakalian, M. R. (2003). Imipramine vs. sertraline in panic disorder: 24 week treatment completers. *Annals of Clinical Psychiatry*, **15**, 171–180.

Mavissakalian, M. R., & Perel, J. M. (1999) Long-term maintenance and discontinuation of imipramine therapy in panic disorder with agoraphobia. *Archives of General Psychiatry*, **56**, 821–827.

Mavissakalian, M. R., & Perel, J. M. (2002). Duration of imipramine therapy and relapse in panic disorder and agoraphobia. *Journal of Clinical Psychopharmacology*, **22**, 294–299.

McGrath, P. J., Quitkin, F. M., Klein, D. F. (1995). Bromocriptine treatment of relapses seen during selective serotonin re-uptake inhibitor treatment of depression. *Journal of Clinical Psychopharmacology*, **15**, 289–291.

McNally, R. J. (1994). *Panic Disorder: a Critical Analysis*. New York, NY: Guilford Press.

Michelson, D., Allgulander, C., Dantendorfer, K., *et al.* (2001). Efficacy of usual antidepressant dosing regimens in panic disorder: randomized, placebo controlled trial. *British Journal of Psychiatry*, **179**, 514–518.

Mitte, K. (2005). A meta-analysis of the efficacy of psycho- and pharmacotherapy in panic disorder with and without agoraphobia. *Journal of Affective Disorders*, **88**, 27–45.

Modigh, K., Westberg, P., & Eriksson, E. (1992). Superiority of clomipramine over imipramine in the treatment of panic disorder: a placebo-controlled trial. *Journal of Clinical Psychopharmacology*, **12**, 251–261.

Nadiga, D. N., Hensley, P. L., & Uhlenuth, E. H. (2003). Review of the long-term effectiveness of cognitive behavioral therapy compared to medications in panic disorder. *Depression and Anxiety*, **17**, 58–64.

Ninan, P. T. (1997). Issues in the assessment of treatment response in panic disorder with special reference to fluvoxamine. *Journal of Clinical Psychiatry*, **58** (Suppl. 5), 24–31.

Öst, L.-G. (1987). Applied relaxation: description of a coping technique and review of controlled studies. *Behaviour Research and Therapy*, **25**, 397–409.

Öst, L.-G., Westling, B. E., & Hellstrom, K. (1993). Applied relaxation, exposure in vivo and cognitive methods in the treatment of panic disorder with agoraphobia. *Behavior Research and Therapy*, **31**, 383–394.

Otto, M. W., Pollack, M. H., Sachs, G. S., *et al.* (1993). Discontinuation of benzodiazepine treatment: efficacy of cognitive–behavioral therapy for patients with panic disorder. *American Journal of Psychiatry*, **150**, 1485–1490.

Otto, M. W., Tuby, K. S., Gould, R. A., Mclean, R. Y. S., & Pollack, M. H. (2001). An effect-size analysis of the relative efficacy and tolerability of serotonin selective reuptake inhibitors for panic disorder. *American Journal of Psychiatry*, **158**, 1989–1992.

Otto, M. W., Hong, J. J., & Safran, S. A. (2002). Benzodiazepine discontinuation difficulties in panic disorder: conceptual model and outcome for cognitive behavioral therapy. *Current Pharmaceutical Design*, **8**, 75–80.

Otto, M. W., Bruce, S. E., & Deckersbach, T. (2005). Benzodiazepine use, cognitive impairment, and cognitive behavioral therapy for anxiety disorders: issues in the treatment of a patient in need. *Journal of Clinical Psychiatry*, **66** (Suppl. 2), 34–38.

Pollack, M. H. (2002). New advances in the management of anxiety disorders. *Psychopharmacology Bulletin*, **36** (4 Suppl.), 79–94.

Pollack, M. H., Worthington, J. J., & Otto, M. W. (1996). Venlafaxine for panic disorder: results from a double-blind, placebo controlled study. *Psychopharmacology Bulletin*, **32**, 667–670.

Pollack, M. H., Otto, M. W., Worthington, J. J., Manfro, G. G., & Wolkow, R. (1998). Sertraline in the treatment of panic disorder. *Archives of General Psychiatry*, **55**, 1010–1016.

Pollack, M. H., Simon, N. M., & Worthington, J. J. (2003). Combined paroxetine and clonazepam treatment strategies compared to paroxetine monotherapy for panic disorder. *Journal of Psychopharmacology*, **17**, 276–282.

Pollack, M. H., Lepola, U., Koponen, H., *et al.* (2007a). A double blind study of the efficacy of venlafaxine extended release, paroxetine, and placebo in the treatment of panic disorder. *Depression and Anxiety*, **24**, 1–14.

Pollack, M., Mangano, R., Entsuah, R., Tzanis, E., & Simon, N. M. (2007b). A randomized controlled trial of venlafaxine ER and paroxetine in the treatment of outpatients with panic disorder. *Psychopharmacology*, **194**, 233–242.

Rapaport, M. H., Wolkow, R., Rubin, A., *et al.* (2001). Sertraline treatment of panic disorder: Results of a long term study. *Acta Psychiatrica Scandinavica*, **104**, 289–298.

Rickels, K., Schweizer, E., Weiss, S., & Zavodnick, S. (1993). Maintenance drug treatment of panic disorder. II. Short and long term outcome after drug taper. *Archives of General Psychiatry*, **50**, 61–68.

Rosenbaum, J. F., Moroz, G., & Bowden, C. L. (1997). Clonazepam in the treatment of panic disorder with or without agoraphobia: a dose response study of efficacy, safety and discontinuance. *Journal of Clinical Psychopharmacology*, **17**, 390–400.

Schweizer, E., Patterson, W., & Rickels, K. (1993) Double blind, placebo controlled study of a once-a-day, sustained-release preparation of alprazolam for the treatment of panic disorder. *American Journal of Psychiatry*, **150**, 1210–1215.

Sharp, D. M., Power, K. G., & Simpson, R. J. (1996). Fluvoxamine, placebo and cognitive behavioral therapy used alone and in combination in the treatment of panic disorder and agoraphobia. *Journal of Anxiety Disorders*, **10**, 219–242.

Sheehan, D. V., Ballenger, J., & Jacobsen, G. (1980). Treatment of endogenous anxiety with phobic, hysterical and hypochondriacal symptoms. *Archives of General Psychiatry*, **37**, 51–59.

Sheehan, D. V., Burnham, D. B., Iyengar, M. K., Perera, P. (2005). Efficacy and tolerability of controlled release paroxetine in the treatment of panic disorder. *Journal of Clinical Psychiatry*, **66**, 34–40.

Shear, M. K., Brown, T. A., Barlow, D. H., *et al.* (1997). Multicenter collaborative panic disorder severity scale. *American Journal of Psychiatry*, **154**, 1571–1575.

Shear, M. K., Frank, E., Rucci, P., *et al.* (2001a). Panic-agoraphobic spectrum: reliability and validity of assessment instruments. *Journal of Psychiatric Research*, **35**, 59–66.

Shear, M. K., Rucci, P., Williams, J., *et al.* (2001b). Reliability and validity of Panic Disorder Severity Scale: replication and extension. *Journal of Psychiatric Research*, **35**, 293–296.

Simon, N. M., Safren, S. A., Otto, M. W., *et al.* (2002). Longitudinal outcome with pharmacotherapy in a naturalistic study of panic disorder. *Journal of Affective Disorders*, **69**, 201–208.

Soumerai, S. B., Simoni-Wastila, L., & Singer, C. (2003). Lack of relationship between long-term use of benzodiazepines and escalation to high dosages. *Psychiatric Services*, **54**, 1006–1011.

Spiegel, D. A., & Bruce, T. J. (1997). Benzodiazepines and exposure-based cognitive behavior therapies for panic disorder: conclusions from combined treatment trials. *American Journal of Psychiatry*, **154**, 773–781.

Spiegel, D. A., Bruce, T. J., Gregg, S. F., & Nuzzarello, A. (1994) Does cognitive behavioral therapy assist slow taper discontinuation in panic disorder? *American Journal of Psychiatry*, **151**, 876–881.

Stahl, S. M., Gergel, I., & Li, D. (2003). Escitalopram in the treatment of panic disorder: a randomized, double-blind, placebo controlled trial. *Journal of Clinical Psychiatry*, **54**, 1322–1327.

Susman, J. S., & Klee, B. (2005). The role of high potency benzodiazepines in the treatment of panic disorder. Primary care companion. *Journal of Clinical Psychiatry*, **7**, 5–11.

Tesar, G. E., Rosenbaum, J. E., Pollack, M. H., *et al.* (1991). Double blind, placebo controlled comparison of clonazepam and alprazolam for panic disorder. *Journal of Clinical Psychiatry*, **52**, 69–76.

Tiller, J. W., Bouwer, C., & Behnke, K. (1999). Moclobemide and fluoxetine for panic disorder. International Panic Disorder Study Group. *European Archives of Psychiatry and Clinical Neuroscience*, **249** (Suppl. 1), S7–10.

Uhlenhuth, E. H., Balter, M. B., Ban, T. A., & Yang, K. (1999). International study of expert judgment on therapeutic use of benzodiazepines and other psychotherapeutic medications, VI: trends in recommendations for the pharmacotherapy of anxiety disorders, 1992–1997. *Depression and Anxiety*, **9**, 107–116.

van Apeldoorn, F. J., van Hout, W. J. P. J., Mersch, P. P. A., *et al.* (2008). Is a combined therapy more effective than either CBT or SSRI alone? Results of a multicenter trial on panic disorder with or without agoraphobia. *Acta Psychiatrica Scandinavia*, **117**, 260–270.

van Vliet, I. M., Den Boer, J. A., Westenberg, H. G., & Slaap, B. R. (1996). A double-blind comparative study of brofaromine and fluvoxamine in outpatients with panic disorder. *Journal of Clinical Psychopharmacology*, **16**, 299–306.

Wade, A. G., Lepola, U., & Koponen, H. J. (1997). The effect of citalopram in panic disorder. *British Journal of Psychiatry*, **170**, 549–553.

Weissman, M. M., Klerman, G. L., Markowitz, J. S., & Ouellette, R. (1989) Suicidal ideation and suicide attempts in panic disorder and attacks. *New England Journal of Medicine*, **31**, 1209–1214.

Westen, D., & Morisson, K. (2001). A multidimensional meta-analysis of treatments for depression, panic and generalized anxiety disorder: an empirical examination of the status of empirically supported therapies. *Journal of Consulting and Clinical Psychiatry*, **69**, 875–899.

Wilkinson, G., Balestrieri, M., Ruggeri, M., & Bellantuono, C. (1991). Meta-analysis of double-blind placebo controlled trials of antidepressants and benzodiazepines for patients with panic disorders. *Psychological Medicine*, **21**, 991–998.

Chapter 26

Treatment of late-life generalized anxiety disorder

Laszlo A. Papp, Ethan E. Gorenstein, Jan Mohlman

26.1 Introduction

Patients with generalized anxiety disorder (GAD) suffer from "excessive anxiety and worry" that is difficult to control for at least six months (DSM-IV-TR: American Psychiatric Association 2000). They experience motor tension, autonomic hyperactivity, and hypervigilance. GAD is a highly disabling illness, often complicated by multiple comorbidities, most commonly depression and other anxiety disorders (Papp 2010). Comorbid GAD is common in psychiatric and medical conditions, and it is associated with substantially increased disability and medical cost (Kessler *et al.* 1999). The prominent somatic symptoms of GAD lead many patients to seek help first from non-mental-health specialists (Papp 2004). The GAD diagnosis is often missed or delayed, and, if correctly diagnosed, the condition frequently remains untreated. Even with adequate treatment, partial response with residual symptoms is common, and relapse rates are high (Yonkers *et al.* 2000).

GAD is also one of the most common anxiety disorders in late life, with a prevalence of 7% in the community (Beekman *et al.* 1998). The severe disability associated with late-life GAD is comparable to, but independent of, the frequently comorbid depression (Kessler *et al.* 1999). Still, effective and acceptable treatments for late-life GAD are lacking (Flint 2005). In addition to GAD, the rate of significant anxiety problems or "anxiety syndromes" that do not reach the threshold of an anxiety disorder may be as high as 20% among the elderly (Sheikh 1991). This chapter will focus on the specific problems encountered in treating late-life GAD. Treatment guidelines for GAD in the general adult population are briefly presented for the purpose of comparison.

26.2 Treatment of adults with generalized anxiety disorder

Both psychotherapy and pharmacotherapy have been found effective in randomized controlled clinical trials for patients with GAD. Given their comparable efficacy, a non-pharmacological treatment is usually preferable and also is favored by most patients (Riedel-Heller *et al.* 2005). However, those who view their GAD as a "medical," non-psychiatric condition are more likely to choose medications over psychotherapy.

Cognitive–behavioral therapy (CBT) is the most well-established psychotherapy for GAD (Lang 2004). Approximately one-half of the patients completing this relatively short-term (typically 12-week) manualized treatment are considered responders (Hunot *et al.* 2007). As detailed later in this chapter, the most common elements of CBT are didactic information about anxiety and instruction in self-monitoring of anxiety, relaxation training, imaginal relaxation, cognitive therapy, worry behavior prevention, problem solving, and gradual exposure to anxiety-provoking stimuli (Butler *et al.* 1987, Deberry *et al.* 1989, Gorenstein *et al.* 1999).

Several medications with varied pharmacology and mechanisms of action seem effective for approximately one-half to two-thirds of patients (Hidalgo *et al.* 2007). The relatively few head-to-head comparative medication trials have rarely shown differential efficacy, so the choice among the many efficacious agents is usually made based on potential side effects and individual patient characteristics (Papp 1999).

Combining CBT with pharmacotherapy is a common clinical practice in the treatment of most anxiety disorders. Study findings of the value of this strategy are mixed. The conclusion of one review (Westra & Stewart 1998) was that combined therapy has no clear

Anxiety Disorders: Theory, Research, and Clinical Perspectives, ed. Helen Blair Simpson, Yuval Neria, Roberto Lewis-Fernández, Franklin Schneier. Published by Cambridge University Press. © Cambridge University Press 2010.

advantage over CBT alone. Combined therapy may be more justified, however, in conditions where CBT produces only limited benefits. As described below, rather than starting with "mandated" combined treatment, we advocate a flexible model that begins with CBT and, after a few weeks, gives patients the option to add pharmacotherapy or to continue with CBT alone. This flexible model is also preferable because adding a second treatment only upon evidence of inadequate response to the first may spare patients from burdens of a potentially unnecessary combination.

26.3 Pharmacotherapy

Benzodiazepines, the traditional pharmacological option for GAD, have been gradually replaced by antidepressants as first-line anxiolytics. Long-term use of benzodiazepines can be problematic, and relapse rate upon discontinuation is high. Nevertheless, they can be useful when the need for immediate benefits outweighs their risks, which include development of tolerance, emergence of withdrawal symptoms when lowering the dose, and cognitive impairment. They are also useful when the side effects of the alternatives, such as antidepressants, are unacceptable (e.g., weight gain, sexual dysfunction). Data do not support the advantage of any one benzodiazepine over the others, and clinical response does not correlate with dose or plasma level. A daily equivalent of 15–25 mg of diazepam in divided doses is usually sufficient to relieve most symptoms in the majority of GAD patients. Both somatic and, to a lesser extent, psychic anxiety symptoms respond within the first week of treatment. Tolerance to the sedative effects of benzodiazepines develops quickly, but the anti-anxiety effect of a given dose is usually well maintained over time.

The 5-HT$_{1A}$ agonist buspirone was promoted as an alternative to benzodiazepines, but clinical experience has been disappointing (Enkelmann 1991). While buspirone is safe and less likely to induce drowsiness than benzodiazepines, the initial side effects of nausea, dizziness, and gastrointestinal irritation may be problematic. The onset of action is delayed for an average of 4–5 weeks, effect sizes are relatively low, and dropout rates are high in buspirone trials for GAD (Gould et al. 1997). Due to the fact that buspirone, like the benzodiazepines, does not have established antidepressant effects, comorbid or emergent depressive symptoms should further justify the use of antidepressants. The theory that GAD may represent a prodromal state toward major depressive disorder, or alternatively, that GAD and major depressive disorder may represent different symptomatic expressions of the same underlying pathophysiological condition (Andrews et al. 2008), while controversial, would also argue for antidepressants as preventive treatment.

In the absence of contraindications, the currently recommended first-line medication is a selective serotonin reuptake inhibitor (SSRI), with or without as-needed benzodiazepines or beta-blockers to provide immediate benefits during the 4–5 weeks until the antidepressant becomes effective. In spite of side effects such as agitation, nausea, and anorexia or weight gain, some argue that SSRIs may be superior to all other existing anti-anxiety medications. SSRIs seem to improve both psychic and somatic symptoms of GAD (Davidson et al. 2005).

There is strong evidence that the serotonin–norepinephrine reuptake inhibitor (SNRI) venlafaxine is also efficacious for GAD. While it resembles cyclic antidepressants, venlafaxine is largely devoid of anticholinergic and cardiovascular side effects. The reported elevation in blood pressure is less likely on low doses (Thase 1998), and the initial nausea usually responds to more gradual dose increase. Venlafaxine has also outperformed buspirone and placebo (Entsuah et al. 1998). The SNRI duloxetine has also received US Food and Drug Administration (FDA) approval for GAD indication.

SSRIs and SNRIs have replaced tricyclic (and heterocyclic) antidepressants (TCAs) with proven efficacy for GAD as first-line agents. Increased initial anxiety seen with TCAs may be related to their other side effects such as dry mouth, constipation, sedation, and positional hypotension. Typical and atypical antipsychotics, given their serious side effects (movement and metabolic disorders) and unproven benefits for GAD, should be strictly limited to use by expert psychopharmacologists for the most serious and treatment-resistant cases (Leucht et al. 2009).

26.4 Pharmacotherapy for late-life GAD

Pharmacotherapy for older patients requires both flexibility and creativity. These patients tend to be highly sensitive to the physiological and psychological effects of medications; many take multiple agents, and the addition and discontinuation of psychoactive medications complicate their already complex medical management. Treatment resistance is common;

older patients are reluctant to add new medications to their already complicated regimen, and many do not even fill their prescriptions (Frank & Kupfer 2003). The presence of an anxiety disorder only increases their resistance to altering an already complex regimen for chronic physical conditions. Patient education, including specific cognitive–behavioral strategies (e.g., fostering choice, control, etc.), could significantly improve adherence and consequently improve the efficacy of pharmacotherapy (Papp 2007).

As a general precaution, any medication use in the elderly should contain a number of special provisions. First, because memory impairment and confusion may affect adherence (Mohlman 2005), clear instructions, simplified drug regimens, and reminders of drug adherence should be included. Second, because most anxiolytics are associated with neurocognitive side effects, regular assessment of cognitive functions is essential throughout treatment (Mohlman & Gorman 2005). Third, due to significantly altered drug metabolism and an increased potential for toxicity, the principle of "starting low and going slow" should be observed, while also making allowance for great flexibility in dosing. Fourth, given that non-psychiatric medical and psychiatric comorbidity are both more common and more complex in the elderly compared to the general population, close attention to initial assessment and ongoing monitoring of comorbid conditions is particularly important.

Pharmacotherapy remains the most widely used treatment for managing late-life anxiety (Gorenstein et al. 1997). Use of anxiolytic drugs increases with age (Salzman 1985, Rifkin 1989). Earlier surveys showed that as many as 20% of the non-institutionalized elderly and 30% of the medically hospitalized elderly were using benzodiazepines (Shaw & Opit 1976, Salzman 1991). More recent data have suggested that current prevalence of benzodiazepine use has declined to about 10%, frequently only on an as-needed basis, and probably subtherapeutic and below the recommended dose (Hanlon et al. 1998). Less frequent use of anxiolytics may reflect a trend of switching to less effective and more problematic drugs (Krasucki et al. 1999), but more likely it is due to the general acceptance and use of novel antidepressants (Salzman et al. 2001).

Findings in younger, mixed-age adult populations are used to guide treatment of GAD in older adults under age 65. These studies suggest that older patients under the age of 65 are not that different from younger adults with respect to pharmacodynamics and pharmacokinetics. Therefore, recommended doses for patients under the age of 65 are comparable to those for younger adults.

Data from medication trials in late-life depression, while also not extensive, are informative as well (Charney et al. 2003). It seems that cyclic antidepressants have only limited utility in the elderly; the associated anticholinergic side effects may result in tachycardia and/or cardiac conduction delay in addition to urinary hesitancy or retention, constipation, and cognitive impairment. Cyclic antidepressants are also associated with falls and cerebrovascular insufficiency secondary to orthostatic hypotension (Richelson 1993). Trazodone may be better tolerated, but it may exacerbate pre-existing ventricular irritability (Pohl et al. 1986) and it can induce priapism and orthostatic hypotension (Ellison et al. 1990).

The literature on the pharmacologic management of anxiety in older patients is fairly meager (Papp 1999, Lenze et al. 2005). Benzodiazepines have established efficacy in anxious elderly patients (Salzman 1991). The undisputed benefits of benzodiazepine treatment include rapid onset, effective symptom relief, wide margin of safety, and relative absence of side effects. Due to concerns about dependence, withdrawal, and cognitive impairment, utilization is declining, but benzodiazepines remain the most frequently used anxiolytic drugs in the elderly. While claims of benzodiazepine-induced amnesia, memory impairment due to chronic use, and increased incidence of hip fractures in the elderly have been challenged (Lucki et al. 1986, Gorenstein et al. 1994, Hanlon et al. 1998, Wang et al. 2001), the long-term use of benzodiazepines in the elderly remains controversial.

As discussed above, the 5-HT$_{1A}$ agonist buspirone was considered an alternative to benzodiazepines, but its side effects (nausea, dizziness, and gastrointestinal irritation) are especially troublesome in the elderly. Antihistamines such as diphenhydramine and hydroxyzine are also used as alternatives. The side effects of excessive daytime sedation, irritability, cognitive impairment, and ataxia, however, make these drugs particularly problematic in the elderly. Antihistamines can be lethal in overdose (Stoudemire & Moran 1993). Also as discussed earlier, antipsychotics are rarely justifiable for the treatment of GAD in general. They are even more problematic for the elderly (US Food and Drug Administration 2005), and are almost never indicated in the treatment of late-life GAD.

As noted above for younger adults, SSRIs have become first-line agents in the treatment of depression and in most anxiety disorders for the elderly as well. SSRIs are largely free of the adverse psychomotor and autonomic effects of TCAs, and they appear to be safer for the elderly. Paroxetine, the first SSRI with an indication for the treatment of GAD, has advantages for the elderly, including lack of initial agitation (Mulsant *et al.* 1999) and, surprisingly, relatively low risk of weight gain in GAD patients (Rocca *et al.* 1997). Citalopram is favored due to the virtual absence of drug–drug interactions, an important concern for the elderly with comorbid medical problems. Escitalopram, the active isomer of citalopram, seems better tolerated by the elderly (Burke *et al.* 2003), with better, or at least comparable, efficacy and fewer side effects (Goodman *et al.* 2005, Moore *et al.* 2005).

In the first controlled study of an SSRI in patients with late-life anxiety disorders, mainly GAD, citalopram was significantly more efficacious than placebo (Lenze *et al.* 2005). It was well tolerated; the only clinically significant side effect reported was sedation. Another recent study showed benefits of sertraline for anxiety in elderly patients (Schuurmans *et al.* 2006). Paroxetine had the highest incidence of discontinuation symptoms in comparison to sertraline and fluoxetine (Rosenbaum *et al.* 1998), while citalopram caused no meaningful discontinuation symptoms in patients switched to placebo after eight weeks of treatment (Markowitz *et al.* 2000).

In the most recent large-scale, randomized controlled trial of an SSRI in late-life GAD, 177 patients age 60 or older were randomized to 12 weeks of escitalopram 10–20 mg per day or placebo (Lenze *et al.* 2009). In the completer analysis, the response rate to escitalopram (69%) was significantly greater than that of placebo (51%), and escitalopram treatment resulted in greater improvement in anxiety symptoms and role functioning. Escitalopram was well tolerated, with only a 3% rate of dropout due to adverse effects. However, the intent-to-treat analysis showed no significant difference in response rates between escitalopram and placebo, demonstrating again that older patients benefit less from treatments that have proven efficacy for younger populations.

Venlafaxine is also well tolerated by the elderly (Schatzberg 2000): effect sizes in older and younger GAD patients seem comparable (Katz *et al.* 2002), and 90% of responders who continued taking the extended-release version were able to control GAD for six months (Gelenberg *et al.* 2000, Sheehan 2001). As a dual-mechanism agent, venlafaxine may be particularly advantageous in patients with comorbid GAD and depression (Silverstone & Ravindran 1999). Our own experience with venlafaxine in late-life GAD is limited but promising (Papp *et al.* 1998). Several of our elderly patients respond to low-dose venlafaxine with only mild, transient side effects. Given its similarity to venlafaxine and preliminary evidence of a favorable side effect profile, duloxetine, the second marketed SNRI in the USA, may be a good choice as well.

26.5 Psychosocial treatment

CBT is the best-supported psychosocial treatment for anxiety disorders in younger adults, as well as the best potential alternative to medications. Basic principles and techniques, described below, are similar across age cohorts (Table 26.1). Elements and modules are emphasized and tailored for specific age groups and symptoms. Treatment manuals have been developed, and studies are ongoing to test their efficacy and identify necessary and sufficient components.

Psychosocial treatments have many advantages over pharmacotherapy in older patients (see above), and studies have begun to examine the efficacy and acceptability of CBT for late-life GAD (Stanley *et al.* 1996, 2003, Mohlman *et al.* 2003, Wetherell *et al.* 2003, Gorenstein *et al.* 2005). These studies consistently demonstrate improvement, but caveats apply. First, standard CBT is about 50% more effective for younger adults than it is for the elderly. Second, unlike younger adults, older patients do not show significantly better response to group-administered CBT than to supportive psychotherapy (Stanley *et al.* 1996). Third, over a third of the patients drop out, and less than a third of the completers show clinically significant improvement. In sum, existing biological and psychosocial methods of treating anxiety, although effective for younger adults, are lacking when applied to the elderly. Novel approaches are required to meet their needs.

26.5.1 Cognitive–behavioral therapy for late-life GAD

We designed and published an enhanced and modified late-life-specific form of CBT (Gorenstein *et al.* 1999). In addition to the standard components (relaxation training, cognitive restructuring, behavioral skills training, in-vivo exposure), it also includes (1) specialized cognitive–behavioral guidelines for managing anxiety due to physical conditions and coping with

Table 26.1. Modules in CBT for late-life GAD

Module	Description
Psychoeducation and awareness module	Explanation of tripartite model of anxiety (physiological, cognitive, and behavioral components); treatment principles and procedure; self-monitoring of symptoms; charting of numerical mood ratings; weekly reading assignments
Relaxation skills	Training in slow, diaphragmatic breathing and progressive deep muscle relaxation
Cognitive skills	Role of thinking in anxiety (thoughts as hypotheses, logical errors, alternative explanations with emphasis on health/medical anxiety, adaptive/rational self-statements, thought stopping)
Behavioral skills	Daily schedule/structure; worry behavior prevention; problem solving; regular social activity (senior center, volunteer job, continuing education, etc.); sleep hygiene; problem solving (contingencies of old age, potential disability and/or death [spouse or self])
Skills application	Monitoring progress and follow-up of all modules; in-vivo exposure (counter-conditioning model); hierarchy construction; graduated exposure
Final sessions	Summary of therapeutic principles, plans for maintaining gains, and continued practice
Maintenance CBT	Seven sessions over six months; written self-monitoring is reviewed, skills, applications updated

medical/physical comorbidity; (2) problem-solving approaches for increasing social support and social involvement to counter social isolation; (3) daily activity structuring to address idleness, which can contribute to anxiety; (4) problem solving to address anxiety over contingencies of old age, such as potential disability and/or death (spouse or self).

Since publishing our initial CBT protocol for general dissemination, we have added other features designed to increase homework adherence, strengthen memory, and facilitate use of techniques. The methods include (1) weekly reading assignments in a CBT workbook, (2) graphing exercises in which patients chart numerical mood ratings at each session, (3) midweek phone calls for the first four weeks to facilitate homework adherence, (4) written summaries of session content and assignments following each therapy session, and (5) a homework adherence requirement of no more than three missed assignments. The enhancements boosted response rate by about 35% (Mohlman *et al.* 2003).

26.5.2 Flexible, multimodal treatments

We tested another version of CBT for late-life GAD, specifically designed for patients who wanted to decrease their medication use (Gorenstein *et al.* 1999). Its components were (1) training in relaxation/breathing, (2) cognitive restructuring, (3) behavioral skills training (including worry behavior prevention, problem solving, and daily structure), (4) naturalistic exposure, (5) withdrawal management skills training, and (6) sleep hygiene training.

Forty-three patients over age 65 who desired to discontinue anxiolytic treatment of GAD were randomized to taper of anxiolytics with medical management alone or with augmentation of medical management by 13 weeks of CBT. Patients who deteriorated clinically discontinued taper and were re-stabilized on their anxiolytic. This study showed that the addition of CBT resulted in more improvement in anxiety and depression compared to medication management alone. CBT responders were significantly more likely to discontinue medication than CBT non-responders. Half of the patients receiving CBT to help taper off anxiolytics, however, ultimately chose to continue on medication (Gorenstein *et al.* 2005). Some of the non-responders to CBT increased their doses.

We are currently studying flexible approaches to combining CBT and pharmacotherapy treatments as an initial treatment for late-life GAD. Given elderly anxiety patients' apprehension about medication, a combined treatment that entails an initial trial with CBT alone seems particularly appropriate. In a group of 30 consecutive elderly respondents to our generic advertisements for "anxiety treatment," all preferred psychotherapy over medication as the initial treatment. However, this resistance was not absolute. We also found that these patients were more likely to accept pharmacotherapy if their initial preference was considered and addressed during the treatment process.

Accordingly, in our current, manualized, modular CBT protocol, the emphasis is on patient choice among treatment modalities. The components of the CBT are delivered in dedicated sessions, with follow-up procedures specified for each module. The clinician may alter the ordering of the modules while maintaining a clinical checklist to insure that all components of all modules are completed. Optimally, patients attend two sessions per week for the first four weeks and one session per week for the next eight weeks, for a total of 16 sessions over 12 weeks. The integrated illness model (psychological and biological) as the theoretical basis of both treatments is presented before the first CBT session, and the option to add medication later is discussed. After the first eight sessions of CBT, the medication option is revisited.

A prerequisite for successfully combining CBT with medication in a flexible, multimodal treatment model is the presentation of an integrated view of the illness at the very beginning of the treatment. Both biological and psychological theories and manifestations should be discussed, conveying that the two perspectives are not mutually exclusive, but rather complementary, and that addressing both can be beneficial. Misperceptions and biases, potential side effects of medications, and pros and cons of CBT versus adding or tapering medication should be addressed. It is important to convey "therapeutic equipoise," to explain that the therapist does not have an allegiance to either approach and to create an atmosphere of support rather than persuasion.

The discussion should include available data/information on the expected outcome of continued CBT following full or partial response to acute CBT, the anticipated likelihood of success if CBT is supplemented or replaced with medication, as well as the potential benefits of tapering medication with the help of targeted CBT. Significant leeway should be given to the patient in deciding the sequence and timing of these interventions (e.g., medication can be introduced before, during, or after CBT; medication taper should be tailored and flexible; frequency and content of CBT sessions can vary; etc.). In all cases, the patient should make the final choice.

26.6 Summary and treatment guidelines

The treatment of GAD is challenging in general, and particularly in the elderly. Given the comparable efficacy of psychotherapy and/or medications, both are reasonable alternatives for most patients. In choosing and implementing treatment, flexibility is key; considering the preference of patients can significantly improve the outcome. A modular, multimodal approach that begins with CBT and offers optional pharmacotherapy seems to appeal to most patients and addresses the high dropout rates reported in studies with mandated treatment assignments.

With this in mind, after ruling out "organic" abnormalities (e.g., cardiovascular, gastrointestinal,

neurological, etc.), treatment selection should be based on several factors, including comorbidity (both psychiatric and medical), prior treatments, course, family history, personality disorders/traits, and very importantly, patient's choice and need for control. Since GAD is a chronic, frequently lifelong condition, treatment should probably be continued indefinitely but perhaps intermittently. Intermittent, brief treatments may prove to be the best long-term strategy (Rickels & Schweitzer 1998). In all pharmacotherapy, the lowest dosage of medication that controls the patient's symptoms should be prescribed. Slow, gradual taper of medication may be attempted after one year in symptom-free patients (Rickels & Schweizer 1990). Recurrence should be re-treated promptly. Treatments of longer duration seem to confer the benefits of improved functioning, fewer residual symptoms, and lower relapse rates, but it is unknown whether the type of treatment (i.e., pharmacological, psychological, or the combination of the two) matters in conferring the long-term benefits.

Patients with predominantly somatic symptoms and/or early-onset GAD may require ongoing pharmacotherapy, while those with primarily excessive worry and/or late-onset GAD may be better controlled by regularly practiced CBT techniques. Insomnia is a frequent symptom of GAD and should be addressed specifically, either by selecting a sedating antidepressant given at bedtime or a hypnotic like zolpidem and/or by adding the "sleep hygiene" module of a CBT package. Because it is not known what is required for the proper long-term clinical management of GAD, patients who have responded to either CBT or medication should be scheduled for follow-up appointments at increasing intervals in order to continually monitor the course of illness.

CBT could be augmented with as-needed benzodiazepines (e.g., lorazepam, alprazolam, clonazepam) and/or beta-blockers (e.g., propranolol, atenolol) to facilitate exposure and to tone down autonomic arousal, but, because of their wider therapeutic range, antidepressants are generally more beneficial than benzodiazepines.

References

American Psychiatric Association (2000). *Diagnostic and Statistical Manual of Mental Disorders*, 4th edn, text revision (DSM-IV-TR). Washington, DC: American Psychiatric Association.

Andrews, G., Anderson, T. M., Slade, T., & Sunderland, M. (2008). Classification of anxiety and depressive disorders: problems and solutions. *Depression and Anxiety*, **25**, 274–281.

Beekman, A. T., Bremmer, M. A., Deeg, D. J., *et al.* (1998). Anxiety disorders in later life: a report from the Longitudinal Aging Study Amsterdam. *International Journal of Geriatric Psychiatry*, **13**, 717–726.

Burke, W. J., de Swart, J., & Rothschild, T. (2003). Safety of escitalopram in the treatment of elderly patients. Paper presented at the Annual Meeting of the American Association for Geriatric Psychiatry, Honolulu, Hawaii, March 2003.

Butler, G., Cullington, A., Hibbut, G., Klimes, I., & Gelder, M. (1987). Anxiety management for persistent generalized anxiety. *British Journal of Psychiatry*, **151**, 535–542.

Charney, D. S., Reynolds, C. F., & Lewis, L. (2003). Depression and bipolar support alliance consensus statement on the unmet needs in diagnosis and treatment of mood disorder in late life. *Archives of General Psychiatry*, **60**, 664–672.

Davidson, J., Bose, A., & Wang, Q. (2005). Safety and efficacy of escitalopram in the long term treatment of generalized anxiety disorder. *Journal of Clinical Psychiatry*, **66**, 1441–1446.

Deberry, S., Davis, S., & Reinhard, K. E. (1989). A comparison of meditation relaxation and cognitive/behavioral techniques for reducing anxiety and depression in a geriatric population. *Journal of Geriatric Psychiatry*, **22**, 231–247.

Ellison, J. M., Milofsky, J. E., & Ely, E. (1990). Fluoxetine-induced bradycardia and syncope in two patients. *Journal of Clinical Psychiatry*, **51**, 385–386.

Enkelmann, R. (1991). Alprazolam versus buspirone in the treatment of outpatients with generalized anxiety disorder. *Psychopharmacology*, **105**, 428–432.

Entsuah, R., Derivan, A. T., Haskins, T., *et al.* (1998). Double-blind placebo-controlled study of once daily venlafaxine extended release and buspirone. New Research Program and Abstract of the Annual Meeting of the American Psychiatric Association, June 1998, Toronto, Canada. NR644: 241.

Flint, A. J. (2005). Generalized anxiety disorder in elderly patients: epidemiology, diagnosis and treatment options. *Drugs and Aging*, **22**, 101–14

Frank, E., & Kupfer, D. J. (2003). Progress in the therapy of mood disorders: scientific support. *American Journal of Psychiatry*, **160**, 1277–1285.

Gelenberg, A. J., Lydiard, R. B., Rudolph, R. L., *et al.* (2000). Efficacy of venlafaxine extended-release capsules in nondepressed outpatients with generalized anxiety disorder: a six-month randomized controlled trial. *JAMA*, **283**, 3082–3088.

Goodman, W. K., Bose, A., & Wang, Q. (2005). Treatment of generalized anxiety disorder with escitalopram: pooled results from double-blind, placebo-controlled trials. *Journal of Affective Disorders*, **87**, 161–167.

Gorenstein, C., Bernik, M. A., & Pompeia, S. (1994). Differential acute psychomotor and cognitive effects of diazepam on long-term benzodiazepine users. *International Clinical Psychopharmacolpgy*, **9**, 145–153.

Gorenstein, E. E., Papp, L. A., & Kleber, M. S. (1997). Psychosocial treatment of benzodiazepine dependence and anxiety in later life. Paper presented at the 1997 Annual Meeting of the Association for Advancement of Behavior Therapy, Miami, FL.

Gorenstein, E. E., Papp, L. A., & Kleber, M. S. (1999). Cognitive–behavioral treatment of anxiety in later life. *Cognitive and Behavioral Practice*, **6**, 305–319.

Gorenstein, E. E., Papp, L. A., Kleber, M. S., *et al.* (2005). Cognitive–behavioral therapy for management of anxiety and medication taper in older adults. *American Journal of Geriatric Psychiatry*, **13**, 901–909

Gould, R. A., Otto, M. N., Pollack, M. H., & Yap, L. (1997). Cognitive behavioral and pharmacological treatment of generalized anxiety disorder: a preliminary meta-analysis. *Behavior Therapy*, **28**, 285–305.

Hanlon, J. T., Horner, R. D., Schmader, K. E., *et al.* (1998). Benzodiazepine use and cognitive function among community-dwelling elderly. *Clinical Pharmacology and Therapeutics*, **64**, 684–692.

Hidalgo, R. B., Tupler, L. A., & Davidson, J. R. (2007). An effect size analysis of pharmacologic treatments for generalized anxiety disorder. *Journal of Psychopharmacology*, **21**, 864–872.

Hunot, V., Churchill, R., Silva de Lima, M., & Teixeira, V. (2007). Psychological therapies for generalised anxiety disorder. *Cochrane Database of Systematic Reviews*, (1), CD001848.

Katz, R., Reynolds, C. F., Alexopoulos, G. S., & Hackett, D. (2002). Venlafaxine ER as a treatment for generalized anxiety disorder in older adults: pooled analysis of five randomized placebo-controlled clinical trials. *Journal of the American Geriatric Society*, **50**, 18–24.

Kessler, R. C., DuPont, R. L., Berglund, P., & Wittchen, H. (1999). Impairment in pure and comorbid generalized anxiety disorder and major depression at 12 months in two national surveys. *American Journal of Psychiatry*, **156**, 1915–1923.

Krasucki, C., Howard, R., & Mann, A. (1999). Anxiety and its treatment in the elderly. *International Psychogeriatrics*, **11**, 25–45.

Lang, A. J. (2004). Treating generalized anxiety disorder with cognitive behavioral therapy. *Journal of Clinical Psychiatry*, **65** (Suppl. 13), 14–19.

Lenze, E. J., Mulsant, B. H., Shear, M. K., *et al.* (2005). Efficacy and tolerability of citalopram in the treatment of late-life anxiety disorders: results from an 8-week randomized, placebo-controlled trial. *American Journal of Psychiatry*, **162**, 146–150.

Lenze, E. J., Rollman, B. L., Shear, M. K., *et al.* (2009). Escitalopram for older adults with generalized anxiety disorder: a randomized controlled trial. *JAMA*, **301**(3), 295–303.

Leucht, S., Corves, C., Arbter, D., *et al.* (2009). Second-generation versus first-generation antipsychotic drugs for schizophrenia: a meta-analysis. *Lancet*, **373**, 31–41.

Lucki, I., Rickels, K., & Geller, A. M. (1986). Chronic use of benzodiazepines and psychomotor and cognitive test performance. *Psychopharmacology*, **88**, 426–433.

Markowitz, J. S., DeVane, C. L., Liston, H. L., & Montgomery, S. A. (2000). An assessment of selective serotonin reuptake inhibitor discontinuation symptoms with citalopram. *International Clinical Psychopharmacology*, **15**, 329–333.

Mohlman, J. (2005). Does executive dysfunction affect treatment outcome in late-life mood and anxiety disorders? *Journal of Geriatric Psychiatry and Neurology*, **18**, 97–108.

Mohlman, J., & Gorman, J. M. (2005). The role of executive functioning in CBT: a pilot study with anxious older adults. *Behavior Research and Therapy*, **43**, 447–465.

Mohlman, J., Gorenstein, E. E., Kleber, M., *et al.* (2003). Standard and enhanced cognitive–behavior therapy for late-life generalized anxiety disorder: two pilot investigations. *American Journal of Geriatric Psychiatry*, **11**, 24–32.

Moore, N., Verdoux, H., & Fantino, B. (2005). Prospective, multicentre, randomized, double-blind study of the efficacy of escitalopram versus citalopram in outpatient treatment of major depressive disorder. *International Clinical Psychopharmacology*, **20**, 131–137.

Mulsant, B. H., Pollock, B. G., Nebes, R. D., *et al.* (1999). A double-blind randomized comparison of nortriptyline and paroxetine in the treatment of late-life depression: 6-week outcome. *Journal of Clinical Psychiatry*, **60** (Suppl. 20), 16–20.

Papp, L. A. (1999). Somatic treatment of anxiety disorders. In H. I. Kaplan & B. J. Sadock, eds., *Comprehensive Textbook of Psychiatry*, 7th edn. Baltimore, MD: Williams & Wilkins.

Papp, L. A. (2004). Generalized anxiety disorder: evaluation and treatment. In Spitzer & First (Eds.), *Treatment Companion to the DSM-IV-TR Case Book*. Washington DC: American Psychiatric Press.

Papp, L. A. (2007). Pharmacotherapy of stress and anxiety. In P. M. Lehrer, R. L. Woolfolk, & W. E. Sime, eds., *Principles and Practice of Stress Management*, 3rd edn. New York, NY: Guilford Press.

Papp, L. A. (2010). Phenomenology of generalized anxiety disorder. In D. J. Stein, E. Hollander, & B. O. Rothbaum, eds., *Textbook of Anxiety Disorders*, 2nd edn. Washington, DC: American Psychiatric Publishing.

Papp, L. A., Sinha, S. S., Martinez, J. M., *et al.* (1998). Low-dose venlafaxine treatment in panic disorder. *Psychopharmacology Bulletin*, **34**, 207–209.

Pohl, R., Bridges, M., & Rainey, J. M. (1986). Effects of trazodone and desipramine on cardiac rate and rhythm in a patient with preexisting cardiovascular disease. *Journal of Clinical Psychopharmacology*, **6**, 380–381.

Richelson, E. (1993). Review of antidepressants in the treatment of mood disorders. In D. L. Dunner, ed., *Current Psychiatric Therapy*. Philadelphia, PA: Saunders.

Rickels, K., & Schweizer, E. (1990). The clinical course and long-term management of generalized anxiety disorder. *Journal of Clinical Psychopharmacology*, **10** (3 Suppl.), 101S–110S.

Rickels, K., & Schweizer, E. (1998). The spectrum of generalized anxiety disorder in clinical practice: The role of short-term, intermittent treatment. *British Journal of Psychiatry*, **34**, 49–54.

Riedel-Heller, S. G., Matschinger, H., & Angermeyer, M. C. (2005). Mental disorders: who and what might help? Help-seeking and treatment preferences of the lay public. *Social Psychiatry and Psychiatric Epidemiology*, **40**, 176–174.

Rifkin, A. (1989). Benzodiazepine use and abuse by patients at outpatient clinics. *American Journal of Psychiatry*, **146**, 1331–1332.

Rocca, P., Fonzo, V., Scotta, M., Zanalda, E., & Ravizza, L. (1997). Paroxetine efficacy in the treatment of generalized anxiety disorder. *Acta Psychiatrica Scandinavia*, **95**, 444–450.

Rosenbaum, J. F., Fava, M., Hoog, S. L., Ascroft, R. C., & Krebs, W. B. (1998). Selective serotonin reuptake inhibitor discontinuation syndrome: a randomized clinical trial. *Biological Psychiatry*, **44**, 75–76.

Salzman, C. (1985). Geriatric psychopharmacology. *Annual Review of Medicine*, **36**, 217–228.

Salzman, C. (1991). Pharmacologic treatment of the anxious elderly patient. In C. Salzman & B. D. Lebowitz, eds., *Anxiety in the Elderly*. New York, NY: Springer.

Salzman, C., Goldenberg, I., Bruce, S. E., & Keller, M. B. (2001). Pharmacologic treatment of anxiety disorders in 1989 versus 1996: results from the Harvard/Brown Anxiety Disorders Research Program. *Journal of Clinical Psychiatry*, **62**, 149–152.

Schatzberg, A. F. (2000). Multicenter trials with Effexor. 13th European College of Neuropsychopharmacology (ECNP) Congress, Brussels.

Schuurmans, J., Comijs, H., Emmelkamp, P. M., *et al.* (2006) A randomized, controlled trial of the effectiveness of cognitive–behavioral therapy and sertraline versus a waitlist control group for anxiety disorders in older adults. *American Journal of Geriatric Psychiatry*, **14**, 255–263.

Shaw, S. M., & Opit, L. J. (1976). Need for supervision in the elderly receiving long-term prescribed medication. *British Medical Journal*, **1**, 505–507.

Sheehan, D. V. (2001). Attaining remission in generalized anxiety disorder: venlafaxine extended release comparative data. *Journal of Clinical Psychiatry*, **62** (Suppl. 19), 26–31.

Sheikh, J. I. (1991). Anxiety rating scales for the elderly. In C. Salzman & B. D. Lebowitz, eds., *Anxiety in the Elderly*. New York, NY: Springer.

Silverstone, P. H., & Ravindran, A. (1999). Once-daily venlafaxine extended release (XR) compared with fluoxetine in outpatients with depression and anxiety. Venlafaxine XR 360 Study Group. *Journal of Clinical Psychiatry*, **60**, 795–796.

Stanley, M. A., Beck, J. G., & Glassco, J. D. (1996). Treatment of generalized anxiety in older adults: a preliminary comparison of cognitive–behavioral and supportive approaches. *Behavior Therapy*, **27**, 565–581.

Stanley, M. A., Hopko, D. R., Diefenbach, G. J., *et al.* (2003). Cognitive–behavior therapy for late-life generalized anxiety disorder in primary care: preliminary findings, *American Jouranl of Geriatric Psychiatry*, **11**, 92–96.

Stoudemire, A., & Moran, M. G. (1993). Psychopharmacologic treatment of anxiety in the medically ill elderly patient: Special considerations. *Journal of Clinical Psychiatry*, **54** (Suppl.), 27–33.

Thase, M. E. (1998). Effects of venlafaxine on blood pressure: a meta-analysis of original data from 3744 depressed patients. *Journal of Clinical Psychiatry*, **59**, 502–508.

US Food and Drug Administration (2005). Public Health Advisory. Deaths with Antipsychotics in Elderly Patients with Behavioral Disturbances. www.fda.gov/Drugs/DrugSafety/PublicHealthAdvisories/UCM053171 (accessed February 2010).

Wang, P. S., Bohn, R. L., Glynn, R. J., Mogun, H., & Avorn, J. (2001). Hazardous benzodiazepine regimens in the elderly: effects of half-life, dosage, and duration on risk of hip fracture. *American Journal of Psychiatry*, **158**, 892–898.

Westra, H. A., & Stewart, S. H. (1998). Cognitive behavioural therapy and pharmacotherapy: complementary or contradictory approaches to the treatment of anxiety? *Clinical Psychology Review*, **18**, 307–340.

Wetherell, J. L., Gatz, M., & Craske, M. G. (2003). Treatment of generalized anxiety disorder in older adults. *Journal of Consulting & Clinical Psychology*, **71**, 31–40.

Yonkers, K. A., Dyck, I. R., Warshaw, M., & Keller, M. B. (2000). Factors predicting the clinical course of generalized anxiety disorder. *British Journal of Psychiatry*, **176**, 544–549.

Childhood anxiety disorders: best treatment options and practice

Hilary B. Vidair, Moira A. Rynn

27.1 Introduction

Growing up with an anxiety disorder that interferes with everyday life activities and enjoyment can be a painful and exhausting experience, both for the child and for his or her caregivers. Unfortunately, anxiety disorders often are not identified, and when they are, the most appropriate treatment may not be available or provided. It is necessary to differentiate developmentally appropriate childhood anxiety and the clinical presentation of impairing anxiety disorders. We provide a brief overview of how to identify normal from abnormal anxiety in childhood, review evidence-based treatment options, present our recommendations for best practice, and propose directions for future anxiety treatment research.

27.2 Child anxiety: what is normal and what is not

Most children experience some developmentally appropriate fear or worry. For example, many infants fear strangers or loud noises, while toddlers can be afraid of separation from their parents or of monsters. Five- and six-year-olds worry about their physical well-being, while school-age children are more concerned with school performance, social ability, natural events (e.g., hurricane), and illnesses (Muris *et al.* 1998a). In middle childhood, worries can multiply about a variety of issues, perhaps because children develop more complex cognitive abilities (Vasey *et al.* 1994). Adolescents' concerns usually focus on social competence and evaluation, independent functioning, and academic performance.

Anxiety becomes a clinical disorder when: (1) the child avoids age-appropriate activities (e.g., going to school or a party), (2) it interferes with developmentally appropriate functioning or challenges (e.g., playing with others or academic performance), (3) it causes the child and/or family a considerable amount of distress, and/or (4) when the child experiences impairing anxiety over a long period of time. Thus, when differentiating between non-clinical and clinical levels of child anxiety, we assess: (1) Does the fear relate to a specific situation or occur spontaneously? (2) Is the intensity of anxiety developmentally appropriate or disproportionate to the situation? (3) Is anxiety constant or increasing despite receiving reassurance?

Ten anxiety disorders are listed in DSM-IV-TR (American Psychiatric Association 2000). Nine – i.e., specific phobia (SP), generalized anxiety disorder (GAD), obsessive–compulsive disorder (OCD), social anxiety disorder (SAD, also known as social phobia), panic disorder (PD) with and without agorophobia, agorophobia without a history of PD, acute stress disorder, posttraumatic stress disorder (PTSD) – are common to both children and adults, while separation anxiety disorder (SepAD) is specific to children. One general criterion for anxiety disorders is that symptoms interfere with the child's functioning or cause clinically significant distress. The disorder must not be due to a medical condition or the physiological effects of a substance, and it must occur outside the confines of another disorder.

Like patterns of worry, anxiety disorders tend to follow a developmental progression. Younger children are more likely to experience SepAD, which involves excessive distress related to separating from a primary caregiver or leaving home. SP also tends to begin at a young age and includes fear of a particular animal, blood/injection/injury, natural environment (e.g., water, heights), situation (e.g., elevators), or other (e.g., vomiting, costumed characters). GAD is more common in school-age children and involves difficulty controlling excessive worry in several areas such as

Anxiety Disorders: Theory, Research, and Clinical Perspectives, ed. Helen Blair Simpson, Yuval Neria, Roberto Lewis-Fernández, Franklin Schneier. Published by Cambridge University Press. © Cambridge University Press 2010.

school, family, health, and peer interactions. OCD is also likely to begin in middle childhood and includes impairing, distressful, or time-consuming obsessions or compulsions.

SAD and PD are more likely to occur in adolescence. SAD includes a clear and persistent fear of being evaluated in social and performance situations, particularly with peers. PD includes repetitive, unexpected panic attacks with associated behavioral changes or concern about additional attacks and their implications. Finally, PTSD can occur only after experiencing, witnessing, or confronting a traumatic event with symptoms including repetitive, intrusive recollections; avoidance and numbing; and sleep disturbances.

Anxiety is the most common type of childhood disorder (Anderson *et al.* 1987), with prevalence rates ranging from 6% to 20% (e.g., Costello *et al.* 2004). For child and adolescent OCD, prevalence rates are between 0.5% and 2% (Barrett *et al.* 2008). PTSD prevalence rates vary depending on population, methodology, and type of traumatic event (American Academy of Child and Adolescent Psychiatry 1998) but have been found to be as high as 24–34.5% in urban communities (Breslau *et al.* 1991, Berman *et al.* 1996). Anxiety disorders can be chronic or remit, but those who have had one anxiety diagnosis often experience the onset of another anxiety disorder (Keller *et al.* 1992) as well as later problems including adult anxiety and depressive disorders (Pine *et al.* 1998), substance abuse/dependence (Compton *et al.* 2007), and suicidality (Boden *et al.* 2006).

27.3 Evidence-based treatments for child and adolescent anxiety

Cognitive–behavioral therapy (CBT), behavior therapy (BT), and medications have all been found to be effective for the treatment of childhood anxiety. CBT programs include a variety of techniques such as psychoeducation, somatic management, cognitive restructuring, problem solving, exposure, and relapse prevention (for descriptions, see Velting *et al.* 2004). Behavior therapy focuses predominantly on behavioral change via techniques such as imaginal and in-vivo exposure and social skills training rather than on the modification of maladaptive thoughts. Below is an overview of published randomized clinical trials (RCTs) through 2008, including CBT, BT, and psychopharmalogical treatments for child and adolescent anxiety disorders (see Table 27.1 for details, and

for studies of school refusal and alternative delivery modes, including the Internet and bibliotherapy). All studies reviewed compared treatment to a wait list, psychosocial or pill placebo, or other active treatment; crossover designs are excluded. All studies included participants who met DSM criteria for at least one anxiety disorder, with the exception of the PTSD studies, which included RCTs focused on trauma with at least 85% of the sample meeting PTSD criteria. No RCTs have assessed CBT, BT, or medication for PD, agoraphobia, or acute stress disorder.

27.3.1 Multiple anxiety disorders

27.3.1.1 CBT trials

Twenty-one RCTs assessed the effects of CBT or BT on a range of childhood anxiety disorders, most commonly GAD, SepAD, and SAD. These three disorders are often comorbid, occur in familial patterns, share comparable symptoms, and respond similarly to psychosocial and medication interventions (Velting *et al.* 2004). Twelve RCTs for these disorders compared individual, group, and/or family CBT to a wait list, and all indicated that CBT/BT was significantly more effective. Of these, five trials compared one active treatment to a wait list (Table 27.1).

Kendall and colleagues developed the first individual manualized CBT treatment, Coping Cat, consisting of two parts: (1) skills training (e.g., identifying feelings and physical symptoms, relaxation, modifying maladaptive cognitions into "coping self-talk," problem solving, self-evaluation/reinforcement) and (2) imaginal/in-vivo exposure and skills practice. In two RCTs, significantly more children receiving Coping Cat no longer met criteria for a primary anxiety disorder at post-treatment as compared to those in the wait list (i.e., 64% vs. 5% in Kendall 1994, and 53% vs. 6% in Kendall *et al.* 1997). Results were maintained at one year in both studies and at approximately 3.35 years in the first study (Kendall & Southam-Gerow 1996). Approximately 7.4 years after the 1997 study, over 80% of children no longer had their primary anxiety diagnosis (Kendall *et al.* 2004). Treatment responders had less reported substance use at long-term follow-up, suggesting that early intervention for child anxiety may prevent later problems.

Barrett and colleagues (1996) developed a family anxiety management group as an adjunct to an Australian adaptation of Coping Cat (Coping Koala)

Table 27.1. Randomized controlled trials using cognitive–behavioral therapy (CBT) and medication for child and adolescent anxiety disorders

Study	Treatment modality	Overall results	Overall follow-up
MULTIPLE ANXIETY DISORDERS			
CBT			
Kendall 1994 $n = 47$; 9–13 y.o. AD, OAD, SepAD	ICBT vs. WL; 16 sessions	ICBT > WL	Maintained at 1, 3.35 yrs (Kendall & Southam-Gerow 1996)
Barrett *et al.* 1996 $n = 79$; 7–14 y.o. OAD, SepAD, SAD	ICBT vs. ICBT+FAM vs. WL; 12 sessions	ICBT+FAM > ICBT > WL	Maintained at 6, 12 mos; CBT groups equal at 6 yrs (Barrett *et al.* 2001)
Kendall *et al.* 1997 $n = 94$; 9–13 y.o. AD, OAD, SepAD	ICBT vs. WL; 16–20 sessions	ICBT > WL	Maintained at 1, 7.4 yrs (Kendall *et al.* 2004)
Barrett 1998 $n = 60$; 7–14 y.o. OAD, SepAD, SAD	GCBT vs. GCBT+FAM vs. WL; 12 sessions	GCBT+FAM > GCBT > WL; groups equal in diagnostic recovery	Maintained at 1 yr
Cobham *et al.* 1998 $n = 67$; 7–14 y.o. GAD, OAD, SepAD, SAD, agoraphobia	GCBT vs. GCBT+PAM; 10 sessions	Child-only anxiety: GCBT = GCBT+PAM; child + parent anxiety: GCBT+PAM > GCBT	Maintained at 6, 12 mos
Mendlowitz *et al.* 1999 $n = 68$; 7–12 y.o. Anxiety disorders	GCBT vs. PGCBT vs. GCBT+PGCBT; 12 sessions (65% WL before randomization)	GCBT = PGCBT = GCBT+PGCBT > WL	Generally maintained at 6–7 yrs (Manassis *et al.* 2004)
Silverman *et al.* 1999b $n = 56$; 6–16 y.o. GAD, OAD, SAD	GCBFT vs. WL; 12 sessions	GCBFT > WL	Maintained at 3, 6, 12 mos
Silverman *et al.* 1999a $n = 81$; 6–16 y.o. Majority SP	CM vs. SC vs. EST; 10 sessions	CM = SC = EST; SC superior on diagnostic recovery	Groups equal at 3, 6, 12 mos
Flannery-Schroeder & Kendall 2000 $n = 37$; 8–14 y.o. GAD, SepAD, SAD	GCBT vs. ICBT vs. WL; 18 sessions	GCBT = ICBT > WL	Maintained at 3 mos
Muris *et al.* 2001 $n = 36$; 8–13 y.o. GAD, SepAD, SAD	GCBT vs. ICBT; 12 sessions	GCBT = ICBT	N/A
Shortt *et al.* 2001 $n = 71$; 6–10 y.o. GAD, SepAD, SAD	Family GCBT vs. WL; 10 sessions + 2 boosters	Family GCBT > WL	Maintained at 1 yr
Ginsburg & Drake 2002 $n = 12$; 14–17 y.o. GAD, SAD, SP	School-based GCBT vs. attention support group; 10 sessions	School-based GCBT > attention support group	N/A
Manassis *et al.* 2002 $n = 78$; 8–12 y.o. GAD, PD, SepAD, SAD, SP	GCBT vs. ICBT; 12 sessions (stable medication allowed)	GCBT = ICBT	Global improvement maintained at 1 yr
Muris *et al.* 2002 $n = 30$; 9–12 y.o. GAD, SepAD, SAD	GCBT vs. ED vs. no treatment; 12 sessions	GCBT > ED = no treatment	N/A
Nauta *et al.* 2003 $n = 79$; 7–18 y.o. GAD, PD, SepAD, SAD	ICBT vs. ICBT + cognitive parent training vs. WL; 12 sessions	ICBT = ICBT + cognitive parent training > WL	Maintained at 3 mos
Rapee *et al.* 2006 $n = 267$; 6–12 y.o. Anxiety disorders but not PTSD	GCBT vs. bibliotherapy vs. WL; 9 sessions (stable medication allowed)	GCBT > bibliotherapy > WL	Maintained at 3 mos
Spence *et al.* 2006 $n = 72$; 7–14 y.o. GAD, SepAD, SAD, SP	GCBT+P vs. GCBT+P + Internet vs. WL; 10 child/6 parent sessions + 2 boosters	GCBT+P = GCBT+P + Internet > WL	Maintained at 6, 12 mos
Wood *et al.* 2006 $n = 40$; 6–13 y.o. GAD, SepAD, SAD	CBFT vs. ICBT; 12–16 sessions (stable medication allowed)	CBFT > ICBT on clinician ratings; groups equal on diagnostic recovery	N/A
Liber *et al.* 2008 $n = 127$; 8–12 y.o. GAD, SepAD, SAD, SP	GCBT vs. ICBT; 17 sessions (stable ADHD medication allowed)	GCBT = ICBT	N/A
March *et al.* 2008 $n = 73$; 7–12 y.o. GAD, SepAD, SAD, SP	Internet CBT vs. WL; 10 child, 6 parent sessions + 2 boosters	Internet CBT > WL on clinician ratings; groups equal on diagnostic recovery	Maintained at 6 mos

Table 27.1 (cont.)

Study	Treatment modality	Overall results	Overall follow-up
Kendall *et al.* 2008 $n = 161$; 7–14 y.o. GAD, SAD, SP	ICBT vs. CBFT vs. family EST	ICBT = CBFT > family EST; both parents anxiety: CBFT > ICBT	Groups equal at 1 yr
Medication			
Simeon *et al.* 1992 $n = 30$; 8–17 y.o. AD, OAD	Alprazolam (0.5–3.5 mg/day) vs. PBO; 4 wks (after 1 wk PBO)	Alprazolam = PBO	Maintained after 2 wks PBO & 6 wks
RUPP Anxiety Study Group 2001 $n = 128$; 6–17 y.o. GAD, SepAD, SAD	FVM (50–300 mg/day) vs. PBO; 8 wks (after failed ST; ST throughout study)	FVM > PBO	Maintained in FVM responders (RUPP Anxiety Study Group 2002)
Birmaher *et al.* 2003 $n = 74$; 7–17 y.o. GAD, SepAD, SAD	Fluoxetine (20 mg/day) vs. PBO; 12 wks	Fluoxetine > PBO for GAD, SAD; Fluoxetine = PBO for SepAD	Maintained at 1 yr (Clark *et al.* 2005)
Comparing CBT and medication			
Walkup *et al.* 2008 $n = 488$; 7–17 y.o. GAD, SepAD, SAD	ICBT (14 sessions) vs. SRT (25–200 mg/day) vs. ICBT+SRT vs. PBO; 12 wks	ICBT+SRT > ICBT = SRT > PBO	N/A
GENERALIZED ANXIETY DISORDER (GAD)			
Medication			
Rynn *et al.* 2001 $n = 22$; 5–17 y.o.	SRT (25–50 mg/day) vs. PBO; 9 wks (PT except CBT allowed)	SRT > PBO	N/A
Rynn *et al.* 2007 $n = 320$; 6–17 y.o.	Venlafaxine (37.5–225 mg/day) vs. PBO (stable PT allowed)	Venlafaxine > PBO	N/A
SOCIAL ANXIETY DISORDER (SAD)			
CBT			
Beidel *et al.* 2000 $n = 67$; 8–12 y.o.	SET-C vs. academic skills group	SET-C > academic skills group	Maintained at 6 mos; 3 yrs (Beidel *et al.* 2005); 5 yrs (Beidel *et al.* 2006)
Spence *et al.* 2000 $n = 50$; 7–14 y.o.	GCBT vs. GCBT+P vs. WL; 12 sessions + 2 boosters	GCBT = GCBT+P > WL	Maintained at 6 mos; 1 yr
Gallagher *et al.* 2003 $n = 23$; 8–11 y.o.	GCBT vs. WL; 3 sessions	GCBT = WL	GCBT > WL at 3 wks
Baer & Garland 2005 $n = 12$; 13–18 y.o.	Group SET-C for adolescents vs. WL; 12 sessions (medication allowed)	Group SET-C for adolescents > WL	N/A
Medication			
Wagner *et al.* 2004 $n = 322$; 8–17 y.o.	Paroxetine (10–50 mg/day) vs. PBO; 16 wks	Paroxetine > PBO	N/A
March *et al.* 2007 $n = 293$; 8–17 y.o.	Venlafaxine ER (37.5–225 mg/day) vs. PBO; 16 wks	Venlafaxine > PBO	N/A
Comparing CBT and medication			
Beidel *et al.* 2007 $n = 122$; 7–17 y.o.	Fluoxetine (10–40 mg/day) vs. SET-C vs. PBO; 12 wks	SET-C > Fluoxetine > PBO; SET-C superior for social skills/competence	Maintained at 1 yr
SPECIFIC PHOBIA (SP)			
CBT			
Cornwall *et al.* 1996 $n = 24$; 7–10 y.o. Darkness	Emotive image therapy vs. WL; 6 sessions	Emotive image therapy > WL	Maintained at 3 mos
Muris *et al.* 1998b $n = 26$; 8–17 y.o. Spider	EMDR vs. IVE vs. computerized exposure; 1 session + 1 IVE session	IVE > EMDR > computerized exposure; EMDR+IVE = IVE	N/A

Table 27.1 (cont.)

Study	Treatment modality	Overall results	Overall follow-up
Dewis et al. 2001 n = 28, 10–17 y.o. Spider	Exposure therapy vs. computerized exposures vs. WL; 3 sessions	Exposure therapy > computerized exposures > WL	Maintained at 1 mo
Öst et al. 2001 n = 60; 7–17 y.o. 50% Animal, 50% Other	IVE vs. IVE + parent vs. WL; 1 session	IVE = IVE + parent > WL	Maintained at 1 yr
OBSSESSIVE–COMPULSIVE DISORDER (OCD)			
CBT			
Barrett et al. 2004 n = 77; 7–17 y.o.	GCBFT vs. CBFT vs. WL; 14 sessions + 2 boosters (stable medication allowed)	GCBFT = CBFT > WL	Maintained at 3, 6 mos
Storch et al. 2007 n = 40; 7–17 y.o.	Intensive CBFT vs. weekly CBFT; 14 sessions (stable medication allowed)	Intensive CBFT = weekly CBFT; intensive > weekly on CGI-S	Groups equal at 3 mos
Bolton & Perrin 2008 n = 20; 8–17 y.o.	Intensive E/RP vs. WL; 10 sessions	Intensive E/RP > WL	Maintained at 14 wks
Medication			
DeVeaugh-Geiss et al. 1992 n = 60; 10–17 y.o.	CMI (25–200 mg/day) vs. PBO; 8 wks	CMI > PBO	Maintained after 1 yr extension of CMI
March et al. 1998 n = 187; 6–17 y.o.	SRT (max. 200 mg/day) vs. PBO; 12 wks	SRT > PBO	Maintained after 1 yr extension of SRT (Cook et al. 2001)
Geller et al. 2001 n = 103; 7–17 y.o.	Fluoxetine (20–60 mg/day) vs. PBO; 13 wks	Fluoxetine > PBO	N/A
Riddle et al. 2001 n = 120; 8–17 y.o.	FVM (50–200 mg/day) vs. PBO; 10 wks	FVM > PBO	N/A
Liebowitz et al. 2002 n = 43; 8–17 y.o.	Fluoxetine (20–80 mg/day) vs. PBO; 8wks acute, then 8 wks maintenance	fluoxetine = PBO at 8 wks; fluoxetine > PBO at 16 wks	N/A
Geller et al. 2003 n = 193; 8–17 y.o.	Paroxetine (10–60 mg/day) vs. PBO; 16 wks (after 16 wks paroxetine)	Paroxetine = PBO	N/A
Geller et al. 2004 n = 203; 7–17 y.o.	Paroxetine (10–50 mg/day) vs. PBO; 10 wks	Paroxetine > PBO	N/A
Comparing CBT and medication			
de Haan et al. 1998 n = 22; 8–18 y.o.	BT (12 sessions) vs. CMI (25–200 mg/day); 12 wks	CYBOCS: BT > CMI; symptom frequency: BT = CMI	At 3 mos, 7 non-responders improved with BT or BT+ CMI
Neziroglu et al. 2000 n = 10; 10–17 y.o.	FVM (50–200 mg/day) vs. FVM+BT (20 sessions); 52 wks (after failed BT and 10 wks FVM)	FVM+BT > FVM	Maintained at 2 yrs
Pediatric OCD Treatment Study Team 2004 n = 112; 7–17 y.o.	ICBT (14 sessions) vs. SRT (25–200 mg/day) vs. ICBT+SRT vs. PBO; 12 wks	CYBOCS: ICBT+SRT > ICBT = SRT > PBO; remission: ICBT+SRT = ICBT, SRT = PBO	N/A
Asbahr et al. 2005 n = 40; 9–17 y.o.	GCBT (12 sessions) vs. SRT (25–200 mg/day); 12 wks	GCBT = SRT	GCBT > SRT at 9 mos

Table 27.1 (cont.)

Study	Treatment modality	Overall results	Overall follow-up
POSTTRAUMATIC STRESS DISORDER (PTSD)			
CBT			
Ahrens & Rexford 2002 N = 38, 15–18 y.o. 100% met criteria for PTSD	CPT vs. WL; 8 sessions	CPT > WL	N/A
Cohen *et al.* 2004 n = 229; 8–14 y.o. 89% met criteria for PTSD	TF-CBT vs. child-centered therapy (both included parent sessions); 12 Sessions	TF-CBT > child centered therapy for children and parents	N/A
Smith *et al.* 2007 n = 24, 8–18 y.o. 100% met criteria for PTSD	ICBT with parent involvement vs. WL; 10 sessions	ICBT with parent involvement > WL	Maintained at 6 mos
Comparing CBT plus medication or placebo			
Cohen *et al.* 2007 n = 24, 10–17 y.o. 92% met criteria for PTSD	TF-CBT (12 sessions) + SRT (50–200 mg/day) vs. TF-CBT+PBO; 12 wks (TF-CBT includes parent sessions)	TF-CBT+SRT = TF-CBT+PBO	N/A
SCHOOL REFUSAL			
CBT			
King *et al.* 1998 n = 34; 5–15 y.o. Most had anxiety disorders	ICBT+PTT vs. WL; 6 sessions	ICBT+PTT > WL	Maintained at 3 mos
Last *et al.* 1998 n = 56; 6–17 y.o. All had anxiety disorders	ICBT vs. EST; 12 sessions	CBT = EST	Maintained at 4 wks
Heyne *et al.* 2002 n = 61; 7–14 y.o. All had anxiety disorders	ICBT vs. ICBT+PTT vs. PTT; 8 sessions	ICBT = ICBT+PTT = PTT; ICBT+PTT = PTT > ICBT on attendance	Groups equal at 4.5 mos
Medication			
Gittleman-Klein & Klein 1971 n = 35; 6–14 y.o. Most had anxiety disorders	IMP (100–200 mg/day) vs. PBO; 6 wks (with parent instruction)	IMP > PBO	N/A
Berney *et al.* 1981 n = 51; 9–14 y.o.	CMI (40–75 mg/day) vs. PBO; 12 wks (all received concurrent PT)	CMI = PBO	N/A
Bernstein *et al.* 1990 n = 24; 7–18 y.o. 65% SepAD or OAD	Alprazolam (0.75–4.0 mg/day) vs. IMP (50–175 mg/day) vs. PBO; 8 wks (all received concurrent PT)	Alprazolam = IMP = PBO	N/A
Klein *et al.* 1992 n = 21; 6–15 y.o. All had SepAD	IMP (75–275 mg/day) vs. PBO; 6 wks (after failed BT; BT allowed through treatment)	IMP = PBO	N/A
Comparimg CBT plus medication or placebo			
Bernstein *et al.* 2000 n = 63; 12–18 y.o. All had anxiety disorders, MDD	IMP (mean 182.3 mg/day) +ICBT (8 sessions) vs. PBO+ICBT; 8 wks	IMP+ICBT > PBO+ICBT for attendance, depressive symptoms	Many met diagnostic criteria at 1 yr (Bernstein *et al.* 2001)

AD, avoidant disorder; BT, behavior therapy; CBFT, family CBT; CBT, cognitive–behavioral therapy; CM, exposure-based contingency management; CMI, clomipramine; CPT, cognitive processing therapy; ED, group emotional disclosure; EMDR, eye movement desensitization and reprocessing; E/RP, exposure/response prevention; EST, education support therapy; FAM, family management; FVM, fluvoxamine; GAD, generalized anxiety disorder; GCBT, group CBT; GCBT+P, GCBT + parent sessions; GCBFT, group CBFT; ICBT, individual CBT; IMP, imipramine; IVE, in-vivo exposure; MDD, major depressive disorder; OAD, overanxious disorder; OCD, obsessive–compulsive disorder; PAM, parental anxiety management; PBO, placebo; PD, panic disorder; PGCBT, parent GCBT; PT, psychotherapy; PTSD, posttraumatic stress disorder; PTT, parent/teacher training; SAD, social anxiety disorder; SepAD, separation anxiety disorder; SC, exposure-based cognitive self-control; SET-C, social effectiveness therapy for children; SP, specific phobia; SRT, sertraline; ST, supportive therapy; TF-CBT, trauma-focused ICBT; WL, wait list.

and compared it to Coping Koala alone and to a wait list control. The CBT plus family group was significantly more effective than CBT alone for remission of any anxiety disorder (84% vs. 57%, $p < 0.05$), while both performed significantly better than the wait list and maintained many gains through 12-month follow-up. At six-year follow-up, participants from both CBT groups derived equal benefits (Barrett *et al.* 2001).

Another group of RCTs compared CBT or BT to one of three psychosocial placebos: education support (Silverman *et al.* 1999a), group emotional disclosure (Muris *et al.* 2002), or an attention support group (Ginsburg & Drake 2002). The latter two studies utilized group CBT in school settings and found it performed significantly better than the psychosocial control. In contrast, Silverman and colleagues (1999a) compared exposure-based cognitive self-control, exposure-based contingency management, and education support therapy. There were no significant treatment differences across conditions at post-treatment or through 12-month follow-up. The authors commented on the apparent utility of educational support and suggested designing studies to determine effective mechanisms of action (e.g., familial change after educational support, treatment credibility, non-specific factors).

Eleven RCTs have compared family or group CBT to individual CBT. Seven studies compared CBT with a parent involvement component to child CBT (Table 27.1). The typical recommendation is that clinicians include parents in child anxiety treatment, to address parental challenges such as when to ignore behaviors, how to set limits, and how to utilize positive reinforcement. However, results of these studies are mixed, indicating uncertainty about the benefits of adding a specific parent involvement component. Variability in type of parent participation across trials may account for a lack of consistent results. Four studies compared group and individual CBT (Table 27.1). In all, both conditions were associated with significant child improvement, but neither individual nor group CBT was more effective.

27.3.1.2 Medication trials

Three RCTs assessed the effects of medications for children with a range of anxiety disorders (GAD, SAD, or SepAD). Two focused on the effects of selective serotonin reuptake inhibitors (SSRIs). Birmaher and colleagues (2003) found that significantly more children taking fluoxetine than placebo were much or very much improved (61% vs. 35%, $p = 0.03$); fluoxetine also

led to improved functioning, and it was well tolerated. However, further analyses indicated that only those with SAD or GAD had greater treatment outcomes, and only SAD moderated clinical and functional responses. A one-year extension trial of fluoxetine was offered to all participants, regardless of group (Clark *et al.* 2005). Those who took medication demonstrated superior outcomes as compared to those who did not. No participants reported clinically suicidal thoughts or behavior.

The Research Unit on Pediatric Psychopharmacology Anxiety Study Group (RUPP ASG) (2001) found that fluvoxamine led to significantly greater reductions in anxiety ($p < 0.001$) and higher response rates (76% vs. 29%, $p < 0.001$) compared to placebo in children with GAD, SAD, or SepAD. Abdominal pain was significantly more likely in the medication group, and five children withdrew from this group due to sedation, hyperactivity, or somatic discomfort. Later analysis indicated that participants with SAD ($p < 0.05$) and more severe illness ($p < 0.05$) were less likely to improve, regardless of treatment condition (RUPP ASG 2003). In the six-month open extension phase (RUPP ASG 2002), fluvoxamine responders continued on fluvoxamine (94% maintained their response), fluvoxamine non-responders were switched to fluoxetine (71% responded), and placebo non-responders received fluvoxamine (56% responded).

One RCT assessed the efficacy of the benzodiazepine alprazolam versus placebo for the treatment of overanxious disorder and avoidant disorder (former DSM-III diagnoses). There were no significant differences at post-treatment or through six-week follow-up (Simeon *et al.* 1992). Further research assessing benzodiazepines for children and adolescents should evaluate higher dosages, longer treatment, larger samples, diagnostic specification, and gradual tapering periods.

27.3.1.3 Trial comparing CBT and medication

The largest pediatric anxiety RCT, the Child/Adolescent Anxiety Multimodal Treatment Study (CAMS), compared the efficacy of the CBT manual, Coping Cat alone, sertraline alone, pill placebo, and a combination of Coping Cat and sertraline for 488 children and adolescents with the primary diagnosis of GAD, SepAD, and/or SAD (Walkup *et al.* 2008). Combined treatment led to significantly higher response rates than either CBT or sertraline (81% vs. 60% and 55%, $p < 0.001$), and the monotherapies were not significantly different from each other. All three treatments were superior to placebo (24%, $p < 0.001$). Rates of adverse events did not significantly differ between the sertraline and placebo groups, with few related study withdrawals. The most common side effects in the medication group were headaches, gastric distress, and insomnia. No child attempted suicide, and, across treatment groups, suicidal ideation did not rise above 3.6%.

27.3.2 Generalized anxiety disorder (GAD)

27.3.2.1 Medication trials

Rynn, Siqueland, and Rickels (2001) were the first to examine the effects of medication for children and adolescents with a primary diagnosis of GAD with or without SepAD. Sertraline was safe and efficacious compared to placebo for reducing anxiety symptoms ($p < 0.001$) and global improvement ($p = 0.001$). Rynn and colleagues (2007) conducted two RCTs comparing venlafaxine extended-release (ER), a serotonin–norepinephrine reuptake inhibitor, to placebo for children and adolescents with GAD. In the pooled analysis, medication was superior to placebo for reducing anxiety ($p < 0.001$) and had higher response (69% vs. 48%, $p = 0.004$). The dose was titrated according to weight and response. Although venlafaxine was generally well tolerated, adverse events that occurred at least twice as often as in placebo included asthenia, pain, anorexia, and somnolence. One child withdrew from each condition due to suicidal ideation or behavior, while one child taking medication experienced agitation and confusion. There were statistically significant changes in weight, height, heart rate, blood pressure, and cholesterol level, indicating the importance of monitoring growth, vital signs, and cholesterol throughout treatment.

27.3.3 Social anxiety disorder (SAD)

27.3.3.1 CBT trials

Four RCTs assessed the effects of group CBT or BT for SAD. The largest (Beidel *et al.* 2000) randomly assigned children to either a behavioral treatment program (Social Effectiveness Therapy for Children, SET-C) that included social skills training, peer generalization, and in-vivo exposure or to an "active, but non-specific intervention" (i.e., strategies for studying/taking tests). SET-C was superior on a variety of self-report measures, observation of social interaction, and diagnostic remission (67% vs. 5%, $p < 0.0001$). Gains were maintained through five-year follow-up (Beidel *et al.*

2005, 2006). A smaller trial comparing SET-C for adolescents to a wait list also yielded positive results (Baer & Garland 2005). The two CBT groups in the study by Spence and colleagues (2000) (child-focused and child plus parent involvement) were both superior to a wait list on a variety of measures, including diagnostic remission (87.5% parent and 58% child vs. 7% wait list, $p < 0.001$). There were no significant differences between active treatments. Results were maintained through 12-month follow-up. One small trial found that children who received three sessions of group CBT for SAD did not perform better than those in a wait list until three-week follow-up, suggesting a need for time to practice and master skills (Gallagher *et al.* 2003).

27.3.3.2 Medication trials

Two multisite RCTs examined the effects of medications for childhood SAD. Wagner and collegaues (2004) reported that those taking paroxetine versus placebo were significantly more likely to respond (78% vs. 38%, $p < 0.001$) and to meet criteria for "very much improved" (48% vs. 15%, $p < 0.001$). Adverse events that occurred at least twice as often in the medication group included insomnia, decreased appetite, and vomiting. Four adolescents taking paroxetine reported suicidal ideation or behavior without attempts, compared to none in the placebo. At discontinuation, nausea, dizziness, and vomiting were twice as likely in the paroxetine group.

March and colleagues (2007) compared venlafaxine ER to placebo and found those receiving venlafaxine had more reduction in their social anxiety symptoms ($p = 0.001$) and higher response rates (56% vs. 37%). Both groups (90% venlafaxine and 81% placebo) reported mild to moderate adverse events, which usually resolved. Almost 6% on medication lost a clinically significant amount of weight. During the tapering period, three participants taking venlafaxine ER reported suicidal ideation, compared to none in the placebo.

27.3.3.3 Trial comparing CBT and medication

Beidel and colleagues (2007) compared group SET-C, fluoxetine, and pill placebo in children and adolescents with SAD. While both active treatments performed better than placebo, those receiving SET-C as compared to fluoxetine or placebo had significantly higher rates of response (79% vs. 36% vs. 6%, $p < 0.001$) and diagnostic remission (53% vs. 21% vs. 3%, $p < 0.005$). SET-C was also the only treatment superior to placebo for increasing social skills and social competence. No severe adverse events occurred, yet some taking fluoxetine experienced moderate side effects (e.g., diarrhea). Treatment gains were maintained at one year.

27.3.4 Specific phobia (SP)

27.3.4.1 CBT trials

Four RCTs examined the effects of behavior therapy for childhood SP. Cornwall and colleagues (1996) found that emotive imagery therapy (i.e., systematic desensitization) was significantly better than a wait list for reducing children's fear of the dark at post-treatment and three-month follow-up. Two RCTs found in-vivo exposure therapy for specific phobia of spiders superior to other conditions (Muris *et al.* 1998b, Dewis *et al.* 2001). Finally, Öst and colleagues (2001) found that one-session in-vivo exposure therapy (with or without a parent present) performed significantly better than a wait list for various child and adolescent phobias, with results maintained at one year. No medication studies have targeted childhood SP.

27.3.5 Obsessive–compulsive disorder (OCD)

27.3.5.1 CBT trials

Three RCTS examined the effects of CBT for child and adolescent OCD. Barrett and colleagues (2004) compared individual and group, family-based CBT (i.e., child, parent, and sibling sessions, including child anxiety management, cognitive training, and exposure and response prevention) to a wait list and found both active conditions led to significantly more diagnostic remission (88% and 76% vs. 0%, $p < 0.001$) and reductions in symptom severity. However, the two treatments were not different from each other, and both CBT groups sustained their treatment gains through six-month follow-up. Storch and colleagues (2007) compared intensive and weekly individual, family-based CBT (including cognitive training and exposure and response prevention) and found slight advantages of intensive treatment at post-treatment but no significant differences at three-month follow-up. Finally, Bolton and Perin (2008) found intense exposure plus response prevention (ERP) superior to a wait-list condition, with findings maintained approximately 14 weeks later.

27.3.5.2 Medication trials

Seven RCTs have examined the effects of medications for childhood OCD. One multisite study compared clomipramine (tricyclic antidepressant) to placebo (DeVeaugh-Geiss *et al.* 1992). Clomipramine led to significantly greater reductions in OCD symptom severity than placebo (e.g., 37% vs. 8%, $p < 0.05$). Overall, clomipramine was well tolerated but associated with four discontinuations (due to anticholinergic effects). Many participants remained on clomipramine treatment for one year and demonstrated further symptom improvement.

Six trials compared the effects of different SSRIs versus pill placebo in OCD. March and colleagues (1998) found that sertraline led to significantly more treatment responders (42% vs. 26%, $p = 0.02$) and reduction in symptom severity (e.g., $p = 0.005$). Cook and colleagues (2001) conducted a one-year extension of sertraline (for participants from either group) and found that 67% of the sample responded to treatment, with 85% of initial responders maintaining their improvement and 43% of initial non-responders demonstrating a response. Two RCTs compared fluoxetine to placebo. Geller and colleagues (2001) found that fluoxetine led to significantly more treatment responders (49% vs. 25%, $p = 0.030$) and improvement in symptom severity ($p = 0.026$) than placebo. Liebowitz and colleagues (2002) found no significant differences between fluoxetine and placebo after eight weeks; however, after another eight weeks, fluoxetine led to significantly more improvement in OCD symptoms ($p = 0.009$) and more treatment responders (57% vs. 27%, $p = 0.047$). Riddle and colleagues (2001) found that fluvoxamine was significantly more effective in reducing OCD symptoms than placebo (25% vs. 14%, $p < 0.05$), while differences in frequency of treatment response approached significance (42% vs. 26%, $p = 0.065$). Adverse events reported as due to the SSRIs were similar across studies and included headache, nausea, weight loss, insomnia, and agitation.

The two largest RCTs for pediatric OCD compared paroxetine to placebo. Geller and colleagues (2003) randomized responders to a 16-week open trial of paroxetine to either continued medication or placebo. While no significant differences existed between groups at post-treatment, about half of this sample had comorbid psychiatric disorders, which were associated with lower response rates and greater relapse than those with OCD only ($p < 0.05$). In a 10-week study that randomized entrants to paroxetine or placebo from the start, Geller and colleagues (2004) found that paroxetine led to significantly more improvement in OCD symptoms than placebo ($p = 0.002$) and more treatment responders (65% vs. 41%, $p = 0.002$). One participant taking medication had suicidal thoughts. Nausea and vomiting upon discontinuation were twice as likely in the paroxetine group.

27.3.5.3 Trials comparing CBT and medication

Four RCTs compared CBT and medication for childhood OCD (Table 27.1). The largest, the Pediatric OCD Treatment Study (POTS), compared CBT alone (including cognitive training and exposure and response prevention), sertraline alone, their combination, and pill placebo (Pediatric OCD Treatment Study Team 2004). The combined intervention was significantly better at reducing symptoms than the other three conditions ($p = 0.008$ CBT alone, $p = 0.006$ sertraline alone, $p = 0.001$ placebo), while CBT and sertraline were both better than placebo ($p = 0.003$ CBT, $p = 0.007$ sertraline) but not significantly different from each other ($p = 0.80$). With regards to the proportion of patients achieving clinical remission, the combination treatment and CBT were not significantly different (54% and 39%, $p = 0.42$), and medication did not differ from placebo (21% and 4%, $p = 0.10$). Therefore, clinicians should first consider treating OCD with an adequate course of CBT. If that is not effective, adding an SSRI could provide enhanced treatment response.

27.3.6 Posttraumatic stress disorder (PTSD)

27.3.6.1 CBT trials

While numerous RCTs have been conducted on childhood trauma (Silverman *et al.* 2008), only two focused solely on children with PTSD. Ahrens and Rexford (2002) found that cognitive processing therapy (cognitive restructuring and exposure to narratives of trauma) was significantly more efficacious than a wait list for reducing depression and posttraumatic stress symptoms (PTSS) in incarcerated adolescent males diagnosed with PTSD. Smith and colleagues (2007) compared CBT (including cognitive restructuring, stimulus discrimination, behavioral experiments, and parent involvement) to a wait list for pediatric PTSD and found CBT superior for improving functioning and diagnostic recovery while reducing PTSS, anxiety, and depressive symptoms. Treatment gains were maintained at six months.

One large RCT compared trauma-focused CBT (including coping skills training, exposure to trauma narratives, cognitive processing, and parent sessions) and child-centered therapy (i.e., usual community treatment) for children with significant PTSS (89% met criteria for PTSD) who had experienced sexual abuse (Cohen *et al.* 2004). Trauma-focused CBT resulted in significantly greater improvements on a variety of outcomes, including child PTSS, depression, behavior problems, and parental depression. Significantly more children in the child-centered group had PTSD at posttreatment (46% vs. 21%, $p < 0.001$).

27.3.6.2 Trial comparing CBT plus medication or placebo

Cohen and colleagues (2007) compared the effects of trauma-focused CBT in conjunction with sertraline or a placebo for girls who had been sexually abused and were experiencing PTSD (92%) or PTSS. Both groups resulted in significant improvement in PTSD and were generally equal at posttreatment, suggesting such children should try CBT before being prescribed medication.

27.3.7 Summary of RCTs

Over the past 15 years, the methodological rigor utilized for CBT, BT, and psychopharmacological studies has increased, and larger and larger RCTs for childhood anxiety disorders have been conducted. The data from these studies have shown that there are three efficacious options for pediatric anxiety: CBT, medication, and their combination.

27.3.7.1 CBT and BT

As reviewed, CBT and BT repeatedly have been found to be more efficacious than wait list in children with mixed anxiety disorders, SAD, SP, OCD, and PTSD. However, several different variants of CBT have been used. Due to Coping Cat's superiority to placebo in CAMS, it is considered a "well-established" treatment, while several other CBT and BT manuals can be considered "probably efficacious" (see Chambless *et al.* 1996, Chambless & Hollon 1998 for criteria). CBT also resulted in better outcomes than placebo or other active treatments in two of three multiple anxiety disorder studies (Ginsburg & Drake 2002, Muris *et al.* 2002) and four studies focused on SAD (Beidel *et al.* 2000), PTSD (Cohen *et al.* 2004), and SP (Muris *et al.* 1998b, Dewis *et al.* 2001). However, no CBT RCTs focused solely on GAD, SepAD, or PD, and none included agoraphobia or acute stress disorder. The effects of individual and group CBT did not differ, and results on the added benefits of involving parents were mixed. Overall, CBT and

BT have demonstrated their ability to maintain gains at follow-up.

27.3.7.2 Medication

As reviewed, SSRIs are useful for treating children and adolescents with GAD, SAD, or OCD. There is also preliminary evidence for using venlafaxine ER for pediatric GAD and SAD. The results for TCAs have been mixed, and they are not used as often as SSRIs because of their safety profile. Benzodiazepines have not demonstrated efficacy for treating child anxiety. No medication RCTs have been conducted for SepAD or SAD alone, or for SP, PD, agoraphobia, or acute stress disorder. Few medication trials have included extensive follow-up periods, but those that have indicate sustained treatment results.

27.3.7.3 Combination treatment: CBT and medication

CAMS (Walkup *et al.* 2008) and POTS (Pediatric OCD Treatment Study Team 2004) demonstrated the efficacy of combining CBT and SSRIs as well as CBT or an SSRI alone for treating certain pediatric anxiety disorders. In both studies, the combined approach was superior to either monotherapy. Theoretical support for the combined approach includes: (1) two treatments may result in faster improvement; (2) comorbid diagnoses or symptoms may respond to different treatments; and (3) for partial responders, augmenting the first treatment with another intervention can increase treatment effects (March 2002). However, one RCT focused on treating pediatric SAD found that group BT (SET-C) performed significantly better than an SSRI (Beidel *et al.* 2007).

27.3.7.4 Limitations

While we have made major advances in effective treatment for childhood anxiety, limitations exist. Even in trials where many improved, some did not, and others were still symptomatic. Research is needed to determine how to enhance treatments for partial and non-responders. In addition, most studies did not compare follow-up samples to controls to assess if findings were a result of treatment or maturity, and we do not know the long-term effects of chronic medication treatment for children and adolescents. Finally, since all RCTs began with children over age six, we cannot assume that these interventions are generalizable to younger children.

27.4 Best clinical practice

The studies summarized above support the use of CBT and medications in the treatment of childhood anxiety disorders. However, merging science and practice is necessary to achieve a high standard of care for children and their families. When an anxious child is referred, potential benefits and risks of evidence-based treatment options should be discussed, to help families make educated decisions. Some may not be willing to consider medication, while others may prefer it. Finding a CBT clinician can be challenging. We suggest families consider medication when a child's symptoms are in the moderate to severe range, where they cannot function, cannot engage in CBT, or have not improved after 8–12 weeks of CBT. We remind skeptical families that they are seeking help because child anxiety has become problematic, and suggest they view treatment as an experiment that can be changed or stopped.

27.4.1 Best CBT practice

Best CBT and BT practice is grounded in learning theory and is framed as collaboration among the child, family, and clinician. In CBT, children are taught to think of automatic thoughts as hypotheses, find evidence to support or refute them, and respond to maladaptive thoughts. Cartoons reflecting the child's interests or role models with blank thought bubbles can be utilized to illustrate these concepts. For successful exposure therapy, we urge clinicians to work outside of the office (e.g., conducting exposure for school refusal on school grounds). Homework should be assigned to reinforce concepts between sessions. Clinicians should continually review techniques to help prevent relapse after termination.

27.4.2 Best medication practice

Children should have a physical examination to rule out medical conditions that might be related to anxiety. SSRIs are the first-line treatment, and each is thought to be equally effective. If a child has comorbid depression, one option is fluoxetine, since it has the US Food and Drug Administration (FDA) indication for both pediatric OCD and major depression. Children and families should be educated about possible side effects. Directly addressing children is essential, as they do not always discuss adverse events with their families (e.g., sexual side effects). SSRIs are well tolerated with few side effects and do not require laboratory tests. Venlafaxine ER is considered a second- to third-line treatment option when a child has failed to respond to an SSRI, CBT, or their combination. Using venlafaxine ER requires regular monitoring, because of potential weight and vital-sign changes. Time-limited use of benzodiazepines can be helpful as adjunctive treatment to the SSRIs for moderate to severe somatic symptoms.

The lowest medication dosage is started for the first seven days. If this is tolerated after one week, dosage can be titrated upwards over the next several weeks until there is a treatment response. Once a clinically efficacious dose is reached, it should be maintained for 8–12 weeks and then re-evaluated. The average successful medication dose for children is similar to those of adults, as seen in CAMS (sertraline, 134 mg).

The FDA recommends seeing the child weekly for four weeks and then every other week for four weeks, followed by a medication management session at 12 weeks and then monthly. Once a significant reduction in symptoms has been maintained over one year, a medication-free trial during a low-stress time should be considered. However, if the child begins to relapse, medication should be immediately reinstated (Pine 2002). If a child does not respond, another SSRI can be considered.

27.4.2.1 FDA warning

In 2004, the FDA placed a "black box" warning on all antidepressant medications, publicizing a two-fold increased risk for suicidal thinking or behavior in children and adolescents taking this medication as compared to placebo. The warning stated that clinicians should closely monitor children taking these medications for a worsening of depression, suicidal thoughts/behavior, or agitation, particularly in the first few months of treatment and when changing dosages. This warning was based on the FDA review of RCTs that assessed the use of antidepressant medications for pediatric depression, anxiety, and other psychiatric disorders. No one completed suicide in these studies; however, the only medications currently approved by the FDA for treating pediatric anxiety disorders are for OCD, and they include clomipramine, fluoxetine, fluvoxamine, and sertraline.

27.5 Future directions

We highlight five innovative areas. First, RCTs should use more behavioral outcomes and observable measures of changes in functioning (e.g., assessment of conversational skills after treatment for social anxiety disorder) and parent–child interactions, as well as physiological measures of change such as blood pressure and heart rate during behavioral tasks, rather than the numerous subjective paper-and-pencil tests.

Self-reports can be biased by factors such as social desirability and treatment expectations, while parent reports may be impacted by parental psychopathology or ignorance about children's internal symptoms. Research on treatment for childhood anxiety would benefit from a return to assessment of observable change.

Second, findings from attention bias studies may inform more basic research on how to change neural pathways related to anxiety, which may impact future treatment. A variety of imaging studies indicate that attention bias differentiates humans with and without anxiety, and primates can be trained to shift these biases. Of interest would be studies to determine how primate training changes brain development and behavior. Such work could lead to innovative treatment procedures focused on changing neural circuitries directly related to threat-oriented behavior. For example, computer training of attentional biases toward ambiguous threats could be offered as an adjunct to CBT (Pine *et al.* 2009).

Third, children whose parents suffer from a psychiatric disorder are significantly more at risk for an anxiety disorder (e.g., Weissman *et al.* 2006). Researchers have indicated that parental psychopathology is associated with poorer treatment outcome for children (Berman *et al.* 2000, Southam-Gerow *et al.* 2001). Only one study has attempted to treat parental symptoms through a specific parent anxiety management component to determine how this impacts treatment outcomes for child anxiety (Cobham *et al.* 1998). Results indicated that CBT plus parental anxiety management significantly increased the efficacy of CBT for children with at least one anxious parent. However, parents who reported anxiety at baseline were not necessarily the same parents who participated, making the relationship between change in parental symptoms and child outcome unclear. Anxiety can also be a precursor for later depression in children of depressed parents (e.g., Weissman *et al.* 2006). The effects of targeting parental psychopathology in addition to treatment for child anxiety must be determined.

Fourth, Leonardo and Hen (2008) have reviewed research on critical periods during development in animals and longitudinal studies of humans. They theorize that children may have a period of plasticity in which they are more sensitive to adverse events, during which exposure may lead to the development of neural circuits of anxiety. Moffit and colleagues (2007) found that family environmental risks (including maternal internalizing symptoms) during childhood were strongly related to adult GAD and GAD with major depression, but not major depression alone, suggesting that anxiety may have a specific developmental critical period. Determining if this critical window exists and who is affected would help us know who is at risk, when, and if we should test early interventions meant to alter the development of anxious neural circuits in some children. Before addressing human pathophysiology, research on animals can manipulate the timing of genetic expression along with environmental challenges at different developmental points to see how this affects them in adulthood (Leonardo & Hen 2008).

Finally, there is a need to study combinations of evidence-based treatments to address the problems of partial and non-responders. Since children with anxiety may have comorbid depression, using treatment strategies from Interpersonal Psychotherapy for Adolescents (IPT-A) (Mufson et al. 2004) in combination with CBT or BT may be beneficial. IPT-A begins with an interpersonal inventory that might provide helpful information, such as who triggers anxiety in a child with social anxiety disorder.

There is also preliminary evidence on using medication to enhance CBT/BT strengths. Basic learning paradigms can lead to novel clinical practice. For example, in order for fears to become extinct, children must learn to discriminate between safe, dangerous, and previously dangerous situations (Pine et al. 2009). In recent studies, D-cycloserine (DCS) administered prior to CBT/BT for adults with different anxiety disorders has been found to enhance the effects of learning fear extinction (Hofmann et al. 2006, Rothbaum 2008, Wilhelm et al. 2008). As children in CBT/BT can have difficulty engaging in exposure exercises, researchers need to examine if augmenting child CBT/BT with DCS enhances the treatment's cognitive effects.

The scientific knowledge base for treating childhood anxiety has made great strides but is still emerging, with a promise of future advances.

Acknowledgments

This chapter was supported by Columbia University's Advanced Center for Intervention and Services Research (ACISR) for Pediatric Psychiatric Disorders, Grant # P30MH071478 from the National Institute of Mental Health. Hilary B. Vidair is a Research Fellow supported by a National Institute of Mental Health T32 National Research Service Award in the Research Training Program in Child and Adolescent Psychiatry at Columbia University's College of Physicians and Surgeons/New York State Psychiatric Institute. The content is solely the responsibility of the authors and does not necessarily represent the official views of the National Institute of Mental Health or the National Institutes of Health.

We would like to thank Maegan Addis and Raashida Edwards for their assistance in the preparation of this chapter.

References

Ahrens, J., & Rexford, L. (2002). Cognitive processing therapy for incarcerated adolescents with PTSD. *Journal of Aggression Maltreatment and Trauma*, **6**, 201–216.

American Academy of Child and Adolescent Psychiatry (1998). Practice parameters for the assessment and treatment of children and adolescents with post traumatic stress disorder. *Journal of the American Academy of Child and Adolescent Psychiatry*, **37** (10S), 4S–26S.

American Psychiatric Association (2000). *Diagnostic and Statistical Manual of Mental Disorders*, 4th edn, text revision (DSM-IV-TR). Washington, DC: American Psychiatric Association.

Anderson, J. C., Williams, S., McGee, R., & Silva, P. A. (1987). DSM-III disorders in preadolescent children. Prevalence in a large sample from the general population. *Archives of General Psychiatry*, **44**, 69–76.

Asbahr, F. R., Castillo, A. R., Ito, L. M., et al. (2005). Group cognitive–behavioral therapy versus sertraline for the treatment of children and adolescents with obsessive–compulsive disorder. *Journal of the American Academy of Child and Adolescent Psychiatry*, **44**, 1128–1136.

Baer, S., & Garland, E. J. (2005). Pilot study of community-based cognitive behavioral group therapy for adolescents with social phobia. *Journal of the American Academy of Child and Adolescent Psychiatry*, **44**, 258–264.

Barrett, P. M. (1998). Evaluation of cognitive–behavioral group treatments for childhood anxiety disorders. *Journal of Clinical Child Psychology*, **27**, 459–468.

Barrett, P. M., Dadds, M. R., & Rapee, R. M. (1996). Family treatment of childhood anxiety: a controlled trial. *Journal of Consulting and Clinical Psychology*, **64**, 333–342.

Barrett, P.M., Duffy, A.L., Dadds, M.R., & Rapee, R.M. (2001). Cognitive–behavioral treatment of anxiety disorders in children: long-term (6-year) follow-up. *Journal of Consulting and Clinical Psychology*, **94**, 135–141.

Barrett, P., Healy-Farrell, L., & March, J. S. (2004). Cognitive–behavioral family treatment of childhood obsessive–compulsive disorder: a controlled trial. *Journal of the American Academy of Child and Adolescent Psychiatry*, **43**, 46–62.

Barrett, P. M., Farrell, L., Pina, A. A., Peris, T. S., & Piacentini, J. (2008). Evidence-based psychosocial treatments for child and adolescent obsessive–

compulsive disorder. *Journal of Clinical Child and Adolescent Psychology*, **37**, 131–155.

Beidel, D. C., Turner, S. M., & Morris, T. L. (2000). Behavioral treatment of childhood social phobia. *Journal of Consulting and Clinical Psychology*, **68**, 1072–1080.

Beidel, D. C., Turner, S. M., Young, B. J., & Paulson, A. (2005). Social effectiveness therapy for children: three-year follow-up. *Journal of Consulting and Consulting Clinical Psychology*, **73**, 721–725.

Beidel, D. C., Turner, S. M., & Young, B. J. (2006). Social effectiveness therapy for children: five years later. *Behavior Therapy*, **37**, 416–425.

Beidel, D. C., Turner, S. M., Sallee, F. R., *et al.* (2007). SET-C versus fluoxetine in the treatment of childhood social phobia. *Journal of the American Academy of Child and Adolescent Psychiatry*, **46**, 1622–1632.

Berman, S. L., Kurtines, W. M., Silverman, W. K., & Serafini, L. T. (1996). The impact of exposure to crime and violence on urban youth. *American Journal of Orthopsychiatry*, **66**, 329–336.

Berman, S. L., Weems, C. F., Silverman, W. K., & Kurtines, W. M. (2000). Predictors of outcome in exposure-based cognitive and behavioral treatments for phobic and anxiety disorders in children. *Behavior Therapy*, **31**, 713–731.

Berney, T., Kolvin, I., Bhate, S. R., Garside, R. F., Jeans, J., Kay, B., & Scarth, L. (1981). School phobia: a therapeutic trial with clomipramine and short-term outcome. *British Journal of Psychiatry*, **138**, 110.

Bernstein, G. A., Garfinkel, B. D., & Borchardt, C. M. (1990). Comparative studies of pharmacotherapy for school refusal. *Journal of the American Academy of Child and Adolescent Psychiatry*, **29**, 773–781.

Bernstein, G. A., Borchardt, C. M., Perwien, A., *et al.* (2000). Imipramine plus cognitive–behavioral therapy in the treatment of school refusal. *Journal of the American Academy of Child and Adolescent Psychiatry*, **39**, 276–283.

Bernstein, G. A., Hektner, J. M., Borchardt, C. M., & McMillan, M. H. (2001). Treatment of school refusal: one-year follow-up. *Journal of the American Academy of Child and Adolescent Psychiatry*, **40**, 206–213.

Birmaher, B., Axelson, D. A., Monk, K., *et al.* (2003). Fluoxetine for the treatment of childhood anxiety disorders. *Journal of the American Academy of Child and Adolescent Psychiatry*, **42**, 415–423.

Boden, J. M., Fergusson, D. M., & Horwood, L. J. (2006). Anxiety disorders and suicidal behaviours in adolescence and young adulthood: findings from a longitudinal study. *Psychological Medicine*, **37**, 431–440.

Bolton, D., & Perrin, S. (2008). Evaluation of exposure with response-prevention for obsessive compulsive disorder in childhood and adolescence. *Journal of Behavior Therapy and Experimental Psychiatry*, **39**, 11–22.

Breslau, N., Davis, G. C., Andreski, P., & Peterson, E. (1991). Traumatic events and posttraumatic stress disorder in an urban population of young adults. *Archives of General Psychiatry*, **48**, 216–222.

Chambless, D. L., & Hollon, S. D. (1998). Defining empirically supported therapies. *Journal of Consulting and Clinical Psychology*, **66**, 7–18.

Chambless, D. L., Sanderson, W. C., Shoham, V., *et al.* (1996). An update on empirically validated treatments. *Clinical Psychologist*, **49**, 5–18.

Clark, D. B., Birmaher, B., Axelson, D., *et al.* (2005). Fluoxetine for the treatment of childhood anxiety disorders: open-label, long-term extension to a controlled trial. *Journal of the American Academy of Child and Adolescent Psychiatry*, **44**, 1263–1270.

Cobham, V. E., Dadds, M. R., & Spence, S. H. (1998). The role of parental anxiety in the treatment of childhood anxiety. *Journal of Consulting and Clinical Psychology*, **66**, 893–905.

Cohen, J. A., Deblinger, E., Mannarino, A. P., & Steer, R. A. (2004). A multisite randomized controlled trial for children with sexual abuse-related PTSD symptoms. *Journal of the American Academy of Child and Adolescent Psychiatry*, **43**, 393–402.

Cohen, J. A., Mannarino, A. P., Perel, J. M., & Staron, V. (2007). A pilot randomized controlled trial of combined trauma-focused CBT and sertraline for childhood PTSD symptoms. *Journal of the American Academy of Child and Adolescent Psychiatry*, **46**, 811–819.

Compton, W. M., Thomas, Y. F., Stinson, F. S., & Grant, B. F. (2007). Prevalence, correlates, disability, and comorbidity of DSM-IV drug abuse and dependence in the United States: results from the National Epidemiologic Survey on Alcohol and Related Conditions. *Archives of General Psychiatry*, **64**, 566–576.

Cook, E. H., Wagner, K. D., March, J. S., *et al.* (2001). Long-term sertraline treatment of children and adolescents with obsessive–compulsive disorder. *Journal of the American Academy of Child and Adolescent Psychiatry*, **40**, 1175–1181.

Cornwall, E., Spence, S. H., & Schotte, D. (1996). The effectiveness of emotive imagery in the treatment of darkness phobia in children. *Behaviour Change*, **13**, 223–229.

Costello, E. J., Egger, H. L., & Angold, A. (2004). Developmental epidemiology of anxiety disorders. In T. H. Ollendick & J. S. March, eds., *Phobic and Anxiety Disorders in Children and Adolescents*. New York, NY: Oxford University Press.

de Haan, E., Hoogduin, K. A. L., Buitelaar, J. K., & Keijsers, G. (1998). Behavior therapy versus clomipramine for the treatment of obsessive–compulsive disorder in children and adolescents. *Journal of the American Academy of Child and Adolescent Psychiatry*, **37**, 1022–1029.

DeVeaugh-Geiss, J., Moroz, G., Biederman, J., *et al.* (1992). Clomipramine hydrochloride in childhood and adolescent obsessive–compulsive disorder: a multicenter trial. *Journal of the American Academy of Child and Adolescent Psychiatry*, **31**, 45–49.

Dewis, L. M., Kirkby, K. C., Martin, F., *et al.* (2001). Computer-aided vicarious exposure versus live graded exposure for spider phobia in children. *Journal of Behavior Therapy and Experimental Psychiatry*, **32**, 17–27.

Flannery-Schroeder, E. C., & Kendall, P. C. (2000). Group and individual cognitive–behavioral treatments for youth with anxiety disorders: a randomized clinical trial. *Cognitive Therapy and Research*, **24**, 251–278.

Gallagher, H. M., Rabian, B. A., & McCloskey, M. S. (2003). A brief group cognitive–behavioral intervention for social phobia in childhood. *Journal of Anxiety Disorders*, **18**, 459–479.

Geller, D. A., Hoog, S. L., Heiligenstein, J. H., *et al.* (2001). Fluoxetine treatment for obsessive–compulsive disorder in children and adolescents: a placebo-controlled clinical trial. Fluoxetine Pediatric OCD Study Team. *Journal of the American Academy of Child and Adolescent Psychiatry*, **4**, 773–779.

Geller, D. A., Biederman, J., Stewart, S. E., *et al.* V. (2003). Which SSRI? A meta-analysis of pharmacotherapy trials in pediatric obsessive–compulsive disorder. *American Journal of Psychiatry*, **160**, 1919–1928.

Geller, D. A., Wagner, K. D., Emslie, G., *et al.* (2004). Paroxetine treatment in children and adolescents with obsessive–compulsive disorder: a randomized, multicenter, double-blind, placebo-controlled trial. *Journal of the American Academy of Child and Adolescent Psychiatry*, **43**, 1387–1396.

Ginsburg, G. S., & Drake, K. L. (2002). School-based treatment for anxious African-American adolescents: a controlled pilot study. *Journal of the American Academy of Child and Adolesent Psychiatry*, **41**, 768–775.

Gittelman-Klein, R., & Klein, D. F. (1971). Controlled imipramine treatment of school phobia. *Archives of General Psychiatry*, **25**, 204–207.

Heyne, D., King, N., Tonge, B., *et al.* (2002). Evaluation of child therapy and caregiver training in the treatment of school refusal. *Jounal of the Academy of Child Adolescents and Psychiatry*, **41**, 687–695.

Hofmann S. G., Meuret, A. E., Smits, J. A. J., *et al.* (2006). Augmentation of exposure therapy for social anxiety disorder with d-cycloserine. *Archives of General Psychiatry*, **63**, 298–304.

Keller, M. B., Lavori, P. W., Wunder, J., *et al.* (1992). Chronic course of anxiety disorders in children and adolescents. *Jounal of the American Academy of Child Adolescents and Psychiatry*, **31**, 595–599.

Kendall, P. C. (1994). Treating anxiety disorders in children: results of a randomized clinical trial. *Jounal of Consulting and Clinical Psychology*, **62**, 100–110.

Kendall, P. C., & Southam-Gerow, M. A. (1996). Long-term follow-up of a cognitive–behavioral therapy for anxiety-disordered youth. *Journal of Consulting and Clinical Psychology*, **64**, 724–730.

Kendall, P. C., Flannery-Schroeder, E., Panichelli-Mindel, S. M., *et al.* (1997). Therapy for youths with anxiety disorders: a second randomized clinical trial. *Journal of Consulting and Clinical Psychology*, **65**, 366–380.

Kendall, P. C., Safford, S., Flannery-Schroeder, E., & Webb, A. (2004). Child anxiety treatment: outcomes in adolescence and impact on substance use and depression at 7.4-Year follow-up. *Journal of Consulting and Clinical Psychology*, **72**, 276–287.

Kendall, P. C., Hudson, J.L., Gosch, E., Flannery-Schroeder, E., & Suveg, C. (2008). Cognitive–behavioral therapy for anxiety disordered youth: a randomized clinical trial evaluating child and family modalities. *Journal of Consulting and Clinical Psychology*, **76**, 282–297.

King, N. J., Tonge, B. J., Heyne, D., *et al.* (1998). Cognitive-behavioral treatment of school-refusing children: a controlled evaluation. *Journal of the American Academy of Child and Adolescent Psychiatry*, **37**, 395–403.

Klein, R. G., Koplewicz, H. S., & Kanner, A. (1992). Imipramine treatment of children with separation anxiety disorder. *Journal of the American Academy of Child and Adolescent Psychiatry*, **31**, 21–28.

Last, C. G., Hansen, C., & Franco, N. (1998). Cognitive-behavioral treatment of school phobia. *Journal of the American Academy of Child and Adolescent Psychiatry*, **37**, 404–411.

Leonardo, E., & Hen, R. (2008). Anxiety as a developmental disorder. *Neuropsychopharmacology*, **33**, 134–140.

Liber, J. Van Widenfelt, B. M., Utens, E. M., *et al.* (2008). No differences between group versus individual treatment of childhood anxiety disorders in a randomised clinical trial. *Journal of Child Psychology and Psychiatry*, **49**, 886–893.

Liebowitz, M. R., Turner, S. M., Piacentini, J., *et al.* (2002). Fluoxetine in children and adolescents with OCD: a placebo-controlled trial. *Journal of the American Academy of Child and Adolescent Psychiatry*, **41**, 1431–1438.

Manassis, K., Mendlowitz, S. L., Scapillato, D., *et al.* (2002). Group and individual cognitive–behavioral therapy for childhood anxiety disorders: a randomized trial. *Journal of the American Academy of Child and Adolescent Psychiatry*, **41**, 1423–1430.

Manassis, K., Avery, D., Butalia, S., & Mendlowitz, S. (2004). Cognitive–behavioral therapy with childhood anxiety disorders: functioning in adolescence. *Depression and Anxiety*, **19**, 209–216.

March, J. S. (2002). Combining medication and psychosocial treatments: an evidence-based medicine approach. *International Review of Psychiatry*, **14**, 155–163.

March, J. S., Biederman, J., Wolkow, R., *et al.* (1998). Sertraline in children and adolescents with obsessive–compulsive disorder: a multicenter randomized controlled trial. *JAMA*, **280**, 1752–1756.

March, J. S., Entush, A. R., Rynn, M., Albano, A. M., & Tourian, K. A. (2007). A randomized controlled trial of venlafaxine ER versus placebo in pediatric social anxiety disorder. *Biological Psychiatry*, **62**, 1149–1154.

March, S., Spence, S. H., & Donovan, C. L. (2008). The efficacy of an internet-based cognitive–behavioral therapy intervention for child anxiety disorders. *Journal of Pediatric Psychology*, **34**, 474–487.

Mendlowitz, S. L., Manassis, K., Bradley, S., *et al.* (1999). Cognitive–behavioral group treatments in childhood anxiety disorders: the role of parental involvement. *Journal of the American Academy of Child and Adolescent Psychiatry*, **38**, 1223–1229.

Moffitt, T., Caspi, A., Harrington, H., *et al.* (2007). Generalized anxiety disorder and depression: childhood risk factors in a birth cohort followed to age 32. *Psychological Medicine*, **37**, 441–452.

Mufson, L., Dorta, K. P., Moreau, D., & Weissman, M. M. (2004). *Interpersonal Psychotherapy for Depressed Adolescents*, 2nd edn. New York, NY: Guilford Press.

Muris, P., Meesters, C., Merckelbach, H., Sermon, A., & Zwakhalen, S. (1998a). Worry in normal children. *Journal of the American Academy of Child and Adolescent Psychiatry*, **37**, 703–710.

Muris, P., Merckelbach, H., Holdrinet I., Sijsenaar M. (1998b). Treating phobic children: effects of EMDR versus exposure. *Journal of Counseling and Clinical Psychology*, **66**, 193–198.

Muris, P., Mayer, B., Bartelds, E., Tierney, S., & Bogie, N. (2001). The revised version of the screen for child anxiety related emotional disorders (SCARED-R): treatment sensitivity in an early intervention trial for childhood anxiety disorders. *British Journal Clinical Psychology*, **40**, 323–336.

Muris, P., Meesters, C., & van Melick, M. (2002). Treatment of childhood anxiety disorders: a preliminary comparison between cognitive–behavioral group therapy and a psychological placebo intervention. *Journal of Behavior Therapy and Experimental Psychiatry*, **33**, 143–158.

Nauta, M. H., Scholing, A., Emmelkamp, P. M., & Minderaa, R. B. (2003). Cognitive–behavioral therapy for children with anxiety disorders in a clinical setting: no additional effect of a cognitive parent training. *Journal of the American Academy of Child and Adolescent Psychiatry*, **42**, 1270–1278.

Neziroglu, F., Yaryura-Tobias, J. A., Walz, J., & Mckay, D. (2000). The effect of fluvoxamine and behavior therapy on children and adolesecents with obsessive–compulsive disorder. *Journal of Child and Adolescent Psychopharmacology*, **10**, 295–306.

Öst, L.-G., Svensson, L., Hellstrom, K., & Lindwall, R. (2001). One-session treatment of specific phobias in youths: a randomized clinical trial. *Journal of Consulting and Clinical Psychology*, **69**, 814–824.

Pediatric OCD Treatment Study Team (2004). Cognitive–behavior therapy, sertraline, and their combination for children and adolescents with obsessive–compulsive disorder: the Pediatric OCD Treatment Study (POTS) randomized controlled trial. *JAMA*, **292**, 1969–1976.

Pine, D. S. (2002). Treating children and adolescents with selective serotonin reuptake inhibitors: how long is appropriate? *Journal of Child and Adolescent Psychopharmacology*, **12**, 189–203.

Pine, D. S., Cohen, P., Gurley, D., Brook, J., & Ma, Y. (1998). The risk for early-adulthood anxiety and depressive disorders in adolescents with anxiety and depressive disorders. *Archives of General Psychiatry*, **55**, 56–64.

Pine, D. S., Helfinstein, S. M., Bar-Haim, Y., Nelson, E., & Fox, N. A. (2009). Challenges in developing novel treatments for childhood disorders: lessons from research on anxiety. *Neuropsychopharmacology*, **34**, 213–228.

Rapee, R. M., Abbott, M. J., & Lyneham, H. J. (2006). Bibliotherapy for children with anxiety disorders using written materials for parents: a randomized controlled trial. *Journal of Consulting and Clinical Psychology*, **74**, 436–444.

Research Unit on Pediatric Psychopharmacology Anxiety Study Group (2001). Fluvoxamine for the treatment of anxiety disorders in children and adolescents. *New England Journal of Medicine*, **344**, 1279–1285.

Research Unit on Pediatric Psychopharmacology Anxiety Study Group (2002). Treatment of Pediatric Anxiety Disorders: an open-label extension of the research units on pediatric psychopharmacology anxiety study. *Journal of Child and Adolescent Psychopharmacology*, **12**, 175–188.

Research Unit on Pediatric Psychopharmacology Anxiety Study Group (2003). Searching for moderators and mediators of pharmacological treatment effects in children and adolescents with anxiety disorders. *Journal of the American Academy of Child and Adolescent Psychiatry*, **42**, 13–21.

Riddle, M. A., Reeve, E. A., Yaryura-Tobias, J. A., *et al.* (2001). Fluvoxamine for children and adolescents with obsessive–compulsive disorder: a randomized, controlled, multicenter trial. *Journal of the American Academy of Child and Adolescent Psychiatry*, **40**, 222–229.

Rothbaum, B. (2008). Critical parameters for d-cycloserine enhancement of cognitive–behaviorial therapy for obsessive–compulsive disorder. *American Journal of Psychiatry*, **165**, 293–296.

Rynn, M. A., Siqueland, L., & Rickels, K. (2001). Placebo-controlled trial of sertraline in the treatment of children with generalized anxiety disorder. *American Journal of Psychiatry*, **158**, 2008–2014.

Rynn, M. A., Riddle, M. A., Yeung, P. P., & Kunz, N. R. (2007). Efficacy and safety of extended-release venlafaxine in the treatment of generalized anxiety disorder in children and adolescents: two placebo-controlled trials. *American Journal of Psychiatry*, **164**, 290–300.

Shortt, A., Barrett, P., & Fox, T. (2001). Evaluating the FRIENDS program: a cognitive–behavioral group treatment for anxious children and their parents. *Journal of Clinical Child Psychology*, **30**, 525–535

Silverman, W. K., Kurtines, W. M., Ginsburg, G. S., *et al.* (1999a). Contingency management, self-control, and education support in the treatment of childhood phobic disorders: a randomized clinical trial. *Journal of Consulting and Clinical Psychology*, **67**, 675–687.

Silverman, W. K., Kurtines, W. M., Ginsburg, G. S., *et al.* (1999b). Treating anxiety disorders in children with group cognitive–behaviorial therapy: a randomized clinical trial. *Journal of Consulting and Clinical Psychology*, **67**, 995–1003.

Silverman, W. K., Ortiz, C. D., Viswesvaran, C., *et al.* (2008). Evidence-based psychosocial treatments for children and adolescents exposed to traumatic events. *Journal of Clinical Child and Adolescent Psychology* **37**, 156–183.

Simeon, J. G., Ferguson, H. B., Knott, V., *et al.* (1992). Clinical, cognitive, and neurophysiological effects of alprazolam in children and adolescents with overanxious and avoidant disorders. *Journal of the American Academy of Child and Adolescent Psychiatry*, **31**, 29–36.

Spence, S. H., Donovan, C., & Brechman-Toussaint, M. (2000). The treatment of childhood social phobia: the effectiveness of a social skills training-based, cognitive-behavioral intervention, with and without parental involvement. *Journal of Child Psychology and Psychiatry, and Allied Disciplines*, **41**, 713–726.

Spence, S. H., Holmes, J., March, S., & Lipp, O. (2006). The feasibility and outcome of clinic plus internet delivery of cognitive–behavior therapy for childhood anxiety. *Journal of Consulting and Clinical Psychology*, **74**, 614–621.

Smith, P., Yule, W., Perrin, S., *et al.* (2007). Cognitive-behavioral therapy for PTSD in children and adolescents: a preliminary randomized controlled trial. *Journal of the American Academy of Child and Adolescent Psychiatry*, **46**, 1051–1061.

Southam-Gerow, M. A., Kendall, P. C., & Weersing V. R. (2001). Examining outcome variability: correlates of treatment response in a child and adolescent anxiety clinic. *Journal of Clinical and Child Psychology*, **30**, 422–436.

Storch, E. A., Geffken, G. R., Merlo, L. J., *et al.* (2007). Family-based cognitive–behavioral therapy for pediatric obsessive–compulsive disorder: comparison of intensive and weekly approaches. *Journal of the American Academy of Child Adolescent Psychiatry*, **46**, 469–478.

Vasey, M. W., Crnic, K. A., & Carter, W. G. (1994). Worry in childhood: a developmental perspective. *Cognitive Therapy and Research*, **18**, 529–549.

Velting, O. N., Setzer, N. J., & Albano, A. M. (2004). Update on and advances in assessment and cognitive-behavioral treatment of anxiety disorders in children and adolescents. *Professional Psychology Research and Practice*, **35**, 42–54.

Wagner, K. D., Berard, R., Stein, M. B., *et al.* (2004). A multicenter, randomized, double-blind, placebo-controlled trial of paroxetine in children and adolescents with social anxiety disorder. *Archives of General Psychiatry*, **61**, 1153–1162.

Walkup, J. T., Albano, A. M., Piacentini, J., *et al.* (2008). Cognitive behavioral therapy, sertraline, or a combination in childhood anxiety. *New England Journal of Medicine*, **359**, 2753–2766.

Weissman, M. M., Wickramaratne, P., Nomura, Y., *et al.* (2006). Offspring of depressed parents: 20 years later. *American Journal of Psychiatry*, **163**, 1001–1008.

Wilhelm, S., Buhlmann, U., Tolin, D. F., *et al.* (2008). Augmentation of behavior therapy with d-cycloserine for obsessive–compulsive disorder. *American Journal of Psychiatry*, **165**, 335–341.

Wood, J. J., Piacentini, J. C., Southam-Gerow, M., Chu, B., & Sigman, M. (2006). Family Cognitive behavioral therapy for child anxiety disorders. *Journal of the American Academy of Child and Adolescent Psychiatry*, **45**, 314–321.

28.1 Introduction

Brain stimulation represents a growing family of interventions that alter brain function using electrical fields that are either directly applied or indirectly induced using rapidly alternating magnetic fields. Brain stimulation techniques include transcranial electrical approaches (e.g., electroconvulsive therapy, ECT), magnetic approaches (e.g., transcranial magnetic stimulation, TMS), and surgical approaches (e.g., vagus nerve stimulation, VNS; and deep brain stimulation, DBS) (Table 28.1). These modalities differ in their means of application, focality, invasiveness, mechanism of action, side-effect profile, and clinical spectrum. They have in common the use of electrical stimulation to modulate neuronal functioning. Here we review research to date on these approaches in the treatment of anxiety disorders and discuss how this work may advance knowledge and test hypotheses about the neural circuitry underlying anxiety disorders.

28.2 Electroconvulsive therapy (ECT)

Electroconvulsive therapy (ECT) uses pulsed electrical fields applied to the scalp to induce a generalized seizure. Abundant literature supports the efficacy of ECT as a highly successful therapy for patients with major depressive disorder (MDD), especially with the psychotic subtype, melancholia, and catatonia. However, there is limited controlled evidence regarding its use in patients with anxiety or the many disorders in which anxiety is prominent (Carney et al. 1965, Pande et al. 1988). Early investigators considered "neurotic" depression, in which symptoms of somatic anxiety are prominent, to predict poor response to ECT (Hobson 1953, Roberts 1959, Carney et al. 1965, Mendels, 1965), although some modern studies have failed to replicate these findings (Abrams et al.

1973, Abrams 1982, Zimmerman et al. 1986, Prudic et al. 1989, Sobin et al. 1996). In a large group (n = 253) of unipolar depressed patients referred for ECT, Rasmussen and colleagues (2004) found that somatic anxiety and hypochondriasis, as reflected in items 11 and 15 of the Hamilton Rating Scale for Depression (HAM-D), correlate negatively with likelihood of sustained remission. Patients with high combined scores on those two items had a sustained remission rate less than half of that shown by those with low combined scores.

In contrast, eight patients with comorbid MDD and panic disorder improved with ECT (Figiel et al. 1992). Before ECT was begun, each subject's panic disorder and depression were rated as at least markedly ill. After receiving ECT, all eight showed improvement in their depression. In addition, none of the eight patients reported having a panic attack from the time of their fourth ECT treatment until discharge, which occurred after 7–16 days.

Case reports suggest that ECT might be helpful in the treatment of refractory obsessive–compulsive disorder (OCD) as well. Mellman and Gorman (1984) reported the case of a man with OCD without evidence of depression who responded to ECT but not to medication treatments. An open trial of ECT conducted in nine subjects who met DSM-III criteria for OCD showed an initial reduction in symptomatology that lasted from one to four months (Khanna et al. 1988). Maletzky and colleagues (1994) reviewed their experience with ECT in 32 patients meeting DSM-III-R criteria for OCD. All patients had received extensive behavioral and cognitive therapy and pharmacotherapy prior to the initiation of ECT without apparent benefit. Following ECT, most subjects showed considerable improvement in obsessive–compulsive symptoms, which was maintained up to one year after ECT.

Anxiety Disorders: Theory, Research, and Clinical Perspectives, ed. Helen Blair Simpson, Yuval Neria, Roberto Lewis-Fernández, Franklin Schneier. Published by Cambridge University Press. © Cambridge University Press 2010.

Table 28.1. Brain stimulation techniques tested for the treatment of anxiety disorders

Electroconvulsive therapy (ECT)	Convulsive electrical current stimulation of the cerebral cortex
Transcranial magnetic stimulation (TMS)	Subconvulsive electromagnetic-induced stimulation of the cerebral cortex
Vagus nerve stimulation (VNS)	Implanted, battery-operated stimulation of the left vagus nerve
Deep brain stimulation (DBS)	Implanted, battery-operated stimulation of deep brain structures

Strassnig and colleagues (2004) presented the case of a 39-year-old female patient who chronically suffered from both Tourette syndrome (TS) and OCD. After a course of nine electroconvulsive treatments, her symptoms resolved fairly rapidly. Monthly outpatient ECT sessions were successful in sustaining remission of both disorders for more than a year. Fukuchi and colleagues (2003) reported a case of a 36-year-old pregnant woman with severe OCD successfully treated by ECT. During the pregnancy, severe obsessions of contamination and compulsive washing appeared, so severely that she was unable to lie down, endangering the life of the fetus. Since pharmacotherapy was ineffective, ECT was performed in cooperation with her obstetrician, along with fetal heart monitoring throughout the procedure. During the second ECT, late deceleration of the fetal heart rate occurred, but rapid intravenous administration of ritodrine led to the cessation of abnormal uterine contraction. Two courses of ECT markedly diminished her symptoms, and she delivered a healthy infant without complications. The authors concluded that ECT can be an alternative treatment for pregnant patients with OCD.

Uncontrolled case series suggest that ECT also may be an effective treatment for patients with refractory depression and co-occurring posttraumatic stress disorder (PTSD). Using a retrospective chart review, Watts (2007) examined the outcome of 26 patients with MDD and co-occurring PTSD who received a course of ECT. The patients received either suprathreshold right unilateral ECT, bilateral ECT, or a combination of both. Patients receiving ECT had a significant reduction in the symptoms of major depression and some amelioration in PTSD symptoms.

In conclusion, the literature on the use of ECT for anxiety disorders that are primary or comorbid with depression is limited to small case series and naturalistic chart reviews. These reports suggest encouraging results but need to be followed up with controlled trial evidence to evaluate the efficacy of ECT in these conditions. The American Psychiatric Association practice guidelines do not yet recommend ECT as a treatment for OCD (Koran *et al.* 2007).

28.3 Transcranial magnetic stimulation (TMS)

Transcranial magnetic stimulation (TMS) is a non-invasive means of stimulating focal regions of the brain using rapidly alternating magnetic fields. Since its introduction in 1985, TMS has been used to study localization of brain functions, functional connectivity, and pathophysiology of neuropsychiatric disorders. TMS was recently approved by the US Food and Drug Administration (FDA) for the treatment of depression, and its potential for treatment of other psychiatric disorders is under active study. After a short description of the mechanism of TMS, we then review the state of knowledge about the therapeutic potential of TMS in anxiety disorders.

28.3.1 TMS and rTMS background

TMS is performed by placing an electromagnetic coil on the scalp. High-intensity current is rapidly turned on and off in the coil through the discharge of a capacitor. This produces a time-varying magnetic field that lasts for about 100–200 microseconds. The magnetic field strength is about 1.5–2 tesla (about the same intensity as the static magnetic field used in clinical magnetic resonance imaging, MRI) at the surface of the coil, but the strength of the magnetic field drops off exponentially with distance from the coil. The proximity of the brain to the time-varying magnetic field results in current flow in neural tissue and membrane depolarization.

The ability of TMS to activate functional circuits is easily demonstrated when one places the coil on the scalp over the primary motor cortex. A single TMS pulse of sufficient intensity causes involuntary movement in the muscle represented by that region of cortex through activation of the corticospinal tract. Thus, a TMS pulse produces a powerful but brief magnetic field that passes through the skin, soft tissue, and skull, which induces electrical current in neurons, causing depolarization that then has behavioral effects. The minimum magnetic field intensity needed to produce motor movement is known as the individual motor threshold. The motor threshold is used to individualize the intensity of TMS for each subject.

Repeated application of TMS pulses at regular intervals is called repetitive TMS (rTMS). The physiological effects of rTMS depend upon the site and frequency of stimulation. If the stimulation occurs faster than once per second (> 1 Hz) it is referred to as high-frequency rTMS, and can result in excitatory physiologic changes. If on the contrary the frequency is low (≤ 1 Hz), it is referred to as low-frequency rTMS and can have an inhibitory effect on brain excitability. rTMS carries a risk of seizure, and that risk is higher with high-frequency rTMS. Guidelines to reduce this risk include appropriate screening of subjects for seizure risk factors, titrating the individual motor threshold, and limiting rTMS dosage (Wassermann 1998, Belmaker *et al.* 2003).

rTMS was recently approved by the FDA for the treatment of unipolar major depressive disorder in adults who have failed to respond to one antidepressant medication of adequate dosage and duration in the current episode. The use of rTMS in other conditions is still considered investigational.

28.3.2 rTMS in the treatment of anxiety disorders

The ability to focally alter cortical excitability provides the potential to modulate cortical circuitry for therapeutic benefit in anxiety disorders and other conditions. The focality of the effects also presents a challenge to clinical application, since it is necessary to know the circuitry of the underlying disorder to guide where and how to stimulate in order to produce clinical benefit. Limited studies have been conducted on the therapeutic applications of rTMS in anxiety disorders. A number of neuroimaging studies have shown elevated right-sided activity in the frontal and hippocampal–parahippocampal regions in experimental fear paradigms and in anxiety disorders (van den Heuvel *et al.* 2005, Morinaga *et al.* 2007, Alvarez *et al.* 2008). These findings have led to the hypothesis that low-frequency rTMS of the right prefrontal cortex may be helpful in dampening that lateralized hyperexcitability and improving anxiety symptoms. Therefore, some of the studies have tested low-frequency rTMS of the right prefrontal cortex, although other studies have targeted other brain regions and used high-frequency rTMS.

28.3.2.1 Generalized anxiety disorder (GAD)

Data on rTMS in generalized anxiety disorder (GAD) are limited to one clinical trial (Bystritsky *et al.* 2008).

This pilot study used functional magnetic resonance imaging (fMRI) to guide the placement of the electromagnetic coil and then stimulated the right dorsolateral prefrontal cortex (DLPFC), the brain region in which every patient showed a significant cluster of activation during a gambling task. The researchers used an fMRI-activation gambling task that in a previous study had shown to reliably produce prefrontal activation as well as elevation in anxiety and apprehension in healthy individuals (Hsu *et al.* 2005). Ten participants completed six sessions of low-frequency (1 Hz) rTMS over the course of three weeks, stereotactically directed to the prefrontal location. Overall, rTMS was associated with significant decreases in anxiety as measured by the Hamilton Rating Scale for Anxiety (HAM-A). At endpoint, six (60%) of the 10 participants who completed the study showed reductions of 50% or more on the HAM-A and had a Clinical Global Impression–Improvement (CGI-I) scale score of one ("very much improved") or two ("much improved"); those six subjects also met criteria for remission (HAM-A score less than eight). This study suggests that fMRI-guided rTMS treatment may be a beneficial technique for the treatment of GAD. However, it was an open trial, and the sophisticated pretreatment and treatment technologies used could have enhanced the placebo response. Thus, further research is needed to determine whether the inhibitory 1 Hz rTMS is indeed effective in treating GAD, or whether different frequencies and/or locations might be more effective.

28.3.2.2 Panic disorder

In an open case study of a patient with panic disorder, 1 Hz rTMS delivered to the right DLPFC produced a reduction of panic symptoms and a marked improvement of anxiety (Zwanzger *et al.* 2002). Symptoms of anxiety decreased 78%, and panic/agoraphobia symptoms decreased 59%, with long-lasting improvements at one-month follow-up. Interestingly, rTMS caused reduction in cholecystokinin tetrapeptide (CCK-4)-induced panic attacks, which was associated with blunting of the CCK-4-induced elevation of adrenocorticotropic hormone (ACTH) and cortisol.

In another open case series, Garcia-Toro and colleagues (2002) demonstrated a modest clinical improvement in three patients with treatment-resistant panic disorder treated with 10 rTMS sessions (1 Hz, 110% motor threshold, 30 trains, 60-second duration) to the right DLPFC. Alternating right DLPFC 1 Hz rTMS with left DLPFC 20 Hz rTMS failed to produce further benefits. Another patient treated with right frontal 1 Hz rTMS for nine sessions did not report any change. When switched to left frontal high-frequency rTMS for 20 sessions, the patient reported a significant improvement in panic symptoms and markedly decreased agoraphobia. Her Panic Disorder Severity Scale (PDSS) baseline score was 20 (severe panic disorder), and her endpoint PDSS score was three. At one month and three months after rTMS treatment had been stopped, her PDSS score remained at three (Guaiana *et al.* 2005).

We recently reported a case series of six patients with panic disorder and comorbid MDD showing improvements in both panic and depression with motor cortex excitability decreases after two weeks of 1 Hz rTMS to the right DLPFC (Mantovani *et al.* 2007a). We are conducting a sham-controlled four-week trial of right DLPFC low-frequency rTMS in the treatment of panic and comorbid depression to follow up on these findings.

A sham-controlled study was done to assess whether rTMS would facilitate the effect of serotonin reuptake inhibitors (SRIs) in patients with panic disorder (Prasko *et al.* 2007). Fifteen patients completed the study. Both the active and the sham group improved, leading to the conclusion that low-frequency rTMS administered over the right DLPFC after 10 sessions did not differ from sham rTMS added to SRIs in patients with panic disorder.

28.3.2.3 Posttraumatic stress disorder (PTSD)

Two patients with treatment-resistant PTSD and elevated baseline cerebral metabolism on positron emission tomography (PET) were successfully treated by low-frequency rTMS. In particular, 1 Hz rTMS to the right DLPFC reduced posttraumatic symptoms and reversed the cerebral hypermetabolism, most markedly in the right prefrontal cortex (McCann *et al.* 1998).

In line with symptom provocation studies that have demonstrated significantly greater activity in brain regions associated with motor preparedness in response to threat, Grisaru and colleagues (1998) applied 0.3 Hz rTMS bilaterally on the motor cortex of PTSD patients. PTSD scores improved transiently; however, these results may underestimate the value of such an approach, since the parameters of stimulation were overly conservative (lower frequency, only 60 pulses per day).

Rosenberg and colleagues (2002) hypothesized that left frontal rTMS (either 1 or 5 Hz, 90% of motor threshold, total 6000 stimuli) could mimic

the beneficial effect of antidepressant medications in patients with combat PTSD and comorbid major depression. Seventy-five percent of patients showed at least a 50% decrease in depressive symptoms but minimal improvement in PTSD. The antidepressant effects were stable at two-month follow-up.

Finally, in a double-blind sham-controlled trial, Cohen and colleagues (2004) reported beneficial effects in PTSD core symptoms (i.e., re-experiencing, avoidance) and anxiety from 10 Hz to the right DLPFC but not from 1 Hz or sham rTMS. The frequency specificity of these effects, demonstrated in the context of a well-controlled study, offers strong support that rTMS is worth exploring further in the treatment of PTSD.

In a preliminary report, rTMS was combined with exposure therapy for PTSD (Osuch *et al.* 2009). Nine subjects with chronic, treatment-refractory PTSD were studied in a placebo-controlled, within-subject crossover design of right DLPFC rTMS (1 Hz) and sham rTMS with imaginal exposure therapy. PTSD symptoms, serum prolactin and thyroxine (T_4), and 24-hour urine epinephrine were assessed. Active rTMS showed a larger effect size of improvement for hyperarousal symptoms compared to sham. In addition, 24-hour urinary norepinephrine and serum T_4 increased while serum prolactin decreased. The authors concluded that active low-frequency rTMS coupled with exposure therapy may have symptomatic and physiological effects. This interesting work opens the possibility that rTMS coupled with behavioral therapy could have value in anxiety disorders. Whether the rTMS was a priming response to behavioral therapy or acting in some other synergistic fashion is yet to be determined.

28.3.2.4 Obsessive–compulsive disorder (OCD)

Convergent neurophysiological data suggest that cognitive impairment and "intrusive" and repetitive behaviours in OCD may be a consequence of a reduction of cortico-subcortical inhibitory phenomena and a higher than normal level of cortical excitability (Rossi *et al.* 2005). Using TMS, Greenberg and colleagues (1998, 2000) tested whether deficient intracortical inhibition exists in OCD. They found that OCD patients, like those with Tourette syndrome (TS) (Ziemann *et al.* 1997), had markedly decreased intracortical inhibition. Those with "tic-related" OCD showed the most profound deficit in intracortical inhibition. Additionally, OCD subjects had lower resting and active motor thresholds than normal volunteers.

Imaging studies of OCD implicate hyperactivity in a circuit involving prefrontal cortex and basal ganglia.

To test whether modulating activity in this network could influence OCD symptoms, Greenberg and colleagues (1997) administered rTMS (80% motor threshold, 20 Hz for two seconds per minute for 20 minutes) to the right lateral prefrontal, left lateral prefrontal, and a midoccipital (control) site on separate days in a blinded trial. Compulsive urges decreased significantly for eight hours after right lateral prefrontal rTMS. A short-lasting, modest, and non-significant reduction in compulsive urges occurred after left lateral prefrontal rTMS.

Other studies have examined the possible therapeutic effects of rTMS in OCD. A double-blind study using right prefrontal 1 Hz rTMS and a less focal coil (a circular one instead of the figure-eight coil) failed to find statistically significant effects greater than sham (Alonso et al. 2001). In contrast, an open study in a group of OCD patients refractory to standard treatments who were randomly assigned to right or left prefrontal high-frequency rTMS found that clinically significant and sustained improvement was observed in a third of their patients (Sachdev et al. 2001). More recently Prasko and colleagues (2006) and Sachdev and colleagues (2007) found that either low- or high-frequency rTMS administered over the left DLPFC did not differ from sham (placebo).

Given the evidence for deficient intracortical inhibition in OCD, the use of low-frequency rTMS, which has been reported to be inhibitory on motor cortex excitability (Chen et al. 1997), may be a fruitful avenue to explore as a putative treatment. Furthermore, given the evidence of supplementary motor area (SMA) hyperactivation in OCD (Yücel et al. 2007), low-frequency rTMS to SMA may be worth examining.

To test the potential value of low-frequency rTMS to SMA, we performed an open-label study on 10 patients with treatment-resistant OCD and TS (Mantovani et al. 2006). OCD symptoms improved by an average of 29%, and improvements were significantly correlated with increases in right-hemisphere motor threshold and normalization of baseline hemispheric asymmetry of cortical excitability. Sustained benefit was seen at three-month follow-up. Subsequently, we reported clinical benefit in two more cases of comorbid OCD and TS (Mantovani et al. 2007b).

While these open-label data were encouraging, whether improvements would be evident in a sham-controlled design was still unknown. Therefore, we performed a randomized sham-controlled trial of SMA stimulation in the treatment of resistant OCD

and found that response rate (defined as a ≥ 25% decrease on the Yale–Brown Obsessive Compulsive Scale, YBOCS) was 67% with active and 22% with sham rTMS after four weeks of daily treatment. At four weeks, patients receiving active rTMS showed on average a 25% reduction in the YBOCS, while those who received sham had on average a 12% decrease on the same scale. In patients who received eight weeks of active rTMS, OCD symptoms improved from 28.2 (SD = 5.8) to 14.5 (SD = 3.6). In those randomized to active rTMS, motor threshold measures on the right hemisphere increased significantly over time. At the end of four weeks of rTMS, the abnormal hemispheric laterality found in the group randomized to active rTMS normalized (Mantovani et al. 2010).

28.3.2.5 Future directions for rTMS

Future work with rTMS in anxiety disorders could examine the potential utility of other stimulation paradigms with (1) a better localization of the brain region in individual patients using MRI; (2) more robust neuromodulatory action, such as theta burst stimulation (TBS); and (3) the use of coils able to reach deeper brain structures (Levkovitz et al. 2007, Di Lazzaro et al. 2008). The combination of rTMS with behavioral interventions (as illustrated by Osuch et al. 2009) could also be explored.

28.4 Vagus nerve stimulation (VNS)

The vagus nerve is composed mostly of sensory afferents carrying information to the nucleus tractus solitarius (NTS), which sends projections along three pathways: (1) an autonomic feedback loop, (2) direct projections to the medullary reticular formation, and (3) ascending projections to the forebrain. The latter travels via the parabrachial nucleus (PBN) and locus ceruleus (LC), which have direct connections with the forebrain, thalamus, hypothalamus, amygdala, and stria terminalis, regions important in the modulation of emotions (George et al. 1997, Van Bockstaele et al. 1999).

In vagus nerve stimulation (VNS), an electrical pulse generator is implanted in the left chest wall and delivers electrical signals via a bipolar lead to an electrode that is wrapped around the left vagus nerve in the neck (Amar et al. 1998). The pulse generator is programmed telemetrically. Initial reports of emotional changes in patients receiving VNS for the treatment of epilepsy prompted speculation that VNS may have applications in psychiatric disorders (Harden et al.

1999, Elger *et al.* 2000). In support of this hypothesis, there are reports that VNS increases central noradrenergic, serotonergic, and dopaminergic neurotransmission (Krahl *et al.* 1998, Jobe *et al.* 1999, Carpenter *et al.* 2004) and that like other effective psychotropic therapies, VNS alters frontal, limbic (particularly the cingulate), and thalamic blood flow (Henry *et al.* 1999, Devous *et al.* 2001, Conway *et al.* 2002). Lomarev and colleagues (2002) found that depending upon the frequency of stimulation, VNS increased BOLD-fMRI response in the orbitofrontal cortex, frontal pole, hypothalamus, left pallidum, and, less significantly, the thalamus, confirming the previous study by Bohning and colleagues (2001).

The adverse effects of VNS are those associated with the surgical implantation and those that are related to the stimulation, including pain, coughing, vocal cord paralysis, hoarseness, nausea, and, very rarely, infection. The majority of these are transient and are described by most patients as moderate (Schachter & Saper 1998).

28.4.1 VNS in the treatment of anxiety

Researchers have long known that the vagus nerve is involved in modulating autonomic functions. The vagus is actually a mixed nerve composed of about 80% afferent sensory fibers carrying information from the head, neck, thorax and abdomen to the brain (Foley & DuBois 1937). The James–Lange theory of emotion states that the experience of emotion depends upon the perception of autonomic signals. The current view, largely based on the work of Schachter and Singer (1962), stresses the importance of the cognitive interpretation of events but does not dismiss the importance of perception of autonomic arousal. Thus, signals of autonomic arousal are transmitted via the vagus to the brain, where the arousal is interpreted and given emotional valance.

Chavel and colleagues (2003) reported that epileptic patients responding to VNS were also significantly less anxious. Rush and colleagues (2000) also noted a possible effect of VNS on anxiety, having assessed several quality-of-life measures (including anxiety) in depressed patients being treated with VNS. Of the 30 patients assessed by Rush and colleagues, nine also suffered from agitation, 10 reported psychic anxiety, and 11 reported somatic anxiety. All patients reported improvements in agitation (73% reduction), psychic anxiety (50% reduction), and somatic anxiety (36% reduction). These results led to an open trial for VNS

for the treatment of anxiety disorders in a group of 10 patients suffering from OCD, PTSD, and panic disorder. At 10 weeks, all patients reported some improvement, with a mean reduction of 23% in anxiety as measured by the Hamilton Rating Scale for Anxiety (George *et al.* 2003). Despite these findings, there are no published case reports or open trials of VNS in specific anxiety disorders.

28.5 Deep brain stimulation (DBS)

The evidence that chronic high-frequency electrical stimulation of the brain results in clinical benefits similar to those achieved by surgical lesioning (Benabid *et al.* 1987, 1991) has transformed the use of functional neurosurgery for the treatment of movement disorders and has opened the door for the potential uses of deep brain stimulation (DBS) in psychiatric disorders (Gross & Lozano 2000). DBS involves delivering a current using implanted quadripolar electrodes connected to a battery-powered pulse-generating device. Stimulation can be adjusted by varying electrode selection and polarity and by altering frequency, amplitude, and pulse width. Thalamic DBS for intractable tremor has virtually replaced ablative lesions (Benabid *et al.* 1996), and DBS of the subthalamic nucleus (STN) or globus pallidus internus has largely replaced pallidotomy for Parkinson's disease (Kumar *et al.* 2000). Studies have begun to examine the utility of DBS for dystonia (Coubes *et al.* 2000, Yianni *et al.* 2003), epilepsy (Hodaie *et al.* 2002), obsessive–compulsive disorder (Gabriels *et al.* 2003), and depression (Aouizerate *et al.* 2004).

Serious adverse effects of the surgical procedure for DBS include intracerebral hemorrhage (less than 2% of cases), which can result in a range of deficits and even death. Confusion is a more common perioperative adverse effect. The stimulation itself can result in speech disturbances, paresthesias, eye movement difficulties, and motor contractions. The mechanism of action is still under evaluation, but it may be related to direct disruption of neuronal activity, increased GABA-mediated inhibitory neurotransmission, or stimulation-induced modulation of pathological network activity (McIntyre *et al.* 2004).

28.5.1 DBS in the treatment of obsessive–compulsive disorder (OCD)

Stereotactic lesioning has been of some benefit in severe, intractable OCD cases (Schmidek & Sweet

1995, Greenberg *et al.* 2003), suggesting that DBS of these surgical targets may have a clinical role as an alternative to lesioning (Devinsky *et al.* 1995, Zald & Kim 1996). Therefore, several investigators have examined the effects of DBS for the treatment of OCD.

Researchers have used different brain targets. For example, Gabriels and colleagues (2003) investigated the impact of DBS in the anterior limbs of the internal capsules in three patients with chronic, severe, treatment-resistant OCD and found improvement in two cases. In four other OCD patients with DBS implanted bilaterally in the anterior limbs of the internal capsules, chronic DBS significantly improved obsessional and compulsive symptoms in three out of the four patients (Cosyns *et al.* 2003). In two patients with leads placed bilaterally in the anterior limbs of the internal capsules, Abelson and colleagues (2005) found dramatic benefits to mood, anxiety, and OCD symptoms in one patient during blinded study and open, long-term follow-up. A second patient showed moderate benefit during open follow-up.

In another study, Aouizerate and colleagues (2004) examined the utility of DBS of the ventral caudate nucleus in a patient with intractable severe OCD and concomitant major depression. Depression and anxiety improved six months after the start of stimulation, and remission of OCD was observed after one year, with a progressive increase in the level of functioning. No neuropsychological deterioration was observed.

At the present time, DBS of the ventral (anterior internal) capsule/ventral striatum (VC/VS) is the primary location under investigation for severe OCD. Six patients enrolled in a DBS trial for OCD underwent positron emission tomography to measure regional cerebral blood flow (rCBF) in the right hemisphere; the rCBF measured during acute DBS at high frequency was then compared with that measured during DBS at low-frequency and off (control) conditions. On the basis of neuroanatomical knowledge about the VC/VS and neuroimaging data on OCD, the authors predicted that acute DBS at this target would result in modulation of activity within the frontal-basal ganglia–thalamic circuit, the brain circuit implicated in the pathogenesis of OCD. In a comparison of acute high-frequency DBS with control conditions, the authors found significant activation of the orbitofrontal cortex, anterior cingulate cortex, striatum, globus pallidus, and thalamus, as hypothesized (Rauch *et al.* 2006).

Greenberg and colleagues (2006) reported the long-term effects of VC/VS DBS in eight patients for 36 months. Group YBOCS scores decreased from 34.6 (SD = 0.6) (severe) at baseline to 22.3 (SD = 2.1) (moderate) at 36 months. Four of eight patients had a 35% or more decrease in YBOCS severity at 36 months; in two patients, scores declined between 25 and 35%. Global Assessment of Functioning scores improved from 36.6 (SD = 1.5) at baseline to 53.8 (SD = 2.5) at 36 months. Depression and anxiety also improved, as did self-care, independent living, and work, school, and social functioning. Surgical adverse effects included an asymptomatic hemorrhage, a single seizure, and a superficial infection. Psychiatric adverse effects included transient hypomanic symptoms and worsened depression and OCD when DBS was interrupted by stimulator battery depletion. This open study found promising long-term effects of DBS in highly treatment-resistant OCD.

Recently, Greenberg and colleagues (2010) reported the results obtained by psychiatric neurosurgery teams in the United States and Europe on VC/VS DBS for severe and highly treatment-resistant OCD. Combined long-term results in 26 OCD patients revealed clinically significant symptom reductions and functional improvement in about two-thirds. Mean YBOCS scores decreased after stimulation onset from 34.0 (SD = 0.5) to 20.9 (SD = 2.4) at 36 months. This degree of improvement was apparent by the third month of active stimulation, when the mean YBOCS had declined to 21.0 (SD = 1.8). Overall, 73% of patients had at least a 25% YBOCS improvement at last follow-up; a large majority of these patients improved at least 35%. DBS was well tolerated overall, and adverse effects were overwhelmingly transient. Based on these results, the FDA recently approved a humanitarian device exemption for DBS in severe OCD.

Patients implanted more recently tended to show greater improvement. The main factor accounting for these gains appears to be the refinement of the implantation site. Initially, an anterior–posterior location based on anterior capsulotomy lesions was used. In an attempt to improve results, more posterior sites were investigated, resulting in the current target, at the junction of the anterior capsule, anterior commissure, and posterior ventral striatum.

Although DBS has been applied at several locations along the rostral–caudal extent of the anterior limb of the internal capsule and/or the adjacent striatum, the most common surgical approach in OCD has been to target the VC/VS. Fibers within the cortico-striatal-thalamo-cortical (CSTC) networks hypothesized as central to the therapeutic effects of lesions or DBS

Table 28.2. Brain stimulation in the treatment of anxiety disorders: summary

Reference	Diagnosis	n	Treatment	Outcome
Rush et al. (2000)	GAD/MDD	30	VNS	Patients reported 73% improvement in agitation, 50% in psychic anxiety and 36% in somatic anxiety after 10 weeks of VNS
Chavel et al. (2003)	Epilepsy/GAD	29	VNS	17 patients reported >50% reduction in seizures and a >50% reduction on BAI at 24 months of VNS
Rasmussen et al. (2004)	GAD/MDD	253	ECT	Somatic anxiety correlates negatively with likelihood of sustained remission to ECT.; patients with anxiety had a much lower sustained remission rates to ECT
Bystritsky et al. (2008)	GAD	10	rTMS	6 patients reported >50% reduction on HAM-A after 6 right DLPFC 1 Hz rTMS sessions
Figiel et al. (1992)	Panic disorder	8	ECT	Patients reported no panic attack from their fourth ECT treatment
Garcia-Toro et al. (2002)	Panic disorder	3	rTMS	Patients reported a modest improvement of panic after 10 right DLPFC 1 Hz rTMS sessions
Zwanzger et al. (2002)	Panic disorder	1	rTMS	Patient reported 78% decrease of anxiety and 59% reduction of panic and agoraphobia after 10 right DLPFC 1 Hz rTMS sessions
Guaiana et al. (2005)	Panic disorder	1	rTMS	Patient reported PDSS = 3 after 20 left DLPFC 10 Hz rTMS sessions
Mantovani et al. (2007a)	Panic disorder	6	rTMS	5 patients reported >50% reduction on PDSS after 10 right DLPFC 1 Hz rTMS sessions
Prasko et al. (2007)	Panic disorder	15	rTMS	Patients reported 35% or 50% reduction on PDSS after 10 active or sham right DLPFC 1 Hz rTMS sessions
Grisaru et al. (1998)	PTSD	10	rTMS	Patients reported significant improvement on IES avoidance, anxiety and somatization after 1 bilateral motor cortex 0.3 Hz rTMS session
McCann et al. (1998)	PTSD	2	rTMS	Patients reported significant improvement on PTSD Symptom Scale after 17–30 right DLPFC 1 Hz rTMS sessions
Rosenberg et al. (2002)	MDD/PTSD	12	rTMS	9 patients reported >50% reduction on HAM-D and minimal improvement in PTSD after 10 left DLPFC 1 or 5 Hz rTMS sessions
Cohen et al. (2004)	PTSD	24	rTMS	10 patients reported >30% reduction on CAPS after 10 left DLPFC 10 Hz rTMS sessions; no change was reported after 10 left DLPFC 1 Hz rTMS sessions (8 patients), or sham (6 patients)
Osuch et al. (2009)	PTSD	9	rTMS	Patients reported improvement on hyperarousal (CAPS) after 20 right DLPFC 1 Hz rTMS sessions and ET; no change was reported after sham and ET
Watts (2007)	MDD/PTSD	26	ECT	Patients reported >50% reduction on MADRS, and >20 on PCL after 10–15 ECT sessions
Mellman & Gorman (1984)	OCD	1	ECT	Patient reported remission after 10 bilateral ECT
Khanna et al. (1988)	OCD	6	ECT	Patients reported improvement up to 1–4 months after ECT
Maletzky et al. (1994)	OCD	32	ECT	Patients reported a considerable improvement up to 1 year after ECT
Greenberg et al. (1997)	OCD	12	rTMS	Patients reported reduction in compulsions after 1 right PFC 20 Hz rTMS session
Alonso et al. (2001)	OCD	18	rTMS	10 patients reported 15% improvement on YBOCS after 18 active right DLPFC 1 Hz rTMS sessions; 8 patients reported no change after sham
Sachdev et al. (2001)	OCD	12	rTMS	Patients reported >30% reduction on YBOCS after 10 right or left DLPFC 10 Hz rTMS sessions
Fukuchi et al. (2003)	OCD	1	ECT	Patient reported marked improvement after two courses of ECT

Table 28.2 (cont.)

Reference	Diagnosis	n	Treatment	Outcome
Cosyns et al. (2003)	OCD	4	DBS	3 patients reported acute reduction of obsessive–compulsive symptoms after bilateral DBS in the anterior limbs of the internal capsules
Gabriels et al. (2003)	OCD	3	DBS	2/3 patients reported >35% reduction on YBOCS after 33 months bilateral DBS in the anterior limbs of the internal capsules
George et al. (2003)	Panic disorder, PTSD, OCD	10	VNS	Patients with panic disorder, PTSD, and OCD reported 23% reduction on HAM-A at 10 weeks of VNS
Aouizerate et al. (2004)	OCD	1	DBS	Patient reported remission after 12–15 months of DBS of the ventral caudate nucleus
Strassnig et al. (2004)	OCD	1	ECT	Patient reported remission after 9 ECT
Abelson et al. (2005)	OCD	4	DBS	2 patients reported >35% reduction on YBOCS after 1 and 2 years bilateral DBS in the anterior limbs of the internal capsules
Greenberg et al. (2006)	OCD	8	DBS	Patients reported 35% reduction on YBOCS after 3 years ventral capsule/ventral striatum DBS
Mantovani et al. (2006)	OCD	10	rTMS	Patients reported 29% reduction on YBOCS after 10 SMA 1 Hz rTMS sessions
Prasko et al. (2006)	OCD	30	rTMS	Patients reported a 20% reduction on YBOCS after 10 right DLPFC 1 Hz rTMS sessions or sham
Baker (2007)	OCD	1	DBS	Patient reported 42% reduction on YBOCS after 1 year bilateral DBS in the anterior limbs of the internal capsules
Sachdev et al. (2007)	OCD	18	rTMS	5/18 patients reported >40% reduction on YBOCS after 10 left DLPFC 10 Hz rTMS sessions or sham
Mantovani et al. (2007b)	OCD	2	rTMS	Patients reported >20% reduction on YBOCS after 10 SMA 1 Hz rTMS sessions
Greenberg et al. (2010)	OCD	26	DBS	Patients reported 39% reduction on YBOCS after 3 years ventral capsule/ventral striatum DBS
Mantovani et al. (2010)	OCD	18	rTMS	6/9 patients reported >25% reduction on YBOCS after 20 SMA 1 Hz rTMS sessions, 2/9 responded to sham

BAI, Beck Anxiety Inventory; CAPS, Clinician-Administered PTSD Scale; DBS, deep brain stimulation; DLPFC, dorsolateral prefrontal cortex; ECT, electroconvulsive therapy; GAD, generalized anxiety disorder; HAM-A, Hamilton Rating Scale for Anxiety; HAM-D, Hamilton Rating Scale for Depression; IES, Impact of Events Scale; MADRS, Montgomery–Asberg Depression Rating Scale; MDD, major depressive disorder; OCD, obsessive–compulsive disorder; PDSS, Panic Disorder Severity Scale; PTSD, posttraumatic stress disorder; rTMS, repetitive TMS; SMA, supplementary motor area; TMS, transcranial magnetic stimulation; VNS, vagus nerve stimulation; YBOCS, Yale–Brown Obsessive Compulsive Scale.

(Rauch 2003) become more compact as they course posteriorly toward the thalamus, to which they connect via the inferior thalamic peduncle (Kopell et al. 2004, Velasco et al. 2006). The VC/VS may thus represent a node of CSTC circuits that is readily targeted for modulation by DBS.

28.6 Conclusions

Brain stimulation techniques for the treatment of anxiety disorders remain investigational and are not yet used in routine clinical practice. Most of the positive findings are based on small samples in short-term trials (Table 28.2). Larger, placebo-controlled trials are needed. However, in addition to the usual concerns about sample comparability and the reliability of assessment, brain stimulation studies encounter two unique methodological issues: (1) the creation of an effective sham (placebo) condition and (2) the decision of what parameters to use.

Sham-controlled trials represent the gold standard for establishing the efficacy of an intervention. An adequate placebo should be plausible and inactive, and it should simulate as closely as possible the ancillary effects of the treatment. In TMS, progress has been made: the initial way the coil was angled off the head so that the magnetic field stimulates scalp muscles but does not enter the brain was proven to exert some effects on the brain (Lisanby et al. 2001); as a result, new sham coils have been designed to blind both subject and treater by either making active TMS feel more like sham, or by making sham feel more like active. The plausibility of these sham systems is being systematically evaluated, and such approaches will likely afford better blinding for clinical trials than former approaches. In VNS and DBS it might be difficult to eliminate side effects related to the stimulation itself (e.g., VNS may cause voice alteration, vocal cord paralysis, neck or throat pain, dyspnea, coughing, and nausea; DBS may result in speech disturbances, paresthesias, eye movement difficulties, and motor contractions); these side effects can potentially unblind patient and treater. By refining the surgical procedures and minimizing side effects, it may be possible to maintain the blind and to rigorously test the clinical efficacy of both VNS and DBS.

With regards to the stimulation parameters, a large number of variables must be taken into account, such as stimulation frequency and intensity, treatment duration, site of stimulation, and method of site localization. As a result, only a limited range of these myriad parameters have been explored. Dose finding and mechanistic studies are extremely important to guide the ultimate clinical use of these interventions in the treatment of anxiety disorders. Multicenter trials sponsored both by industry and by the National Institute of Mental Health are presently under way to address some of these questions.

Despite these methodological issues, initial studies suggest that rTMS, VNS, and DBS can exert a variety of both short- and long-term anxiolytic effects. On the optimistic side, they raise the possibility that focal modulation of cortical and subcortical excitability can have therapeutic properties in anxiety disorders and may prove informative about the anatomy and physiology of the neural systems involved in achieving therapeutic effects. At the clinical level, since their adverse-effect profile can be benign, they may ultimately offer a less invasive alternative to already established somatic interventions (e.g., ECT and neurosurgery) for severe or treatment-resistant anxiety conditions.

References

Abelson, J. L., Curtis, G. C., Sagher, O., et al. (2005). Deep brain stimulation for refractory obsessive–compulsive disorder. *Biological Psychiatry*, **57**, 510–516.

Abrams, R. (1982). Clinical prediction of ECT response in depressed patients. *Psychopharmacology Bulletin*, **18**, 48–50.

Abrams, R., & Taylor, M. A. (1973). Anterior bifrontal ECT: a clinical trial. *British Journal of Psychiatry*, **122**, 587–590.

Alonso, P., Pujol, J., Cardoner, N., et al. (2001). Right prefrontal repetitive transcranial magnetic stimulation in obsessive–compulsive disorder: a double-blind, placebo-controlled study. *American Journal of Psychiatry*, **158**, 1143–1145.

Alvarez, R. P., Biggs, A., & Chen, G. (2008). Contextual fear conditioning in humans: cortical-hippocampal and amygdala contributions. *Journal of Neuroscience*, **28**, 6211–6219.

Amar, A. P., Heck, C. N., Levy, M. L., et al. (1998). An institutional experience with cervical vagus nerve trunk stimulation for medically refractory epilepsy: rationale, technique, and outcome. *Neurosurgery*, **43**, 1265–1280.

Aouizerate, B., Cuny, E., Martin-Guehl, C., et al. (2004). Deep brain stimulation of the ventral caudate nucleus in the treatment of obsessive–compulsive disorder and major depression. Case report. *Journal of Neurosurgery*, **101**, 682–6.

Baker, K. B., Kopell, B. H., Malone, D., et al. (2007). Deep brain stimulation for obsessive–compulsive disorder. Using functional magnetic resonance imaging and electrophysiological techniques: technical case report. *Neurosurgery*, **61** (5 Suppl. 2), E367–368.

Belmaker, B., Fitzgerald, P., George, M.S., et al. (2003). Managing the risks of repetitive transcranial stimulation. *CNS Spectrums*, **8**, 489.

Benabid, A. L., Pollak, P., Louveau, A., Henry, S., & de Rougemont, J. (1987). Combined (thalamotomy and stimulation) stereotactic surgery of the VIM thalamic nucleus for bilateral Parkinson disease. *Applied Neurophysiology*, **50**, 344–346.

Benabid, A. L., Pollak, P., Gervason, C., et al. (1991). Long-term suppression of tremor by chronic stimulation of the ventral intermediate thalamic nucleus. *Lancet*, **337**, 403–406.

Benabid, A. L., Pollak, P., Gao, D., et al. (1996). Chronic electrical stimulation of the ventralis intermedius nucleus of the thalamus as a treatment of movement disorders. *Journal of Neurosurgery*, **84**, 203–214.

Bohning, D. E., Lomarev, M. P., Denslow, S., et al. (2001). Feasibility of vagus nerve stimulation-synchronized blood oxygenation level-dependent functional MRI. *Investigations in Radiology*, **36**, 470–479.

Bystritsky, A., Kaplan, J. T., Feusner, J. D., et al. (2008). A preliminary study of fMRI-guided rTMS in the treatment of generalized anxiety disorder. *Journal of Clinical Psychiatry*, **69**, 1092–1098.

Carney, M. W. P., Roth, M., & Garside, R. F. (1965). The diagnosis of depressive syndromes and the prediction of ECT response. *British Journal of Psychiatry*, **111**, 659–674.

Carpenter, L. L., Moreno, F. A., Kling, M. A., et al. (2004). Effect of vagus nerve stimulation on cerebrospinal fluid monoamine metabolites, norepinephrine, and gamma-aminobutyric acid concentrations in depressed patients. *Biological Psychiatry*, **56**, 418–426.

Chavel, S. M., Westerveld, M., & Spencer, S. (2003). Long-term outcome of vagus nerve stimulation for refractory partial epilepsy. *Epilepsy and Behavior*, 4, 302–309.

Chen, R., Classen, J., Gerloff, C., *et al.* (1997). Depression of motor cortex excitability by low frequency transcranial magnetic stimulation. *Neurology*, 48, 1398–1403.

Cohen, H., Kaplan, Z., Kotler, M., *et al.* (2004). Repetitive transcranial magnetic stimulation of the right dorsolateral prefrontal cortex in posttraumatic stress disorder: a double-blind, placebo-controlled study. *American Journal of Psychiatry*, 161, 515–524.

Conway, C. R., Chibnall, J. T., Li, X., & George, M. S. (2002). Changes in brain metabolism in response to chronic vagus nerve stimulation in depression. *Biological Psychiatry*, 51, 8S–544.

Cosyns, P., Gabriels, L., & Nuttin, B. (2003). Deep brain stimulation in treatment refractory obsessive compulsive disorder. *Verhandelingen – Koninklijke Academie voor Geneeskunde van België*, 65, 385–399, discussion 399–400.

Coubes, P., Roubertie, A., Vayssiere, N., Hemm, S., & Echenne, B., (2000). Treatment of DYT1-generalised dystonia by stimulation of the internal globus pallidus. *Lancet*, 355, 2220–2221.

Devinsky, O., Morrell, M. J., & Vogt, B. A. (1995). Contributions of anterior cingulated cortex to behaviour. *Brain*, 118, 279–306.

Devous, M. D. (2001). Effects of VNS on regional cerebral blood flow in depressed subjects. vagus nerve stimulation (VNS) for treatment-resistant depression. Satellite Symposium in conjunction with the 7th World Congress of Biological Psychiatry. Berlin, Germany.

Di Lazzaro, V., Pilato, F., Dileone, M., *et al.* (2008). The physiological basis of the effects of intermittent theta burst stimulation of the human motor cortex. *Journal of Physiology*, 586, 3871–3879.

Elger, G., Hoppe, C., Falkai, P., Rush, A. J., & Elger, C. E. (2000). Vagus nerve stimulation is associated with mood improvements in epilepsy patients. *Epilepsy Research*, 42, 203–210.

Figiel, G. S., Zorumski, C. F., Doraiswamy, P. M., Mattingly, G. W., & Jarvis, M. R. (1992). Simultaneous major depression and panic disorder: treatment with electroconvulsive therapy. *Journal of Clinical Psychiatry*, 53, 12–15.

Foley, J. O., & DuBois, F. (1937). Quantitative studies of the vagus nerve in the cat. I. The ratio of sensory and motor studies. *Journal of Computative Neurology*, 67, 49–67.

Fukuchi, T., Okada, Y., Katayama, H., *et al.* (2003). A case of pregnant woman with severe obsessive-compulsive disorder successfully treated by modified-electroconvulsive therapy. *Seishin Shinkeigaku Zasshi*, 105, 927–932.

Gabriels, L., Cosyns, P., Nuttin, B., Demeulemeester, H., & Gybels, J. (2003). Deep brain stimulation for treatment-refractory obsessive–compulsive disorder: psychopathological and neuropsychological outcome in three cases. *Acta Psychiatria Scandinavia*, 107, 275–282.

Garcia-Toro, M., Salva Coll, J., Crespi Font, M. *et al.* (2002). Panic disorder and transcranial magnetic stimulation. *Actas Espanolas de Psiquiatria*, 30, 221–224.

George, M. S., Post, R. M., Ketter, T. A., Kimbrell, T. A., & Speer, A. M. (1997). Neural mechanisms of mood disorders. *Current Review of Mood and Anxiety Disorders*, 1, 71–83.

George, M. S., Rush, A. J., Sackeim, H. A., & Marangell, L. B. (2003). Vagus nerve stimulation (VNS): utility in neuropsychiatric disorders. *International Journal of Neuropsychopharmacology*, 6, 73–83.

Greenberg, B. D., George, M. S., Dearing, J., *et al.* (1997). Effects of prefrontal repetitive transcranial magnetic stimulation (rTMS) in obsessive–compulsive disorder: a preliminary study. *American Journal of Psychiatry*, 154, 867–869.

Greenberg, B. D., Ziemann, U., Harmon, A., Murphy, D. L., & Wassermann, E. M. (1998). Decreased neuronal inhibition in cerebral cortex in obsessive–compulsive disorder on transcranial magnetic stimulation. *Lancet*, 352, 881–882.

Greenberg, B. D., Ziemann, U., Cora-Locatelli, G., *et al.* (2000). Altered cortical excitability in obsessive–compulsive disorder. *Neurology*, 54, 142–147.

Greenberg, B. D., Price, L. H., Rauch, S. L., *et al.* (2003). Neurosurgery for intractable obsessive–compulsive disorder and depression: critical issues. *Neurosurgery Clinics of North America*, 14, 199–212.

Greenberg, B. D., Malone, D. A., Friehs, G. M., *et al.* (2006). Three-year outcomes in deep brain stimulation for highly resistant obsessive–compulsive disorder. *Neuropsychopharmacology*, 31, 2384–2393.

Greenberg, B. D., Gabriels, L. A., Malone, D. A., *et al.* (2010). Deep brain stimulation of the ventral internal capsule/ventral striatum for obsessive–compulsive disorder: worldwide experience. *Molecular Psychiatry*, 15, 64–79.

Grisaru, N., Amir, M., Cohen, H., & Kaplan, Z. (1998). Effects of transcranial magnetic stimulation in post-traumatic stress disorder: a preliminary study. *Biological Psychiatry*, 44, 52–55.

Gross, R. E., & Lozano, A. M. (2000). Advances in neurostimulation for movement disorders. *Neurological Research*, 22, 247–258.

Guaiana, G., Mortimer, A. M., & Robertson, C. (2005). Efficacy of transcranial magnetic stimulation in panic disorder: a case report. *Australian and New Zealand Journal of Psychiatry*, 39, 1047.

Harden, C. L., Pulver, M. C., Nikolov, B., Halper, J. P., Labar, D. R. (1999). Effect of vagus nerve stimulation on mood in adult epilepsy patients. *Neurology*, **52** (Suppl. 2), A238–P03122.

Henry, T. R., Votaw, J. R., Pennell, P. B., *et al.* (1999). Acute blood flow changes and efficacy of vagus nerve stimulation in partial epilepsy. *Neurology*, **52**, 1166–1173.

Hobson, R. F. (1953). Prognostic factors in electric convulsive therapy, *Journal of Neurology, Neurosurgery, and Psychiatry*, **16**, 275–281.

Hodaie, M., Wennberg, R. A., Dostrovsky, J. O., & Lozano, A. M. (2002). Chronic anterior thalamus stimulation for intractable epilepsy. *Epilepsia*, **43**, 603–608.

Hsu, M., Bhatt, M., Adolphs, R., Tranel, D., & Camerer, C. F. (2005). Neural systems responding to degrees of uncertainty in human decision-making. *Science*, **310**, 1680–1683.

Jobe, P. C., Dailey, J. W., & Wernicke, J. F. (1999). A noradrenergic and serotonergic hypothesis of the linkage between epilepsy and affective disorders. *Critical Reviews in Neurobiology*, **13**, 317–356.

Khanna, S., Gangadhar, B. N., Sinha, V., Rajendra, P. N., & Channabasavanna, S. M. (1988). Electroconvulsive therapy in obsessive–compulsive disorder. *Convulsive Therapy*, **4**, 314–320.

Kopell, B. H., Greenberg, B., & Rezai, A. R. (2004). Deep brain stimulation for psychiatric disorders. *Journal of Clinical Neurophysiology*, **21**, 51–67.

Koran, L. M., Hanna, L. G., Hollander, E., *et al.* American Psychiatric Association (2007). Practice guideline for the treatment of patients with obsessive-compulsive disorder. *American Journal of Psychiatry*, **164** (7 Suppl.), 1–56.

Krahl, S. E., Clark, K. B., Smith, D. C., & Browning, R. A. (1998). Locus coeruleus lesions suppress the seizure-attenuating effects of vagus nerve stimulation. *Epilepsia*, **39**, 709–714.

Kumar, R., Lang, A. E., Rodriguez-Oroz, M. C., *et al.* (2000). Deep brain stimulation of the globus pallidus pars interna in advanced Parkinson's disease. *Neurology*, **55** (12 Suppl. 6), S34–S39.

Levkovitz, Y., Roth, Y., Harel, E. V., *et al.* (2007). A randomized controlled feasibility and safety study of deep transcranial magnetic stimulation. *Clinical Neurophysiology*, **118**, 2730–2744.

Lisanby, S. H., Gutman, D., Luber, B., Schroeder, C., & Sackeim, H. A. (2001). Sham TMS: intracerebral measurement of the induced electrical field and the induction of motor-evoked potentials. *Biological Psychiatry* **49**, 460–463.

Lomarev, M., Denslow, S., Nahas, Z., *et al.* (2002). Vagus nerve stimulation (VNS) synchronized BOLD fMRI suggests that VNS in depressed adults has frequency/dose dependent effects. *Journal of Psychiatric Research*, **36**, 219–227.

Maletzky, B., McFarland, B., & Burt, A. (1994). Refractory obsessive compulsive disorder and ECT. *Convulsive Therapy*, **10**, 34–42.

Mantovani, A., Lisanby, S. H., Pieraccini, F., *et al.* (2006). Repetitive transcranial magnetic stimulation (rTMS) in the treatment of obsessive–compulsive disorder (OCD) and Tourette's syndrome (TS). *International Journal of Neuropsychopharmacology*, **9**, 95–100.

Mantovani, A., Lisanby, S. H., Pieraccini, F., *et al.* (2007a). Repetitive transcranial magnetic stimulation (rTMS) in the treatment of panic disorder (PD) with comorbid major depression. *Journal of Affective Disorders*, **102**, 277–280.

Mantovani, A., Leckman, J. F., Grantz, H., *et al.* (2007b). Repetitive transcranial magnetic stimulation of the supplementary motor area in the treatment of Tourette syndrome: report of two cases. *Clinical Neurophysiology*, **118**, 2314–2315.

Mantovani, A., Simpson, H. B., Fallon, B. A., Rossi, S., & Lisanby, S. H. (2010). Randomized sham-controlled trial of repetitive transcranial magnetic stimulation in treatment-resistant obsessive–compulsive disorder. *International Journal of Neuropsychopharmacology*, **13**, 217–227.

McCann, U. D., Kimbrell, T. A., Morgan, C. M., *et al.* (1998). Repetitive transcranial magnetic stimulation for post-traumatic stress disorder. *Archives of General Psychiatry*, **55**, 276–279.

McIntyre, C. C., Savasta, M., Kerkerian-Le Goff, L., & Vitek, J. L. (2004). Uncovering the mechanism(s) of action of deep brain stimulation: activation, inhibition, or both. *Clinical Neurophysiology*, **115**, 1239–1248.

Mellman, L. A., & Gorman, J. M. (1984). Successful treatment of obsessive–compulsive disorder with ECT. *American Journal of Psychiatry*, **141**, 596–597.

Mendels, J. (1965). Electroconvulsive therapy and depression: I. The prognostic significance of clinical factors, *British Journal of Psychiatry*, **111**, 675–681.

Morinaga, K., Akiyoshi, J., Matsushita H., *et al.* (2007). Anticipatory anxiety-induced changes in human lateral prefrontal cortex activity. *Biological Psychology*, **74**, 34–38.

Osuch, E. A., Benson, B. E., Luckenbaugh, D. A., *et al.* (2009). Repetitive TMS combined with exposure therapy for PTSD: a preliminary study. *Journal of Anxiety Disorders*, **23**, 54–59.

Pande, A. C., Krugler, T., Haskett, R. F., Greden J. F., Grunhaus, L. J. (1988). Predictors of response to electroconvulsive therapy in major depression, *Biological Psychiatry*, **24**, 91–93.

Prasko, J., Pasková, B., Záleský, R., *et al.* (2006). The effect of repetitive transcranial magnetic stimulation (rTMS) on symptoms in obsessive compulsive disorder. A randomized, double blind, sham controlled study. *Neuro-Endocrinology Letters*, **27**, 327–332.

Prasko, J., Záleský, R., Bares, M., *et al.* (2007). The effect of repetitive transcranial magnetic stimulation (rTMS) add on serotonin reuptake inhibitors in patients with panic disorder: a randomized, double blind sham controlled study. *Neuro-Endocrinology Letters*, **28**, 33–38.

Prudic, J., Devanand, D. P., Sackeim, H. A., Decina, P., & Kerr, B. (1989). Relative response of endogenous and non-endogenous symptoms to electroconvulsive therapy. *Journal of Affective Disorders*, **16**, 59–64.

Rasmussen, K. G., Snyder, K. A., Knapp, R. G., *et al.* (2004). Relationship between somatization and remission with ECT. *Psychiatry Research*, **129**, 293–295.

Rauch, S. L. (2003). Neuroimaging and neurocircuitry models pertaining to the neurosurgical treatment of psychiatric disorders. *Neurosurgery Clinics of North America*, **14**, 213–223, vii–viii.

Rauch, S. L., Dougherty, D. D., Malone, D., *et al.* (2006). A functional neuroimaging investigation of deep brain stimulation in patients with obsessive–compulsive disorder. *Journal of Neurosurgery*, **104**, 558–565.

Roberts, J. (1959) Prognostic factors in the electroshock treatment of depressive states, *Journal of Mental Science*, **105**, 693–702.

Rosenberg, P. B., Mehndiratta, R. B., Mehndiratta, Y. P., *et al.* (2002). Repetitive transcranial magnetic stimulation treatment of comorbid posttraumatic stress disorder and major depression. *Journal of Neuropsychiatry and Clinical Neurosciences*, **14**, 270–276.

Rossi, S., Bartalini, S., Ulivelli, M., *et al.* (2005). Hypofunctioning of sensory gating mechanisms in patients with obsessive–compulsive disorder. *Biological Psychiatry*, **57**, 16–20.

Rush, A. J., George, M. S., Sackeim, H. A., *et al.* (2000). Vagus nerve stimulation (VNS) for treatment-resistant depressions: a multicenter study. *Biological Psychiatry*, **47**, 276–286.

Sachdev, P. S., McBridge, R., Loo, C. K., *et al.* (2001). Right versus left prefrontal transcranial magnetic stimulation for obsessive–compulsive disorder: a preliminary investigation. *Journal of Clinical Psychiatry*, **62**, 981–984.

Sachdev, P. S., Loo, C. K., Mitchell, P. B., McFarquhar, T. F., & Malhi, G. S. (2007). Repetitive transcranial magnetic stimulation for the treatment of obsessive compulsive disorder: a double-blind controlled investigation. *Psychological Medicine*, **37**, 1645–1649.

Schachter, S. & Singer, J. E. (1962). Cognitive, social and physiological determinants of emotional state. *Psychological Review*, **69**, 379–399.

Schachter, S. C., & Saper, C. B. (1998). Vagus nerve stimulation. *Epilepsia*, **39**, 677–686.

Schmidek, H. H., & Sweet, W. H., eds. (1995). *Operative Neurosurgical Techniques*, 4th edn. Philadelphia, PA: Saunders.

Sobin, C., Predict, J., Devanand, D. P., Nobler, M. S., & Sackeim, H. A. (1996). Who responds to electroconvulsive therapy? A comparison of effective and ineffective forms of treatment. *British Journal of Psychiatry*, **169**, 322–328.

Strassnig, M., Riedel, M., & Müller, N. (2004). Electroconvulsive therapy in a patient with Tourette's syndrome and co-morbid obsessive compulsive disorder. *World Journal of Biological Psychiatry*, **5**, 164–166.

Van Bockstaele, E. J., Peoples, J., & Valentino, R. J. (1999). Anatomic basis for differential regulation of the rostrolateral peri-locus coeruleus region by limbic afferents. *Biological Psychiatry*, **46**, 1352–1363.

van den Heuvel, O. A., Veltman, D. J., Groenewegen, H. J., *et al.* (2005). Disorder-specific neuroanatomical correlates of attentional bias in obsessive–compulsive disorder, panic disorder, and hypochondriasis. *Archives of General Psychiatry*, **62**, 922–933.

Velasco, M., Velasco, F., Jimenez, F., *et al.* (2006). Electrocortical and behavioral responses elicited by acute electrical stimulation of inferior thalamic peduncle and nucleus reticularis thalami in a patient with major depression disorder. *Clinical Neurophysiology*, **117**, 320–327.

Wassermann, E. M. (1998). Risk and safety of repetitive transcranial magnetic stimulation: report and suggested guidelines from the International Workshop on the Safety of Repetitive Transcranial Magnetic Stimulation, June 5–7, 1996. *Electroencephalography and Clinical Neurophysiology*, **108**, 1–16.

Watts, B. V. (2007). Electroconvulsive therapy for comorbid major depressive disorder and posttraumatic stress disorder. *Journal of ECT*, **23**, 93–95.

Yianni, J., Bain, P., Giladi, N., *et al.* (2003). Globus pallidus internus deep brain stimulation for dystonic conditions: a prospective audit. *Movement Disorders*, **18**, 436–442.

Yücel, M., Harrison, B. J., Wood, S. J., *et al.* (2007). Functional and biochemical alterations of the medial frontal cortex in OCD. *Archives of General Psychiatry*, **64**, 946–955.

Zald, D. H., & Kim, S. W. (1996). Anatomy and function of the orbital frontal cortex: II. Function and relevance to obsessive–compulsive disorder. *Journal of Neuropsychiatry and Clinical Neuroscience*, **8**, 249–261.

Ziemann, U., Paulus, W., & Rothenberger, A. (1997). Decreased motor inhibition in Tourette's disorder: evidence from transcranial magnetic stimulation. *American Journal of Psychiatry*, **154**, 1277–1284.

Zimmerman, M., Coryell, W., Pfohl, B., Corenthal, C., & Stangl, D. (1986). ECT response in depressed patients with and without a DSM-III personality disorder. *American Journal of Psychiatry*, **143**, 1030–1032.

Zwanzger, P., Minov, C., Ella, R., *et al.* (2002). Transcranial magnetic stimulation for panic. *American Journal of Psychiatry*, **159**, 315–316.

Chapter 29

Complementary and alternative medicine approaches to the treatment of anxiety

Sapana R. Patel, Anthony J. Tranguch, Philip R. Muskin

29.1 Introduction

Western biomedicine approaches healing as related to either the body or the mind, as if they were in isolation from each other. In this conception, illness is external, following a disease-oriented model. In contrast, Eastern medicine views the mind and body as unified and approaches healing as an internal process. As we adopt Eastern medicine into Western society, alternative practices to address both physical and mental health problems are becoming widely employed. These "non-traditional practices," from the perspective of conventional Western biomedicine, have been termed *complementary and alternative medicine* (CAM). CAM is typically divided into two broad categories: complementary medicine – approaches used along with conventional biomedicine – and alternative medicine – approaches used instead of conventional biomedicine.

CAM approaches are diverse and abundant, and they are grouped by the National Center for Complementary and Alternative Medicine (NCCAM) of the National Institutes of Health into four general domains: (1) mind–body medicine, (2) biologically based practices, (3) manipulative and body-based practices, and (4) energy medicine. Kessler and colleagues (2001) found that people with anxiety and depressive disorders use CAM therapies more frequently than conventional mental health therapies. Almost nine out of ten patients with self-defined "anxiety attacks" seen by a psychiatrist also use some type of complementary and alternative therapy to treat their anxiety. Predictors of CAM use include poor general health, anxiety, chronic pain, and higher education. Additional motivations for CAM use include compatibility with the person's worldviews regarding health and illness, fears about conventional medical treatments, and concern that suffering will not be sufficiently relieved by conventional approaches (Astin 1998, Testerman *et al.*

2004). The strength of the scientific evidence supporting CAM therapies varies tremendously, and questions remain regarding efficacy and safety for some treatments. This chapter will review the four general domains of CAM therapies for anxiety disorders.

29.2 Mind–body medicine

Mind–body interventions constitute a major portion of overall CAM use, with about 17% of adults in the United States utilizing such approaches in 2002 (Barnes *et al.* 2004). Intervention strategies for anxiety disorders include meditation, yoga and yogic breathing exercises, and psychotherapy-based interventions. Despite the large body of research on mind–body techniques, limitations in study design and methodological rigor constrain the quality of the scientific evidence and the generalizability of efficacy results.

Using mind–body interventions to treat anxiety disorders requires some background information on the stress-response system. Many people with traumatic experiences, panic attacks, phobias, and generalized anxiety disorder (GAD) experience a "fight or flight" response that is repeatedly set off by signals misinterpreted as threatening in the absence of actual danger. The fight-or-flight response activates the autonomic nervous system (ANS), which comprises two primary branches, the sympathetic nervous system (SNS) and the parasympathetic nervous system (PNS). The SNS stimulates physiological alterations, including increases in heart rate, cardiac stroke volume, and vasoconstriction, consistent with somatic tension. In contrast, the PNS produces the opposite physiologic effects to achieve a more relaxed somatic state. In people who suffer from anxiety disorders, the PNS is underactive while the SNS is overactive (Beauchaine 2001). Mind–body techniques such as meditation and yoga can activate the relaxation response (i.e., excite

Anxiety Disorders: Theory, Research, and Clinical Perspectives, ed. Helen Blair Simpson, Yuval Neria, Roberto Lewis-Fernández, Franklin Schneier. Published by Cambridge University Press. © Cambridge University Press 2010.

the PNS) or reduce the stress response (i.e., suppress the SNS). In the treatment of anxiety disorders, it is important to augment PNS control and to increase the flexibility of the entire stress-response system.

29.2.1 Meditation

Meditation has been defined as "self-regulation of attention, in the service of self-inquiry, in the here and now" (Maison *et al.* 1995). Meditation techniques can be classified according to their focus. Some focus on the general field of perception ("background" perception), leading to an experience referred to by some as "mindfulness;" others focus on a preselected specific object/image/phrase/breath and are called "concentrative" (e.g., transcendental) meditation. There are also techniques that shift between the field and the object (Pérez de Albéniz & Holmes 2000). Four out of five randomized controlled trials (RCTs) found that concentrative meditation produced effects equivalent to other forms of relaxation (Thomas & Abbas 1978, Raskin *et al.* 1980, Lehrer *et al.* 1983, Wilson 2000). The improvement was superior to remaining on a wait list (control group) but not to sitting meditation (Lehrer *et al.* 1983, Wilson 2000). In contrast, Boswell and Murray (1979) reported no difference between transcendental meditation, relaxation, and two control groups: an anti-relaxation group (simultaneous active walking and concentrating on problems) and a no-treatment control.

A Cochrane review of RCTs in which meditation was used as an intervention for anxiety disorders identified studies comparing meditation versus conventional biomedical treatments (Krisanaprakornkit *et al.* 2006). Due to the small number of studies eligible for this review, the efficacy of meditation for anxiety disorders was inconclusive. A factor to consider in reviewing all such research is whether the participants regularly practiced the techniques. Failure to demonstrate differences may be secondary to a true lack of effect or to non-adherence by study participants.

29.2.2 Mindfulness-based stress reduction

Mindfulness-based stress reduction (MBSR) is an eight-week intensive stress reduction and relaxation intervention that employs mindfulness meditation (Kabat-Zinn 1990). Research on MBSR and other mindfulness-based treatments for anxiety disorders has increased in the past decade. In a small RCT, Lee and colleagues (2007) investigated the effectiveness of MBSR versus an educational control in 46 patients with

anxiety disorders. Results showed significant decreases in all anxiety scale scores for the meditation-program group compared with patients in the educational program. A review of controlled studies (*n* = 15) of MBSR for the treatment of anxiety and depression found no evidence for the efficacy of MBSR in reliably reducing anxiety symptoms (Toneatto & Nguyen 2007). These studies show that mindfulness meditation may provide some short-term benefit in the treatment of anxiety. However, research on MBSR is limited to case reports (Patel *et al.* 2007) and pilot studies with small sample sizes (Kabat-Zinn *et al.* 1992, Evans *et al.* 2008, Yook *et al.* 2008). Thus, this area requires further validation using well-designed and controlled studies with larger samples and objective measures.

29.2.3 Yoga

Yoga refers to traditional physical and mental disciplines originating in India. Major classic branches of yoga include Raja yoga, Karma yoga, Jnana yoga, Bhakti yoga, and Hatha yoga. There are over 15 types of yogas – including Iyengar, Kundalini, and Vinyasa yoga – that have become popular in Western culture. Although each yoga practice consists of different techniques and postures, most yoga practice consists of four components: gentle stretching, exercises for breath control (*pranayama*), postures (*asanas*), and meditation (Ernst 2001). While many clinicians recommend yoga for relief of psychological symptoms, research evidence on its efficacy is very limited.

One non-randomized study showed that yoga was superior to diazepam for GAD (Sahasi *et al.* 1989). In a randomized trial, test anxiety was treated with a set of yoga exercises combined with either autosuggestion, progressive muscle relaxation, or a control talking session (Broota & Sangvhi 1994). Yoga treatment was found to be superior to both relaxation and control treatments on only one outcome measure.

One 12-month study compared the efficacy of Kundalini yoga (*n* = 12) against that of a control therapy based on relaxation and mindfulness meditation (*n* = 10) for the treatment of obsessive–compulsive disorder (OCD). Kundalini yoga consists of different combinations of bodily postures, expressive movements and utterances, breathing patterns, and degrees of concentration (Arambula *et al.* 2001, Shanahoff-Khalsa 2003). The group that practiced Kundalini yoga showed a significant mean reduction (– 38.4%) on the Yale–Brown Obsessive Compulsive Scale (YBOCS) compared to the control group (– 13.9%), and no adverse events were reported (Shannahoff-Khalsa *et al.* 1999). Subsequently, both groups merged for an additional year of the Kundalini program, and the 11 completers had a mean improvement of 70.1% on YBOCS compared to baseline (Shanahoff-Khalsa 2003).

Kirkwood and colleagues (2005) conducted a systematic review of yoga as a treatment for anxiety symptoms and disorders and found positive results reported for the eight studies meeting inclusion criteria, although there were many methodological inadequacies. Although promising, the current evidence for the efficacy of yoga for the treatment of anxiety disorders remains inconclusive.

29.2.4 Yogic breathing exercises

Yogic breathing is a method for balancing the autonomic nervous system and influencing psychological stress and stress-related disorders (Raghuraj & Telles 2008). Sudarshan Kriya yoga (SKY) is a comprehensive course on yogic breathing that has been promoted for the treatment of stress and anxiety. The clinical applications of and guidelines for SKY on stress, anxiety, and depression may be found in several articles by Brown and colleagues (Brown & Gerbarg 2005, Brown *et al.* 2008).

In a rater-blind, randomized, wait-list-controlled study of 30 disabled Australian Vietnam veterans with posttraumatic stress disorder (PTSD), those who participated in a five-day course on SKY showed significantly greater reductions on the Clinician-Administered PTSD Scale (CAPS) than those in the wait-list control group (Brown & Gerbarg 2005). CAPS scores were significantly reduced ($p < 0.01$) by an average of 30 points compared to baseline following the SKY intervention.

29.2.5 EMDR

Eye movement desensitization and reprocessing (EMDR) is a psychotherapy for PTSD (Shapiro 1989) that integrates elements of cognitive–behavioral, psychodynamic, experiential, interpersonal, and somatic psychotherapies and combines them with alternating eye movements or other sensory, bilateral stimulation in order to process and resolve maladaptive traumatic memories and responses (Shapiro 2001). A recent Cochrane review judged EMDR, individual and group trauma-focused cognitive–behavioral therapies (CBTs), and stress management as efficacious treatments for PTSD (Bisson & Andrew 2007). Based on controlled evidence, EMDR qualified for the highest level of efficacy and research support for the treatment

of trauma-related disorders and has been included in national and international PTSD practice guidelines, such as those of the American Psychiatric Association and the International Society for Traumatic Stress Studies (Spates *et al.* 2009).

29.2.6 Hypnosis

Hypnosis involves elements of absorption, imagination, focused attention, dissociation, and heightened suggestibility, during which the hypnotist suggests changes in sensations, perceptions, thoughts, feelings, or behaviors (Spiegel & Spiegel 2004). The procedure of hypnosis entails client preparation, followed by an "induction" and subsequent deepening of a hypnotic state. Once a trance-like state has been achieved, suggestions are made for various therapeutic changes (e.g., anxiety reduction); the client is then re-alerted back into normal consciousness. Although hypnosis is generally a benign process, infrequent side effects have been observed, including drowsiness, confusion, dizziness, headaches, nausea, anxiety, dissociation, depression, and false memories (Yapko 2003). The American Medical Association and the American Psychiatric Association endorsed hypnosis as an acceptable treatment modality more than 40 years ago. In the last decade, a growing body of EEG, PET, and fMRI studies has demonstrated that measurable and reproducible phenomena occur during hypnosis (reviewed in Jamieson 2007).

Hypnosis may be used as an adjunct to other psychotherapies, including CBT (Alladin 2008) and psychoanalysis (Watkins 1992). A meta-analysis of 18 studies using hypnosis as an adjunct to CBT showed additional improvement in at least 70% of clients compared to CBT without hypnosis augmentation (Kirsch *et al.* 1995), although many of these studies had methodological limitations (Schoenberger 2000). Adding hypnosis to CBT in patients with acute stress disorder improved response after six months in a controlled trial (Bryant *et al.* 2005). Hypnotherapy for PTSD fared as well as desensitization and psychodynamic psychotherapies and better than wait-list control in one large study (Brom *et al.* 1989). Some experts favor using adjunctive hypnosis to treat PTSD (Cardeña *et al.* 2009), while several studies of specific phobias show that hypnosis has similar efficacy to CBT (Marks *et al.* 1968, Horowitz 1970, Spiegel *et al.* 1981).

29.2.7 Implications for clinical practice

In clinical practice, it is important for clinicians (1) to educate anxiety disorder patients about the relationship

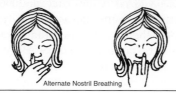

Alternate Nostril Breathing

Figure 29.1 Alternate nostril breathing.

Close the right nostril with your right thumb and inhale through the left nostril. Do this to the count of four seconds. Immediately close the left nostril with your right ring finger and little finger and at the same time remove your thumb from the right nostril, and exhale through this nostril. Do this to the count of eight seconds, completing a half round. Inhale through the right nostril to the count of four seconds. Close the right nostril with your right thumb, and exhale through the left nostril to the count of eight seconds. This completes one full round.

Recommendation: 10 to 20 minutes of ANB twice a day plus as needed for anxiety. Five to ten minutes of ANB prior to meditation enhances meditative or prayer practices. Using a certain number of counts for each breath phase produces different effects. For example, most beginners find that slowly counting to four during inspiration and six during expiration is comfortable and beneficial.

between imbalances in the stress-response system and resulting symptoms, (2) to understand the connection between breathing practice and regulation of the fight-or-flight response, and (3) to explore the ways in which mind–body techniques may help adjust imbalances and manage anxiety. Since patients with anxiety disorders often seek immediate relief, it can be helpful for clinicians to show them how breathing techniques can alleviate anxiety within minutes. For example, alternate nostril breathing (ANB) is a simple breathing practice than can be quickly efficacious (Figure 29.1). When patients experience rapid physical relaxation and mental calming, they may become more motivated to work with their breath.

Multimodal programs that include yoga postures, breathing practices, relaxation techniques, group processes, and psychoeducation are particularly beneficial for reducing stress. For these multimodal programs, understanding patients' treatment preferences and primary mode of anxiety expression can be helpful in tailoring a specific mind–body approach for each patient. Kabat-Zinn and colleagues (1997) report that patients prefer meditation techniques that focus on objects of attention that differ most from their dominant mode of anxiety expression. Instruments such as the Cognitive Somatic Anxiety Questionnaire (Schwartz *et al.* 1978) can help characterize patients' dominant mode of anxiety expression, which can range from high cognitive/low somatic to high somatic/low cognitive. Part of learning mind–body practice is incorporating lifestyle changes. Ordering the introduction of techniques based on patients' preference may help them achieve a sense of mastery and increase the likelihood of incorporating these practices into their daily routine. Inviting patients to talk about their experiences with mind–body techniques brings important material into the treatment. A clinician who helps patients process these experiences verbally is helping the patient gain the most from them.

Clinicians should also be aware of precautions and contraindications in using mind–body techniques in the treatment of anxiety disorders. It is important to control anxiety as quickly as possible, thereby avoiding reinforcement of the stress response, which could otherwise lead to exhaustion, depression, and/or avoidance behaviors. Patients who tend to hyperventilate need preparation before taking a yoga breathing course to avoid inducing a panic attack. Since both fast- and slow-breathing techniques will be taught during this approach, patients can simply learn to decrease their respirations to a medium or slow rate should they begin to feel anxious during the fast-breathing component. If patients begin to experience light-headedness, paresthesias, or cramping in their hands or feet, they can exhale less forcefully to avoid releasing too much carbon dioxide. Patients can be assured that these controlled breath techniques are different from uncontrolled hyperventilation, and that the breath training will help to reduce their anxiety (Brown *et al.* 2008).

29.3 Biologically based practices

The CAM domain of biologically based practices for the treatment of anxiety disorders includes a wide range of dietary supplements such as botanicals (e.g., kava), animal-derived extracts, vitamins (e.g., inositol), minerals, fatty acids, amino acids, proteins, and functional foods. Many studies of these supplements have been performed, yet none has been proven efficacious. Nevertheless, there are several supplements for which early studies have yielded positive or encouraging results. Extensive reviews of CAM approaches to mental health problems have been carried out by Lake and Spiegel (2007) and Brown and colleagues (2009).

29.3.1 Kava

Kava is extracted from *Piper methysticum* (a member of the pepper family) and is a traditional beverage throughout the Pacific Basin. In Western countries, kava extract pills (100 mg three times a day) are marketed for the treatment of anxiety and insomnia. The active ingredients of kava are the kavalactones (at least 15 have been identified), which modulate a range of neurotransmitter systems, including serotonin, norepinephrine, dopamine, glutamine, and GABA, as well as block actions at sodium channels and calcium channels. These activities presumably account for the anxiolytic, sedative, intoxicant, analgesic, and anticonvulsant properties of kava.

Although kava has the relatively best evidence for the treatment of anxiety among the herbal remedies, its efficacy remains debated. A recent Cochrane review (Pittler & Ernst 2003), which included 11 clinical trials with a total of 645 participants, and a meta-analysis of six studies (Witte *et al.* 2005) both concluded that kava extract appeared to be an effective symptomatic treatment option for anxiety. Conversely, a subsequent meta-analysis of three randomized placebo-controlled double-blind trials found no significant effects of

kava on GAD (Connor *et al.* 2006). However, most treatments in this meta-analysis typically lasted four weeks, whereas a 25-week study showed that therapeutic effects start in the eighth week (Volz & Kieser 1997).

The safety of kava is controversial. The Cochrane review (Pittler & Ernst 2003) noted that most adverse events were mild, transient, and infrequent, with a 2% incidence of common side effects, including gastrointestinal issues, headaches, allergic reactions, and photosensitivity. However, less frequent adverse reactions included drowsiness, intoxication, abuse, dependency, facial swelling, scaly rash, dyspnea, hematuria, EKG changes, restlessness, tremor, and hepatitis. Due to several cases of liver failure, the US Food and Drug Administration (FDA) and Centers for Disease Control and Prevention (CDC) have issued warnings of potential liver toxicity due to kava. Kava should be avoided in pregnancy and should not be combined with alcohol or sedatives. In general, caution should be used when considering treatment with kava.

29.3.2 Inositol

Inositol is part of the B-vitamin complex (B_8), and it functions as an intracellular second messenger, stimulating cyclic AMP. Approximately one gram of inositol is consumed daily in the average human diet. As a dietary supplement, inositol has been used for anxiety management. In one RCT, ingestion of inositol 12 g/day was superior to placebo for the treatment of panic disorder (Benjamin *et al.* 1995), and in another RCT, efficacy of inositol 20 g/day in reducing panic was comparable to that of the selective serotonin reuptake inhibitor (SSRI) fluvoxamine (Luvox) 150 mg/day (Palatnik *et al.* 2001). Two RCTs of inositol 18 g/day for treatment-refractory OCD showed that inositol alone might have positive effects on OCD, but it does not augment SSRI therapy (Fux *et al.* 1996, 1999). In a PTSD study with a short treatment duration and a small sample size, inositol did not differ from placebo (Kaplan *et al.* 1996). Although the side effects of inositol tend to be minimal (e.g., gas and loose stools), adherence could be an issue, since therapeutic doses require 18 large 650 mg pills daily (11.7 g/day). Larger and longer-term trials are required to confirm inositol's efficacy in OCD and panic disorder.

29.3.3 Passion flower

The genus *Passiflora* consists of about 500 species of flowering plants collectively known as passion flowers. The leaves and roots of the species *Passiflora incarnata* have a long history among North American natives. The leaves are cultivated to make an infusion tea, which is used to treat anxiety, insomnia, hysteria, pain, and epilepsy. Passion flower contains the dehydroflavone chrysin, which binds to benzodiazepine receptors, and it also contains beta-carbolin harmala alkaloids that are monoamine oxidase inhibitors (MAOIs) with antidepressant properties. In one double-blind randomized placebo-controlled trial of 36 GAD patients, 45 drops/day of passiflora tincture was compared to 30mg/day of the benzodiazepine oxazepam; a marked reduction in anxiety was noted in both groups (Akhondzadeh *et al.* 2001). A recent Cochrane review indicated that larger studies are needed to confirm whether passiflora's anti-anxiety effects are scientifically supported (Miyasaka *et al.* 2007).

29.3.4 Valerian

Of the 200 valerian species, the one most commonly used is *Valeriana officinalis*. The dried root of the valerian plant has been used primarily as a remedy for insomnia since antiquity. The sleep-promoting and anxiolytic properties of valerian are thought to be mediated through its binding to $GABA_A$ receptors, although the exact mechanism remains unknown. A recent review revealed only one study of valerian for anxiety that met Cochrane standards (Miyasaka *et al.* 2006). Valerian use is generally safe for short periods (4–6 weeks), but longer-term use has not been studied. Other than its unpleasant taste, valerian is generally well tolerated, with minimal hangover side effects on high doses (> 600 mg) and occasional stomach aches, headaches, dizziness, night terrors, or apathy. There have been no cases of habituation or abuse, only one case of reported withdrawal, and debatable cases of hepatitis or dystonia. Valerian should be avoided in hepatic disease or pregnancy.

29.3.5 GABA

Gamma-aminobutyric acid (GABA) is one of the major inhibitory neurotransmitters in the mammalian central nervous system. It is involved in the regulation of cardiovascular control, the immune system, and several hormonal systems (e.g., pituitary). Enhancement of GABA activity reduces anxiety and stabilizes mood. One study demonstrated that GABA could produce positive changes in EEG brain waves associated with relaxation as well as enhance immunity, as measured by salivary immunoglobulin A (IgA) levels (Abdou *et al.* 2006). Pregabalin is a synthetic structural analogue of GABA used to treat epilepsy and neuropathic pain. Several RCTs confirm that the efficacy of pregabalin in the treatment of moderate-to-severe GAD is comparable to that of lorazepam, alprazolam, and venlafaxine (Bandelow *et al.* 2007). Treatment with pregabalin generally requires at least one week prior to the onset of anxiolytic effects. Pregabalin is generally well tolerated, producing occasional dizziness, sedation, or headaches. Risk for cognitive clouding, abuse, or dependence is lower than with benzodiazepines.

29.3.6 5-Hydroxytryptophan

A biochemical precursor of serotonin, the amino acid 5-hydroxy-L-tryptophan (5-HTP) is made naturally by the human body, although it can be consumed as a dietary supplement extracted from the plant *Griffonia simplicifolia*. Imbalances in serotonergic pathways are implicated in depressive disorders and some anxiety disorders. In a double-blind placebo-controlled trial, panic disorder patients ($n = 24$) received a single 200 mg dose of 5-HTP or placebo and were exposed to a panic-inducing carbon dioxide challenge (Schruers *et al.* 2002). Patients in the 5-HTP arm showed significantly fewer panic symptoms than the placebo group. An eight-week double-blind placebo-controlled trial with mixed anxiety disorder patients (GAD, OCD, panic disorder with or without agoraphobia) ($n = 45$) that compared 5-HTP (up to 150 mg/day), clomipramine (up to 150 mg/day), and placebo yielded indeterminate results (Kahn *et al.* 1987). An open, uncontrolled study of patients ($n = 10$) with GAD, agoraphobia, or panic disorder showed anxiety reduction with 5-HTP and carbidopa (Kahn & Westenberg 1985). Conversely, a small study of treatment-refractory OCD showed no improvement with the addition of 5-HTP to an SSRI (Blier & Bergeron 1996). Although the FDA has raised concerns about eosinophilia–myalgia syndrome (a potentially fatal condition) due to 5-HTP contaminants, no definitive cases of toxicity have emerged in the last 24 years (Das *et al.* 2004), and prescription-grade 5-HTP is available.

29.4 Manipulative and body-based therapies

Manipulative and body-based practices encompass several heterogeneous CAM interventions and therapies. These include massage therapy, reflexology, acupressure, and other practices in which the client's body is manipulated in various ways to achieve improvements in physical health and mental well-being.

29.4.1 Massage

In a given year, 2–14% of US adults receive some form of massage therapy (National Center for Complementary and Alternative Medicine 2004a). Massage is the practice of soft-tissue manipulation for physical, functional, and/or psychological purposes. There are over 80 different massage modalities (e.g., shiatsu, Swedish). Massage therapy has few adverse effects, although contraindications to its use include deep venous thrombosis, wounds, burns, infections, eczema, fractures, and osteoporosis. Research has shown that the benefits of massage include reduced trait anxiety and depression; temporarily reduced blood pressure, heart rate, and state anxiety; and pain relief (Moyer *et al.* 2004). The positive effects of massage include significant changes in cortisol (31% average decrease in salivary or urinary levels), serotonin (28% average increase in urinary levels), and dopamine (31% average increase in urinary levels) (Field *et al.* 2005).

Although there are currently no studies looking at the role of massage therapy for anxiety disorders, there are numerous studies examining the benefits of massage in anxiety states secondary to various medical conditions. A recent systematic review using Cochrane principles identified 10 trials using massage in cancer patients that met inclusion criteria; results suggested that massage might reduce anxiety in the short term, but larger, better-designed trials with longer follow-up periods are needed to establish efficacy (Wilkinson *et al.* 2008). In psychiatric populations, the data on the effects of massage are positive but limited. Compared to standard treatments, both a study of young adult psychiatric inpatients (Garner *et al.* 2008) and an RCT of 24 female adolescent inpatients with bulimia nervosa (Field *et al.* 1998) showed adjunctive massage produced immediate reduction in anxiety and cortisol levels.

29.5 Energy therapies

"Energy medicine" includes putative ("subtle") energies, which have defied measurement by reproducible methods (National Center for Complementary and Alternative Medicine 2004b). Belief in subtle energies supposes that humans contain vital energies, including energy pathways (the "meridian" system and related acupoints), energy centers ("chakras"), and energy systems ("biofields"). Practices that involve altering or manipulating putative energies include acupuncture and acupressure, Qigong, Reiki, and several methods falling under the term "energy psychology" (EP). Many of these practices involve some form of mechanical stimulation to rebalance the subtle energies, which are believed to be unbalanced in various disorders and disease states.

29.5.1 Acupuncture

Acupuncture is a traditional Chinese treatment using needles, which are inserted at specific points of the body, then either manipulated or electrically stimulated. Traditional Chinese theory posits that acupuncture corrects the imbalances of the yin and yang forces that circulate along channels in the body; balance of these forces is thought to be necessary for good health. One review of acupuncture for anxiety symptoms and disorders (Pilkington *et al.* 2006) identified four RCTs for the treatment of GAD, but results were inconclusive due to the lack of details on methodology and insufficient data about efficacy of this technique. Two subsequent RCT's comparing acupuncture to active controlled treatments (breathing retraining and group CBT) found statistically significant differences, in favor of acupuncture, suggesting that acupuncture might be useful in treating symptoms of anxiety and depression (Gibson *et al.* 2007, Hollifield *et al.* 2007). Although both studies have design and sample-size limitations, they provide preliminary evidence for a beneficial effect of acupuncture, and suggest the need for larger studies using more rigorous methodology.

29.5.2 Energy psychology approaches

Energy psychology (EP) comprises over a dozen different methods. Thought field therapy (TFT), the parent EP method, posits that dysfunctional thoughts, emotions, and behaviors create disturbances in the flow of subtle energies ("thought fields"), which in turn reinforce the disordered states (Callahan & Trubo 2002). By tapping on or stimulating key acupoints along the meridians while holding the negative thoughts in mind and verbalizing positive affirmations, this process corrects disturbed energies and restores physical and mental health. The emotional freedom technique (EFT) is a simplification of TFT and has become the most popular and accessible of the EP approaches (Feinstein *et al.* 2005). Despite the proliferation of various EP approaches, there are few scientifically sound research studies confirming their efficacy. One study of 39 patients with PTSD (Carbonell & Figley 1999)

Table 29.1. Reliable online resources for CAM

US government resources (National Institutes of Health)

National Center for Complementary and Alternative Medicine (NCCAM)
http://nccam.nih.gov
US government site that provides thorough descriptions of complementary and alternative therapies and description of the research sites on CAM that it sponsors.

Office of Cancer Complementary and Alternative Medicine (OCCAM)
http://www.cancer.gov/CAM
The Office of Cancer Complementary and Alternative Medicine (OCCAM) coordinates and enhances the activities of the National Cancer Institute (NCI) in the arena of complementary and alternative medicine (CAM).

Medline Plus – Alternative Medicine – Herbal Medicine, National Library of Medicine
http://www.nlm.nih.gov/medlineplus/complementaryandalternativemedicine.html
MedlinePlus directs to information to help answer health questions. MedlinePlus brings together information from NLM, the National Institutes of Health (NIH), and other government agencies and health-related organizations.

Office of Dietary Supplements
http://dietary-supplements.info.nih.gov/databases/ibids.html
The International Bibliographic Information on Dietary Supplements (IBIDS) is a database of published, international, scientific literature on dietary supplements, including vitamins, minerals, and botanicals. IBIDS is produced by the Office of Dietary Supplements (ODS) to assist the public, healthcare providers, educators, and researchers in locating credible, scientific information on dietary supplements. It contains more than 419,000 scientific citations and abstracts.

Health science libraries

Cochrane Library
http://www.thecochranelibrary.com
Published monthly/quarterly on DVD-ROM and the Internet. Residents in a number of countries or regions can access the *Cochrane Library* online for free through special schemes. Contains more than 5000 reports of randomized controlled trials and more than 60 systematic reviews in CAM

Rosenthal Center for CAM – Columbia University
http://www.rosenthal.hs.columbia.edu
This site includes information regarding research and practice of complementary and alternative medicine in women's health and geriatrics. Focuses on the development and support of research and training sites. Provides links to organizations. Identifies training programs. Includes clinical studies, prospective outcome research, and field investigations.

Consortium of Academic Health Centers for Integrative Medicine
http://www.imconsortium.org
The Consortium of Academic Health Centers for Integrative Medicine website offers information and resources on CAM at the academic, clinical and research level at 44 highly esteemed academic medical centers.

M. D. Anderson Cancer Center's Complementary/Integrative Medicine Education Resources (CIMER)
http://www.mdanderson.org/departments/cimer
This is a revised and updated site that contains evidence-based reviews of complementary or alternative cancer therapies as well as links to other authoritative resources. Detailed scientific reviews are provided to assist healthcare professionals in guiding patients who would like to integrate these therapies with conventional treatments.

Non-profit and other web-based information services

Bandolier
http://www.medicine.ox.ac.uk/bandolier/booth/booths/altmed.html
Bandolier is a print and Internet journal about health care, using evidence-based medicine techniques to provide advice about particular treatments/diseases for health care professionals and consumers. Over 75 summaries on the effectiveness of CAM therapies.

The Natural Pharmacist
http://www.tnp.com
A site that carries scientific information on herbs and nutritional supplements. It also has information that can be researched on drug–herb-supplement interactions.

Consumer Lab Reports
http://www.consumerlab.com
ConsumerLab.com is the leading provider of independent test results and information to help consumers and healthcare professionals evaluate health, wellness, and nutrition products. It publishes results of its tests in comprehensive reports at www.consumerlab.com, which receives over three million visits per year from consumers and health professionals.

Epocrates
http://www.epocrates.com/products/online
Epocrates, Inc. develops clinical information and decision support tools that enable healthcare professionals to find answers more quickly and confidently at the point of care. This website contains information on alternative medicine and drug interactions.

Table 29.2 Approach to CAM integration (Eisenberg 1997)

Step 1	Identify principal symptoms and maintain symptom diary
Step 2	Discuss patient preferences and expectations
Step 3	Review issues of safety and efficacy
Step 4	Identify suitable licensed CAM providers
Step 5	Provide key questions for patient to discuss with provider during CAM consultation
Step 6	Schedule follow-up visit to review treatment plan
Step 7	Provide documentation in the medical record

compared TFT to EMDR, traumatic incident reduction, and visual/kinesthetic disassociation. All four approaches showed positive improvements. In one study, 35 subjects with phobias of small animals were randomized to receive one session of EFT or diaphragmatic breathing; the EFT group exhibited significantly greater improvement following the session, and improvement was maintained at six-month and nine-month follow-up visits (Wells *et al.* 2003).

29.6 Summary

We have outlined a broad range of CAM approaches for the treatment of anxiety symptoms and disorders. In clinical practice, we find that mind–body techniques are easily accessible and simple to learn, can be carried out in practitioners' offices, have low risk of adverse effects, and can be combined with pharmacotherapy (Muskin 2000).

Research on mind–body techniques such as EMDR and hypnosis is encouraging, while studies on yoga and meditation are limited by poor study designs and limited sample sizes. Although the CAM domain of biologically based therapies includes a wide range of dietary supplements, no single supplement has been proven efficacious in a compelling way; there is some evidence of efficacy for kava, inositol and 5-HTP. Caution is advised when using certain dietary supplements, because of their side effects or limited safety. Acupuncture and massage show some preliminary evidence of efficacy in the treatment of anxiety symptoms. Although the most controversial of CAM practices (National Center for Complementary and Alternative Medicine 2004b), energy therapies are gaining popularity in the United States and have recevied increased research interest. Research on acupuncture and energy psychology approaches shows preliminary evidence of beneficial effects.

Future studies must recruit larger sample sizes as well as utilize a randomized controlled trial design with blinding of treatments (where feasible), longer follow-up periods, and intention-to-treat analyses. Clinicians should remain alert for reliable updates as new information becomes available on evidence-based treatments. This can be done by searching databases such as Medline, the Cochrane Collaboration, and the NCCAM website for information on the latest research on each CAM modality discussed in this chapter. In addition, key references are provided in Table 29.1.

29.6.1 Talking to patients about CAM

Patients who use CAM services for mental health problems face difficulties in communication and coordination of care with conventional medical providers (Druss & Rosenheck 1999). Given the frequent use of CAM approaches and the potential for drug interactions with herbal treatments, we suggest that clinicians routinely enquire about patients' use of CAM and confirm that its use is consistent with safe and responsible medical practice. Eisenberg's (1997) approach (Table 29.2) aids in exploring CAM use with patients; it emphasizes patient safety, guided by the principle of "do no harm," and uses shared decision-making approaches.

29.6.2 Healthcare professionals

Clinicians and trainees are often subject to severe work stress and are vulnerable to burnout. Some may even develop anxiety, insomnia, or depression. Mind–body practices can provide a healthy method to relieve physical and emotional tension. For mental health providers, yoga and meditation are simple to learn, enhance the ability to remain calm during challenging sessions, enhance alertness and mental focus, and improve energy. Clinicians who receive instruction in mind–body practices are also better equipped to make appropriate referrals, work with challenging patients, and help patients overcome obstacles to maintaining regular practice over time, thus achieving the maximum benefit from the addition of CAM in their treatment.

References

Abdou, A. M., Higashiguchi, S., Horie, K., *et al.* (2006). Relaxation and immunity enhancement effects of gamma-aminobutyric acid (GABA) administration in humans. *Biofactors*, **26**, 201–208.

Akhondzadeh, S., Naghavi, H. R., Vazirian, M,. *et al.* (2001). Passionflower in the treatment of generalized anxiety: a pilot double-blind randomized controlled trial with oxazepam. *Journal of Clinical Pharmacy and Therapeutics*, **26**, 363–367.

Alladin, A. (2008). *Cognitive Hypnotherapy: an Integrated Approach to the Treatment of Emotional Disorders.* Chichester: Wiley.

Arambula, P., Peper, E., Kawakami, M., & Gibney, K.H. (2001). The physiological correlates of Kundalini yoga meditation: a study of a yoga master. *Applied Psychophysiology and Biofeedback*, **26**, 147–53.

Astin J.A. (1998) Why patients use alternative medicine. *JAMA*, **279**, 1548–1553.

Bandelow, B., Wedekind, D., & Leon, T. (2007). Pregabalin for the treatment of generalized anxiety disorder: a novel pharmacologic intervention. *Review of Neurotherapeutics*, **7**, 769–781.

Barnes, P.M., Powell-Griner, E., McFann, K., & Nahin, R.L. (2004). Complementary and alternative medicine use among adults: United States, 2002. *CDC Advance Data Report*, **343**.

Beauchaine, T.P. (2001). Vagal tone, development, and Gray's motivational theory: toward an integrated model of autonomic nervous system functioning in psychopathology. *Development and Psychopathology*, **13**, 183–214.

Benjamin, J., Levine, J., Fux, M., *et al.* (1995). Double-blind, placebo-controlled, crossover trial of inositol treatment for panic disorder. *American Journal of Psychiatry*, **152**, 1084–1086.

Bisson, J., & Andrew, M. (2007). Psychological treatment of post-traumatic stress disorder (PTSD). *Cochrane Database of Systematic Reviews*, (3), CD003388.

Blier, P., & Bergeron, R. (1996). Sequential administration of augmentation strategies in treatment-resistant obsessive–compulsive disorder: preliminary findings. *International Clinical Psychopharmacology*, **11**, 37–44.

Boswell, P. C., & Murray, E. J. (1979). Effects of meditation on psychological and physiological measures of anxiety. *Journal of Consulting Clinical Psychology, 47*, 606–607.

Brom, D., Kleber, R. J., & Defares, P. B. (1989). Brief psychotherapy for posttraumatic stress disorders. *Journal of Consulting and Clinical Psychology*, **57**, 607–612.

Broota, A., & Sanghvi, C. (1994). Efficacy of two relaxation techniques in examination anxiety. Special section: relaxation techniques and psychological management. *Journal of Personality and Clinical Studies*, **10**, 29–35.

Brown, R. P., & Gerbarg, P. L. (2005). Sudarshan Kriya yogic breathing in the treatment of stress, anxiety, and depression. Part II – clinical applications and guidelines. *Journal of Alternative and Complementary Medicine*, **11**, 711–717.

Brown, R. P., Gerbarg, P. L., & Muskin, P. R. (2008). Alternative treatments in psychiatry. In A. Tasman, J. Kay, & J. C. Lieberman, eds., *Psychiatry*, 3rd edn. London: Wiley, pp. 2318–2353.

Brown, R. P., Gerbarg, P. L., & Muskin, P. R. (2009). *How to Use Herbs, Nutrients and Yoga in Mental Health Care.* New York, NY: Norton.

Bryant, R. A., Moulds, M. L., Guthrie, R. M., & Nixon, R. D. (2005). The additive benefit of hypnosis and cognitive–behavioral therapy in treating acute stress disorder. *Journal of Consulting and Clinical Psychology*, **73**, 334–340.

Callahan, R., & Trubo, R. (2002). *Tapping the Healer Within: Using Thought-Field Therapy to Instantly Conquer your Fears, Anxieties, and Emotional Distress.* New York, NY: McGraw-Hill.

Carbonell, J. L., & Figley, C. (1999). A systematic clinical demonstration of promising PTSD treatment approaches. *Traumatology*, **5**, 32–48.

Cardeña, E., Maldonado, J. R., van der Hart, O., & Spiegel, D. (2009). Hypnosis. In E. B. Foa, T. M. Keane, M. J. Friedman, & J. A. Cohen, eds., *Effective Treatments for PTSD: Practice Guidelines from the International Society for Traumatic Stress Studies*, 2nd edn. New York, NY: Guilford Press.

Connor, K. M., Payne, V., & Davidson, J. R. (2006). Kava in generalized anxiety disorder: three placebo-controlled trials. *International Clinical Psychopharmacology*, **21**, 249–253.

Das, Y. T., Bagchi, M., Bagchi, D., & Preuss, H. G. (2004). Safety of 5-hydroxy-l-tryptophan. *Toxicology Letters*, **150**, 111–122.

Druss, B. G., & Rosenheck, R. A. (1999). Associations between use of unconventional therapies and conventional medical therapies. *JAMA*, **282**, 651–656.

Eisenberg, D. M. (1997). Advising patients who seek alternative medical therapies. *Annals of Internal Medicine*, **127**, 61–69.

Ernst, E. (2001). Yoga (section 3). In E. Ernst, ed., *The Desktop Guide to Complementary and Alternative Medicine: an Evidence-Based Approach.* Edinburgh: Mosby, pp. 76–78.

Evans, S., Ferrando, S., Findler, M., *et al.* (2008). Mindfulness-based cognitive therapy for generalized anxiety disorder. *Journal of Anxiety Disorders*, **22**, 716–721.

Feinstein, D., Eden, D., & Craig, G. (2005). *The Promise of Energy Psychology: Revolutionary Tools for Dramatic Personal Change.* New York, NY: Jeremy P. Tarcher/Penguin.

Field, T., Schanberg, S., Kuhn, C., *et al.* (1998). Bulimic adolescents benefit from massage therapy. *Adolescence*, **33**, 555–563.

Field, T., Hernandez-Reif, M., Diego, M., Schanberg, S., & Kuhn, C. (2005). Cortisol decreases and serotonin and dopamine increase following massage therapy. *International Journal of Neuroscience*, **115**, 1397–1413.

Fux, M., Levine, J., Aviv, A., & Belmaker, R. H. (1996). Inositol treatment of obsessive–compulsive disorder. *American Journal of Psychiatry*, **153**, 1219–1221.

Fux, M., Benjamin, J., & Belmaker, R. H., (1999). Inositol versus placebo augmentation of serotonin reuptake inhibitors in the treatment of obsessive–compulsive disorder: a double-blind cross-over study. *International Journal of Neuropsychopharmacology*, **2**, 193–195.

Garner, B., Phillips, L. J., Schmidt, H. M., et al. (2008). Pilot study evaluating the effect of massage therapy on stress, anxiety and aggression in a young adult psychiatric inpatient unit. *Australian and New Zealand Journal of Psychiatry*, **42**, 414–422.

Gibson D., Bruton A., Lewith G. T., & Mullee M. (2007). Effects of acupuncture as a treatment for hyperventilation syndrome a pilot, randomized crossover trial. *Journal of Alternative and Complementary Medicine*, **13**, 39–46.

Hollifield, M., Sinclair-Lian, N., Warner, T. D., & Hammerschlag R. (2007). Acupuncture for posttraumatic stress disorder: a randomized controlled pilot trial. *Journal of Nervous and Mental Disease*, **195**, 504–513.

Horowitz, S. L. (1970). Strategies within hypnosis for reducing phobic behavior. *Journal of Abnormal Psychology*, **75**, 104–112.

Jamieson, G. A. (2007). *Hypnosis and Conscious States: the Cognitive Neuroscience Perspective*. Oxford: Oxford University Press.

Kabat-Zinn, J. (1990). *Full Catastrophe Living: Using the Wisdom of your Body and Mind to Face Stress, Pain and Illness*. New York, NY: Bantam Doubleday Dell.

Kabat-Zinn, J., Massion, A.O., Kristellar, J., et al. (1992). Effectiveness of a meditation-based stress reduction program in the treatment of anxiety disorders. *American Journal of Psychiatry*, **149**, 936–943.

Kabat-Zinn, J., Chapman, A., & Salmon, P. (1997). Relationship of cognitive and somatic components of anxiety to patient preference for different relaxation techniques. *Mind Body Medicine*, **2**, 101–109.

Kahn, R. S., & Westenberg, H. G. (1985). L-5-hydroxytryptophan in the treatment of anxiety disorders. *Journal of Affective Disorders*, **8**, 197–200.

Kahn, R. S., Westenberg, H. G., Verhoeven, W. M., Gispen-de Wied, C. C., & Kamerbeek, W. D. (1987). Effect of a serotonin precursor and uptake inhibitor in anxiety disorders; a double-blind comparison of 5-hydroxytryptophan, clomipramine and placebo. *International Clinical Psychopharmacology*, **2**, 33–45.

Kaplan, Z., Amir, M., Swartz, M., & Levine, J. (1996). Inositol treatment of post-traumatic stress disorder. *Anxiety*, **2**, 51–52.

Kessler, R.C., Soukup, J., Davis, R. B., et al. (2001). The use of complementary and alternative therapies to treat anxiety and depression in the United States. *American Journal of Psychiatry*, **158**, 289–294.

Kirkwood, G., Rampes, H., Tuffrey, V., et al. (2005). Yoga for anxiety: a systematic review of the research evidence. *British Journal of Sports Medicine*, **39**, 884–891.

Kirsch, I., Montgomery, G., & Sapirstein, G. (1995). Hypnosis as an adjunct to cognitive–behavioral psychotherapy: a meta-analysis. *Journal of Consulting and Clinical Psychology*, **63**, 214–220.

Krisanaprakornkit, T., Krisanaprakornkit, W., Piyavhatkul, N., & Laopaiboon, M. (2006). Meditation therapy for anxiety disorders. *Cochrane Database of Systematic Reviews*. (1), CD004998.

Lake, J. H., & Spiegel, D., eds. (2007). *Complementary and Alternative Treatments in Mental Health Care*. Washington DC: American Psychiatric Press.

Lee, S. H., Ahn, S. C., Lee, Y. J., et al. (2007). Effectiveness of a meditation-based stress management program as an adjunct to pharmacotherapy in patients with anxiety disorder. *Journal of PsychosomaticResearch*, **62**, 189–195.

Lehrer, P. M., Woolfolk, R. L., Rooney, A. J., McCann, M. B., & Carrington, P. (1983). Progressive relaxation and meditation: a study of psychophysiological and therapeutic differences between two techniques. *Behaviour Research and Therapy*, **21**, 651–662.

Maison, A., Herbert, J. R., Werheimer, M. D., & Kabat-Zinn, J. (1995). Meditation, melatonin and breast/prostate cancer: hypothesis and preliminary data. *Medical Hypotheses*, **44**, 39–46.

Marks, I. M., Gelder, M. G., & Edwards, G. (1968). Hypnosis and desensitization for phobias: a controlled prospective trial. *British Journal of Psychiatry*, **114**, 1263–1274.

Miyasaka, L. S., Atallah, A. N., & Soares, B. G. (2006). Valerian for anxiety disorders. *Cochrane Database of Systematic Reviews*, (4), CD004515.

Miyasaka, L. S., Atallah, A. N., & Soares, B. G. (2007). Passiflora for anxiety disorder. *Cochrane Database of Systematic Reviews*, (1), CD004518.

Moyer, C. A., Rounds, J., & Hannum, J. W. (2004) A meta-analysis of massage therapy research. *Psychological Bulletin*, **130**, 3–18.

Muskin P. R., ed. (2000). *Complementary and Alternative Medicine and Psychiatry*. Washington, DC: American Psychiatric Association.

National Center for Complementary and Alternative Medicine (NCCAM) (2004a). *Backgrounder: Manipulative and Body-based Practices: an Overview*. Bethesda, MD: NCCAM.

National Center for Complementary and Alternative Medicine (NCCAM) (2004b). *Backgrounder: Energy Medicine: an Overview*. Bethesda, MD: NCCAM.

Palatnik, A., Frolov, K., Fux, M., & Benjamin, J. (2001). Double-blind, controlled, crossover trial of inositol versus fluvoxamine for the treatment of panic disorder. *Journal of Clinical Psychopharmacology*, **21**, 335–339.

Patel, S. R., Carmody, J., & Simpson, H. B. (2007). Adapting mindfulness based stress reduction for the treatment of obsessive compulsive disorder: a case report. *Cognitive and Behavioral Practice*, **14**, 375–380.

Pérez de Albéniz, A., & Holmes J. (2000). Meditation: concepts, effects and uses in therapy. *International Journal of Psychotherapy*, **5**, 49–59.

Pilkington, K., Rampes, H., & Richardson, J. (2006). Complementary medicine for depression. *Expert Review of Neurotherapeutics*, **6**, 1741–1751.

Pittler, M. H., & Ernst, E. (2003). Kava extract for treating anxiety. *Cochrane Database of Systematic Reviews*, (1), CD003383.

Raghuraj, P., & Telles, S. (2008) Immediate effect of specific nostril manipulating yoga breathing practices on autonomic and respiratory variables. *Applied Psychophysiology and Feedback*, **33**, 65–75.

Raskin, M., Bali, L. R., & Peeke, H. V. (1980). Muscle biofeedback and transcendental meditation. A controlled evaluation of efficacy in the treatment of chronic anxiety. *Archives of General Psychiatry*, **37**, 93–97.

Sahasi, G., Mohan, D., & Kacker, C. (1989). Effectiveness of yogic techniques in the management of anxiety. *Journal of Personality and Clinical Studies*, **5**, 51–55.

Schoenberger, N. E. (2000). Research on hypnosis as an adjunct to cognitive–behavioral psychotherapy. *International Journal of Clinical and Experimental Hypnosis*, **48**, 154–169.

Schruers, K., van Diest, R., Overbeek, T., & Griez, E. (2002). Acute l-5-hydroxytryptophan administration inhibits carbon dioxide-induced panic in panic disorder patients. *Psychiatry Research*, **113**, 237–243.

Schwartz, G. E., Davidson, R. J., & Goleman, D. J. (1978) Patterning of cognitive and somatic processes in the self-regulation of anxiety: effects of meditation versus exercises. *Psychosomatic Medicine*, **40**, 321–328.

Shannahoff-Khalsa, D. S. (2003). Kundalini yoga meditation techniques for the treatment of obsessive–compulsive and OC spectrum disorders. *Brief Treatment Crisis Intervention*, **3**, 369–82.

Shannahoff-Khalsa, D. S., Ray, L. E., Levine, S., *et al.* (1999). Randomized controlled trial of yogic meditation techniques for patients with obsessive–compulsive disorder. *CNS Spectrum*, **4**, 34–47.

Shapiro, F. (1989). Efficacy of the eye movement desensitization: a new treatment for post-traumatic stress disorder. *Journal of Behavior Therapy and Experimental Psychiatry*, **20**, 211–217.

Shapiro, F. (2001). *Eye Movement Desensitization and Reprocessing: Basic Principles, Protocols, and Procedures*, 2nd edn. New York, NY: Guilford Press.

Spates, C. R., Koch, E., Cusack, K., Pagoto, S., & Waller, S. (2009). Eye movement desensitization and reprocessing. In E. B. Foa, T. M. Keane, M. J. Friedman, & J. A. Cohen, eds., *Effective Treatments for PTSD: Practice Guidelines from the International Society for Traumatic Stress Studies*, 2nd edn. New York, NY: Guilford Press.

Spiegel, D., Frischholz, E. J., Maruffi, B., & Spiegel, H. (1981). Hypnotic responsivity and the treatment of flying phobia. *American Journal of Clinical Hypnosis*, **23**, 239–247.

Spiegel, H., & Spiegel, D. (2004). *Trance and Treatment: Clinical Uses of Hypnosis*, 2nd edn. Washington DC: American Psychiatric Publishing.

Testerman, J. K., Morton, K. R., Mason, R. A., & Ronan, A. M. (2004). Patient motivations for using complementary and alternative medicine. *Complementary Health Practice Review*, **9**, 81–92.

Thomas, D., & Abbas, K. A. (1978). Comparison of transcendental meditation and progressive relaxation in reducing anxiety. *British Medical Journal*, **2**, 1749.

Toneatto, T., & Nguyen, L. (2007). Does mindfulness meditation improve anxiety and mood symptoms? A review of the controlled research. *Canadian Journal of Psychiatry*, **52**, 260–266.

Volz, H. P., & Kieser, M. (1997). Kava-kava extract WS 1490 versus placebo in anxiety disorders – a randomized placebo-controlled 25-week outpatient trial. *Pharmacopsychiatry*, **30**, 1–5.

Watkins, J. G. (1992). *Hypnoanalytic Techniques: the Practice of Clinical Hypnosis, Volume II*. New York, NY: Irvington.

Wells, S., Polglase, K., Andrews, H. B., Carrington, P., & Baker, A. H. (2003). Evaluation of a meridian-based intervention, emotional freedom techniques (EFT), for reducing specific phobias of small animals. *Journal of Clinical Psychology*, **59**, 943–966.

Wilkinson, S., Barnes, K., & Storey, L. (2008). Massage for symptom relief in patients with cancer: systematic review. *Journal of Advanced Nursing*, **63**, 430–439.

Wilson, H. B. (2000). The specific effects model: relaxation and meditation effects on cognitive and somatic anxiety. Unpublished dissertation, Ohio University, Athens, Ohio.

Witte, S., Loew, D., & Gaus, W. (2005). Meta-analysis of the efficacy of acetonic kava-kava extract WS*1490 in patients with non-psychotic anxiety disorders. *Phytotherapy Research*, **19**, 183–188.

Yapko, M. (2003). *Trancework*, 3rd edn. New York, NY: Brunner-Routledge.

Yook, K., Lee, S. H., Ryu, M., *et al.* (2008). Usefulness of mindfulness based cognitive therapy in the treatment of insomnia in patients with anxiety disorders: a pilot study. *Journal of Nervous and Mental Disease*, **196**, 501–503.

Chapter 30

The treatment of anxiety disorders in primary care

Mayumi Okuda, Sharaf S. Khan, Ana Alicia De La Cruz, Carlos Blanco

30.1 Introduction

Anxiety disorders are common in primary care, affecting approximately 10% of patients (Sartorius *et al.* 1996). During a one-year period, approximately 84% of adults with a probable anxiety disorder receive care in a primary care setting. However, the quality of the care received is often limited. Only 18% receive appropriate pharmacotherapy and 11% appropriate counseling (Young *et al.* 2001). In university-affiliated primary care practices, the rate of appropriate treatment for anxiety disorders may be higher, around 40%, although the proportion of patients who receive adequate dosage and duration is only around 25%, and the rate of counseling is only 10% (Stein *et al.* 2004).

This chapter reviews the treatment of anxiety disorders in primary care. Topics explored include medication effectiveness (e.g., sertraline, venlafaxine, pregabalin, herbal medication) and use of psychosocial interventions (e.g., cognitive–behavioral therapy, lifestyle modification therapy). We also describe studies that implement organizational and educational interventions aimed at improving quality of care for anxiety disorders in primary care, such as the collaborative care model. The chapter ends with some considerations about future directions in the treatment of anxiety disorders in primary care.

30.2 Pharmacological treatments

At present, selective serotonin reuptake inhibitors (SSRIs) and serotonin–norepinephrine reuptake inhibitors (SNRIs) are considered the first-line pharmacological treatment for anxiety disorders. However, few studies have examined pharmacological agents specifically in primary care settings. We first discuss studies that evaluate pharmacological agent monotherapy, followed by studies combining medication and psychotherapy or embedded in integrated models of care. To date, only two studies have examined the effect of medication monotherapy in the treatment of primary care patients with anxiety disorders. Both studies have been conducted in patients with generalized anxiety disorder (GAD).

Lader and colleagues (1998) conducted a double-blind, parallel-group multicenter study to compare the effectiveness of a four-week course of hydroxyzine, buspirone, or placebo in patients with GAD. The study, which included 244 patients from 62 primary care centers in France and the United Kingdom, was designed to test earlier findings (Darcis *et al.* 1996) regarding the efficacy of hydroxyzine in the treatment of GAD. Patients were randomly allocated to receive fixed doses of hydroxyzine (50 mg/day), buspirone (20 mg/day), or placebo. At baseline, the mean Hamilton Rating Scale for Anxiety (HAM-A) score was 26.5. At study endpoint, the mean HAM-A improvement was 10.8 points on hydroxyzine, 8.8 points on buspirone, and 7.2 points on placebo. Only the difference between placebo and hydroxyzine was statistically significant. Thirty-one participants dropped out, with no significant differences across groups. No withdrawal symptoms were associated with hydroxyzine or buspirone discontinuation. Reported side effects included somnolence (9.9% for hydroxyzine, 4.9% for buspirone, and none in the placebo group), headache and migraine (6.1% for buspirone, 4.9% for hydroxyzine, 1.2% for placebo), and dizziness (6.1% for buspirone, 0 % for hydroxyzine, 2.5% in the placebo group). Whether differences in the rates of side effects across treatment reached statistical significance was not reported.

In the second study, Montgomery and colleagues (2006) conducted a six-week, double-blind randomized controlled trial on the efficacy and safety of pregabalin in 421 outpatients with moderate-to-severe GAD. The study was carried out at 52 primary care and 24 psychiatric centers in Austria, Belgium, Germany, the Netherlands,

Anxiety Disorders: Theory, Research, and Clinical Perspectives, ed. Helen Blair Simpson, Yuval Neria, Roberto Lewis-Fernández, Franklin Schneier. Published by Cambridge University Press. © Cambridge University Press 2010.

and the United Kingdom. Patients were randomly assigned to either 400 or 600 mg/day of pregabalin, 75 mg/day of venlafaxine, or placebo. All three active treatments resulted in significantly greater improvements in HAM-A total score at endpoint than placebo. The response rate (defined as ≥ 50% reduction in HAM-A total score at endpoint) was significantly greater for pregabalin 400 mg/day and for venlafaxine than for the other two groups. Using Clinical Global Impression (CGI) scale definitions of greater-than-minimal response, all three active treatments had significantly higher response rates than placebo. All three active treatment groups also showed significantly greater improvement in Hamilton Rating Scale for Depression (HAM-D) total scores compared to placebo.

The study reported that the most common side effect was dizziness (pregabalin 23% at 400 mg/day and 26% at 600 mg/day, venlafaxine 12%, placebo 7%). Somnolence was also common, reported with pregabalin (13% at 400 mg/day, 14% at 600 mg/day), venlafaxine (4%), and placebo (3%). The level of significance of these findings was not reported. Discontinuation rates due to adverse effects were 20% in the venlafaxine group, 6% in the pregabalin 400 mg/day group, 14% in the pregabalin 600 mg/day group, and 10% in the placebo group. The attrition rate due to discontinuations associated with adverse effects was significantly greater in the venlafaxine 75 mg/day group than in the pregabalin 400 mg/day group. This study was limited by the lack of longer follow-up periods.

30.3 Pharmacotherapy and cognitive–behavioral therapy (CBT)

Haug and colleagues conducted a 24-week trial that examined the efficacy of sertraline or CBT-based exposure therapy, alone or in combination, for the treatment of social anxiety disorder (SAD) (Haug *et al.* 2000, Blomhoff *et al.* 2001). Patients with SAD of greater than one year's duration and at least moderate severity (CGI ≥ 3) were recruited from 41 primary care centers in Norway and Sweden. Patients were randomly assigned to four different groups: exposure therapy plus sertraline (*n* = 98), exposure therapy plus placebo (*n* = 98), general care plus sertraline (*n* = 96), or general care plus placebo (*n* = 95). The doses of sertraline ranged from 50 to 150 mg/day.

General care was limited to a discussion of clinical history, psychoeducation on SAD, and provision of general support by the primary care physician (PCP).

Patients receiving exposure therapy identified their goals for the therapy as well as 1–3 target complaints, each scored on a scale of 1–4 based on prevalence. The therapy itself consisted of eight sessions (each lasting 15–20 minutes) and homework.

Exposure therapy plus placebo, exposure therapy plus sertraline, and general care plus sertraline were significantly superior to general care plus placebo in decreasing target complaint scores at weeks 12 and 24. The largest reductions occurred in the exposure therapy plus sertraline group. This trial defined treatment response as a reduction of at least 50% from baseline in symptom burden, assessed on the Social Phobia Scale, an endpoint Clinical Global Impression–Social Phobia (CGI-SP) overall severity score of three or more ("no mental illness" to "mild severity"), and a CGI-SP overall improvement score of "very much" or "much improved" (≤ 2). To be considered responders, patients had to meet all criteria. The CGI-SP computed overall severity and improvement through performance on four subscales, which included anxiety attacks, avoidance, performance anxiety, and disability. At week 24, significantly more sertraline-treated patients than non-sertraline treated patients were considered responders. There was no significant difference between exposure therapy and non-exposure-treated patients. Combined exposure therapy plus sertraline (45%) and general care plus sertraline (40%) were associated with significantly higher response rates than general care plus placebo (24%). Significantly more patients in the combined exposure plus sertraline group met response criteria compared to general care plus placebo by week 12.

In this study, sertraline – either with general care or in combination with exposure therapy – was effective in the treatment of SAD. Findings for exposure therapy plus placebo approached, but did not reach, statistical significance. Since no interaction between sertraline and exposure therapy was found, the study suggested additive effects of the two active treatments.

The trial was followed by analysis of the longitudinal effects of these interventions 28 weeks after the 24-week treatment was administered (i.e., week 52) (Haug *et al.* 2003). Patients who had received exposure therapy plus placebo or general care plus placebo had additional significant improvement on social phobia scores at week 52 compared to scores at the end of the treatment period (week 24). The exposure therapy plus sertraline group and the general care plus sertraline group maintained their gains by week 52 compared to scores at week 24, except in scores on a measure of impairment, the 36-Item Short Form Survey (SF-36), in which there was significant deterioration at week 52. This follow-up suggests that exposure therapy, sertraline, and the combination of the two were all effective treatments for SAD. Limitations of this study included the fact there were no direct group comparisons, that the PCPs evaluated their own patients, and that there was no registry of relapses during follow-up.

30.4 Integrated treatments

Several alternatives to usual care have been explored in the treatment of mental disorders in primary care, including strategies that seek to overcome patient, physician, and process-of-care barriers. These strategies have focused mainly on depression (Katon *et al.* 1995, 1996, 1999, Lin *et al.* 1999, Gilbody *et al.* 2003) rather than on anxiety disorders. One of these interventions is the chronic care model, which provides chronic illness management within primary care (Wagner *et al.* 2001, Bodenheimer *et al.* 2002) based on improvement in six interrelated components: self-management support, clinical information systems, delivery system redesign, decision support, healthcare organization resources, and community resources. The goal is to produce system reform in which informed, activated patients interact with prepared, proactive practice teams. In this model, patients typically remain under the care of their PCP, who is assisted by a care manager working in consultation with a mental-health expert (typically a psychiatrist). Provision of care also includes restructuring of practice through continuous clinical assessments and the addition of resources to help increase the patients' self-management (e.g., psychoeducation, motivational enhancement).

Roy-Byrne and colleagues (2001) tested the effects of a collaborative care (CC) intervention on 115 patients with panic disorder (PD) drawn from three primary care clinics in Seattle, Washington. Patients were randomized to CC (*n* = 57) or usual care (UC) (*n* = 58). Patients in the CC group received an initial psychiatric visit, in which they were prescribed paroxetine starting at 10 mg daily and increasing subsequently as tolerated. Two follow-up telephone calls and a second visit were offered to address problems with adverse side effects or other clinical issues. No formal CBT was given, but patients were encouraged to expose themselves, as tolerated, to feared or avoided situations. Extended care (i.e., telephone calls, extra sessions for selected patients) was also implemented for CC patients. Between months 3 and 12, psychiatrists

followed up five times with CC patients over the phone. CC patients were also given educational materials with information about PD and medication; this information was also emphasized during psychiatrist visits. The psychiatrist made all the medication adjustments. The PCP received a typed consultation note after each psychiatric visit. UC patients only received pharmacotherapy from their PCP, who received the results of an initial psychiatric diagnostic assessment (to eliminate non-recognition of panic and associated disorders as a factor in outcome) and could offer specialty mental-health referrals as needed.

Assessments of panic, anxiety sensitivity, depression, and disability were performed at three, six, nine, and 12 months. Adequacy of pharmacotherapy was rated from patient self-reports during these assessments using an algorithm based on a review of efficacy studies. Patients were classified as adherent if they reported taking the medication for at least 25 days in the previous month. Patient satisfaction with the care received for emotional problems was also assessed. Fifty-one percent of the patients in the study had major depression, and 43% and 39% had comorbid GAD or SAD, respectively. At three months, and again at six months, significantly more CC patients received an adequate dose of an appropriate medication and showed greater treatment adherence than UC patients. These differences were no longer significant at nine and 12 months.

Compared to UC patients, those receiving the CC intervention reported lower overall panic severity on the Panic Disorder Severity Scale (PDSS) at six months. Compared to UC patients, CC patients had significantly lower scores on the Anxiety Sensitivity Index (ASI) at three-, six-, and 12-month follow-ups. CC patients also showed significant improvement in role functioning at 12-month follow-up. At six- and 12-month follow-up, significantly more CC than UC patients were satisfied or very satisfied with the quality of care they had received for emotional problems. Overall, results indicated that, compared to UC, the CC intervention for patients with PD resulted in stronger adherence to pharmacotherapy, greater clinical and functional improvement, and higher treatment satisfaction. These differences were most consistent and pronounced during the first six months of the study, which might be explained by the more intensive care provided in the CC intervention. Although the study provided useful information, it had some limitations. A small number of sites were used, limiting its generalizability. Subjects were given medication free of charge, which does not reflect the care provided in most primary care settings, and they did not receive any form of psychotherapy.

In a subsequent study, Roy-Byrne and colleagues (2005) tested the effectiveness of combined pharmacotherapy and CBT for PD. Patients were drawn from university-affiliated primary care clinics in Seattle, San Diego, and Los Angeles. Patients were randomized to receive UC ($n = 113$) or an intervention following a CC model ($n = 119$). PCPs received a one-hour didactic session on PD. The intervention consisted of a combination of an algorithm-based pharmacotherapy provided by the PCP with guidance from a psychiatrist, and up to six sessions (across 12 weeks) of modified CBT for primary care (some sessions could be conducted over the telephone). CBT providers were behavioral health specialists with minimal or no CBT experience. The specialists were trained to deliver a shortened version of evidence-based CBT (six sessions plus six brief follow-up telephone contacts; the telephone follow-ups each lasted 15–30 minutes). The behavioral health specialist also relayed information from the consulting psychiatrist to the PCP. Patients receiving the intervention received a workbook and a video about the disorder and its treatment. The algorithm began with dose titration of an SSRI for at least six weeks, unless the subject had already failed trials of two SSRIs, in which case alternative antidepressants (e.g., SSNIs, tricyclic antidepressants) or adjunctive medications (e.g., benzodiazepines) were used first.

Remission was defined as meeting all three of the following criteria: no panic attacks in the past month; minimal anticipatory anxiety about panic (0–1 on a three-point scale); and an agoraphobia subscale score of 10 or less (range 0–40) (Marks & Matthews 1979). Response was defined as an Anxiety Sensitivity Index (ASI) score < 20. Other measures assessed included change over time in the World Health Organization Disability Scale (WHODS) and 12-Item Short Form Survey (SF-12) scores.

The proportion of guideline-concordant pharmacotherapy use increased from baseline in both groups and did not differ statistically at any point. Significantly more patients in the intervention group responded and remitted at each assessment point over 12 months. After 12 months, over 63% of patients responded in the intervention group, compared to 38% in the UC group, and 29% of the intervention patients remitted, compared to 16% in the UC group. These results suggest that the CC intervention was significantly more effective than

UC for PD in primary care. The study used a more generalizable sample, required that patients pay for their medication, and used relatively inexperienced therapists to provide CBT and coordinate management. Limitations of the study include the facts that all care was delivered in university settings, CBT was provided free of charge, and many patients did not adhere to the entire CBT program.

Rollman and colleagues (2005) examined the effects of a randomized telephone-based CC intervention for PD or GAD. The study included patients from four primary care practices in the Pittsburgh area, Pennsylvania. Patients were randomly assigned to either telephone-based CC ($n = 116$) or to UC ($n = 75$). The intervention involved non-mental-health professionals who worked as care managers. These care managers telephoned each intervention patient and conducted a detailed mental-health assessment, provided psychoeducation, assessed the patient's treatment preferences, monitored treatment response, and informed physicians of the patient's care preferences and progress through an electronic medical record. Patients in the CC group could choose a combination of treatment components: a workbook detailing self-management skills for PD or GAD, a guideline-based trial of anxiolytic pharmacotherapy, or referral to a community mental-health specialist. In addition, the principal investigators of the study conducted weekly 60- to 75-minute case review sessions at which care managers presented all patients (new and ongoing), constantly tracking the full group's progress. Principal investigators would give pharmacotherapy suggestions or recommended referrals if warranted. Care managers would then communicate these recommendations to the PCPs and the patients. Care managers followed up on patients' adherence and clinical response by telephone at regular intervals, and also referred patients to specific sections in the workbooks, reviewed lesson plans, performed exercises and confirmed patients' understanding of the materials. The care manager informed PCPs of patients' progress, recommended modifications, and offered them other types of assistance. The PCPs were always free to accept or reject the recommendations.

When compared to UC patients, intervention patients reported a significantly higher rate of pharmacotherapy use only at the two-month follow-up. The proportion of patients who reported visiting a mental-health specialist did not differ between the groups. Intervention and UC patients had similar rates of office and telephone contacts with their physicians. At 12-month follow-up, patients randomized to the intervention reported a greater reduction of anxiety symptoms, which correlated with a drop of 3.6 points in the structured interview guide for HAM-A. At 12 months, improvement was also statistically significant in the PDSS and HAM-D scores, and in the SF-12 mental-component summary score. Intervention patients also reported improved employment patterns. Telephone-based CC for PD and GAD was more effective than UC in the treatment of anxiety symptoms. The study did not employ costly health professionals to deliver the intervention and was able to demonstrate that the intervention was associated with a significant reduction in anxiety and depressive symptoms and with improved mental health-related quality of life and employment patterns without increasing the number of physician contacts over the course of a year. The study was limited by the exclusion of patients with high risk of alcohol use disorder, and by the fact that the study relied on patients' self-reported use of mental-health specialists, with no confirmation. Finally, 95% of the study's patients were Caucasians, limiting its generalizability.

Price and colleagues (2000) compared the efficacy of an integrated care model in the treatment of GAD. A matched-cohort experimental design was used to compare outcomes for the integrated model ($n = 68$) to UC ($n = 69$). The integrated care model was implemented in the Family Practice Department at the Westminster medical office of Kaiser Permanente of Colorado, and a non-randomized matched control group of patients was drawn from the General Internal Medicine Department at the same site. Two Ph.D.-level mental-health specialists worked with the PCPs at the intervention medical clinic. These specialists worked as curbside consultants to the PCPs and coordinated treatment plans (attended meetings to discuss difficult cases, provided patient education, coordinated referrals, and followed up treatment progress and adherence). Treatment options included medication, CBT (ideally 4–6 sessions but with no rigid limits), or both. The patient, psychologist, and PCP jointly formulated the treatment plan. The team could also consult with a liaison psychiatrist (on site two hours/week and available for telephone consultation). UC patients received treatment as usual (i.e., pharmacotherapy) and could be referred to the mental health department.

Patients were assessed with the Shedler Quick PsychoDiagnostics Panel (QPD), SF-12, and the panic subscale of the Symptom Checklist 90 (SCL-90).

Patients were assessed for anxiety symptom remission at three- and six-month follow-ups. At baseline, 77.8% of the intervention group and 61.4% of the UC group had anxiety scores greater than 10 (clinically significant) on the QPD. At six months, the intervention group had a significantly lower mean anxiety score than the UC group (5.81 vs. 7.93 on the QPD). Intervention patients were significantly satisfied with their treatment. Limitations in this study include the fact that patients were not randomized to control or intervention groups, and there were some baseline differences between the groups. In addition, unaccounted-for differences could exist in part due to patient self-selection of a family physician instead of a general internist. The study did not examine long-term effects of this intervention.

30.5 Other approaches

Lambert and colleagues (2007) conducted a 16-week unblinded, randomized controlled trial comparing the effects of an occupational-therapy-led lifestyle intervention for PD versus UC. Patients were recruited from 15 primary care centers in the east of England. After stratification for the presence/absence of agoraphobia and lifestyle factors, patients were randomized to the occupational-therapy-led lifestyle approach ($n = 57$) or to UC ($n = 60$). The intervention aimed to promote positive lifestyle changes and addressed four areas: diet, fluid intake, exercise, and habitual drug use (caffeine, alcohol, nicotine). The intervention group received 10 sessions over a 16-week period. The sessions involved a lifestyle review, education, suggestions for specific lifestyle changes, and ongoing monitoring.

At baseline, over 85% of patients in both study arms had moderate-to-severe anxiety according to the Beck Anxiety Inventory (BAI) (range 0–63, minimal 0–7, mild 8–15, moderate 16–25, severe 26–63). After 20 weeks, only 20% of the intervention patients experienced severe anxiety, although this rose to 30% after 10 months. In the UC group, the level of severe anxiety dropped to 55% after 20 weeks and was further reduced to 40% after 10 months. After 20 weeks, 64% of lifestyle arm patients were panic-free in the previous month, compared with 40% in the UC group. At the end of treatment, significantly more patients receiving lifestyle intervention reported improvement in anxiety, but at 10-month follow-up between-group differences were not statistically significant. Approximately 66% of patients incorporated positive lifestyle changes and were able to maintain improvements in their anxiety symptoms. The approach did not seem effective in the long term, as one-third of the intervention group returned to their previous lifestyle and anxiety patterns after 10 months.

Schreuders and colleagues (2007) investigated the effectiveness of problem-solving therapy for primary care patients with mental health problems. A randomized controlled trial was conducted in 12 primary care centers in Amsterdam, the Netherlands. Patients were allocated to either UC plus problem-solving treatment provided by a nurse (4–6 sessions) ($n = 88$) or UC ($n = 87$). There were no significant differences between groups in the anxiety subscale of the Hospital Anxiety and Depression Scale at the three-month endpoint assessment. The study suggested that problem-solving treatment added little to UC.

Van Boeijen and colleagues (2005a) conducted a 12-week randomized controlled trial comparing the effectiveness of three forms of individual treatment based on cognitive–behavioral principles. Patients with GAD and/or PD were recruited from 46 primary care centers in the Netherlands. PCPs and therapists were trained through meetings and supervision and were randomized to the different treatment forms. The first form of treatment consisted of "self-help," which was delivered as a manual with cognitive techniques in addition to five 20-minute sessions where the PCP assessed and reinforced patients' achievements and motivated them to continue using the manual. The second group was offered twelve 45-minute sessions of CBT. The third group received guideline-assisted treatment consisting of a simple form of CBT. The physician was free to choose the number of sessions and could refer the patient for relaxation exercises or psychiatric treatment for medication. The main outcome measure used was the Spielberger Anxiety Inventory. The three treatments did not differ significantly in reducing anxiety and associated symptoms. Most of the improvement was observed in the first 12 weeks. About half the patients were treated with antidepressants or referred to secondary care instead. The limitations of this study include the fact that since the physicians found the feasibility of "guidelines" to be low, the sample size in this group only reached half of what was intended, making it difficult to draw conclusions based on the results.

30.6 Self-help

A systematic review of the efficacy of self-help manuals for anxiety disorders in primary care identified six studies (van Boeijen *et al.* 2005b). Overall, study samples were small and had high rates of dropout. Furthermore, the studies differed in the diagnosis included, criteria used, design, and duration of the intervention and follow-up periods. Some studies compared a self-help manual with a waiting list or UC. Two studies did not find significant differences between a manual and waiting list, or a manual and UC (Milne & Covitz 1988, Donnan *et al.* 1990); one of these studies used a very small sample (less than 10 patients per group) (Milne & Covitz 1988), and the other had a moderate quality score (Donnan *et al.* 1990). Two studies showed superior outcomes for the use of self-help manuals (White 1995, Sorby *et al.* 1991). Two other studies evaluated the use of manuals compared to different levels of contact (Sharp *et al.* 2000, Kupshik & Fisher 1999). One of the latter studies (Sharp *et al.* 2000) found that CBT on a standard contact basis (six hours) had greater efficacy than self-help alone. In general, the review suggested that manuals had larger effects when administered with increased contacts and guidance. Thus, there is still insufficient information on the efficacy of these approaches.

30.7 Complementary and alternative treatments: herbal medicine

Although several studies have been conducted on the use of valerian and passiflora in the treatment of anxiety disorders, there is general agreement that not enough evidence exists to draw conclusions on the efficacy of either compound (Miyasaka *et al.* 2006, 2007, Ernst 2007). Meta-analyses have reported a common finding: there are so few valid studies to include in these analyses that they include a mix of relevant randomized and quasi-randomized controlled trials of the compound (at any dose or method of administration) for patients with anxiety disorders (Miyasaka *et al.* 2006, 2007).

30.8 Future directions

While progress has been made in the treatment of depression in primary care, moving from efficacy to effectiveness studies to multifaceted interventions aimed at quality improvement, much less work has been done in the field of anxiety disorders. This has led to the development of different approaches to enhance primary care that typically involve the participation of other specialists. The combination of professional and organizational interventions appears to be the most promising. However, determining which components of these integrated interventions are responsible for the beneficial effects, and the best combination of components, is still a subject of future research.

Most of the studies described above found varying levels of adherence across a number of different therapeutic alternatives (e.g., pharmacotherapy, CBT). Motivational interviewing has been explored as a strategy for addressing this problem, as it focuses on preparing the client for change and, as a result, is highly complementary to alternatives like CBT (Westra 2004). Further research into the mediators of adherence to the different alternatives and components of integrated models of care treatments is also needed.

In addition, most studies have only evaluated short-term effects. Some therapeutic approaches might have long-term effects while others appear to have only temporary benefits. Another issue is the limited number of anxiety disorders studied. Ongoing research is currently trying to overcome this issue. The CALM study (Sullivan *et al.* 2007) is one of the largest to date ($n = 1042$); it will test the efficacy of CBT and/or a medication in the treatment of anxiety in primary care and will include patients with GAD, SAD, PD, and PTSD recruited from four national sites. The study uses a "stepped care" approach and allows patient choice of treatment. Patients will first be treated by their PCP, and only incomplete responders or those at a high risk of relapse or in a chronic condition will receive a second "step" of care. This model of care could be more cost-effective than the present CC approaches, and could address the hesitancy to adopt CC models because of their increased costs. The study will measure outcomes at six, 12, and 18 months.

Some of the studies described in this chapter did not employ costly, highly trained, or experienced professionals to deliver the interventions. The development of interventions involving the participation of these and other types of health professionals should also be the focus of research. Finally, while initial cost-effectiveness studies have suggested positive results (Katon *et al.* 2002), future research should also focus on the evaluation of the feasibility and implementability of these interventions in large healthcare systems.

References

Blomhoff, S., Haug, T. T., Hellstrom, K., *et al.* (2001). Randomized controlled general practice trial of sertraline, exposure therapy and combined treatment in generalized social phobia. *British Journal of Psychiatry*, **179**, 23–30.

Bodenheimer, T., Wagner, E. H., & Grumback, K. (2002). Improving primary care for patients with chronic illness. *JAMA*, **288**, 1775–1779.

Darcis, T., Ferreri, M., Natens, J., *et al.* (1996). A multicentre double-blind placebo-controlled study investigating the anxiolytic efficacy of hydroxyzine in patients with generalized anxiety. *Human Psychopharmacology*, **10**, 181–187.

Donnan, P., Hutchinson, A., Paxton, R., Grant, B., & Firth, M. (1990). Self-help materials for anxiety: a randomized controlled trial in general practice. *British Journal of General Practice*, **40**, 498–501.

Ernst, E. (2007). Herbal remedies for depression and anxiety. *Advances in Psychiatric Treatment*, **13**, 312–316.

Gilbody, S., Whitty, P., Grimshaw, J., & Thomas, R. (2003). Educational and organizational interventions to improve the management of depression in primary care: a systematic review. *JAMA*, **289**, 3145–3151.

Haug, T. T., Hellstrom, K., Blomhoff, S., *et al.* (2000). The treatment of social phobia in general practice. Is exposure therapy feasible? *Family Practice*, **17**, 114–118.

Haug, T. T., Blomhoff, S., Hellstrom, K., *et al.* (2003). Exposure therapy and sertraline in social phobia: 1 year follow-up of a randomized controlled trial. *British Journal of Psychiatry*, **182**, 312–318.

Katon, W., Von Korff, M., Lin, E., *et al.* (1995). Collaborative management to achieve treatment guidelines: impact on depression in primary care. *JAMA*, **273**, 1026–1031.

Katon, W., Robinson, P., Von Korff, M., *et al.* (1996). A multifaceted intervention to improve treatment of depression in primary care. *Archives of General Psychiatry*, **53**, 924–932.

Katon, W., Von Korff, M., Lin, E., *et al.* (1999). Stepped collaborative care for primary care patients with depression. *Archives of General Psychiatry*, **56**, 1109–1115.

Katon, W., Roy-Byrne, P., Russo, J., & Cowley, D. (2002). Cost-effectiveness and cost offset of a collaborative care intervention for primary care patients with panic disorder. *Archives of General Psychiatry*, **59**, 1098–1104.

Kupshik, G. A., & Fisher, C. R. (1999). Assisted bibliotherapy: effective, efficient treatment for moderate anxiety problems. *British Journal of General Practice*, **49**, 47–48.

Lader, M., & Scotto, J. (1998). A multicentre double-blind comparison of hydroxyzine, buspirone and placebo in patients with generalized anxiety disorder. *Psychopharmacology*, **139**, 402–406.

Lambert, R. A., Harvey, I., & Poland, F. (2007). A pragmatic, unblinded randomised controlled trial comparing an occupational therapy-led lifestyle approach and routine GP care for panic disorder treatment in primary care. *Journal of Affective Disorders*, **99**, 63–71.

Lin, E. H., Simon, G. E., Katon, W. J., *et al.* (1999). Can enhanced acute-phase treatment of depression improve long-term outcomes? A report of randomized trials in primary care. *American Journal of Psychiatry*, **156**, 643–645.

Marks, I. M., & Matthews, A. M. (1979). Brief standard self-rating for phobic patients. *Behaviour Research and Therapy*, **17**, 263–267.

Milne, D., & Covitz, F. (1988). A comparative evaluation of anxiety management materials in general practice. *Health Education Journal*, **47**, 67–69.

Miyasaka, L. S., Atallah, A. N., & Soares B. G. (2006). Valerian for anxiety disorders. *Cochrane Database of Systematic Reviews*, (4), CD004515.

Miyasaka, L. S., Atallah, A. N., & Soares B. G. (2007). Passiflora for anxiety disorder. *Cochrane Database of Systematic Reviews*, (1), CD004518.

Montgomery, S. A., Tobias, K., Zornberg, G. L., Kasper, S., & Pande, A. C. (2006). Efficacy and safety of pregabalin in the treatment of generalized anxiety disorder: a 6-week, multicenter, randomized, double-blind, placebo-controlled comparison of pregabalin and venlafaxine. *Journal of Clinical Psychiatry*, **67**, 771–782.

Price, D., Beck, A., Nimmer, C., & Bensen, S. (2000). The treatment of anxiety disorders in a primary care HMO setting. *Psychiatric Quarterly*, **71**, 31–45.

Rollman, B. L., Belnap, B. H., Mazumdar, S., *et al.* (2005). A randomized trial to improve the quality of treatment for panic and generalized anxiety disorders in primary care. *Archives of General Psychiatry*, **62**, 1332–1341.

Roy-Byrne, P. P., Katon, W., Cowley, D. S., & Russo, J. (2001). A randomized effectiveness trial of collaborative care for patients with panic disorder in primary care. *Archives of General Psychiatry*, **58**, 869–876.

Roy-Byrne, P. P., Craske, M. G., Stein, M. B., *et al.* (2005). A randomized effectiveness trial of cognitive–behavioral therapy and medication for primary care panic disorder. *Archives of General Psychiatry*, **62**, 290–298.

Sartorius, N., Ustun, T.B., Lecubrier, Y., & Wittchen, H. U. (1996). Depression comorbid with anxiety: results from the WHO study on psychological disorders in primary health care. *British Journal of Psychiatry Supplement*, (30), 38–43.

Schreuders, B., Marwijk, H. V., Smit, J., *et al.* (2007). Primary care patients with mental health problems: outcome of

a randomized controlled trial. *British Journal of General Practice*, **57**, 886–891.

Sharp, D. M., Power, K. G., & Swanson, V. (2000). Reducing therapist contact in cognitive behaviour therapy for panic disorder and agoraphobia in primary care: global measures of outcome in a randomised controlled trial. *British Journal of General Practice*, **50**, 963–968.

Sorby, N. G., Reavley, W., & Huber, J. W. (1991). Self help programme for anxiety in general practice: controlled trial of an anxiety management booklet. *British Journal of General Practice*, **41**, 417–420.

Stein, M. B., Sherbourne, C. D., Craske, M. G., *et al.* (2004). Quality of care for primary care patients with anxiety disorders. *American Journal of Psychiatry*, **161**, 2230–2237.

Sullivan, G., Craske, M. G., Sherbourne, C., *et al.* (2007). Design of the Coordinated Anxiety Learning and Management (CALM) Study: innovations in collaborative care for anxiety disorders. *General Hospital Psychiatry*, **29**, 379–387.

van Boeijen, C. A., van Oppen, P., van Balkom, A. J. L. M., *et al.* (2005a). Treatment of anxiety disorders in primary care practice: a randomized controlled trial. *British Journal of General Practice*, **55**, 763–769.

van Boeijen, C. A., van Oppen, P., van Balkom, A. J. L. M., *et al.* (2005b). Efficacy of self-help manuals for anxiety disorders in primary care: a systematic review. *Family Practice*, **22**, 192–196.

Wagner, E. H., Austin, B. T., Davis, C., *et al.* (2001). Improving chronic illness care: translating evidence into action. *Health Affairs*, **20**, 64–78.

Westra, H. A. (2004). Managing resistance in cognitive behavioral therapy: the application of motivational interviewing in mixed anxiety and depression. *Cognitive Behaviour Therapy*, **33**, 161–175.

White, J. (1995). Stresspac: a controlled trial of a self-help package for the anxiety disorders. *Behavioural and Cognitive Psychotherapy*, **23**, 89–107.

Young, A. S., Klap., R, Sherbourne., C. D., & Wells, K. B. (2001). The quality of care for depressive and anxiety disorders in the United States. *Archives of General Psychiatry*, **58**, 55–61.

Conclusion: gaps in knowledge and future directions

Helen Blair Simpson, Franklin Schneier, Roberto Lewis-Fernández, Yuval Neria

> Progress in the scientific analysis of the human mind demands a joint attack from virtually all of the behavioral sciences, in which the findings of each will force continual theoretical reassessments upon all of the others.
>
> Clifford Geertz, The Interpretation of Cultures (1973)

31.1 Overview

This book presents a selective review of work conducted over the last three decades to advance our understanding of anxiety and anxiety disorders. The chapters illustrate how much we have learned about topics ranging from nosology and clinical assessment to mechanisms and treatments of anxiety disorders. At the same time, there remain significant gaps in our knowledge, and several areas of inquiry are just beginning to be explored. In this final chapter, we highlight some of the most important advances in the field, integrate findings across the chapters, and outline a number of unanswered questions that need to be addressed in future research.

31.2 What is an anxiety disorder?

The last three decades have produced changes in influential models of anxiety and in the classification of anxiety disorders. For example, Glick and Roose (Chapter 5) trace the evolution of psychodynamic models of anxiety from Freudian psychology to contemporary theories. Although these psychodynamic models are unified by their emphasis on anxiety as a response to an anticipated unconscious, intrapsychic danger, the early focus on internal concepts of anxiety is modified in later theories by increasing attention to environmental influences (such as poor parenting) that help shape the developing mind and personality.

Cognitive–behavioral models of anxiety evolved in another direction, as outlined by Hambrick, Comer, and Albano (Chapter 18). Early behavioral models focused on the role of associative learning in fear acquisition. Then the cognitive revolution shifted the focus to the individual's attitudes, attributions, interpretations, and beliefs (i.e., inner cognitive processes). Cognitive–behavioral therapy (CBT) of anxiety disorders integrates these two perspectives: learning theory focuses on environmental contingencies of behavior, while the cognitive focus is on dysfunctional thinking patterns that trigger and maintain fears. Today, CBT theories emphasize that an individual's vulnerability to anxiety is multi-determined by biological, psychological, and environmental factors.

Hofer (Chapter 6) presents an evolutionary perspective on anxiety, where the adaptive function of anxiety is considered from the broader context of conceding advantage or disadvantage to organisms in the process of natural selection. In this paradigm, anxiety disorders may constitute "failed experiments" in the evolutionary struggle – in other words, blind alleys along the pathways to anxiety regulation. These evolutionary models share with psychodynamic and cognitive–behavioral approaches the characterization of anxiety as an adaptive or maladaptive response to internal and external threats. As detailed in Section 3 of this book (and discussed below), biological models of anxiety have arrived at a similar conclusion: an individual's biology interacts with environmental influences over the life course, generating and shaping the expression of anxiety.

As our concepts about anxiety have evolved, the nosology of anxiety disorders has also changed. As described by First and colleagues (Chapter 3), there has been a progressive expansion and specification of the different anxiety disorders in the *Diagnostic and Statistical Manual* (DSM) from DSM-I (1952) to DSM-5 (expected 2013). In turn, the increase in specificity and reliability of these diagnostic criteria has fostered epidemiologic research. As described by Comer and Olfson

Anxiety Disorders: Theory, Research, and Clinical Perspectives, ed. Helen Blair Simpson, Yuval Neria, Roberto Lewis-Fernández, Franklin Schneier. Published by Cambridge University Press. © Cambridge University Press 2010.

(Chapter 2), this research has revealed, somewhat to the field's surprise, that anxiety disorders as a group are more common than any other class of mental illness. Increased reliability of diagnoses has also allowed us to compare the prevalence of anxiety disorders across communities and continents, and across various types of medical and community settings, to search for risk factors that can clarify their etiology and provide entry points for intervention, and to guide neurobiological research to discover brain mechanisms. This process is described by Liebowitz (Chapter 4), who provides a rare first-person account of this progression, within one scientific lifetime, in the study of social anxiety disorder.

As prototypical forms of specific anxiety disorders have been defined, exceptions to these prototypes have been described, leading to attempts to reduce heterogeneity for research and treatment by adding subtypes or altogether new diagnoses (Chapter 4). The progress and challenges of subtyping are described for obsessive–compulsive disorder (OCD) in Chapter 7 and for social anxiety disorder (SAD) in Chapter 8. How various psychopathologies may be quite distinct in their prototypical forms, yet in real life often overlap with each other and with other disorders, has also become clearer. As a result, links between anxiety disorders and other psychopathologies, such as depression (Chapter 9), the somatoform disorders (Chapter 10), and the personality disorders (Chapter 11), are being explored at both the phenomenological and the mechanistic level.

At the same time, this concerted effort toward reliable characterization of phenomenology is revealing the inherent limitations of the descriptive approach to psychiatric disorders. Diagnostic comorbidity is the rule rather than the exception, and the limitations of our knowledge are evidenced by limited specificity of pharmacological treatments, such as between most anxiety and mood disorders. Moving forward, a key challenge for our nosology and our methods of assessment is to integrate emerging data from epidemiology, neurobiology, genetics, developmental and social psychology, sociology, and cultural anthropology with phenomenological description to enhance the validity of diagnoses. How can we develop a nosology that characterizes the anxiety disorders in substantive, descriptive detail while also leaving room for individual and sociocultural variation? Can we develop a nosology that is based on pathophysiology or etiology? In the end, our goals should be: (1) a model of anxiety that incorporates the entire range of contributory factors (e.g., from single genes to sociocultural influences), (2) a nosology that can be used across individuals and cultures, and (3) assessment tools that help clinicians characterize these factors in individual patients and use them to enhance treatment outcome.

31.3 What causes anxiety and anxiety disorders?

There has been an explosion of research into the biological mechanisms that underlie anxiety disorders, as outlined by many of the chapters in Section 3. Because of progress in basic neuroscience, we know more about the cellular and molecular functioning of the brain than ever before. The ongoing development of new technologies (e.g., the ability to alter individual genes in animals, and brain imaging methods that permit exploration of the structure, metabolism, neurochemistry, and functioning of the living human brain) promises continued advances.

These new methods have revealed new layers of complexity. For example, serotonin, a brain neurotransmitter implicated in anxiety disorders, has over a dozen functionally distinct receptors, several of which are described in this book by Richardson-Jones, Leonardo, Hen, and Ahmari (Chapter 14) and by Weisstaub, McOmish, Hanks, and Gingrich (Chapter 15). As described in these chapters, different elements of the serotonin system (e.g., the serotonin transporter; the 5-HT_{1A} and 5-HT_{2A} receptors) all appear to play a role in the development, modulation, and/or treatment of anxiety in animal models. The complexity of the serotonin system is also shared by the other brain neurochemical systems, and there are complex interactions between these systems as well (e.g., the serotonergic and glutamatergic systems, as outlined in Chapter 15). The hope is that delineating the organization of underlying neurobiological systems will create new opportunities for treatment of anxiety disorders by more targeted modulation of these systems.

New methods have also facilitated the search for genes associated with the different anxiety disorders. As reviewed by Nugent, Weissman, Fyer, and Koenen (Chapter 13), after years of candidate gene studies that produced variable and often unreplicated findings, the field has moved to whole-genome association studies, with the hope that this effort will prove more productive and conclusive. The current thinking is that there will be multiple genes with small effects that contribute to vulnerability to anxiety. As a result, there has been a shift toward considering how to map genes to non-diagnostic, dimensional neurobehavioral constructs, including anxiety sensitivity, behavioral inhibition, and neuroticism. This theme resonates with the authors of several chapters of Section 2, who address diagnostic challenges and call for incorporating a neurobehaviorally informed dimensional approach in psychopathological research.

In addition to the focus on neurochemistry and genes, there is also growing interest in identifying brain circuits that underlie the expression of anxiety behaviors and studying how these circuits function (and presumably malfunction) to produce the symptoms we observe. For example, as outlined by Gordon and Adhikari (Chapter 16), we now know from animal studies what parts of the brain generate a learned fear response (e.g., the amygdala and its projections to hypothalamus and brainstem nuclei) and what parts of the brain can extinguish that learned response (e.g., the medial prefrontal cortex [mPFC] and the hippocampus). We also now know that extinction is not the erasure of learned fear, but rather a learning process. As a result, the original fear may re-emerge in response to contextual cues. Brain regions associated with innate anxiety have also been identified (e.g., the ventral hippocampus and the bed nucleus of the stria terminalis), regions that are also tightly connected to the amygdala and the mPFC. This has led to a model of separable but interrelated functional circuits that are involved in learned and innate fears and in the extinction of those fears in animals.

These animal findings have informed functional human imaging studies, and the results suggest that many of the brain regions involved in anxiety in animals serve similar functions in humans. For example, as described by Etkin and Wager (Chapter 17), negative affective reactivity in humans appears to involve "core" limbic circuitry that includes the amygdala. It is modulated by two large-scale distributed systems: (1) a network including prefrontal cortices that is involved in cognitive reappraisal and suppression of emotion via downregulation of amygdala activity and (2) an "affective appraisal system" (including the rostral mPFC and hippocampus) that integrates memories about a situation, information about the internal state of the body, and implications of this context for the future self. As reviewed by Gordon and Adhikari (Chapter 16), successful treatment of some anxiety disorders has resulted in increased mPFC activity and/or decreased amygdala activity, suggesting that changing the functioning of the brain structures involved in extinction of learned fear may underlie the therapeutic response.

These breakthroughs into the neural mechanisms of fear and anxiety in animals have relied on learning paradigms with roots in early behavioral psychology, similar to those that led to the development of modern cognitive–behavioral therapies, as outlined by Hambrick, Comer, and Albano (Chapter 18). Now these neurobiological findings in animals are influencing our human therapies. For example, understanding that fear conditioning and extinction are separable processes clarifies why posttraumatic stress disorder (PTSD) can appear months or even years after exposure to trauma, as new exposure to salient cues may reactivate dormant conditioned fears. These animal findings have also led to one of the first translational success stories in psychopharmacology: a medication (D-cycloserine) found to facilitate extinction learning in animals has been successfully applied to facilitate learning from exposure therapy in humans with anxiety disorders (Chapter 16). As more is uncovered about how these brain circuits generate and modulate innate and learned fear, we anticipate that a new era of pharmacological discovery for anxiety disorders will ensue.

Although the identification of abnormal neurotransmitters, genes, or brain circuits might one day explain how our brain produces the symptoms of anxiety disorders, it will not fully explain what caused an individual to develop this abnormality in the first place. To address etiology, it is increasingly clear that we need to understand the interplay of genetic vulnerability with the environment throughout the course of development. However, this work is still in its infancy. As outlined by Richardson-Jones, Leonardo, Hen, and Ahmari (Chapter 14), study of gene–development interactions in animals is now possible because of the increasingly sophisticated application of genetic knockout, knock-in, and transgenic approaches. For example, these approaches have been used to demonstrate that $5\text{-}HT_{1A}$ receptors play a role in the development of anxiety-related brain circuitry: if these receptors are removed from the forebrain during a critical period of postnatal development, the mouse will develop an anxious phenotype as an adult. However, the relevance of these findings for human anxiety disorders remains unclear.

Environmental influences, which can shape development by a variety of mechanisms including modulation of gene expression, are also critical to understanding why some people end up crippled by anxiety and others remain resilient and functional. Illustrating the complexity, Hofer (Chapter 6) reviews his own and others' pioneering work on developmental pathways to an anxious phenotype in rat pups. Hofer describes two paths to an anxious phenotype – one occurring through repeated selection of genetic alleles over 15 or 20 generations, the other occurring more rapidly through a transgenerational effect on development, in which maternal behavioral interactions affect gene expression within the developing brain systems of her infants and later determine their fear responses (and maternal behavior) as adults. As noted by Hofer, this second pathway provides an elegant non-Lamarckian alternative to the transmission of learned behavior across generations, and a mechanism by which any influence on maternal behavior (e.g., social and cultural factors in humans) might affect the development of the brain.

Several environmental factors of possible importance in the generation of anxiety are detailed in the book, including life stressors (Chapter 19), cultural illness representations (Chapter 12), attachment patterns (Chapter 20), and maternal environment (Chapters 5, 6, and 21). The complexity of studying the interaction of these environmental factors with underlying biological vulnerability cannot be overestimated. For example, while PTSD would appear to be the clearest example of an anxiety disorder with an environmental cause, as it requires exposure to a stressor, stressors of different types and magnitudes can lead to PTSD, as dissected by Dohrenwend (Chapter 19). This suggests that there is a complicated interaction between the stressor and the experience of the stressor, the latter of which is mediated by multiple factors including availability of social support, personality traits, and underlying biological systems (e.g., genes, neural circuitry).

Studies in non-human primates also emphasize the complexity of the interaction of environmental factors with underlying biological vulnerability. For example, Natarajan, Shrestha, and Coplan (Chapter 21) describe the troubling persistent effects of relatively subtle maternal deprivation on a myriad of outcome assessments, including juvenile behavior, neurotransmitter systems, hypothalamic–pituitary axis, and amygdala reactivity. However, they also describe a parallel line of research documenting that mild periodic maternal–infant separations appear to inoculate offspring, reducing anxious behaviors and conferring resilience to subsequent stressors. The parallels in the human literature are striking: as reviewed by Mulhare, Ghesquiere and Shear (Chapter 20), different attachment styles can also either protect or make one vulnerable to anxiety. Likewise, Glick and Roose (Chapter 5) discuss the role of infant temperament and infant–mother empathic failures in the development of the

infant's self, as described in the work on object relations and self psychology. Parent–infant interaction is an area deserving more study and integration of findings across animal and human studies. Learning how to optimize exposure to stressors that facilitate resilience may contribute to the "art" of parenting; experimental investigation in this area offers promise for improving the prevention of anxiety disorders.

Finally, as described by Hinton and Lewis-Fernández (Chapter 12), culture is also a powerful environmental factor, as it influences not only the forms of expression of anxiety symptoms but also their development. For example, Caribbean Latino cultures anticipate that unexpected bad news may be met with the expression of a panic-like emotional fit called an *ataque de nervios* (attack of nerves). This culturally patterned anxiety reaction may contribute to the increased likelihood of panic attacks and panic disorder in this population after sudden stressors, such as the September 11th attacks.

Taken together, this emerging work on environmental factors that underlie the generation and modulation of anxiety and anxiety disorders underscores the challenge in determining what causes anxiety disorders. To understand the interplay between genes, environment, and development, we will need as sophisticated an understanding of environmental factors as of genetic and other neurobiological mechanisms.

31.4 Which treatments work?

As reviewed in Section 4, we now have evidence-based treatments for the anxiety disorders. In particular, cognitive–behavioral therapy (CBT) has been shown to be effective for all of the anxiety disorders. Although the relative contributions of its ingredients (e.g., psychoeducation, cognitive restructuring, exposure, relaxation) are debated, most experts would agree that exposure-based techniques are key. CBT manuals have been developed and published, and these research-based treatments are being disseminated to community clinics and primary care settings (Chapter 30). CBT treatments have also been tailored for children (Chapter 27) and the elderly (Chapter 26) and are in the process of being modified for other specific populations, such as war veterans with PTSD (Chapter 24) and various cultural groups (Chapter 12).

In addition to CBT, the serotonin reuptake inhibitors (SRIs) have a proven broad spectrum of efficacy in large-scale, randomized controlled trials for OCD, PTSD, panic disorder, SAD, and generalized anxiety disorder (GAD). Other classes of medications have proven efficacious for specific disorders (e.g., benzodiazepines for panic disorder, SAD, and GAD but not for OCD or PTSD; buspirone for GAD only; noradrenergic tricyclic antidepressants for panic disorder but not for OCD or SAD). It is believed, but not proven, that these classes of medications work for one disorder but not for another because of underlying differences in pathophysiology.

Comparative trials of CBT and medications have also been conducted within different anxiety disorders in both adults and children (Chapters 22–27). Expectations that the combination of these two potentially complementary approaches might be better than either one alone have not been consistently fulfilled. Findings vary depending on the anxiety disorder, the population (children or adults), and the characteristics of treatments delivered (e.g., intensity of CBT or dose of medication). In general, these trials support the use of CBT and medications as monotherapy and show benefit of combination treatment in specific populations.

While there has been undeniable progress in the development of treatments for anxiety disorders, much remains to be done. Many patients cannot access appropriate treatments. The reasons vary and include patient barriers (e.g., stigma), structural barriers (e.g., lack of insurance), and clinician barriers (e.g., lack of expertise in evidence-based treatments for anxiety disorders). As a result, there remains a large gap between what we know works and what treatments patients actually receive in routine clinical care. The demands of exposure-based treatments and the risks of adverse effects from medications deter others from adequate treatment trials. Even for those who do access treatment, a sizeable minority will not respond, will respond only partially, or will not maintain response. Remission remains the exception.

One obstacle to improving treatment is that, although we know that existing treatments work, we do not know how they work. For example, how SRIs treat symptoms remains a mystery despite decades of investigation. The hypotheses range from restoration of neurotransmitter imbalance to stimulation of neurogenesis. Perhaps the closest we have come to understanding a key mechanism is the observation that exposure-based CBT may work through extinction learning, a process well characterized in animals. It is also worth noting that no new class of medications on the order of SRIs has been highly successful for the treatment of any of the anxiety disorders since the field first "listened to" Prozac (fluoxetine) in the early 1990s.

Important earlier classes that proved useful for anxiety disorders, such as the tricyclics, benzodiazepines, and monoamine oxidase inhibitors (MAOIs), were discovered through serendipity. The hope is that through translational study of normal and pathological anxiety in animals, we will develop a better understanding of what biological abnormalities underlie human anxiety disorders, and this knowledge in turn will lead to novel pharmacological targets and rational drug development. In addition, through a better understanding of how the environment impacts the development of anxiety in a vulnerable host, we may also identify novel psychosocial interventions.

Our current treatments are far from perfect. For example, although we know that our evidence-based treatments work, they only work for some. Within a disorder, we are generally unable to predict who will respond to what and when they will respond, which is the essential information we need in order to deliver personalized medical care. Moreover, when our first-line evidence-based treatments do not work, there is relatively little evidence to guide selection of second-line treatments. Should a non-responder to a single course of an SRI receive sequential trials of other SRIs, medication of a different class, or CBT? Lack of data regarding such common scenarios leaves the clinician in a quandary over how to proceed.

Another problem for the clinician is that our evidence-based treatments are usually developed and tested in the prototypical anxiety disorder patient. However, many patients present with not just one diagnosis, but with multiple psychiatric and medical diagnoses requiring different treatments. For example, comorbid depression is extremely common among treatment-seeking patients with anxiety disorders, yet few studies have assessed its impact on treatment (Chapter 9). While personalized medicine has been designated a new frontier for research, market forces push in the opposite direction, toward one-size-fits-all treatments that can be widely disseminated at relatively low cost. The need for cultural adaptations of psychosocial treatments (Chapter 12) and engagement approaches to pharmacotherapy is often minimized in this scenario, despite the growing evidence of their efficacy.

The limitations of our current treatments have spurred investigation of a variety of novel approaches. Promising medications based on new theories of underlying brain mechanisms of anxiety disorders are being tested (e.g., glutamatergic agents in OCD, as described in Chapter 22). Modifications or augmentations of CBT have been developed (e.g., attention training, acceptance and commitment therapy, motivational interviewing). Complementary medicine approaches such as yoga, meditation, and herbal treatments are being studied (Chapter 29), as are brain stimulation techniques (Chapter 28), including vagal nerve stimulation, transcranial stimulation, and deep brain stimulation (DBS). To date, data supporting the efficacy of DBS is strongest in treatment-refractory OCD, probably because the brain circuits underlying OCD are best delineated. Finally, as mentioned above, CBT is being combined with medications in novel ways (e.g., using D-cycloserine to facilitate extinction learning during exposure exercises in CBT).

Despite all of these advances, we still fall short of predictably effective therapies, and we remain a long way from prevention. To accomplish the latter, we will need to understand not only the pathophysiology of these disorders but also their developmental trajectories. Early intervention in childhood is an important yet challenging approach that needs more study. How exposure to a traumatic event gives rise to PTSD in some individuals and not others provides the most obvious natural laboratory for identifying resiliency factors that may prevent anxiety disorders from developing into a chronic condition, and it is being actively investigated as a possible basis for resiliency-enhancing treatment (Chapter 24). The range of therapeutic avenues to pursue will grow with our understanding of the mechanisms that mediate the emergence of anxiety disorders.

31.5 Concluding remarks

There have been significant advances in the field of anxiety and anxiety disorders over the last three decades. These advances have built upon the framework of an increasingly reliable and evidence-based nosology and standardized methods of assessment. Enormous technological innovations have permitted us to study mechanisms of the genome and its interaction with the environment and to image neural and chemical activity in the living brains of animals and humans. In parallel, improvements in design and conduct of randomized clinical trials in both children and adults have helped provide the evidence that support the effectiveness of our current treatments.

Looking ahead, the future holds increasing opportunities to integrate findings across these different areas of research. The potential of an approach that translates findings between basic neuroscience and clinical treatment has already been demonstrated. For example,

increased understanding of the brain circuits that underlie the learning and extinction of fear responses in animals has led to testable ideas for how the human brain learns and extinguishes fear responses, as well as novel treatment approaches. Continued research on the pathophysiology of anxiety disorders has the potential to lead not only to new therapies but also to transform our nosology. We envision a day when such research will yield valid biomarkers of dysfunction in brain systems central to the different anxiety disorders, and that such biomarkers will be used both in animal models (e.g., to dissect cellular and molecular mechanisms) and in clinical settings (e.g., to diagnose, to choose treatments, or to monitor treatment response).

A different type of translation also shows potential: the translation of evidence-based treatments for anxiety disorders into the community. Although still in its infancy, this work has the potential to have a huge impact on public health, because anxiety disorders as a group are the most common psychiatric illness, and most sufferers in the community are not receiving evidence-based care. This line of research holds the promise that effective new treatments developed in research settings (and based on improved understanding of pathophysiology) will no longer take decades to disseminate to the public. It also creates the opportunity for diverse communities to influence what treatments are developed, to help guide the adaptation of promising approaches for specific sociocultural needs, and to exert political pressure needed to overcome disparities in implementation.

Given the increasing sophistication and complexity of each area of study, one challenge for the future will be to maintain collaboration between researchers and clinicians with different types of expertise, so that advances in one area can spur advances in another. Moreover, since time and money are not limitless, areas that are ripe for an interdisciplinary approach will need to be strategically identified and pursued. In our opinion, one of the most exciting and promising areas to pursue both in animal and human studies is the question of how an individual's genetic make-up, developmental trajectory, and environmental influences interact to create an anxious phenotype. We look forward to a day when researchers can explain how these different factors interact to produce (or protect against) dysfunctional anxiety, and when clinicians can assess these relevant factors in individual patients and intervene strategically to provide superior treatment outcomes.

Index